Proprioception and Neuromuscular Control in Joint Stability

Proprioception and Neuromuscular Control in Joint Stability

Scott M. Lephart, PhD, ATC
University of Pittsburgh

Freddie H. Fu, MD,ScD (Hon.)
University of Pittsburgh

Editors

Human Kinetics

Library of Congress Cataloging-in-Publication Data

Proprioception and neuromuscular control in joint stability / [edited by Scott M. Lephart, Freddie H. Fu].
p. cm.
Includes bibliographical references.
ISBN 0-88011-864-4
1. Proprioception. 2. Motor ability. 3. Joints--Pathophysiology. I. Lephart, Scott M., 1961 - II. Fu, Freddie H.

QP454.P77 2000
612.7'5--dc21 99-052106

ISBN 0-88011-864-4

Acquisitions Editor: Loarn Robertson
Developmental Editor: Kent Reel
Assistant Editors: Kim Thoren and Stephan Seyfert
Copyeditor: Judy Peterson
Proofreader: Sarah Wiseman
Graphic Artist: Angela K. Snyder
Cover Designer: Jack Davis
Mac Illustrator: Tom Roberts
Medical Illustrator: Beth Young
Printer: United Graphics

Human Kinetics books are available at special discounts for bulk purchase. Special editions or book excerpts can also be created to specification. For details, contact the Special Sales Manager at Human Kinetics.

Printed in the United States of America

10 9 8 7 6 5 4 3 2 1

Human Kinetics
Web site: http://www.humankinetics.com/

United States: Human Kinetics
P.O. Box 5076
1-800-747-4457
e-mail: humank@hkusa.com

Canada: Human Kinetics
475 Devonshire Road Unit 100
Windsor, ON N8Y 2L5
1-800-465-7301 (in Canada only)
e-mail: humank@hkcanada.com

Europe: Human Kinetics, P.O. Box IW14
Leeds LS16 6TR, United Kingdom
+44 (0)113-278 1708
e-mail: humank@hkeurope.com

Australia: Human Kinetics
57A Price Avenue
Lower Mitcham, South Australia 5062
(08) 82771555
e-mail: humank@hkaustralia.com

New Zealand: Human Kinetics
P.O. Box 105-231, Auckland Central
09-523-3462
e-mail: humank@hknewz.com

Contents

Foreword

During the last 20 years, we have seen enormous improvements in the treatment of many sports injuries. The treatment of severe knee ligament injuries is certainly a prime example. Complete disruption of the anterior cruciate ligament has ceased to be a career- or activity-ending injury, largely through advances in surgical techniques and rehabilitation.

Nevertheless, many important problems in sports medicine remain unsolved and knee ligament injuries illustrate this situation. For example, we know some ACL injuries occur under circumstances that seem innocuous—doing simple maneuvers that the athlete has done hundreds or thousands of times before, such as coming down from a rebound or making a cut. All of us suspect complex neurologic functions like proprioception and fine neuromuscular control play a key role here.

We also know females appear to have a higher incidence of ACL injury than males while doing the same activities. Recent studies have suggested subtle differences in neuromuscular control and function may be one of the causative factors. Other studies have shown teaching athletes at risk how to jump, land, and cut in specific ways may help prevent these ACL injuries. This concept may be equally valuable for athletes who are being rehabilitated following ACL reconstruction.

All of these examples suggest a very important role for proprioception and neuromuscular control. Bringing together 45 experts from all over the world for a 3-day workshop in August 1997 provided a unique opportunity for them to collaborate and share their knowledge with each other. Publishing this material provides the same unique opportunity for all of us to participate in that experience. The American Orthopaedic Society for Sports Medicine (AOSSM), working through its Foundation for Sports Medicine Education and Research (FSMER) is very pleased to have been able to sponsor the workshop from which the material in this monograph was derived.

Douglas W. Brown, MD
President
American Orthopaedic Society for Sports Medicine
March 22, 1999

Contributors and Participants

John Albright, MD†‡
University of Iowa
Department of Orthopaedic Surgery
Iowa City, Iowa

Answorth A. Allen, MD†‡
Instructor in Orthopaedics, Cornell University Medical College
Assistant Attending, Hospital for Special Surgery
New York, New York

Thomas P. Andriacchi, PhD†‡
Rush-Presbyterian, St. Luke's Medical Center
Department of Orthopaedics
Chicago, Illinois

James A. Ashton-Miller, PhD†‡
Biomechanics Research Laboratory
The University of Michigan
Ann Arbor, Michigan

Bernard R. Bach, MD‡
Rush-Presbyterian, St. Luke's Medical Center
Department of Orthopaedics
Chicago, Illinois

Robert L. Barrack, MD‡
Professor of Orthopaedic Surgery
Tulane University School of Medicine
Department of Orthopaedic Surgery
New Orleans, Louisiana

David Beard, PhD, PT†‡
University of Sydney
School of Physiotherapy
Lidcombe, Australia

Mikael Bergenheim, PhD‡
Department of Musculoskeletal Research
National Institution of Working Life
Umeå, Sweden

Bruce D. Beynnon, PhD†‡
Department of Orthopaedics & Rehabilitation
McClure Musculoskeletal Research Center
University of Vermont
Burlington, Vermont

Roland M. Biedert, MD†‡
Sportstraumatology
Institute of Sport Sciences
Swiss Sports School
Magglingen, Switzerland

Kevin P. Black, MD†‡
Hershey Medical Center
Hershey, Pennsylvania

Thomas Bochdansky, MD†‡
Department of Physical Medicine and Rehabilitation
University of Vienna
Vienna, Austria

Andrew W. Brown, MD‡
University of Iowa
Iowa City, Iowa

Charles A. Bush-Joseph, MD‡
Rush-Presbyterian, St. Luke's Medical Center
Department of Orthopaedics
Chicago, Illinois

Edward T. Crowley, ATC‡
University of Iowa
Iowa City, Iowa

Robert D. D'Ambrosia, MD‡
Louisiana State University, Medical Center
New Orleans, Louisiana

Marco Dirks, MD‡
Orthopaedic Group, Inc.
Pawtucket, Rhode Island

M. Djupsjöbacka, PhD‡
Department of Musculoskeletal Research
National Institution of Working Life
Umeå, Sweden

Scott F. Dye, MD†‡
Associate Clinical Professor
University of California, San Francisco
San Francisco, California

Gerold Ebinbechler, PhD‡
Department of Physical Medicine and Rehabilitation
University of Vienna
Vienna, Austria

Lars-Gunnar Elmqvist, MD, PhD‡
Department of Orthopaedics
University Hospital
Umeå, Sweden

Lucio S. Ernlund, MD‡
Sports Medicine Research Fellow
Department of Orthopaedic Surgery
University of Pittsburgh
Pittsburgh, Pennsylvania

Christian Fink, MD†‡
Univ.-Klinik für Unfallchirugie
Innsbruck, Austria

Kelley Fitzgerald, PhD, PT, OCS‡
Department of Physical Therapy
University of Pittsburgh
Pittsburgh, Pennsylvania

Peter J. Fowler, MD, FRCSC†‡
University Hospital
Department of Orthopaedic
London, Ontario Canada

Freddie H. Fu, MD†‡
Silver Professor and Chair, Department of Orthopaedic Surgery
University of Pittsburgh
Pittsburgh, Pennsylvania

Christine Gardner‡
Iowa Spine Research Center
Iowa City, IA

William E. Garrett, Jr., MD, PhD†‡
Chair, Department of Orthopaedic Surgery
University of North Carolina at Chapel Hill
Chapel Hill, NC

Jorge L. Giraldo, MD†‡
Sports Medicine Research Fellow
Neuromuscular Research Laboratory
Department of Orthopaedic Surgery
University of Pittsburgh
Pittsburgh, Pennsylvania

Daniel Gottlieb, MS‡
McClure Musculoskeletal Research Center
Department of Orthopaedics and Rehabilitation
University of Vermont
Burlington, Vermont

Carlos A. Guanche, MD†‡
University of Minnesota
Minneapolis Sports Medicine Center
Minneapolis, MN

Kevin M. Guskiewicz, PhD, ATC†‡
Department of Physical Education, Exercise and Sport Science
University of North Carolina at Chapel Hill
Chapel Hill, North Carolina

Christopher D. Harner, MD†‡
Director, Center for Sports Medicine and Rehabilitation
Department of Orthopaedic Surgery
University of Pittsburgh
Pittsburgh, Pennsylvania

Timothy J. Henry, PhD, ATC†‡
State University of New York at Brockport
Brockport, New York

Timothy E. Hewett, PhD†‡
Cincinnati Sportsmedicine and Orthopaedic Center and the Deaconess Hospital
Cincinnati, Ohio

Debra E. Hurwitz, PhD‡
Rush-Presbyterian, St. Luke's Medical Center
Department of Orthopaedics
Chicago, Illinois

Laura Huston, MS†‡
MedSport
University of Michigan
Ann Arbor, Michigan

Mary Lloyd Ireland, MD†‡
Kentucky Sports Medicine
Lexington, Kentucky

James J. Irrgang, PhD, PT, ATC†‡
Center for Sports Medicine and Rehabilitation
University of Pittsburgh Medicine Center
Pittsburgh, Pennsylvania

Joerg G. Jerosch, MD†‡
Klinik und Poliklinik für Allgemeine Orthopedie
Universität Muenster
Muenster, Germany

Hakan Johansson, MD, PhD†‡
Department of Musculoskeletal Research
National Institution of Working Life
Umeå, Sweden

Donald T. Kirkendall, PhD‡
Departments of Orthopaedic Surgery and Physical and Occupational Therapy
Duke University Medical Center
Durham, North Carolina

Arthur Kleipool, MD†‡
Amsterdam, Netherlands

Josef Kollmitzer, PhD‡
Department of Physical Medicine and Rehabilitation
University of Vienna
Vienna, Austria

Lars Konradsen, MD†‡
Department of Orthopaedic Surgery
Gentofte Hospital
University of Copenhagen, Denmark
Copenhagen, Denmark

Scott M. Lephart, PhD, ATC†‡
Director, Neuromuscular Research Laboratory
Department of Orthopaedic Surgery
University of Pittsburgh
Pittsburgh, Pennsylvania

Ian K.Y. Lo, MD†‡
University Hospital
Department of Orthopaedic
London, Ontario Canada

Barry G. Munn, MD‡
Resident in Orthopaedic Surgery
Director, Adult Reconstructive Surgery
Tulane University School of Medicine
Department of Orthopaedic Surgery
New Orleans, Louisiana

Randy Neri, PT, ATC‡
Center for Sports Medicine and Rehabilitation
University of Pittsburgh Medicine Center
Pittsburgh, Pennsylvania

Frank R. Noyes, MD‡
Cincinnati Sportsmedicine and Orthopaedic Center and the Deaconess Hospital
Cincinnati, Ohio

Jennifer Ocif‡
University of Iowa
Iowa City, Iowa

Louis Osternig, PhD, ATC†‡
Department of Exercise and Movement Science
University of Oregon
Eugene, Oregon

Mark V. Paterno, MS, PT‡
Cincinnati Sportsmedicine and Orthopaedic Center and the Deaconess Hospital
Cincinnati, Ohio

Jonas Pedersen, PhD†‡
Department of Musculoskeletal Research
National Institution of Working Life
Umeå, Sweden

David H. Perrin, PhD, ATC†‡
Chair, Health, Physical and Recreation Education
Curry School of Education
University of Virginia
Charlottesville, Virginia

Danny Pincivero, PhD‡
Eastern Washington University
Cheney, Washington

Roger G. Pollock, MD†‡
New York Orthopaedic Hospital
New York, New York

Malcolm Pope, Dr Med Sci‡
University of Iowa
Iowa City, Iowa

Kathryn Refshauge
University of Sydney
School of Physiotherapy
Lidcombe, Australia

Per A. Renström, MD, PhD†‡
Department of Orthopaedics & Rehabilitation
McClure Musculoskeletal Research Center
University of Vermont
Burlington, Vermont

Michael H. Rieber, MD†‡
Hershey Medical Center
Hershey, Pennsylvania

Bryan L. Riemann, MA, ATC†‡
Neuromuscular Research Laboratory
University of Pittsburgh
Pittsburgh, Pennsylvania

Susan Rozzi, PhD, ATC‡
The College of Charleston
Charleston, South Carolina

Harry E. Rubash, MD‡
Department of Orthopaedic Surgery
University of Pittsburgh Medical Center
Pittsburgh, Pennsylvania

Katherine S. Rudolph, MS, PT†‡
Department of Physical Therapy
University of Delaware
Newark, Delaware

Marc R. Safran, MD†‡
Co-Director, Sports Medicine
Department of Orthopaedic Surgery
Kaiser Permanente, Orange County
Anaheim Hills, California

Sandra J. Shultz, PhD, ATC‡
Curry School of Education
University of Virginia
Charlottesville, Virginia

Lynn Snyder-Mackler, ScD, PT†‡
Department of Physical Therapy
University of Delaware
Newark, Delaware

Moshe Solomonow, PhD‡
Louisiana State University, Medical Center
New Orleans, Louisiana

C. Buz Swanik, PhD, ATC†‡
Temple University
Philadelphia, Pennsylvania

Ivan Vassilev, MD†‡
Arthroskopie Centre
Ubinger, Germany

Geoffrey L. Vaupel, MD‡
Department of Orthopaedics
Davies Medical Center
San Francisco, California

Jon J.P. Warner, MD‡
Orthopaedic Surgery
Harvard Medical School
Cambridge, Massachusetts

Kevin E. Wilk, PT†‡
HealthSouth Sports Medicine and Rehabilitation Center
and American Sports Medicine Institute
Birmingham, Alabama

Edward Wojtys, MD‡
MedSport
University of Michigan
Ann Arbor, Michigan

Savio Woo, PhD†
Department of Orthopaedic Surgery
Musculoskeletal Research Laboratory
University of Pittsburgh Medicine Center
Pittsburgh, Pennsylvania

Pongsak Yuktanandana, MD†‡
Neuromuscular Research Laboratory
University of Pittsburgh
Pittsburgh, Pennsylvania

†Workshop Participant

‡Contributor to Textbook

Preface

The contents of this text include contributions from the participants of the 1997 workshop sponsored by the Foundation for Sports Medicine Education and Research (FSMER) titled "The Role of Proprioception and Neuromuscular Control in the Management and Rehabilitation of Joint Pathology," which was held August 21–23, 1997 in Pittsburgh, Pennsylvania. Thanks to the generous sponsorship of FSMER, 45 international experts convened this three-day workshop with the objective of enhancing the knowledge related to the role of proprioception in joint stability and the effect that joint injury, surgery, and rehabilitation have on this mechanism.

Workshop Premise and Significance

The organizers established the need for the workshop based on the conception of a paradigm describing the role of proprioception and its contribution to joint stability. This rudimentary understanding of a very complex system recently has been the basis for considerable attention being paid to the significance of proprioception in the management of joint pathology. As the following statements will attest, however, the paradigm was not firmly imbedded in significant scientific data and thus is, at the very least, misunderstood and controversial.

Paradigm: Proprioception is related to the senses of position and movement of limbs, as first described by Sherrington. These senses are mediated through peripheral mechanoreceptors located in the joint, muscles, and skin. Proprioceptive sensation relies on simultaneous activity of a number of types of afferent receptors that convert mechanical stimuli to neural signals that are transmitted along afferent pathways to multiple levels within the central nervous system (CNS).

The CNS functions to integrate these afferent signals and ultimately regulates motor commands controlling voluntary muscle activation for performance of complex motor skills along with involuntary motor responses that contribute to joint stability.

Accompanying an injury to articular tissue is a disruption of mechanoreceptors, causing partial deafferentation of the joint.This has been shown to inhibit normal neuromuscular control resulting in diminished joint stabilization, altered patterns of locomotion, and ultimately contributing to repetitive injuries and a progressive decline of the joint (see figure P.1).

The basic understanding of this paradigm led researchers to develop measurement techniques aimed at quantifying the contribution of proprioceptive and neuromuscular mechanisms to normal joint stability and the effects of pathology on their

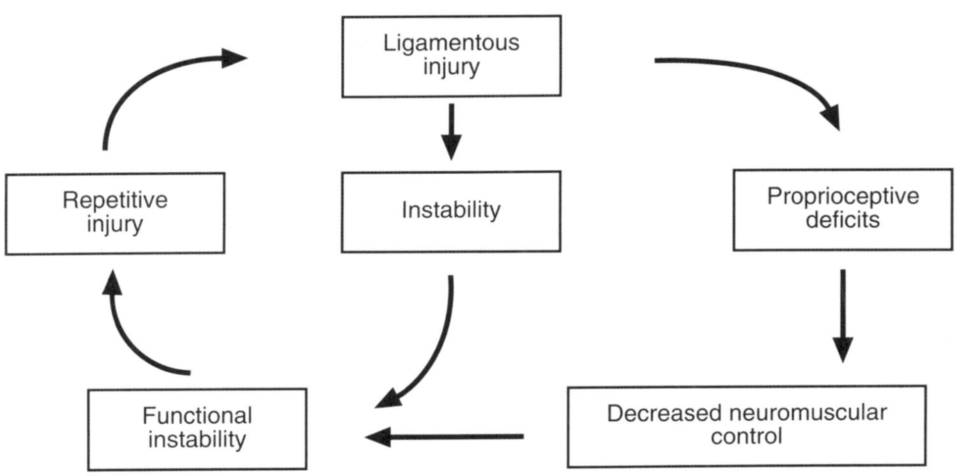

Figure P.1 Paradigm of the pathophysiology of ligament injury on proprioception and neuromuscular control. Reprinted from: Lephart SM, Henry TJ. The physiological basis for open and closed chain rehabilitation for the upper extremity. *J Sport Rehab* 5: 71-87, 1992.

function. However, early instrumentation tended to be crude with limited sensitivity, thus making much of the orthopedic community skeptical of the results being reported and doubtful of the true functional significance of the data. Therefore, the development of enhanced instrumentation that addresses physiologically based hypotheses was viewed as critical, not only to enhance the credibility of the data, but also to demonstrate the true relevance that proprioception and neuromuscular control have on functional joint stability. The lack of solid research capabilities, along with a misunderstanding of the physiological mechanisms of the system, has limited the ability to determine the role surgery and rehabilitation have on restoration of these mechanisms.

To date, the role of surgery relative to the proprioceptive mechanism remains unclear. The few studies that have been reported suggest that surgical intervention may influence joint proprioception and ultimately function, but these studies lack complete acceptance due to the aforementioned limitation in the research setting. The main considerations for surgeons relative to this system include preservation of afferents, promotion of regeneration of mechanoreceptors, and modification of protective reflex arcs in the postoperative patient. Soft tissue tensioning is hypothesized to be important in the efficiency of proprioception and does seem to have a mechanical and physiological basis that would support this hypothesis.

The role of rehabilitation, with respect to the restoration of proprioception and neuromuscular control, is similarly misunderstood. Efforts to improve functional stability in the absence of ligamentous stability have been relatively unsuccessful in those cases where the patient attempts to return to preinjury activities that demand significant joint stability. Attempts to quantify the insufficiency of the dynamic restraint have suggested that reflex-mediated muscle activation is altered following ligament injury, yet little conclusive data exists demonstrating that rehabilitation can induce adequate adaptations to this mechanism to provide functional stability.

It was our belief that, with a better understanding of the basic physiology of this complex system, along with an appreciation for the pathophysiology of articular injury related to the proprioceptive mechanism, improved management strategies for enhancing functional joint stability could be achieved. Given this premise the workshop convened with the following *specific aims:*

1. To review the peripheral somatosensory system and its role in mediating motor control
2. To describe assessment tools that are available to measure proprioception and neuromuscular activity and to enhance the understanding of the effects articular injury has on this mechanism
3. To encourage research to further delineate the contribution of proprioception on dynamic joint stability
4. To enhance the clinician's understanding of restoring proprioception and neuromuscular control to improve joint function
5. To publish this text containing the current knowledge related to the content area and to identify future needs in the area of proprioception and neuromuscular control research as it relates to the management of orthopedic conditions

The workshop participants included a collection of representatives from the areas of basic science research in peripheral afferent physiology, soft tissue biomechanics, applied biomechanics, rehabilitation, and orthopedics who had previously demonstrated scholarship related to proprioceptive and neuromuscular considerations of joint pathology. The participants represented the disciplines of athletic training, biomechanics, engineering, orthopedic surgery, physical therapy, and physiology.

The contents of this text are contributions from each of the invited participants in his or her specific area of research and clinical expertise. The text is divided into four sections including section one : Contribution of the Sensorimotor System to Joint Stability; section two: Effects of Ligament Injury on the Sensorimotor Systems; section three : Special Issues Related to Proprioception and Neuromuscular Control ; section four: Role of Rehabilitation in Reestablishing Proprioception and Neuromuscular Control. The chapters have been organized to provide overviews of the related systems, specific mechanisms of proprioception and neuromuscular control, the processes responsible for joint stability, and the influence of joint pathology and intervention on these mechanisms following injury and disease. The focus of the text is specific to the basic science underlying the sensorimotor system with application to the shoulder, knee, and ankle joints.

Scott M. Lephart, PhD, ATC

Introduction to the Sensorimotor System

Scott M. Lephart, PhD, ATC
Bryan L. Riemann, MA, ATC
Freddie H. Fu, MD

In recent years the orthopedic and sports medicine communities have given considerable attention to the issues surrounding the role of proprioception in mediating muscle function and contributing to joint stabilization. In the general consensus of the participants of the workshop, however, there is confusion across the various disciplines, related to the mechanisms being described and the contribution that proprioception affords to joint homeostasis. This lack of a unified and conclusive body of knowledge, and the absence of a true appreciation of the sensory and motor systems associated with proprioception, has resulted in the inappropriate use of both terminology and the modes for testing the various mechanisms.

This introductory section provides a basis for the terminology used to describe the mechanisms within the nervous and musculoskeletal systems as they relate to proprioception and neuromuscular control. At the end of this section we include a glossary of terms, *Sensorimotor System Terminology*, which define the system and its components. We have attempted to provide definitions based upon the original anatomical and physiological descriptions within which they are embedded. At the very least, the participants in the workshop aspired to produce a common language that will be used for future investigation and reporting of relevant findings related to the sensorimotor system. This section also highlights a few of the contemporary issues and controversies essential to understanding the sensorimotor system, which are detailed in the chapters to follow.

The Sensorimotor System

The term *sensorimotor system* was adopted by the participants to represent the composite of the physiological systems of the complex neurosensory and neuromuscular process, which has been frequently simplified and inappropriately described as *proprioception*. The sensorimotor system describes mechanisms involved in the acquisition of a sensory stimulus and conversion of the stimulus to a neural signal, along with transmission of the signal via afferent pathways to the central nervous system (CNS). Additionally, it describes processing and integration of the signal by the various centers of the CNS and central command generators, as well as the motor responses resulting in muscle activation for locomotion and the performance of functional tasks and joint stabilization (see figure I.1).

The use of the term *proprioception* presented the greatest concern and least consensus among the participants. Generally people agreed that proprioception is often misused to represent many mechanisms and processes within the sensorimotor system, which has resulted not only in misunderstanding but also in some questionable physiological relevance of sensory acquisition and transmission of important information related to joint position and motion. A review of contemporary literature demonstrates that proprioception is often used to describe many of the physiological processes within the sensorimotor system including joint position sense, kinesthesia, balance, reflex muscle activation, and has even been linked to the description of locomotion. Additionally, proprioception has been used inappropriately in the laboratory setting to describe the assessment of most of the variables contained within the sensorimotor system.

As a result of the misuse of the terminology related to the sensorimotor system, we suggest that the nomenclature needs to describe physiological functions, which was the terminology's original intent. Proprioception is inferred from Sherrington's 1906 description of the "proprioceptive system" as the afferent information from "proprio-ceptors" located in the "proprio-ceptive field" that contributes to conscious sensations ("muscle sense"), total posture (postural equilibrium), and segmental posture (joint stability) (29). "Proprio-ceptors" referred to those receptors located in joints, muscles, and tendons that were

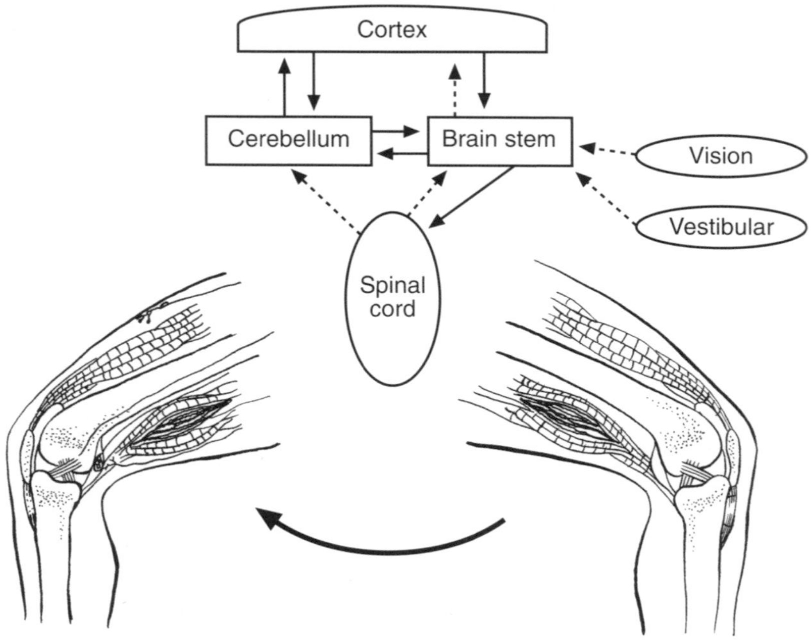

Figure I.1 The sensorimotor system incorporates all of the afferent, efferent and central integration and processing components involved with maintaining functional joint stability. Although visual and vestibular inputs contribute, the peripheral mechanoreceptors are most important from a clinical orthopedic perspective. The peripheral mechanoreceptors (pictured on the lower left) reside in the cutaneous, muscular, joint and ligamentous tissues. Afferent pathways (dotted lines) convey inputs to the three levels of motor control and associated areas such as the cerebellum. Activation of motor neurons may occur in direct response to peripheral sensory input (reflexes) or from descending motor commands, both of which may be modulated and/or regulated by the associated areas (gray lines). Efferent pathways from each of the motor control levels (solid lines) converge upon the alpha and gamma motor neurons located in the ventral aspects of the spinal cord. The contractions by the extrafusal and intrafusal muscle fibers cause new stimuli to be presented to the peripheral mechanoreceptors.

"adapted for excitation consonantly with changes going on in the organism itself." (29)

According to Mathews (23), Sherrington fully described four submodalities of muscle sense in Schafer's *Textbook of Physiology*. These submodalities included those of (1) posture, (2) passive movement, (3) active movement, and (4) resistance to movement. These submodalities are synonymous with contemporary descriptions of joint position sense (posture of segment), kinesthesia (active and passive), and sense of resistance or heaviness.

Sherrington's (29) use of the term "proprioceptive system" and the difficulty with direct interpretation of his writing lead to several descriptions of proprioception, which has contributed to much of the confusion. The source of conflicting interpretations predominantly stems from whether or not proprioception implies the acquisition and transmission of a sensory stimulus inclusively, or if it is ultimately the sensation of this sensory stimulation. The former would suggest that proprioception is the process of presenting the CNS with peripheral data related to joint position, motion, and force that is subsequently processed at conscious and subconscious levels in order to initiate appropriate responses. This would suggest that conscious appreciation of this information is a process other than proprioception relating to the sense of proprioception. The latter interpretation would suggest that proprioception is the conscious perception of the sensation derived from neural afferents related to joint motion, position, and force being processed at the highest centers of the CNS. This definition suggests that afferent acquisition and transmission of the sensory stimulus is some process that only contributes to proprioception.

Our interpretation of Sherrington's work concludes that his implication was that the process termed "proprioception" is referring to all neural inputs originating from joints, muscles, tendons, and associated deep tissue "proprio-ceptors." These proprioceptive signals are projected to the CNS for processing, which ultimately regulates reflexes and motor control (29).

From this interpretation we can derive that proprioception is the acquisition of stimuli by peripheral receptors, as well as the conversion of these mechanical stimuli to a neural signal that is transmitted along afferents pathways to the CNS for processing. Given this elucidation, proprioception defines only the mechanism and process occurring along the afferent (sensory) pathway of the sensorimotor system. Further, this definition suggests that proprioception does not refer to activity related to CNS processing or postprocessing of the sensory signal, and it clearly does not define any activity along the efferent (motor) pathway resulting in a motor response to the original sensory stimulation.

The term *sensorimotor system* progresses Sherrington's description of the proprioceptive system to include a more complex connection between sensory pathways and motor pathways than exclusively reflex. Contemporary research has demonstrated that more of the nervous system is involved (three levels of motor control, basal ganglia, cerebellum), and the reflexive components have been revealed as being more sophisticated (fusimotor integration, supraspinal integration of visual, vestibular, and somatosensory) than previously thought.

Proprioceptive information is a critical source of sensory information for optimal and efficient motor performance (9, 14). It is conveyed to each of the motor control centers (spinal, brain stem, and cerebral cortex) and the associated motor areas (cerebellum and basal ganglia). While the associated areas do not directly control motor neuron activity, they are essential for modulating and regulating the motor commands occurring in each motor center. In addition to being organized in a hierarchical manner, the motor centers are also arranged in parallel (9, 25). Thus, proprioceptive information is supplied to each of these areas, where it undergoes decoding and processing. As one may surmise from the hierarchical and parallel arrangement, each of the motor control centers and associated areas utilizes proprioceptive information differently.

At the highest level of organization, the somatosensory cortex processes proprioceptive information to provide conscious awareness of joint position (joint position sense) and joint motion (kinesthesia). The motor side of the cortex is provided with proprioceptive information emanating directly from the periphery and indirectly via the cerebellum, basal ganglia, and somatosensory cortex (9). It is within the motor areas of the cortex that proprioceptive information is believed to be stored for use with future descending motor commands (22).

The spinal level of motor control integrates and processes proprioceptive information unconsciously to elicit muscle activation through reflex pathways and neural networks. Incoming afferent fibers from peripheral mechanoreceptors enter the spinal cord through the dorsal roots, upon which they often bifurcate. The bifurcations can terminate directly on alpha motor neurons, as in the case of the muscle spindle monosynaptic reflex, or on interneurons connected with more complex reflex networks (polysynaptic) or ascending tract cells. Interneurons provide the basis for the spinal cord's integrative functions. Prime examples, related to enhancing dynamic joint stability, are the polysynaptic interneuronal junctions linking peripheral afferent fibers with gamma motor neurons (1).

Between these two motor control centers, the brain stem integrates proprioceptive signals with afferent information from vestibular and visual centers and other somatosensory inputs to directly control automatic tasks such as postural equilibrium. In addition, the central location of the brain stem within the CNS allows it to function as an indirect relay station between the cortex and spinal cord, as well as a modifier of descending motor commands. Similar to spinal level processing, brain stem processing occurs unconsciously.

Although the cerebellum does not directly control motor neuron activity, it plays an essential role in motor control. The cerebellum receives a continuous inflow of information from peripheral sources, central sensory areas, and motor control areas. The importance of proprioceptive information for cerebellar function is evidenced by its transmission along the fastest ascending tract fibers of the nervous system. An overview of the cerebellum can be found in chapter 4.

Contemporary Issues

Beyond controversies related to defining the sensorimotor system and its constituents, there are a number of contemporary debates relate to the sensory acquisition mechanisms, processing mechanisms, and mechanisms of motor control. Two of the more controversial areas, which are essential to understanding the function of the sensorimotor system and the role related to management and rehabilitation following joint pathology, are the mechanisms by which peripheral afferents transmit sensory information to the CNS and the mechanisms by which the sensory information mediates motor control.

Peripheral Afferents

Proprioception originates from sensory receptors located in joint, muscle, and cutaneous tissue. The relative importance of each receptor to proprioception has long been debated. These mechanosensitive receptors all appear to contribute to the transmission of peripheral information related to joint position and motion as well as muscle tension, and therefore they ultimately regulate muscle activation. Researchers, however, do not conclusively agree upon the mode of sensory acquisition and relative autonomy of the different populations of mechanoreceptors (2, 19).

Speculation on how sensory information from peripheral mechanoreceptors is transmitted to the CNS was originally based on a theory known as labelled lines. The labelled line theory suggests that each type of mechanoreceptor has sensitivity to a single stimulus and transmits individual signals to the CNS for processing (2). However, recent experiments by Johansson and associates support more complex patterns of afferent information transmitted by populations (ensembles) of mechanoreceptors, referred to as ensemble coding (2). This theory suggests that all of the afferents within the ensemble have the capacity to respond to the same stimulus. Research has established that a given ensemble contains afferents with varying ranges of sensitivity and different responses to the same stimulus (8). The combination of these properties gives ensemble coded signals the capacity to furnish more discrete information concerning peripheral stimulation than the traditional labelled line afferents.

The respective contribution of the various peripheral afferents is also controversial. Traditionally, articular mechanoreceptors were thought to initiate protective reflexes directly to alpha motor neurons in response to loads being placed on the joint (28). More recently, some researchers have suggested that articular mechanoreceptors have a very limited functional relevance in mediating reflexes, since they are thought to be activated only under very high loads and physiological end ranges (11). This would suggest that the tenomuscular mechanoreceptors are the only structures that provide proprioceptive information that mediates reflex activity or provides joint position sense. However, Johansson and others recently have suggested that the muscle afferents are indeed the crucial neural element for mediation of muscular control but that muscle spindles are heavily influenced by critical information delivered by articular afferents via the fusimotor system (15). Johansson provides detail of this theory in chapter 1 that describes a sophisticated articular-tenomuscular link called the final common input (1, 18). The final common input theory suggests that muscle spindles integrate peripheral afferent information and transmit a final modified signal that is ultimately responsible for coordinated reflex regulation (1, 18).

Motor Control Mechanisms

We have defined neuromuscular control in this section as the unconscious efferent response to an afferent signal concerning dynamic joint stability. As we have discussed, these motor responses often are the effect of proprioception. The final area that we highlight in this section is the process by which the CNS utilizes the proprioceptive information for the regulation of neuromuscular control (6, 9).

The process by which afferent proprioceptive signals are utilized for motor control can be categorized into either feedback or feedforward control paradigms, which are controversial in terms of the role proprioception plays in maintaining joint stability. The feedback mechanism is characterized by a reactive reflex to imposed forces to the joint (24). The feedforward mechanism is characterized by preactivated muscle control in anticipation of loads or subsequent events (20).

Traditionally, the influence of proprioception over motor control was thought to be a reactive process at the spinal reflex level in response to joint loads, which provided conscious appreciation of position and motion that could be used for fine tuning motor commands for precision movements at the higher centers of the CNS (21). This feedback mechanism is characterized by numerous reflex pathways that continuously adjust muscle activity. This process, however, results in electromechanical time delays, which makes questionable the effectiveness of this reactive process in providing joint stabilization and protection. Therefore, it appears that feedback neuromuscular control mechanisms are best equipped for maintaining posture and regulating slow movement (9).

The feedforward mechanism of motor control suggests that proprioception is a valuable mediator of motor control commands in preparation for anticipated loads or activities that will be encountered. This motor control mechanism implies that an internal model is developed by utilizing information from previous exposures to known conditions. This information is then integrated with ongoing proprioceptive information and is responsible for generating preprogrammed motor commands to achieve a desired outcome (6, 9, 20).

Evaluation of these two motor control mechanisms implies that they are integrated into multiple processes that contribute to motor activation, which results in coordinated motor skills and dynamic joint stabilization, and do not function exclusive of one another. For example, preparatory excitation of the alpha motor nerves is frequently accompanied by activation of the gamma motor nerves, referred to as alpha-gamma coactivation (3, 5, 16, 21, 24). Alpha-gamma coactivation increases the sensitivity of the muscle spindles to stretch, referred to as gain, which heightens the awareness of joint motion and position (4, 16). Additionally, this heightened sensitivity of spindles evokes more vigorous stretch reflexes, which are superimposed onto descending motor commands (5, 27). Sensory information in feedforward motor control is used to evaluate the results and help preprogram future muscle activation strategies. Preactivated muscles, therefore, are stiffer and recognize unexpected joint loads more quickly. A stiffer muscle decreases electromechanical delay and effectively facilitates feedback neuromuscular control mechanisms (4, 5, 12).

Summary

This text provides a basis for understanding the relevance of the sensorimotor system to joint homeostasis. The contributors have detailed what is known definitively about the mechanisms of proprioception and neuromuscular control based on the data available. You will notice that there are many issues upon which the authors disagree, as well as instances where nomenclature, interpretations, and assumptions are conflicting. Most importantly, however, this text illustrates the chasm that exists in our knowledge, which demonstrates the need for future scientific investigation and also provides valuable insights for future research directions and clinical practice.

This section is an introduction both to the text and to our understanding of *Proprioception and Neuromuscular Control in Joint Stability*. Its purpose is to provide an overview of the important issues that will be addressed in detail throughout the text by an international group of experts. This introduction also serves as a basis for future use of the terminology defining the sensorimotor system and is intended to bring cohesiveness to future investigation and the reporting of relevant findings. With the provision of a universal understanding of the relevant language, along with a greater appreciation for the mechanism we are studying, the continued evolution of our knowledge and ultimately our understanding of the "system" is insured.

Sensorimotor System Terminology

The following definitions of nomenclature describe the sensorimotor system:

afferent pathways: Pathways formed by neurons leading to the central nervous system from sensory receptors (30). With respect to the sensorimotor system, this includes (1) the receptor organ and its respective afferent nerve fiber, (2) the synapses within the central nervous system that terminate on alpha motor neurons (monosynaptic reflexes), interneurons (polysynaptic reflexes and patterned responses), and nerve fibers comprising the ascending tracts for supraspinal integration and processing (brain stem, cerebellum, cortical).

afferent (ascending) tracts: A group or bundle of nerve fibers located within the white matter of the spinal cord that carries afferent information toward supraspinal structures (30). The majority of the information concerning the sensorimotor system travels either through the dorsal lateral tracts or the spinocerebellar tracts.

balance: The process of maintaining the center of gravity within the body's base of support (26).

central nervous system processing centers: Spinal—responsible for direct motor responses to sensory information (reflexes) and elementary patterns of motor coordination (rhythmic and central pattern generators). Brain stem—responsible for postural control and many of the automatic and stereotyped movements of the body. Cortical—responsible for initiating and controlling more complex and discrete voluntary movements; commands from the cortex reach the motor neurons either directly (corticospinal tract) or indirectly via brainstem.

chemoreceptors: Sensory receptors responsible for transducing chemical stimuli into neural impulses.

corticospinal tract: Direct descending tract to motor neurons from cortex.

deafferentation: Cutting off neural supply (30); with respect to the sensorimotor system, refers to damage to mechanoreceptors and associated nerve fibers in conjunction with trauma to the joint structures that essentially reduces or eliminates the afferent information arising from the injured structure.

dorsal lateral tracts: Two ascending tracts located in the posterior region of the spinal cord. The majority of sensations traveling in this tract are touch, pressure, and vibration; varying amounts of conscious appreciation of position and kinesthetic sensations have been attributed to this tract (13, 23).

efferent pathways: Pathways formed by neurons leading to an effector from the central nervous system (30). With respect to the sensorimotor system, this includes (1) the initiation level within the central nervous system (spinal, brain stem, cortical),

(2) interneurons and descending tract nerve fibers leading to the ventral roots, and (3) motor neurons (alpha or gamma) terminating on motor endplates.

efferent (descending) tracts: A group of nerve fibers located within the spinal cord that carry efferent information from the supraspinal structures (brain stem and cortex) to spinal cord neural networks (30). With respect to motor control, there are two main pathways from the brainstem (medial and lateral) and one pathway from the cortex (corticospinal).

joint position sense: The submodality of proprioception sense associated with the sense of joint position.

kinesthesia: The submodality of proprioception sense associated with the sensation of joint movement, either from internal forces (active) or external forces (passive).

lateral descending pathways: Influence the motor neurons innervating the distal muscles of the extremities (9). With respect to the sensorimotor system, one tract is most important—the rubrospinal.

mechanism: A response pattern to achieve a result (30); for example, the reflexive responses of the body to maintain or restore joint stability following an imposed joint perturbation represent the mechanism of dynamic joint stability.

mechanoreceptors: Sensory receptors responsible for quantitatively transducing mechanical stimuli occurring in their host tissue into neural impulses (10); with respect to the sensorimotor system, the receptors located on or near the surface of the body that respond to stimuli in the external environment and those responding to stimuli arising within body tissues.

medial descending pathways: Nerve tracts that influence the motor neurons innervating the axial and proximal muscles (9). With respect to the sensorimotor system, the two most important tracts are the vestibulospinal and reticulospinal tracts.

neuromuscular control: The unconscious efferent response to an afferent signal concerning dynamic joint stability.

postural control: The ability to maintain control over posture. Postural control is automatic (conscious activation is not required) and task specific (7); it is accomplished through (1) acquisition of afferent information from somatosensory, visual, and vestibular sources, (2) integration and processing of the afferent information by the central nervous system for the selection and coordination of appropriate motor responses, and (3) execution of the motor commands by the musculoskeletal system.

postural equilibrium: The balanced state of forces and moments acting on the body's center of mass resulting in minimal uniform motion (postural sway) (17); from a clinical perspective, when the body is maintaining the center of gravity within the minimum limits of stability through equalization of forces and optimal alignment of body segments.

process: The series of steps or events that lead to the achievement of specific results (30); in the case of dynamic joint stability, the processes include mechanoreceptor stimulation, neural transmission, integration of the signals by the CNS, transmission of an efferent signal, muscle activation, and force production.

proprioception: Inferred from Sherrington's description of the proprioceptive system as the afferent information from "proprio-ceptors" located in the "proprio-ceptive field" that contributes to conscious sensations ("muscle sense"), total posture (postural equilibrium), and segmental posture (joint stability) (29). Sherrington defined the "proprio-ceptive" field as the "deep" areas of body that were not subjected to stimuli arising either in the external environment ("extero-ceptive field") or the "partially screened" environment of the gastrointestinal tract ("intero-ceptive field"). "Proprio-ceptors" referred to those receptors located in joints, muscles, and tendons that were "adapted for excitation consonantly with changes going on in the organism itself" (29).

reticulospinal tract: Makes excitatory and inhibitory synapses with interneurons; motor neurons involved with movement and postural control originate in reticular formation.

rubrospinal tract: Responsible for contributing to distal extremity muscle control during fine motor movements; originates in the red nucleus.

sensorimotor system: The system of sensory, motor, and central integration and processing components involved with maintaining joint homeostasis during functional activity.

sensory receptor: The specialized neural ending, group of cells, or sense organ that elicits an afferent impulse when stimulated (30). There are five types of sensory receptors located in the body, based on the nature of the stimuli to which they respond: mechanoreceptors, thermoreceptors, chemoreceptors, nociceptors, and electromagnetic receptors (13). Each morphological type of receptor is sensitive only to specific types of stimuli.

somatosensory system: The collection of peripheral sensory receptors responsible for giving rise to afferent information for the perceptions of mechanoreceptive (tactile and proprioceptive), thermoreceptive, and pain sensations (13).

spinocerebellar tracts: Four tracts believed to be responsible for conveying proprioceptive information to the cerebellum originating from muscle, joint, and cutaneous mechanoreceptors utilized for motor control (32).

system: An organized grouping of related structures that perform certain common actions (30); each system of the body has a specific domain in which it contributes to bodily homeostasis.

thermoreceptors: Sensory receptors responsible for transducing temperature stimuli into neural impulses.

vestibulospinal tract: Carries postural control commands from vestibular nuclei.

Testing Terminology

The following definitions of nomenclature are related to laboratory measurement of the sensorimotor system:

closed kinematic chain: Activities in which the distal segment is not free to move (31).

joint position testing: Method of proprioception testing that focuses on an individual's ability to replicate joint angles; may be conducted in either active or passive modes.

kinematics: The study of linear and angular motion independent of the causative forces (7, 33); includes measurement of position, velocity, and acceleration. Measurements are accomplished by tracking the displacement of specific body segments during motion with devices such as high-speed cameras, magnetic fields, and accelerometers.

kinesthesia testing: Method of proprioception testing that focuses on an individual's ability to detect movement of peripheral body segments; may be conducted in either active or passive modes.

kinetics: The study of forces causing movement (7, 33). Measurements may be made directly (e.g., by surgically implanted transducers) or indirectly using load cells and force platforms.

muscle activation measurement: Measurement of muscle activation characteristics (initiation, cessation, and magnitude) through the use of electromyography. Measurements may be taken during reflexive (i.e., joint perturbation), functional (i.e., walking), or voluntary (i.e., maximum voluntary contraction) muscle activation.

muscle performance measurement: Measurement of muscle performance characteristics (torque, work, and power) through use of load cells under varying contractile conditions; isokinetic dynamometry is the most popular method for the assessment of dynamic muscle function.

open kinematic chain: Activities in which the distal segment is free to move (31).

postural control measurement: Measurement of the ability to control posture. Often varying sensory conditions (i.e., foam surface) or mechanical perturbations (i.e., support surface movements) are utilized in attempts to focus on different components of the postural control system. Measurements of postural control can be made by recording center of pressure displacements and forces exerted on a force platform, motion of body segments through kinematic systems, or muscle activation using electromyography.

proprioception testing: Family of testing methods including joint position testing, kinesthesia testing, and sense of effort testing aimed at evaluating the integrity of peripheral mechanoreceptors in conveying proprioceptive sensations (kinesthesia, joint position sense, and sense of force). Models currently available rely on conscious perception; manipulations are often incorporated in attempts to focus on specific receptors (i.e., use of skin anesthesia to reduce cutaneous inputs).

sense of effort testing: Method of proprioception testing that focuses on an individual's ability to replicate torque magnitudes produced by a group of muscles under varying conditions.

References

1. Appleberg B, Hulliger M, Johansson H, Sojka P. Excitation of dynamic fusimotor neurons of the cat triceps surae by contralateral joint afferents. *Brain Res* 160: 529–32, 1979.
2. Bergenheim M, Johansson H, Pedersen J, Öhberg F, Sjölander P. Ensemble coding of muscle stretches in afferent populations containing different types of muscle afferents. *Brain Res* 734: 157–66, 1996.
3. Clark FJ, Burgess PR. Slowly adapting receptors in cat knee joint: Can they signal joint angle? *J Neurophysiol* 38: 1448–463, 1975.
4. Colebatch JG, McCloskey DI. Maintenance of constant arm position or force: Reflex and volitional components in man. *J Physiol* 386: 247–61, 1987.

5. Dietz V, Noth J, Schmidtbleicher D. Interaction between preactivity and stretch reflex in human triceps brachii during landing from forward falls. *J Physiol* 311: 113–25, 1981.
6. Dunn TG, Gillig SE, Ponser SE, Weil N. The learning process in biofeedback: Is it feedforward or feedback. *Biofeedback Self Reg* 11(2): 143–55, 1986.
7. Enoka R. *Neuromechanical basis of kinesiology.* Champaign, IL: Human Kinetics, 1994.
8. Erikson RP. Stimulus coding in topographic and nontopographic afferent modalities: On the significance of the activity of individual sensory neurons. *Psychol Rev* 75: 447–65, 1968.
9. Ghez C. The control of movement. In *Principles of neural science,* E Kandel, J Schwartz, T Jessell, eds. New York: Elsevier Science, 533–47, 1991.
10. Grigg P, Hoffman AH. Calibrating joint capsule mechanoreceptors as in vivo soft tissue load cells. *J Biomechan* 22: 781–85, 1989.
11. Grigg P. Peripheral neural mechanisms in proprioception. *J Sport Rehab* 3: 1–17, 1994.
12. Griller S. A role for muscle stiffness in meeting the changing postural and locomotor requirements for force development by ankle extensors. *Acta Physiol Scand* 86: 92–108, 1972.
13. Guyton AC. *Textbook of medical physiology.* 6th ed. Philadelphia: Saunders, 534–36, 562–64, 588–95, 1981.
14. Hanson Z, Stuart D. Animal solution to problems of movement control: The role of proprioceptors. *Ann Rev Neurosci* 11: 199–223, 1988.
15. Johansson H, Sjölander P, Sojka P. Activity in receptor afferents from the anterior cruciate ligament evoke reflex on fusimotor neurons. *Neurosci Res* 8: 54–59, 1990.
16. Johansson H, Sjölander P, Sojka P. Actions on γ motoneurons elicited by electrical stimulation of joint afferent fibers in the hind limb of the cat. *J Physiol* [London] 375: 137–52, 1986.
17. Johansson R, Magnusson M. Human postural dynamics. *Biomech Eng* 18: 413–37, 1991.
18. Johansson H, Sjölander P, Sojka P. A sensory role for the cruciate ligaments. *Clin Orthop* 268: 161–78, 1991.
19. Johansson H, Bergenheim M, Djupsjobacka M, Sjölander P. A method for analysis of encoding of stimulus separation in ensembles of afferents. *J Neurosci Meth* 63: 67–74, 1995.
20. La Croix JM. The acquisition of autonomic control through biofeedback: The case against an afferent process and a two-process alternative. *Psychophysiol* 18: 573–87, 1981.
21. Leksell L. The action potential and excitatory effects of the small ventral root fibers to skeletal muscle. *Acta Physiol Scand* 10(Suppl 31): 1–84, 1945.
22. Leonard C. *The neuroscience of human movement.* St. Louis: Mosby Year Book, 1998.
23. Mathews P. Where does Sherrington's "muscle sense" originate? Muscles, joints, corollary discharge? *Ann Rev Neuroscience*, 5:89-218, 1992.
24. Merton PA. Speculations on the servocontrol of movement. In *The Spinal Cord,* GEW Wolstenholme, ed. London: Churchill, 247–55, 1953.
25. Mihailoff G, Haines D. Motor system II: Corticofugal systems and the control of movement. In *Fundamental neuroscience,* D. Haines, ed. New York: Churchill Livingstone, 335–46, 1997.
26. Nashner L. Practical biomechanics and physiology of balance. In *Handbook of balance function and testing,* G Jacobson, C Newman, J Kartush, eds. St. Louis: Mosby Year Book, 261–79, 1993.
27. Nichols TR, Houk JC. Improvements in linearity and regulation of stiffness that results from actions of stretch reflex. *J Neurophysiol* 39: 119–42, 1976.
28. Palmar I. Pathophysiology of the medial ligament of the knee joint. *Acta Chir Scand* 115: 312–18, 1958.
29. Sherrington CS. The integrative action of the nervous system. New Haven, CT: Yale University Press, 1906.
30. Thomas C, ed. *Taber's cyclopedic medical dictionary*. Philadelphia: Davis, 1993.
31. Steidler A. *Kinesiology of the human body: Under normal and pathological conditions,* 3d ed. Springfield, IL: Charles C Thomas, 1955.
32. Warren S, Yezierski R, et al. The somatosensory system I: Discriminative touch and position sense. In *Fundamental neuroscience,* D Haines ed. New York: Churchill Livingstone, 220–35, 1997.
33. Winter D. *Biomechanics and motor control of human movement*. New York: Wiley, 1990.

SECTION 1

Contribution of the Sensorimotor System to Joint Stability

Section Leaders: Jonas Pedersen, PhD, and Scott F. Dye, MD

Section Participants: Hakan Johansson, PhD, Roland Biedert, MD,
Kevin Guskiewicz, PhD, ATC, Bryan L. Riemann, MA, ATC,
William Garrett, Jr., MD, PhD, Carlos A. Guanche, MD,
Answorth A. Allen, MD, Kevin P. Black, MD,
Timothy E. Hewett, PhD, and Jon J.P. Warner, MD

This section provides an overview of the mechanisms and processes of the sensorimotor system with specific application to joint stability. The authors present anatomical and physiological reviews of the peripheral and central nervous system, the relationship between the nervous and musculoskeletal systems, and the relationship between static and dynamic joint restraints. Further, the authors describe the effects of selected joint pathology on the restraint mechanisms mediated by the sensorimotor system.

The leading chapters to this section review the basic science of the sensorimotor system. Johansson and associates introduce the role of peripheral afferents in mediating central mechanisms that regulate muscle activation. They describe peripheral afferent histology and physiology and also put forth their hypotheses related to central processing of peripheral afferent information as it contributes to joint stability and muscle coordination. Biedert provides an overview of the subsystems of motor control and discusses the contribution of these respective systems to joint stabilization, followed by an overview by Dye of the role of the cerebellum in regulating motor functions. Guskiewicz and Riemann discuss the contribution of the peripheral somatosensory system on balance and postural control and provide strategies that are employed to maintain balance following lower extremity pathology. Garrett and Kirkendall present motor learning and motor control concepts related to knee joint injuries and pose potential learned strategies that may influence injury to the knee in athletes.

The second area within this section addresses issues specific to the sensorimotor system's role in joint stability. Dye and Vaupel provide an excellent review of the knee joint anatomy and geometry and discuss the role of knee sensory and motor innervation, which contributes to the restraint mechanisms to provide normal joint kinematics. Hewett and associates follow with a presentation of the relationship between various knee pathologies and the resulting kinematic and kinetic alterations.

The next three chapters contain discussion related to the shoulder joint. Ernlund and Warner address the restraint mechanisms of the shoulder and the role of the dynamic force couple in the overall stability of the joint. They further describe the significance of capsular and ligamentous injury related to the resulting imbalance between the dynamic and static restraint mechanisms. Guanche and associates present an overview of the role of shoulder afferents in contributing to both static and dynamic restraint, while Allen discusses the contribution of proprioception to neuromuscular control and joint kinematics.

In the final chapter of this section Black and Reiber present issues related to nerve regeneration. This chapter applies principles of peripheral nerve regeneration to peripheral afferents and discusses the potential of restoration of afferent pathways.

There is considerable agreement that proprioception contributes to joint stability through the mediation of muscle activation. However, research is needed in virtually all areas of basic science in an attempt to determine the physiological mechanisms that acquire and transmit somatosensory information, as well as the organization and activity of central processing. Additionally, the degree to which motor control mechanisms contribute to stability, along with the way they protect articular structures and function following injury, needs to be addressed. The following basic science areas, in particular, warrant studies specifically related to the contribution of the sensorimotor system to joint stability.

Directions for Future Research

1. Study the role of the various mechanoreceptors relative to their respective function in acquisition and transmittal of proprioceptive information, including the levels at which the CNS processes the information and the final outcome of these sensorimotor pathways. Specifically, the role that mechanoreceptive joint afferents have in regulation of the gamma muscle spindle system and, ultimately, in regulation of muscle stiffness needs to be further elucidated.
2. Develop more elaborate paradigms to assess the effects on proprioception resulting from disrupted joint structures, while systematically investigating potential proprioceptive submodalities that are different from the traditional position and movement sense tests.
3. Investigation needs to focus on the physiology and relationships of the somatosensory system at each segment of the kinetic chain that contributes to overall postural and joint stability.
4. The compensatory effects of the entire kinetic chain need to be demonstrated in the presence of pathology and deficits to specific segmental components of the system. These compensatory strategies employed need to be further demonstrated as they relate to static, dynamic, and functional balance following peripheral somatosensory deficits.

5. Determine the mediators of motor control that influence joint stability and then determine the alterations in these mediators that result in failure of the dynamic restraint mechanism and therefore expose the articular structures to injury.
6. Investigate the plasticity of the motor control system that may alter movement strategies and reduce the risk of injury and re-injury.
7. Determine the extent and timing of restoration of proprioception and motor control following injury and surgery, which ultimately influences the restoration of normal gait patterns.
8. The neural patterns of the shoulder capsule need to be delineated. Further, in conditions of recurrent atraumatic instability, the role of augmentation and transfer of neural receptors to enhance afference emanating from the joint needs to be investigated.
9. The effects that thermal agents used in surgical shrinkage procedures have on proprioception need to be investigated.
10. The role of reflex-mediated muscle activation as it relates to loading of articular structures needs to be elucidated, along with its role in shielding articular ligaments from excessive loads.
11. Investigations need to explore the effects of pathology on the neural receptor and the neurochemical signals that are sent by the target organs.
12. Investigations need to begin to establish the link between the basic science neurosensory data and the clinical research data in the normal, pathological, and surgically repaired or rehabilitated joint.

CHAPTER 1

Peripheral Afferents of the Knee: Their Effects on Central Mechanisms Regulating Muscle Stiffness, Joint Stability, and Proprioception and Coordination

Hakan Johansson, MD
Jonas Pedersen, PhD
Mikael Bergenheim, PhD
M. Djupsjöbacka, PhD

Abbreviations Used in the Text

muscle spindle afferent	MSA
anterior cruciate ligament	ACL
posterior cruciate ligament	PCL
medial collateral ligament	MCL
lateral collateral ligament	LCL
posterior articular nerve	PAN

Introduction

In this small review we have tried to cover morphological and physiological characteristics of the joint receptors and the function of these receptors in motor control and proprioception. We have reviewed investigations of several joints, but due to the fact that the knee joint is by far the most investigated, data on the knee joint predominates.

The contribution of joint afferents to motor control and to position and movement sense (proprioception) has been debated among neurophysiologists for many years, and for a couple of decades it has been known that there are nervous end organs in many joint structures. Recently it has also become clear that reflexes from joint afferents may be transmitted via pathways other than those projecting directly to the skeletomotoneurons (α-motoneurons). Thus, the pathways from joint afferents to the muscle spindles via the γ-motoneurons have drawn increasing attention, particularly since the effects on the γ-motoneurons often seem to be more potent and elicited at lower stimulation thresholds.

Since the primary muscle spindle afferents are of great importance for the regulation of muscle stiffness and for position and movement sense, it seems obvious that reflexes from peripheral afferents (e.g., joint afferents) to the γ-muscle spindle system also may be of importance for these functions.

Traditionally in orthopedic literature, relatively little attention has been focused on the articular neuronal structures, while much more interest has been devoted to the bony, ligamentous, and vascular anatomy of different joints. Today, however, much effort is directed to rectifying this imbalance.

Ruffini Receptor Endings in the Knee Joint

Ruffini endings can be found in several knee joint structures. First, they are present in the capsule, where they are more numerous in the superficial layers (42, 44, 46, 61, 62, 106, 143, 144). They can also be found in the cruciate, meniscofemoral, and collateral ligaments (6, 21, 46, 63, 86, 121, 122, 124, 129, 147), and in the menisci (145, 146). Several morphological types of Ruffini endings in different species and tissues have been described (60, 61, 122, 147). Various names have also been used for this type of receptor, such as Golgi-Mazzoni bodies, Meissner corpuscles, basket endings, ball-of-thread endings, bushlike endings and spray endings (46). The Ruffini ending usually consists of a cluster of two to six thinly encapsulated globular corpuscles with a single myelinated parent axon (see figure 1.1*b*). The diameter of the parent nerve fiber varies between 5 and 9 μm (46, 142). The capsule is sometimes complete but is more often incomplete, and it forms capsular septa between the individual cylinders of the nerve endings. The size of this type of receptor may also vary considerably within one joint structure. The Ruffini ending shows a low threshold to mechanical stress and is a slow adapting ending (for references, see 77). Thus, this ending may signal static joint position, intraarticular pressure, and amplitude and velocity of joint rotations (35, 38, 54, 55).

It is also worth mentioning that receptors that are tonically active at intermediate joint angles have been found in several joints, for example, the knee joint (23, 37). It has been suggested that these "midrange" afferents give information concerning joint angles and limb movements (6, 37, 110, 145), and it is likely that many of them arise from Ruffini endings.

Pacinian Corpuscles

Pacinian corpuscles are present in the deeper layers of the capsule (42, 44, 46, 54, 61, 62, 106, 143, 144); the cruciate, meniscofemoral, and collateral ligaments; the extraarticular and intraarticular fat pads of the knee joint (21, 46, 60, 63, 86, 121, 122, 129, 130, 145-147); and the medial meniscus (145, 146).

As with the Ruffini endings, several morphological varieties of Pacinian corpuscles have been described (60, 145), and many different names have been used also for this receptor type, for example, Krause's Endkörperchen, Vater-Pacinian corpuscles, Paciniform corpuscles, simple Pacinian corpuscles, Golgi-Mazzoni bodies, and bulbous corpuscles (46). The Pacinian corpuscles in articular tissues (see figure 1.1*d*) are encapsulated, conical corpuscles that are slightly smaller (20–40 μm wide, 150–250 μm long) than those found in extraarticular tissues (46, 60). Their parent axons are 8–12 μm in diameter (46, 60, 142).

The Pacinian corpuscle demonstrates a low threshold to mechanical stress but, in contrast to the Ruffini ending, rapidly adapts (for references, see 77). Thus, the Pacinian corpuscle is silent during static conditions and when the joint is rotated at constant speed but is very sensitive to acceleration and deceleration (21). Accordingly, these corpuscles behave as pure dynamic mechanoreceptors.

Golgi Tendon Organlike Endings

Golgi tendon organlike endings have been identified in the cruciate ligaments (21, 46, 63, 86, 121, 122, 129, 147), the collateral ligaments (6, 46, 124), and the menisci (145, 146). The Golgi ending, together with the Ruffini ending, belongs to a group called spray endings, which constitute a more or less continuous morphological spectrum of receptors (135); whether the spray endings should be divided into different receptor types is a matter of discussion. However, the largest of the articular mechanoreceptors are usually thinly encapsulated, fusiform corpuscles, which appear to be the articular homologue to the tendon organs of Golgi (see figure 1.1*c*). The diameter of the parent nerve fiber varies between 13 and 17 μm (46, 142, 144).

The Golgi tendon organlike endings are slow adapting, have high thresholds to mechanical stimuli, and are completely inactive in immobile joints (21). Researchers have suggested that, because of their high thresholds, these receptors measure the extremes of the joint's normal movement range (144, 145).

Free Nerve Endings

Free nerve endings are widely distributed throughout most of the articular structures. They can be found in the capsule, where they are evenly spread in all directions (42, 44, 46, 54, 61, 62, 106, 143, 144), the cruciate ligaments (21, 46, 63, 86, 121, 122, 129, 147), and the menisci, where they outnumber other receptor types (145, 146).

A free nerve ending consists of the sensory axon, which lacks a myelin sheath, perineurium, and corpuscle. It has a fine myelinated or unmyelinated axon with a diameter ranging from 0.5 to 5 μm (46, 64, 142, 144) (see figure 1.1*a*). According to an in-

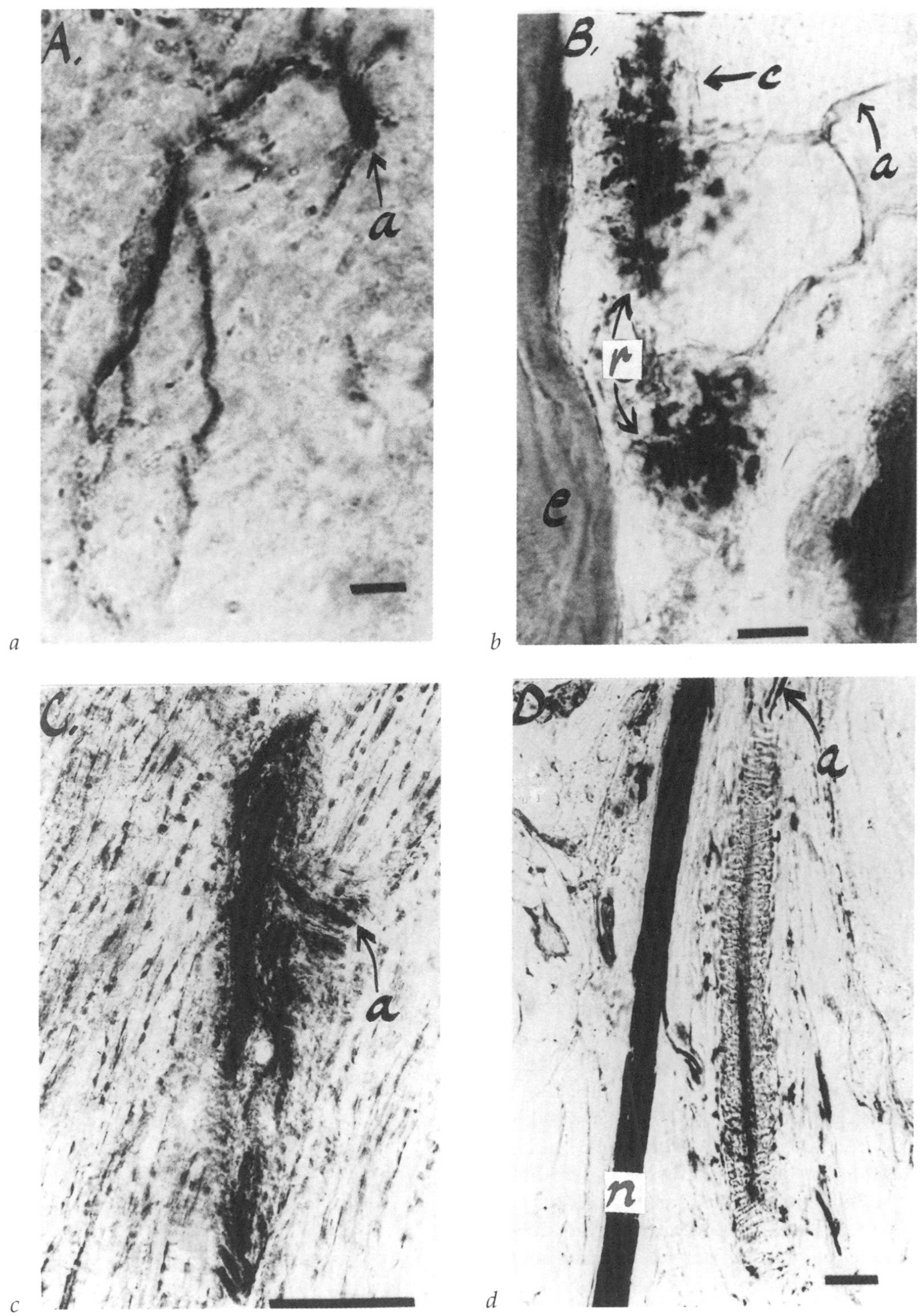

Figure 1.1 Photomicrographs of the different nerve endings found in the cat cruciate ligaments. *(a)* Free nerve endings originating from a single axon (a) in the subsynovial connective tissue of the PCL. *(b)* A Ruffini ending in the ACL close to the epiphysis (e) of tibia. Two corpuscles (r) with fine capsules (c), arising from branches of a single axon (a). *(c)* A Golgi tendon organlike ending within the collagenous substance of the ACL. Note the size of the receptor, the thick axon (a), and the location of the receptor in relation to the orientation of the collagenous fibers. *(d)* A Pacinian corpuscle near a nerve bundle (n) in the superficial layer of the PCL. Note that two axons (a) enter the single corpuscle. Bar in *(a)* = 10 m, b ar in *(b-d)* = 50 μm. (From Ref. 129, with permission.)

vestigation of the ultrastructure of free nerve endings by Heppelmann and others (64), two different types of free nerve endings seem to exist in articular tissues. The two types correlate with group III and group IV afferents. The two types differ in at least four aspects: (i) in the length of their distal branches, (ii) in the number of receptive sites (i.e., beads) per 100 μm axon length, (iii) in mean diameter of axons, and (iv) in the cytoskeletal structure.

The majority of the free nerve endings remain silent during normal conditions but become active when the articular tissue is subjected to damaging mechanical deformations and to certain substances (see 7, 55, 56, 119). Among the free nerve endings are located a considerable number of chemosensitive units. These are activated by certain ions and a number of different biochemical substances such as inflammatory mediators like serotonin, histamine, bradykinin, and prostaglandin (20, 58, 102, 116, 117, 120). It has also been shown that experimentally induced inflammation results in increased activity and in reduced thresholds to mechanical probing and to joint movements of these chemosensitive joint receptors (20, 28, 50, 56, 115, 116, 150).

Segmental Reflexes From Knee Joint Afferents: Effects on α-Motoneurons

Early studies concerning effects evoked on motoneurons by activation of sensory endings in ligaments are rather limited. Some effects on skeletomotor activity were observed when the tension in the MCL (34, 107) or the ACL (59, 100, 133) was selectively increased. However, most of these investigations lack quantitative information on the ligament loading, and more recent studies indeed have indicated that ligament loading, at least at small and moderate loads, does not directly affect the skeletomotor system (5, 53, 108, 109, 133, 134).

Instead, later experiments indicate that a stretch-sensitive receptor in the ACL modulates the EMG response via the α-γ-muscle spindle system, rather than by direct effects on the motoneurons (100).

These experiments are in accordance with results from our laboratory showing potent and frequent effects on the α-γ muscle spindle system, without accompanying direct effects on α-γ motoneurons, during activation of mechanoreceptors in different knee joint ligaments (e.g., 127).

Effects on γ-Motoneurons

It has been known for a long time that reflexes from joint mechanoreceptors contribute considerably to the normal coordination of the muscle activity in posture and movements (43, 44, 46), and it has been proposed that joint afferents influence muscle coordination through the motoneurons (see 34, 46).

Since then, the existence of reflex pathways from knee joint afferents to motoneurons has been demonstrated in a number of studies. By using graded electrical activation of knee joint afferents (mostly in the PAN) it has been shown that both low- and high-threshold joint afferents evoke frequent and strong reflex effects on static and dynamic lumbar motoneurons (16, 57, 78, 123, 139). Recordings from MSAs have revealed that the excitatory reflex effects evoked on motoneurons, by electrical activation of the PAN, are powerful enough to significantly modulate the activity in both primary and secondary MSAs from muscles around the knee joint (79, 97). Although these findings support the suggestion that articular sensory endings can influence motor control and muscle coordination via the muscle spindle system, the use of electrical activation of joint nerves has several distinct limitations—that is, the method allows only crude assessments of the specific tissue and the receptor types from which the joint afferents originate.

A few years ago we developed in our laboratory a method by which fusimotor reflexes elicited by stretch-sensitive sensory endings in cat knee joint ligaments could be assessed (83, 131). In a different series of experiments the intact ligaments (PCL, ACL, MCL, and LCL) were transversely loaded with traction forces of 5 to 40 N, while simultaneous recordings were made from single MSAs from muscles around the knee (73, 80, 83, 127, 131, 132). These muscles were subjected to sinusoidal stretching in order to determine, based on changes in the sinusoidal response of the spindle afferents, the size and character of the induced fusimotor reflex effects (12, 67).

One of the main results of these studies was that potent fusimotor effects regularly were evoked at low levels of ligament loading.

Figure 1.2 shows the responses of an ipsilateral PBSt (posterior biceps and semitendinosus muscles, ipsilateral to the PCL) primary MSA with (*b*) and without (*a*) a 40 N loading of the PCL. Figure 1.2 (*a* and *b*) shows the responses of the spindle afferent (upper traces) to 5 consecutive sinusoidal stretching cycles of the PBSt muscles (lower traces). As can be seen from the figure, the stretching of the PCL considerably increased the mean firing frequency of the primary spindle afferent.

The threshold load for the appearance of fusimotor effects strong enough to influence this spindle afferent was found between 5 and 10 N. Similarly low thresholds were also demonstrated for the LCL, PCL, and ACL (73, 80, 83, 127).

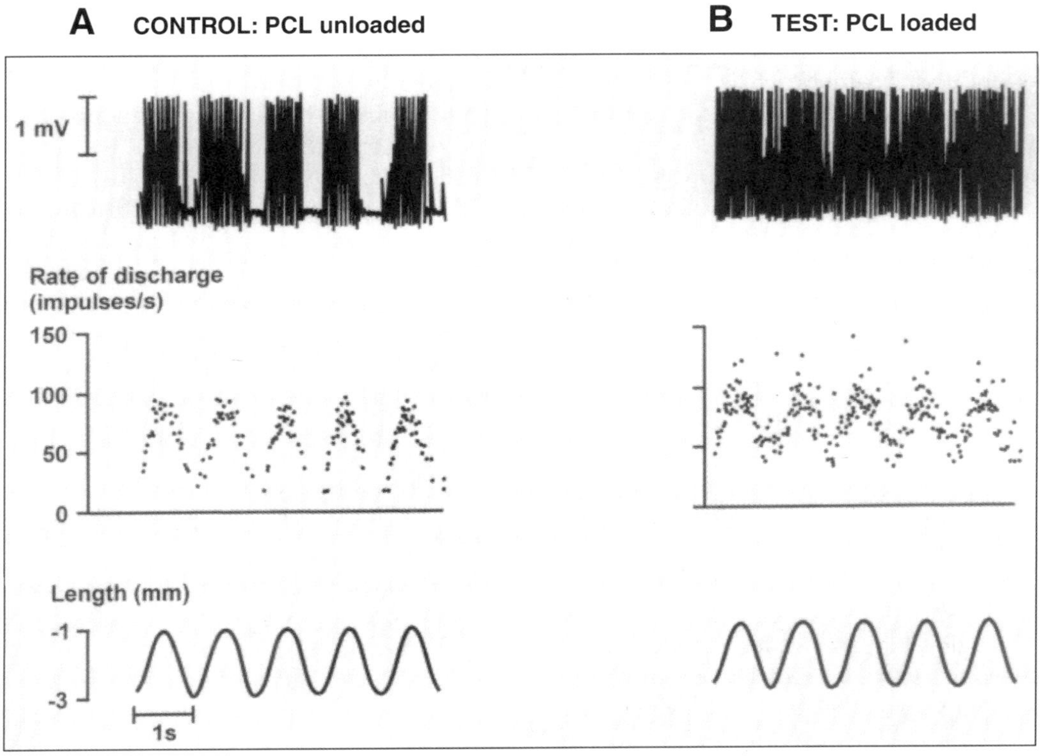

Figure 1.2 Responses of a primary muscle spindle afferent from posterior biceps and semitendinosus muscles (PBSt) to sinusoidal stretching of the receptor-bearing muscle (at 1 Hz, 1 mm) *(a)* without stretch of the PCL and *(b)* during ongoing stretch of the PCL with 40 N. Upper traces: activity of the spindle afferent recorded with a silver electrode from a teased dorsal root filament. Middle traces: display of the rate of discharge. Each dot represents a single action potential. The vertical displacements of the dots are proportional to the reciprocal of the time elapsed since the previous action potential. Lower traces: PBSt muscle length (0 = maximum physiological length). For further details, see text. (From Ref. 131, with permission.)

Small, predominantly dynamic fusimotor effects were elicited at low loads (5–10 N), whereas static fusimotor reflexes dominated at higher loads (20 N). The changes in the fusimotor effects to increased ligament load are likely due to recruitment of stretch-sensitive ligament receptors, which activate previously silent fusimotor neurons or increase the activity in the already active ones (80, 127).

In the cat, ligament loads of 5–10 N could most probably be regarded as low levels of mechanical stress, since loads of 200–300 N have to be applied to the knee joint ligament before they rupture (80, 83, 127, 133). A load of 5–10 N, thus, is comparable to about 1.5 to 5% of the ligament's ultimate strength, which implies a considerable "safety margin," indicating a non-nociceptive origin of the effects found on the α-γ-muscle spindle system. It is worth noting that during normal activities the human ACL is subjected to traction forces amounting to about 25% of that necessary to tear the ligament. Comparable data is still missing for the cat but is available for another quadruped—the goat. In a 1994 study, Holden and others made direct measurements of ACL forces during stance, walking, and trotting. They showed that the ACL was loaded in all three conditions, with the ligament tension positively correlated with the speed of gait. The lowest forces were observed in quiet standing and during the stance phase of gait. In these conditions the maximum magnitude of the ACL force was comparable to about 6% of the ACL's ultimate strength. Thus, these results suggest that the ligament loads needed for reflex activation of the muscle spindle system are low enough to be comparable to loads occurring during normal activities such as stance, walking, and trotting.

In addition to the low threshold of the fusimotor effects, a remarkably high responsiveness to stretch of different knee joints was found among both primary and secondary MSAs, from extensor as well as flexor muscles (73, 80, 83, 127). Moreover, the changes in the sensitivity of the muscle spindles evoked by loading the knee joint ligaments were often of significant magnitudes.

Another principal observation was the considerable degree of complexity in the response patterns found to stimulation of the various knee joint ligaments (43, 73, 80, 83, 127, 131). Thus, the different ligaments often induced fusimotor effects that differed both qualitatively and quantitatively on the individual muscle spindle. Behind these heterogeneous response profiles, however, there was a trend towards a predominance of dynamic fusimotor effects to loading of the ACL; pure static, pure dynamic, and mixtures of static and dynamic effects (with an about even frequency) to loading of the PCL; and pure dynamic or mixed effects to loading of the collateral ligaments.

Integration in the γ-System

Hind limb γ-motoneurons have very complex and individualized receptive profiles with respect to the pattern of reflex effects evoked by electrical stimulation of descending pathways and ipsilateral hind limb nerves (13, 68–70, 78, 84). The potent reflex effects from muscle, skin, and joint afferents and the individualized receptive profiles of the γ-motoneurons are also reflected at the level of the MSAs. This has been demonstrated using natural stimulation of muscle, skin, and joint receptor afferents in the ipsilateral as well as in the contralateral hind limbs (10–12, 43, 68, 73, 80, 83, 131). In order to provide a rationale for these observations, a new hypothesis about the function of the γ-muscle spindle system was proposed, that is, "the final common input" hypothesis (13, 68). This hypothesis advocates that information mediated by the MSAs is shaped, not only by variations in muscle length, but to a large extent also by the signals from descending pathways and from ipsilateral and contralateral peripheral nerves. In other words, descending messages and peripheral receptor information are integrated in the fusimotor neurons and then transmitted to the muscle spindles, where this integrated information undergoes final adjustments according to the ongoing length/tension changes of the parent muscle. Thus, the γ-spindle system is viewed as an integrative system that conveys polymodal feedback to the CNS; due to its intricate reflex regulation, it may be suited to deal with the sophisticated coordination between different muscles and, since there are indications that muscles might be functionally partitioned (141), perhaps also between intramuscular compartments (69).

Muscle Stiffness

Researchers have suggested that polysynaptic reflexes on motoneurons evoked by discharges in articular receptor afferents are responsible for the normal, smooth coordination of muscle tone (45, 56).

In recent studies in our laboratory this concept has gained substantial experimental support (see "Effects on γ-Motoneurons," above). Thus, sensory endings (in ligaments and in joint capsules) with low thresholds to mechanical stimuli exert potent reflex effects simultaneously on the muscle spindle systems of flexor and extensor muscles, and activation of knee ligament receptors can evoke both excitatory and inhibitory effects. Moreover, the relative balance between static and dynamic fusimotor activation, and thereby the alteration of the static and dynamic sensitivity of the muscle spindles, appears to depend on both which knee ligaments are stretched and the amount (and possibly the speed) of stretch. These features of the reflex control of the muscle spindle system from joint-ligament receptors may permit a sophisticated regulation of the muscular activation pattern during various movements and posture.

The total muscle stiffness (change in force/change in length) consists of a reflex-mediated and an intrinsic component (1, 2, 65). While the intrinsic component is dependent on the viscoelastic properties of the muscle and on the number of actomyosin bonds, the reflex-mediated stiffness is determined by the excitability of the α-motoneuron pool. Due to modulation of the reflex-mediated component, the total muscle stiffness has been shown to vary during co-contractions, voluntary dynamic contractions, and rhythmic movements (2, 17, 103, 105). Experiments on humans have demonstrated that the reflex-mediated component can increase the overall stiffness in muscles around the wrist and ankle joints up to 100% (43, 125, 137). Since it is well known that the excitability of the skeletomotoneurons, and hence the reflex-mediated stiffness, to a large extent is dependent on autogenic and heterogenic input from MSAs (3, 66, 103, 104), it would be expected that the fusimotor control of the muscle spindle sensitivity should have an impact on the overall muscle stiffness (2). The importance of the input from MSAs is evident from the fact that half of the total muscle stiffness during contraction levels comparable to standing or phases of walking is caused by the stretch reflex (137). Thus, taking into account the capability of ligament receptors to signal joint positions and movements, and the potent fusimotor effects evoked by these receptors, it seems quite likely that sensory endings in ligaments participate in the regulation of muscle stiffness through their reflex actions on the muscle spindle system (81, 82, 122). Yet, it should be remembered that both motoneurons and interneurons that are influenced by joint receptor discharges also receive input from muscle and cutaneous receptors (29, 82), which implies that it is likely that information from more that one receptor category is involved in the regulation of the reflex-mediated muscle stiffness.

The intrinsic muscle stiffness is largely dependent on the existing actomyosin bonds, which in turn is the result of the level of muscle contraction at a given moment. This stiffness component is thereby caused by the preceding reflex and descending influences on the α-γ-motoneuron pool. As the intrinsic stiffness is always present (but not constant during a movement), it has been regarded as the body's first line of defense against perturbations (1, 2, 125). Thus, if ligament receptors significantly contribute to the control of the reflex-mediated muscle stiffness, then they also will be important for the amount of intrinsic muscle stiffness and, thereby, for the protection of the joint against potentially harmful joint rotations. It has been suggested that a major function of the sensory system of the ligaments in the control of joint stability is to continuously preprogram (both in a spatial and a temporal sense) the intrinsic muscle stiffness through reflex modulation of the reflex-mediated stiffness (81, 82, 122).

Figure 1.3 summarizes the mechanisms by which ligaments can contribute to proprioception and to regulation of joint stability.

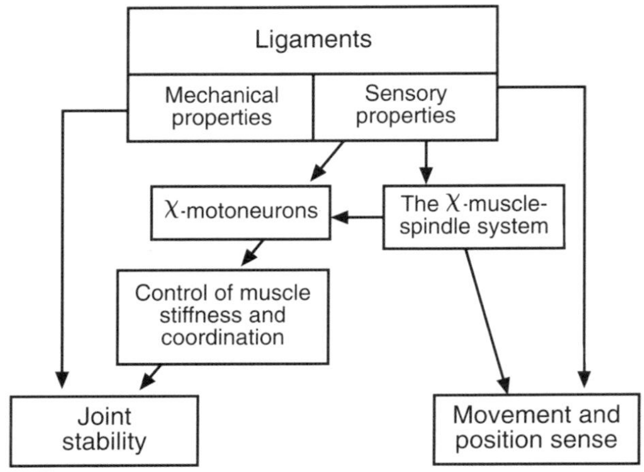

Figure 1.3 Organizational plan of the mechanisms by which ligaments may contribute to regulation of joint stability and to proprioception. (From Ref. 81, with permission.)

Proprioception and Motor Control: Proprioceptive Coding in Ensembles of Afferents

In the research of how peripheral stimuli are encoded in receptor afferent discharges, there has been a strong emphasis on the response properties and maximal sensitivity of single receptors. This line of research to a large extent has been based on the presumption that different stimuli or modalities are separately encoded in specific types of receptor afferents (i.e., the so-called "labelled line" theory). Consequently, receptors in muscles, joints, and the skin have been separated into a number of modality specific categories, for example, temperature, pressure, touch, muscle length, force and chemosensitive receptors.

There are both theoretical and empirical arguments against the belief that as a general rule sensory information is encoded according to traditional modality principles and that such information is transmitted to, and within, various structures in the CNS through private pathways or "labelled lines" (18, 36, 71, 72, 111, 112). The "labelled line" theory relies on the questionable hypothesis that there are decoding mechanisms or algorithms in the CNS that correlate to postulated modalities. This is doubtful, partly since most receptors and neurons seem to be sensitive to different types of stimuli and not only to a specific stimulus.

Another hypothesis on sensory coding is the "ensemble coding" or "population coding" theory, which places the emphasis on encoding in neural populations rather than by individual receptors and "labelled lines" (18, 36, 71, 72, 111, 112). From a teleological point of view, the "ensemble coding" theory has several clear-cut advantages in comparison to the "labelled line" hypothesis (36, 71, 72, 111, 112).

The concept of "ensemble coding" has indeed been discussed over several decades. There are unfortunately still relatively few studies that have addressed the hypothesis in conclusive experiments. Due to the development of novel recording techniques that permit simultaneous recordings of large number of individual afferents, however, and to the application of pattern recognition techniques in the analysis of coding properties in population responses, the concept has lately gained some experimental support (18, 32, 36, 71, 72, 111, 149). Recent experiments conducted in our laboratory (18, 71, 72) revealed that the ensemble responses of primary MSAs had considerably greater ability to discriminate between muscle length stimuli as compared to the response patterns of single spindle afferents. Moreover, the information content in populations of primary MSAs was greatly reduced when the fusimotor innervation of the spindles was eliminated, indicating that the drive is important for the encoding properties in ensembles of MSAs. Another important observation was that the ability to discriminate between passive muscle length inputs was significantly greater in populations containing both primary and secondary MSAs and Golgi tendon organ afferents, as compared to populations containing pure primary spindle afferents (19).

The γ-Muscle Spindle System as a Neural Network

The role of the fusimotor system for the ensemble coding capacity of populations of primary MSAs was discussed earlier (see above). The successive increase in discriminative ability for ensembles of primary MSAs with increasing ensemble size seems to be dependent mainly on the fusimotor drive and is clearly detectable only with simultaneous recordings (18). This may be explained by some of the features of the γ-muscle spindle system. The fusimotor system is influenced by various afferents from the skin, joints, and muscles, and the primary MSAs seem to be affected very individually from these sources (68, 77, 83). The large number of sources influencing the sensitivity of the primary MSAs to different stimuli is likely to increase the amount of situation-specific or nonrandomized response variability in the total population of MSAs over time.

Another feature of the γ-muscle spindle system that is likely to increase the response variability over time, or rather the situation-specific variation in MSA response, is that different muscle spindles in homonymous and heteronomous muscles on both ipsilateral and contralateral sides are connected to each other via the secondary MSAs and the γ-motoneurons (14). Thus, the secondary MSAs project back to the motoneurons that innervate the same and other muscle spindles. These connections seem to constitute a neural network in which each "neuron" (i.e., in this case each individual muscle spindle) is influenced by the activity in the whole network (i.e., the total population of muscle spindles) (69). Such a network may provide a very high-fidelity encoding of mechanical stimuli.

The Role of Muscle and Skin Afferents in Proprioception

For several decades the relative importance of mechanoreceptor input from joints, muscles, and cutaneous tissues to proprioceptive sensations has been a controversial matter. The view has changed over the years, in some periods in favor of muscle receptors, in others in support of articular and cutaneous receptors (122, 128).

Early in the century it was suggested that muscle receptors could play a major part in providing the CNS with proprioceptive cues. This belief was based on the complex morphology and the high sensitivity to mechanical muscle stimuli of muscle receptors like the muscle spindle and the Golgi tendon organ. Over the last three decades this view has been substantially bolstered by a number of experimental results. In animals, muscle afferents were demonstrated to have projections to several supraspinal structures, including the somatosensory cortex and cerebellum (74–76, 88, 89, 92). Activation of muscle receptors by longitudinal vibration of the muscle in a stationary limb was found to induce illusions of joint movements in man (51, 113, 114). Since vibration excites mainly MSAs, these findings indicate that information from these afferents might be especially important for movement sensations. It was also indicated that the frequency of muscle receptor activation (i.e., vibration frequency) was to some extent correlated to the perceived movement velocity (113, 114). Similar movement illusions have been described when an exposed tendon is pulled (whereby tension-sensitive muscle receptors are activated due to increased muscle length) in a stationary limb (95). These observations have lead to the suggestion that the primary MSAs provide relatively more information on limb velocity, whereas secondary MSAs contribute mainly to limb position information (94, 126).

In studies of the ability to detect movements and positions of finger joints, it has been determined that anesthesia of the joint and the skin (i.e., leaving only the muscle afferents unaffected) results in only a partial reduction of the proprioceptive ability (25, 39–41, 47, 52, 96). Other evidence for a major contribution from muscle receptors is the demonstration of disturbed proprioception by muscle loading and the observation that the proprioceptive ability can be enhanced during contractions of muscles around the joint (41, 48, 94). Researchers suggested that the latter finding was caused by increased sensitivity of MSAs due to increased fusimotor activity (8, 9, 41, 48), but it also could be, at least partly, a result of increased feedback from Golgi tendon organs.

In contrast to agreement among researchers on the seemingly clear-cut contribution to proprioception from muscle receptors, there is still an ongoing controversy as to whether or not cutaneous afferents carry specific proprioceptive information. It has long been commonly believed that the main role of afferents from the skin is to enhance the effects of other proprioceptive input. The accuracy of the proprioception of finger joints has been shown to be reduced after skin anesthesia, and it has been suggested that this is due to loss of facilitatory input from cutaneous receptors (25, 39, 40). Since anesthesia of skin areas not directly overlaying the joint induced the same blunting of the proprioception, it was suggested that the facilitatory input from cutaneous afferents is relatively nonspecific. Lately, however, evidence has been reported for a more specific proprioceptive role of cutaneous receptors. Microneurographic recordings from cutaneous afferents emanating from the human wrist and finger joints have shown that receptors located in the dorsal skin have response properties, which potentially can provide information on movements of the hand and fingers (33). This does not necessarily imply, however, that the CNS actually uses the cutaneous input as proprioceptive cues.

The Role of Joint Afferents in Proprioception: Supraspinal Projection of Joint Afferents

By using electrical stimulation of various joint nerves or physiological activation of joint receptors in animals, researchers have shown that joint afferents project to supraspinal centers through several ascending pathways, including the dorsal columns and the spinothalamic, spinoreticular, spinocervical, and spinocerebellar pathways (49, 118). There is also direct evidence that information from joint afferents reaches the cerebral cortex, the cerebellum, the reticular formation, and the thalamus (4, 26, 101). Several of these studies have demonstrated clear-cut projections from low-threshold joint afferents (probably from Ruffini endings). Moreover, a significant number of cerebral neurons, at least in the thalamus, appear to be as sensitive to changes in the joint angle as the slowly adapting low-threshold joint receptors themselves (101). At the cortical level, clear representations of the peripheral topography of joint receptors have been manifested. Thus, it seems fair to conclude that the somatosensory system of the cortex has a good capability to adequately track the activity in joint afferents.

This conclusion has been bolstered by results elicited on human subjects with the use of a microstimulation technique that allows selective excitation of single identified peripheral afferents. In 1990, Macefield and others (93) stimulated 11 single afferents from the wrist or the finger joints and found eight of them to evoke distinct and specific sensations—four induced innocuous deep pressure sensation while the other four induced sensations of joint displacement. The results suggest a potent and secure transmission of joint afferent information to perceptual levels and indicate that the brain might be able to obtain meaningful information on joint movements on the basis of the activation pattern in very few, or perhaps even single, joint afferents (93).

The Role of Joint Afferents in Proprioception: Direct Experimental Support

In addition to the above-described indirect support for a significant proprioceptive function of joint receptors, a number of studies have revealed more explicit evidence for this view. Removal of joint afferent input (by, e.g., local intraarticular injection of anesthetics, nerve blockades, or surgical removal of the joint) has been found to reduce the proprioceptive acuity of different joints (39, 40, 47). Although these findings demonstrate that joint afferents contribute to proprioceptive sensations, they are limited in that no conclusion can be drawn as to the extent to which sensory endings in specific joint structures are involved (i.e., capsule, ligaments, and menisci).

Disturbances in Proprioception Following Knee Ligament Injuries

In attempts to investigate the proprioceptive function of specific joint ligaments, several reports have recently been presented on the proprioceptive ability after ACL disruption. In 1989, Barrack and coworkers observed a statistically significant increase in the threshold to detection of passive motion in ACL-deficient subjects. Essentially the same results were reported in 1992 by Corrigan and others, who, in addition, noted a reduction in static position sense in ACL-deficient knee joints. In 1992, Lephart and coworkers, using a similar experimental approach, demonstrated that the reduction in movement detection ability persists after patellar tendon autograft or allograft ACL reconstruction. A reduced proprioceptive acuity after ACL rupture was also reported in 1991 by Barrett, who measured a significant difference in the ability to actively reproduce a passively guided knee joint position. In this study the position sense was considerably improved, but not fully restored, after reconstruction surgery performed by a modified MacIntosh-Jones method. Somewhat contradictory results were recently reported by Skinner and coworkers (27), who found no differences between the proprioceptive acuity in the ACL-reconstructed and the intact contralateral knee joint when the patients were tested, on average, 31 months after the surgery. The authors suggested that a well-done ACL reconstruction with appropriate rehabilitation could result in a knee joint proprioception that is essentially normal. However, to what extent the proprioceptive ability after an ACL rupture can be fully restored has to be further investigated since it is likely that the proprioceptive ability in the contralateral limb also may be affected after an ipsilateral joint injury (79, 99, 148).

Disturbances in Muscular Activation Following Knee Ligament Injuries

A number of studies have shown more or less inconsistent differences in EMG patterns between ACL-deficient limbs and normal limbs during movements (22, 24, 87, 90, 91, 98, 136). The reason for at least some of the inconsistencies is the fact that the muscular activation patterns have been investigated during very different activities such as, for example, walking, running, cutting, and stair climbing. Yet, in studies where simple activities were assessed the number of contradictory results appears larger than in studies where more demanding tasks were performed. For instance, in 1991 Sinkjær and coworkers (151) reported that during slow horizontal walking ACL-deficient subjects demonstrated no differences in the EMG pattern in comparison to subjects with intact knee joints, but during uphill walking the ligament-deficient subjects showed an earlier recruitment and prolonged activity in muscles around the knee joint (87, 90). The alterations in EMG onset and burst duration were most pronounced in the hamstring and the gastrocnemius muscles. Interestingly, when they compared the coordination patterns and relative levels of activity between a functionally excellent and a functionally poor ACL patient group (according to the Lysholm score), significant differences were observed in both EMG onset and burst duration of the gastrocnemius medialis muscle (see figure 1.4). The EMG profile of patients with poor functional knee joints was in general very similar to that of the control subjects, while the EMG profile of patients with an excellent knee joint function was clearly different (see figure 1.4). These findings demonstrate that the coordination patterns of several muscles around the knee joint are affected by an ACL rupture and that such effects are most clearly manifested in more demanding motor tasks. Sinkjær and Arendt-Nielsen (151) suggested that the altered coordination patterns could be due to a compensatory mechanism that might be essential in the ACL-deficient patient to secure a functional knee joint stability (see also 22, 98, 136).

Kinematic data have indicated also that changes

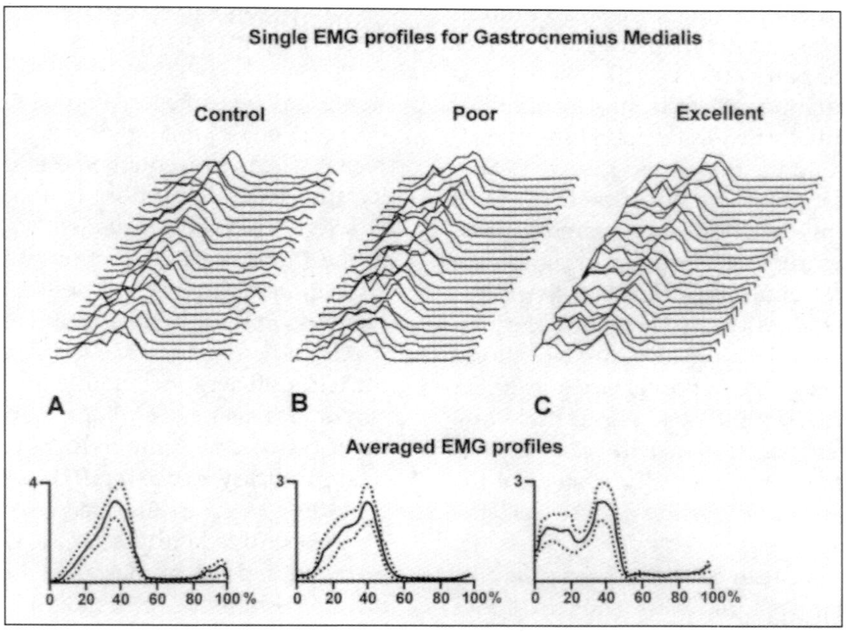

Figure 1.4 Pseudo three-dimensional plots of single EMG profiles and mean EMG profiles from the gastrocnemius medialis muscle. A profile represents rectified and averaged EMG activity over one gait cycle (0–100%) with heel strike at 100%. *(a)* Controls, *(b)* ACL-deficient subject with poor stability, *(c)* ACL-deficient subject with excellent stability. Mean profiles shown with *SD* of the mean. (From Ref. 151, with permission.)

in movement strategies occur as a result of ACL deficiency. Based on angular information from ACL-deficient and uninjured limbs during running at different velocities, McNair and coworkers (98) concluded that the ACL-deficient subjects seem to adopt one of two solutions to the problem introduced by the ligament injury. The overall knee angle in the ACL-deficient limb was increased in one group of subjects, whereas the flexion angle of the injured knee was decreased at footstrike in the other group. Moreover, studies on dogs with unilateral ACL-deficient knee joints have shown that changes in the kinematics are not confined to the unstable joint but also affect the other joints in that limb, the joints in the contralateral limb, as well as the vertical movements of the rump (138). Again, these results may indicate that modification of the movement patterns is functionally important in order to protect the knee joint from giving way and from rapid deterioration in the new sensory and biomechanical situation induced by the ligament rupture.

Functional Joint Stability

Because of the function of ligaments as passive elements opposing and limiting joint move-ments, it commonly is believed that the mechanical properties of the ligaments not only are crucial for passive joint stability but also are primarily responsible for functional joint stability. The "time argument" against protective reflexes has been widely used to support this view. This view, however, disregards the crucial point in the discussion about the importance of muscles in the control of the knee joint stability: the state of the changeable muscle stiffness at the time of the displacement will to a considerable degree determine the load on the joint and thereby the actual stability of the joint at the time of the trauma.

The lack of a strict relationship between the passive stability of a joint (joint laxity determined by clinical laxity tests) and the functional stability has been established in several studies (11). Functional joint stability is determined by the interaction of several factors, including the passive restraint caused by the ligaments and other joint structures, the joint geometry, the friction between the cartilage surfaces, and the load on the joint caused by compression forces resulting from gravity and the muscles acting on the joint. Of all the factors contributing to the functional joint stability, the load imposed on the joint is one of the most important. The knee joint, for instance, is in posture and movement subjected to force and momentum produced by the body weight (gravity), inertia, and muscles. Interaction between these factors results in a joint load/joint reaction force (i.e., in a force that presses the joint surfaces of the femur against those of the tibia). The contribution to the load imposed on joints caused by contraction of the surrounding muscles is considerable and causes a major increase in the stiffness of the joint. For the knee joint, the total load on the joint is increased significantly when there is concomitant antagonist activation (both quadriceps and hamstrings), since this contributes to an equal pressure distribution over the articular surface (15); there are several studies showing that flexor and extensor muscles around the knee joint in man are activated simultaneously (co-contracted) in a wide range of motor activities and movements (11). Thus, during movement, flexor and extensor muscles at the knee cooperate in producing knee joint loading forces, which press together the surfaces of the femur and tibia and thus modify the degree of knee joint stiffness. The fact that simultaneous contraction of agonistic and antagonistic muscles enhances the load imposed on and the stability of the joint stresses the importance of muscle coordination for functional joint stability.

Possible Role of Joint Afferents in Musculoskeletal Pain Syndromes

The effects on secondary MSAs from stretch-sensitive ligament receptors may have especially interesting implications for the regulation of muscle stiffness (43, 50, 53, 83, 109, 127, 140). This is due to the fact that the secondary MSAs, in contrast to the primaries (13), project back to the muscle spindle system, that is, they cause strong effects on static and dynamic motoneurons of both homonymous and heteronymous muscles (14). The secondary spindle afferents may thereby be part of a positive feedback loop (secondary spindle afferents-fusimotor neurons-muscle spindles), which may maintain a high sensitivity of the spindle and a high level of muscle stiffness. It seems also possible that there may exist a certain "threshold" in the activation of the muscle spindle system at which the activity in this positive feedback loop starts working like an amplifier that increases the effect of other inputs.

It has been suggested that this potential "vicious circle" may be involved in the pathophysiological mechanisms behind the onset and spread of muscle

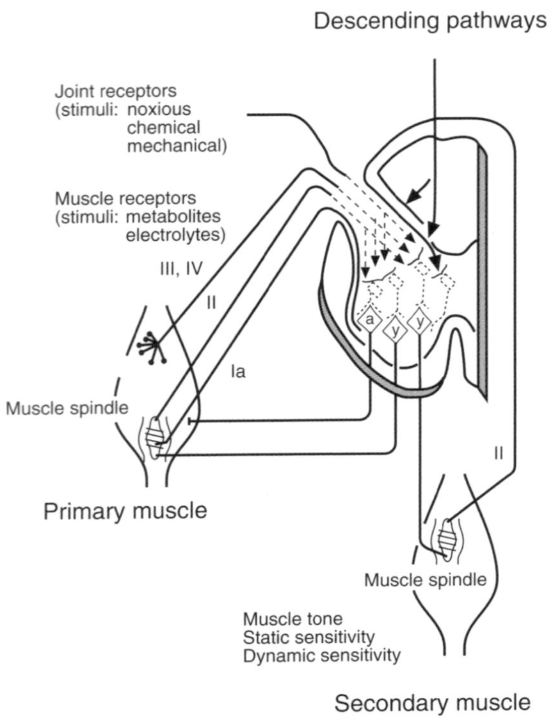

Figure 1.5 The pathophysiological model for possible mechanisms behind the genesis and spread of muscular tension and pain. (From Ref. 85, with permission).

tension and pain in chronic musculoskeletal pain disorders (8, 30, 31, 85). Thus, it is conceivable that, for instance, a whiplash trauma causes a massive afferent input from mechanosensitive and nociceptive sensory endings in ligaments and capsules in the cervical region that triggers the positive feedback circuit, which in turn results in increased muscle stiffness. In this context it should be recalled that the amount of fusimotor excitation seems to be related to the ligament tension (figure 1.5). When the stiffness (or tension) in the muscles is elevated, the production and liberation of ions and metabolites will also be increased (e.g., K ions, lactic acid, arachidonic acid, histamine, and serotonin). These substances are known to activate chemosensitive muscle afferents that, via their reflex effects on fusimotor neurons, further increase the excitatory load on the α-γ- muscle spindle system (e.g., 30, 31). This could tentatively result in a chronic state of high muscle stiffness and pain that is maintained by the positive feedback loop (secondary spindle afferents-fusimotor neurons-muscle spindles) and by the increased activity in the chemosensitive muscle afferents.

References

1. Akazawa K, Aldridge JW, Steeves JD, Stein RB. Modulation of stretch reflexes during locomotion in the mesencephalic cat. *J Physiol* (London) 1982, 329: 553–67.
2. Akazawa K, Milner TE, Stein RB. Modulation of reflex EMG and stiffness in response to stretch of human finger muscle. *J Neurophysiol* 1983, 49: 16–27.
3. Allum JHJ, Mauritz K-H. Compensation for intrinsic muscle stiffness by short-latency reflexes in human triceps surae muscles. *J Neurophysiol* 1984, 52: 797–818.
4. Andersen HT, Körner L, Landgren S, Silfvenius H. Fiber components and cortical projections of the elbow joint nerve in the cat. *Acta Physiol Scand* 1967, 69: 373–82.
5. Andersson S, Stener B. Experimental evaluation of the hypothesis of ligamento-muscular protective reflexes. II: A study in cat using the medial collateral ligament of the knee joint. *Acta Physiol Scand* 1959, 48: 27–49.
6. Andrew BL. The sensory innervation of the medial ligament of the knee joint. *J Physiol* (London) 1954, 123: 241–50.
7. Andrew BL, Dodt E. The deployment of sensory nerve endings at the knee joint of the cat. *Acta Physiol Scand* 1953, 28: 287–96.
8. Aniss AM, Diener H-C, Hore J, Burke D, Gandevia SC. Reflex activation of muscle spindles in human pretibial muscles during standing. *J Neurophysiol* 1990, 64: 671–79.
9. Aniss AM, Diener H-C, Hore J, Gandevia SC, Burke D. Behavior of human muscle receptors when reliant on proprioceptive feedback during standing. *J Neurophysiol* 1990, 64: 661–70.
10. Appelberg B, Hulliger M, Johansson H, Sojka P. Excitation of dynamic fusimotor neurons of the cat triceps surae by contralateral joint afferents. *Brain Res* 1979, 160: 529–32.
11. Appelberg B, Hulliger M, Johansson H, Sojka P. Reflex activation of dynamic fusimotor neurons by natural stimulation of muscle and joint receptor afferent units. In *Muscle Receptors and Movement*, Taylor A, Prochazka A, editors. London: Macmillan, 1981, 149–61.
12. Appelberg B, Hulliger M, Johansson H, Sojka P. Fusimotor reflexes in triceps surae elicited by natural stimulation of muscle afferents from the cat ipsilateral hind limb. *J Physiol* (London) 1982, 329: 211–29.
13. Appelberg B, Hulliger M, Johansson H, Sojka P. Actions on gamma motoneurons elicited by

electrical stimulation of group I muscle afferent fibers in the hind limb of the cat. *J Physiol* (London) 1983, 335: 237–53.
14. Appelberg B, Hulliger M, Johansson H, Sojka P. Actions on gamma motoneurons elicited by electrical stimulation of group II muscle afferent fibers in the hind limb of the cat. *J Physiol* (London) 1983, 335: 255–73.
15. Baratta R, Solomonow M, Zhou BH, Letson ED, Chuinard R, D'Ambrosia R. Muscular coactivation: The role of the antagonistic musculature in maintaining knee stability. *Am J Sports Med* 1988, 16: 113–22.
16. Baxendale RH, Davey NJ, Ellaway PH, Ferrell WR. The interaction between joint and cutaneous afferent input in the regulation of fusimotor neuron discharge. In *Muscle Afferents and Spinal Control of Movement,* Jami L, Pierrot-Deseilligny E, Zytnicki D, editors. Oxford: Pergamon Press, 1992, 95–104.
17. Bennett DJ. Stretch reflex responses in the human elbow joint during a voluntary movement. *J Physiol* (London) 1994, 474: 339–51.
18. Bergenheim M, Johansson H, Pedersen J. The role of the gamma system for improving information transmission in populations of Ia afferents. *Neurosci Res* 1995, 23: 207–15.
19. Bergenheim M, Johansson H, Pedersen J, Öhberg F, Sjölander P. Ensemble coding of muscle stretches in afferent populations containing different types of muscle afferents. *Brain Res* 1996, 734: 157–66.
20. Birrell GJ, McQueen DS, Iggo A, Grubb BD. The effects of 5-HT on articular sensory receptors in normal and arthritic rats. *Br J Pharmacol* 1990, 101: 715–21.
21. Boyd IA. The histological structure of the receptors in the knee joint of the cat correlated with their physiological response. *J Physiol* (London) 1954, 124: 476–88.
22. Branch TP, Hunter R, Donath M. Dynamic EMG analysis of anterior cruciate-deficient legs with and without bracing during cutting. *Am J Sports Med* 1989, 17: 35–41.
23. Burgess PR, Clark FJ. Characteristics of knee joint receptors in the cat. *J Physiol* (London) 1969, 203: 317–35.
24. Ciccotti MG, Kerlan RK, Perry J, Pink M. An electromyographic analysis of the knee during functional activities. II. The anterior cruciate ligament-deficient and reconstructed profiles. *Am J Sports Med* 1994, 22: 651–58.
25. Clark FJ, Burgess RC, Chapin JW, Lipscomb WT. Role of intramuscular receptors in the awareness of limb position. *J Neurophysiol* 1985, 54: 1529–540.
26. Clark FJ, Landgren S, Silfvenius H. Projections to the cat's cerebral cortex from low threshold joint afferents. *Acta Physiol Scand* 1973, 89: 504–21.
27. Co FH, Skinner HB, Cannon WD. Effect of reconstruction of the anterior cruciate ligament on proprioception of the knee and the heel strike transient. *J Orthop Res* 1993, 11: 696–704.
28. Coggeshall RE, Hong KAP, Langford LA, Schaible H-G, Schmidt RF. Discharge characteristics of fine medial articular afferents at rest and during passive movements of inflamed knee joints. *Brain Res* 1983, 272: 185–88.
29. Craig AD, Heppelmann B, Schaible H-G. The projection of the medial and posterior articular nerves of the cat's knee to the spinal cord. *J Comp Neurol* 1988, 276: 279–88.
30. Djupsjöbacka M, Johansson H, Bergenheim M. Influences on the gamma muscle spindle system from muscle afferents stimulated by increased intramuscular concentrations of arachidonic acid. *Brain Res* 1994, 663: 293–302.
31. Djupsjöbacka M, Johansson H, Bergenheim M, Sjölander P. Influences on the gamma muscle spindle system from contralateral muscle afferents stimulated by KCl and lactic acid. *Neurosci Res* 1995, 21: 301–309.
32. Djupsjöbacka M, Johansson H, Bergenheim M, Sandström U. A multichannel hook electrode for simultaneous recording of up to 12 nerve filaments. *J Neurosci Meth* 1994, 52: 69–72.
33. Edin BB, Johansson N. Skin strain patterns provide kinesthetic information to the human central nervous system. *J Physiol* (London) 1995, 487: 243–51.
34. Ekholm J, Eklund G, Skoglund S. On the reflex effects from the knee joint of the cat. *Acta Physiol Scand* 1960, 50: 167–74.
35. Eklund G, Skoglund S. On the specificity of the Ruffini-like joint receptors. *Acta Physiol Scand* 1960, 49: 184–91.
36. Erickson RP. Stimulus coding in topographic and nontopographic afferent modalities: On the significance of the activity of individual sensory neurons. *Psychol Rev* 1968, 75: 447–65.
37. Ferrell WR. The adequacy of stretch receptors in the cat knee joint for signaling joint angle throughout a full range of movement. *J Physiol* (London) 1980, 299: 85–99.
38. Ferrell WR. The effect of acute joint distension on mechanoreceptor discharge in the knee of the cat. *Q J Exp Physiol* 1987, 72: 493–99.

39. Ferrell WR, Craske B. Contribution of joint and muscle afferents to position sense at the human proximal interphalangeal joint. *Exp Physiol* 1992, 77: 331–42.
40. Ferrell WR, Milne SE. Factors affecting the accuracy of position matching at the proximal interphalangeal joint in human subject. *J Physiol* (London) 1989, 411: 575–83.
41. Ferrell WR, Smith A. The effect of loading on position sense at the proximal interphalangeal joint of the human index finger. *J Physiol* (London) 1989, 418: 145–61.
42. Freeman MAR, Wyke B. Reflex innervation of the ankle joint. *Nature* 1965, 207: 196.
43. Freeman MAR, Wyke B. Articular contributions to limb muscle reflexes: The effects of partial neurectomy of the knee joint on postural reflexes. *Br J Surg* 1966, 53: 61–69.
44. Freeman MAR, Wyke B. The innervation of the ankle joint: An anatomical and histological study in the cat. *Acta Anat* (Basel) 1967, 68: 321–33.
45. Freeman MAR, Wyke B. Articular reflexes at the ankle joint: An electromyographic study of normal and abnormal influences of ankle joint mechanoreceptors upon reflex activity in the leg muscles. *Br J Surg* 1967, 54: 990–1001.
46. Freeman MAR, Wyke B. The innervation of the knee joint: An anatomical and histological study in the cat. *J Anat* 1967, 101: 505–32.
47. Gandevia SC, Hall LA, McCloskey DI, Potter EK. Proprioceptive sensation at the terminal joint of the middle finger. *J Physiol* (London) 1983, 335: 507–17.
48. Gandevia SC, McCloskey DI, Burke D. Kinesthetic signals and muscle contraction. *Trends Neurosci* 1992, 15: 62–65.
49. Gardner E, Latimer F, Stilwell D. Central connections for afferent fibers from the knee joint of the cat. *Am J Physiol* 1949, 159: 195–98.
50. Gentle MJ, Thorp BH. Sensory properties of ankle joint capsule mechanoreceptors in acute monoarthritic chickens. *Pain* 1994, 57: 361–74.
51. Gilhodes JC, Roll JP, Tardy-Gervet MF. Perceptual and motor effects of agonist-antagonist muscle vibration in man. *Exp Brain Res* 1986, 61: 395–402.
52. Goodwin GM, McCloskey DI, Matthews PBC. The contribution of muscle afferents to kinesthesia shown by vibration-induced illusions of movement and by the effects of paralyzing joint afferents. *Brain* 1972, 95: 705–48.
53. Grabiner MD, Campbell KR, Hawthorne DL, Hawkins DA. Electromyographic study of the anterior cruciate ligament-hamstrings synergy during isometric knee extension. *J Orthop Res* 1989, 7: 152–55.
54. Grigg P, Hoffman AH. Properties of Ruffini afferents revealed by stress analysis of isolated sections of cat knee capsule. *J Neurophysiol* 1982, 47: 41–54.
55. Grigg P, Hoffman AH, Fogarty KE. Properties of Golgi-Mazzoni afferents in cat knee joint capsule, as revealed by mechanical studies of isolated joint capsule. *J Neurophysiol* 1982, 47: 31–40.
56. Grigg P, Schaible H-G, Schmidt RF. Mechanical sensitivity of group III and IV afferents from posterior articular nerve in normal and inflamed cat knee. *J Neurophysiol* 1986, 55: 635–43.
57. Grillner S, Hongo T, Lund S. Descending monosynaptic and reflex control of gamma motoneurons. *Acta Physiol Scand* 1969, 75: 592–613.
58. Grubb BD, Birrell GJ, McQueen DS, Iggo A. The role of PGE_2 in the sensitization of mechanoreceptors in normal and inflamed ankle joints of the rat. *Exp Brain Res* 1991, 84: 383–92.
59. Grüber J, Wolter D, Lierse W. In vivo study on the proprioceptive function of knee ligaments. *Third Cong. of the Europ Soc of Knee Surg and Arthroscopy*, Amsterdam. 1988, 6.
60. Halata Z. The ultrastructure of the sensory nerve endings in the articular capsule of the knee joint of the domestic cat (Ruffini corpuscles and Pacinian corpuscles). *Kaibogaku Zasshi* 1977, 124: 717–29.
61. Halata Z. Ruffini corpuscle: A stretch receptor in the connective tissue of the skin and locomotion apparatus. *Prog Brain Res* 1988, 74: 221–29.
62. Halata Z, Groth H-P. Innervation of the synovial membrane of the cats joint capsule: An ultrastructural study. *Cell Tissue Res* 1976, 169: 415–18.
63. Halata Z, Haus J. The ultrastructure of sensory nerve endings in human anterior cruciate ligament. *Anat Embryol* (Berlin) 1989, 179: 415–21.
64. Heppelmann B, Messlinger K, Neiss WF, Schmidt RF. Ultrastructural three-dimensional reconstruction of group III and group IV sensory nerve endings ("free nerve endings") in the knee joint capsule of the cat: Evidence for multiple receptive sites. *J Comp Neurol* 1990, 292: 103–16.
65. Hoffer JA, Andreassen S. Limitations in the servoregulation of soleus muscle stiffness in premammillary cats. In *Muscle Receptors and Movement*, Taylor A, Prochazka A, editors. London: Macmillan, 1981, 311–24.
66. Houk JC, Crago PE, Rymer WZ. Function of the spindle dynamic response in stiffness regula-

tion: A predictive mechanism provided by nonlinear feedback. In *Muscle Receptors and Movement,* Taylor A, Prochazka A, editors. London: Macmillan, 1981, 299–309.
67. Hulliger M, Matthews PBC, Noth J. Effects of combining static and dynamic fusimotor stimulation on the response of the muscle spindle primary ending to sinusoidal stretching. *J Physiol* (London) 1977, 267: 839–56.
68. Johansson H. Reflex control of gamma motoneurons. Umeå, Sweden: Umeå University, 1981.
69. Johansson H. Reflex integration in the gamma motor system. In *The Muscle Spindle,* Boyd IA, Gladden MH, editors. London: Macmillan Press, 1985, 297–301.
70. Johansson H. Rubrospinal and rubrobulbospinal influences on dynamic and static gamma motoneurons. *Behav Brain Res* 1988, 28: 97–107.
71. Johansson H, Bergenheim M, Djupsjöbacka M, Sjölander P. Analysis of encoding of stimulus separation in ensembles of muscle afferents. In *Alpha and Gamma Motor Systems,* Taylor A, Gladden M, Durbaba R, editors. New York: Plenum, 1995.
72. Johansson H, Bergenheim M, Djupsjöbacka M, Sjölander P. A method for analysis of encoding of stimulus separation in ensembles of afferents. *J Neurosci Meth* 1995, 63: 67–74.
73. Johansson H, Lorentzon R, Sjölander P, Sojka P. The anterior cruciate ligament: A sensor acting on the gamma muscle spindle systems of muscles around the knee joint. *Neuro Orthoped* 1990, 9: 1–23.
74. Johansson H, Silfvenius H. Axon-collateral activation by dorsal spinocerebellar tract fibers of group I relay cells of nucleus Z in the cat medulla oblongata. *J Physiol* (London) 1977, 265: 341–69.
75. Johansson H, Silfvenius H. Input from ipsilateral proprio- and exteroceptive hind limb afferents to nucleus Z of the cat medulla oblongata. *J Physiol* (London) 1977, 265: 371–93.
76. Johansson H, Silfvenius H. Connections from large, ipsilateral hind limb muscle and skin afferents to the rostral main cuneate nucleus and to the nucleus X region in the cat. *J Physiol* (London) 1977, 265: 395–428.
77. Johansson H, Sjölander P. Neurophysiology of joints. In *Mechanics of Human Joints Physiology, Pathophysiology, and Treatment,* Wright V, Radin EL, editors. New York: Marcel Dekker, 1993, 243–90.
78. Johansson H, Sjölander P, Sojka P. Actions on gamma motoneurons elicited by electrical stimulation of joint afferent fibers in the hind limb of the cat. *J Physiol* (London) 1986, 375: 137–52.
79. Johansson H, Sjölander P, Sojka P. Fusimotor reflexes in triceps surae muscle elicited by natural and electrical stimulation of joint afferents. *Neuro Orthoped* 1988, 6: 67–80.
80. Johansson H, Sjölander P, Sojka P. Activity in receptor afferents from the anterior cruciate ligament evokes reflex effects on fusimotor neurones. *Neurosci Res* 1990, 8: 54–59.
81. Johansson H, Sjölander P, Sojka P. A sensory role for the cruciate ligaments. *Clin Orthop* 1991, 268: 161–78.
82. Johansson H, Sjölander P, Sojka P. Receptors in the knee joint ligaments and their role in the biomechanics of the joint. *CRC Crit Rev Biomed Eng* 1991, 18: 341–68.
83. Johansson H, Sjölander P, Sojka P, Wadell I. Reflex actions on the gamma muscle spindle systems of muscles acting at the knee joint elicited by stretch of the posterior cruciate ligament. *Neuro Orthoped* 1989, 8: 9–21.
84. Johansson H, Sojka P. Actions on gamma motoneurons elicited by electrical stimulation of cutaneous afferent fibres in the hind limb of the cat. *J Physiol* (London) 1985, 366: 343–63.
85. Johansson H, Sojka P. Pathophysiological mechanisms involved in genesis and spread of muscular tension in occupational muscle pain and in chronic musculoskeletal pain syndromes: A hypothesis. *Med Hypotheses* 1991, 35: 196–203.
86. Kennedy JC, Alexander IJ, Hayes KC. Nerve supply of the human knee and its functional importance. *Am J Sports Med* 1982, 10: 329–35.
87. Kålund S, Sinkjær T, Arendt-Nielsen L, Simonsen O. Altered timing of hamstring muscle action in anterior cruciate ligament-deficient patients. *Am J Sports Med* 1990, 18: 245–48.
88. Landgren S, Silfvenius H. Projection to cerebral cortex of group I muscle afferents from the cat's hind limb. *J Physiol* (London) 1969, 200: 353–72.
89. Landgren S, Silfvenius H. Nucleus z, the medullary relay in the projection path to the cerebral cortex of group I muscle afferents from the cat's hind limb. *J Physiol* (London) 1971, 218: 551–71.
90. Lass P, Kaalund S, LeFevre S, Arendt-Nielsen L, Sinkjær T, Simonsen O. Muscle coordination following rupture of the anterior cruciate ligament: Electromyographic studies of 14 patients. *Acta Orthop Scand* 1991, 62: 9–14.
91. Limbird TJ, Shiavi R, Frazer M, Borra H. EMG profiles of knee joint musculature during walking: Changes induced by anterior cruciate ligament deficiency. *J Orthop Res* 1988, 6: 630–38.

92. Lundberg A, Oscarsson O. Functional organization of the dorsal spinocerebellar tract in the cat. VII. Identification of units by antidromic activation from the cerebellar cortex with recognition of five functional subdivisions. *Acta Physiol Scand* 1960, 50: 356–74.
93. Macefield G, Gandevia SC, Burke D. Perceptual responses to microstimulation of single afferents innervating joints, muscles, and skin of the human hand. *J Physiol* (London) 1990, 429: 113–29.
94. McCloskey DI. Differences between the senses of movement and position shown by the effects of loading and vibration of muscles in man. *Brain Res* 1973, 63: 119–31.
95. McCloskey DI, Cross MJ, Honner R, Potter E. Sensory effects of pulling or vibrating exposed tendons in man. *Brain* 1983, 106: 21–37.
96. McCloskey DI, Macefield G, Gandevia SC, Burke D. Sensing position and movements of the fingers. *News Physiol Sci* 1987, 2: 226–30.
97. McIntyre AK, Proske U, Tracey DJ. Afferent fibers from muscle receptors in the posterior nerve of the cat's knee joint. *Exp Brain Res* 1978, 33: 415–24.
98. McNair PJ, Marshall RN, Matheson JA. Gait of subjects with anterior cruciate ligament deficiency. *Clin Biomech* 1989, 4: 243–48.
99. McNair PJ, Wood GA, Marshall RN. Stiffness of the hamstring muscles and its relationship to function in anterior cruciate ligament-deficient individuals. *Clin Biomech* 1992, 7: 131–37.
100. Miyatsu M, Atsuta Y, Watakabe M. The physiology of mechanoreceptors in the anterior cruciate ligament: An experimental study in decerebrate-spinalized animals. *J Bone Joint Surg* (Br) 1993, 75B: 653–57.
101. Mountcastle VB, Poggio GF, Werner G. The relation of thalamic cell response to peripheral stimuli varied over an intensive continuum. *J Neurophysiol* 1963, 26: 807–34.
102. Neugebauer V, Schaible H-G, Schmidt RF. Sensitization of articular afferents to mechanical stimuli by bradykinin. *Pflügers Archiv Eur J Physiol* 1989, 415: 330–35.
103. Nichols TR. The regulation of muscle stiffness: Implications for the control of limb stiffness. *Med Sport Sci* 1987, 26: 36–47.
104. Nichols TR. The organization of heterogenic reflexes among muscles crossing the ankle joint in the decerebrate cat. *J Physiol* (London) 1989, 410: 463–77.
105. Nielsen J, Sinkjær T, Toft E, Kagamihara Y. Segmental reflexes and ankle joint stiffness during co-contraction of antagonistic ankle muscles in man. *Exp Brain Res* 1994, 102: 350–58.
106. Ozaktay AC, Yamashita T, Cavanaugh JM, King AI. A light microscopic study of innervation of the lumbar facet joint capsule. *Soc Neurosci Abst* 1990, 16: 882.
107. Palmer I. Pathophysiology of the medial ligament of the knee joint. *Acta Chir Scand* 1958, 115: 312–18.
108. Petersén I, Stener B. Experimental evaluation of the hypothesis of ligamento-muscular protective reflexes. III. A study in man using the medial collateral ligament of the knee joint. *Acta Physiol Scand* 1959, 48: 51–61.
109. Pope DF, Cole KJ, Brand RA. Physiological loading of the anterior cruciate ligament does not activate quadriceps or hamstrings in the anesthetized cat. *Am J Sports Med* 1990, 18: 595–99.
110. Proske U, Schaible H-G, Schmidt RF. Joint receptors and kinesthesia. *Exp Brain Res* 1988, 72: 219–24.
111. Ray RH, Doetsch GS. Coding of stimulus location and intensity in populations of mechanosensitive nerve fibers of the raccoon. II. Across-fiber response patterns. *Brain Res Bull* 1990, 25: 533–50.
112. Ray RH, Doetsch GS. Coding of stimulus location and intensity in populations of mechanosensitive nerve fibers of the raccoon. I. Single-fiber response properties. *Brain Res Bull* 1990, 25: 517–32.
113. Roll JP, Vedel JP. Kinesthetic role of muscle afferents in man, studied by tendon vibration and microneurography. *Exp Brain Re.* 1982, 47: 177–90.
114. Roll JP, Vedel JP, Ribot E. Alteration of proprioceptive messages induced by tendon vibration in man: A microneurographic study. *Exp. Brain Res.* 1989. 76: 213–22.
115. Schaible H-G, Schmidt RF. Effects of an experimental arthritis on the sensory properties of fine articular afferent units. *J Neurophysiol* 1985, 54: 1109–122.
116. Schaible H-G, Schmidt RF. Time course of mechanosensitivity changes in articular afferents during a developing experimental arthritis. *J Neurophysiol* 1988, 60: 2180–195.
117. Schaible H-G, Schmidt RF. Excitation and sensitization of fine articular afferents from cat's knee joint by prostaglandin E_2. *J Physiol* (London) 1988, 403: 91–104.
118. Schaible H-G, Schmidt RF, Willis WD. Convergent inputs from articular, cutaneous, and

muscle receptors onto ascending tract cells in the spinal cord. *Exp Brain Res* 1987, 66: 479–88.
119. Schaible H-G, Schmidt RF. Responses of fine medial articular nerve afferents to passive movements of knee joint. *J Neurophysiol* 1983, 49: 1118–126.
120. Schepelmann K, Messlinger K, Schaible H-G, Schmidt RF. Inflammatory mediators and nociception in the joint: Excitation and sensitization of slowly conducting afferent fibers of cat's knee by prostaglandin I_2. *Neuroscience* 1992, 50: 237–47.
121. Schultz RA, Miller DC, Kerr CS, Micheli L. Mechanoreceptors in human cruciate ligaments: A histological study. *J Bone Joint Surg* 1984, 1072–1076.
122. Schutte MJ, Dabezies EJ, Zimny ML, Happel LT. Neural anatomy of the human anterior cruciate ligament. *J Bone Joint Surg* 1987, 69A: 243–47.
123. Scott DT, Ferrell WR, Baxendale RH. Excitation of soleus/gastrocnemius gamma motoneurons by group II knee joint afferents is suppressed by group IV joint afferents in the decerebrate, spinalized cat. *Exp Physiol* 1994, 79: 357–64.
124. Sharkey KA, Bray RC. Innervation patterns of collateral knee ligaments as revealed by silver staining and immunohistochemistry. *Soc Neurosci Abst* 1990, 16: 882.
125. Sinkjær T, Toft E, Andreassen S, Hornemann BC. Muscle stiffness in human ankle dorsiflexors: Intrinsic and reflex components. *J Neurophysiol* 1988, 60: 1110–121.
126. Sittig AC, Denier van der Gon JJ, Gielen CCAM. The contribution of afferent information on position and velocity to the control of slow and fast human forearm movements. *Exp Brain Res* 1987, 67: 33–40.
127. Sjölander P, Djupsjöbacka M, Johansson H, Sojka P, Lorentzon R. Can receptors in the collateral ligaments contribute to knee joint stability and proprioception via effects on the fusimotor muscle spindle system? An experimental study in the cat. *Neuro Orthoped* 1994, 15: 65–80.
128. Sjölander P, Johansson H. Sensory endings in ligaments: Response properties and effects on proprioception and motor control. In *Ligaments and Ligamentoplasties,* Yahia L, editor. Berlin: Springer-Verlag, 1997, 39–83.
129. Sjölander P, Johansson H, Sojka P, Rehnholm A. Sensory nerve endings in the cat cruciate ligaments: A morphological investigation. *Neurosci Lett* 1989, 102: 33–38.
130. Skoglund S. Anatomical and physiological studies of knee joint innervation in the cat. *Acta Physiol Scand* 1956, 36: 1–101.
131. Sojka P, Johansson H, Sjölander P, Lorentzon R, Djupsjöbacka M. Fusimotor neurons can be reflexly influenced by activity in receptor afferents from the posterior cruciate ligament. *Brain Res* 1989, 483: 177–83.
132. Sojka P, Sjölander P, Johansson H, Djupsjöbacka M. Influence from stretch-sensitive receptors in the collateral ligaments of the knee joint on the gamma muscle spindle systems of flexor and extensor muscles. *Neurosci Res* 1991, 11: 55–62.
133. Solomonow M, Baratta R, Zhou BH, Shoji H, Bose W, Beck C, et al. The synergistic action of the anterior cruciate ligament and thigh muscles in maintaining joint stability. *Am J Sports Med* 1987, 15: 207–13.
134. Stener B. *Acta Physiol Scand* 1959, 48: 5–26.
135. Stilwell DL. The innervation of deep structures of the hand. *Am J Anat* 1957, 161: 75–99.
136. Tibone JE, Antich TJ, Fanton GS, Moynes DR, Perry J. Functional analysis of anterior cruciate ligament instability. *Am J Sports Med* 1986, 14: 276–84.
137. Toft E, Sinkjaer T, Andreassen S, Larsen K. Mechanical and electromyographic responses to stretch of the human ankle extensors. *J Neurophysiol* 1991, 65: 1402–410.
138. Vilensky JA, O'Connor BL, Brandt KD, Dunn EA, Rogers PI. Serial kinematic analysis of the canine knee after L4-S1 dorsal root ganglionectomy: Implications for the cruciate deficiency model of osteoarthritis. *J Rheumatol* 1994, 21: 2113–117.
139. Voorhoeve PE, van Kanten RW. Reflex behaviour of fusimotor neurons of the cat upon electrical stimulation of various afferent fibers. *Acta Physiol Pharmacol Neerl* 1962, 10: 391–407.
140. Wadell I, Johansson H, Sjölander P, Sojka P, Djupsjöbacka M, Niechaj A. Fusimotor reflexes influencing secondary muscle spindle afferents from flexor and extensor muscles in the hind limb of the cat. *J Physiol* (Paris) 1991 85: 223–34.
141. Windhorst U, Hamm TM, Stuart DG. On the function of muscle and reflex partitioning. *Behav Brain Sci* 1989, 12: 629–81.
142. Wyke B. The neurology of joints. *Ann R Coll Surg* (England) 1967, 41: 25–50.
143. Wyke B. Morphological and functional features of the innervation of the costovertebral

joints. *Folia Morphol* (Praha) 1975, 23: 296–305.
144. Wyke B. The neurology of joints: A review of general principles. *Clin Rheum Dis* 1981, 7: 223–39.
145. Zimny ML. Mechanoreceptors in articular tissues. *Am J Anat* 1988, 182: 16–32.
146. Zimny ML, Albright DJ, Dabezies E. Mechanoreceptors in the human medial meniscus. *Acta Anat* (Basel) 1988, 133: 35–40.
147. Zimny ML, Schutte M, Dabezies E. Mechanoreceptors in the human anterior cruciate ligament. *Anat Rec* 1986, 214: 204–209.
148. Zätterström R, Fridén T, Lindstrand A, Moritz U. The effect of physiotherapy on standing balance in chronic anterior cruciate ligament insufficiency. *Am J Sports Med* 1994, 22: 531–36.
149. Öhberg F, Johansson M, Pedersen J, Djupsjöbacka M. A neural network approach to real-time spike discrimination during simultaneous recording from several multiunit nerve filaments. *J Neurosci Meth* 1996, 64: 181–87.
150. Özaktay AC, Cavanaugh JM, Blagoev DC, Getchell TV, King AI. Effects of a carrageenan-induced inflammation in rabbit lumbar facet joint capsule and adjacent tissues. *Neurosci Res* (New York). 1994, 20: 355–64.
151. Sinkjær T, Toft E, Arendt-Nielsen L. Knee stability and muscle coordination in patients with anterior cruciate ligament injuries: An electromyographic approach. *J Electromyogr Kinesiol* 1991, 1: 209–217.

CHAPTER 2

Contribution of the Three Levels of Nervous System Motor Control: Spinal Cord, Lower Brain, Cerebral Cortex

Roland M. Biedert, MD

Introduction

An organism receives sensory information about its environment through a number of different sensory channels. Information arises through activity of both the peripheral mechanoreceptors as well as visual and vestibular receptors (5, 6). Visual information and vestibular information are analyzed by the central nervous system (CNS) and play an important role in body position and balance. The sensory receptors for proprioception are located in the skin, joints, ligaments, tendons, and muscles (1, 6) (see figure 2.1). They are activated by changes in pressure and movement of soft tissue structures. Their afferent inputs are integrated at all levels of the CNS to generate appropriate motor responses.

The motor systems allow us to move our bodies and limbs and to maintain our posture, our attitude in space. The entire behavioral repertoire is made up of movements and postural adjustments performed to achieve certain goals. The sensory motor systems have to initiate and coordinate all of the specific movements in order to realize these goals. The control of movement and posture is dependent on a continuous flow of sensory information about events in the environment (7).

The motor responses generally fall under three levels of motor control: (a) the *spinal cord* for simple

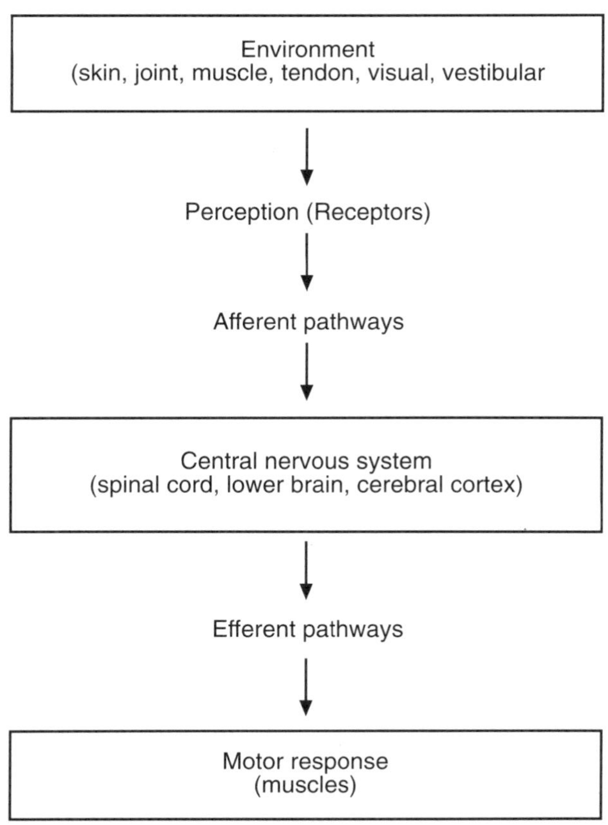

Figure 2.1 Sensory motor system.

reflexes, (b) the *lower regions of the brain* for more complicated responses, and (c) the *cerebral cortex* for control of the most complicated responses (3, 6).

Spinal Cord

The spinal cord is composed of tracts of nerve fibers that allow two-way conduction of nerve impulses. The sensory afferent fibers carry the different signals from the mechanoreceptors to the upper levels (higher centers) of the CNS. The motor efferent fibers from the cerebrum descend down to the end organs (muscles). The spinal cord carries both sensory and motor fibers between the brain and the periphery (9).

Organization for Motor Functions

The cord gray matter is the integrative area for the cord reflexes and other motor functions. The afferent impulses from the mechanoreceptors are conveyed through the sensory posterior roots; from there, every signal travels to a separate destination. One branch of the sensory nerve terminates in the gray matter and elicits local segmental reflexes. Another branch transmits signals to higher levels (brain stem, cerebral cortex) (see figure 2.2) (2).

Each segment of the spinal cord has several million neurons in its gray matter. This substance contains two types of neurons—anterior motor neurons and interneurons.

Anterior Motor Neurons

Located in the anterior horns of the cord gray matter, the anterior motor neurons give rise to the nerve fibers that leave the cord through the anterior roots and innervate the skeletal muscle fibers. The anterior motor neurons consist of two types—*alpha motor neurons* and *gamma motor neurons* (3).

Alpha motor neurons: The large type A alpha (Aα) nerve fibers innervate the large skeletal muscle fibers. All of the muscle fibers innervated by a single motor nerve fiber form a motor unit. Small muscles have few muscle fibers in a motor unit (exact control); large muscles have several hundred muscle

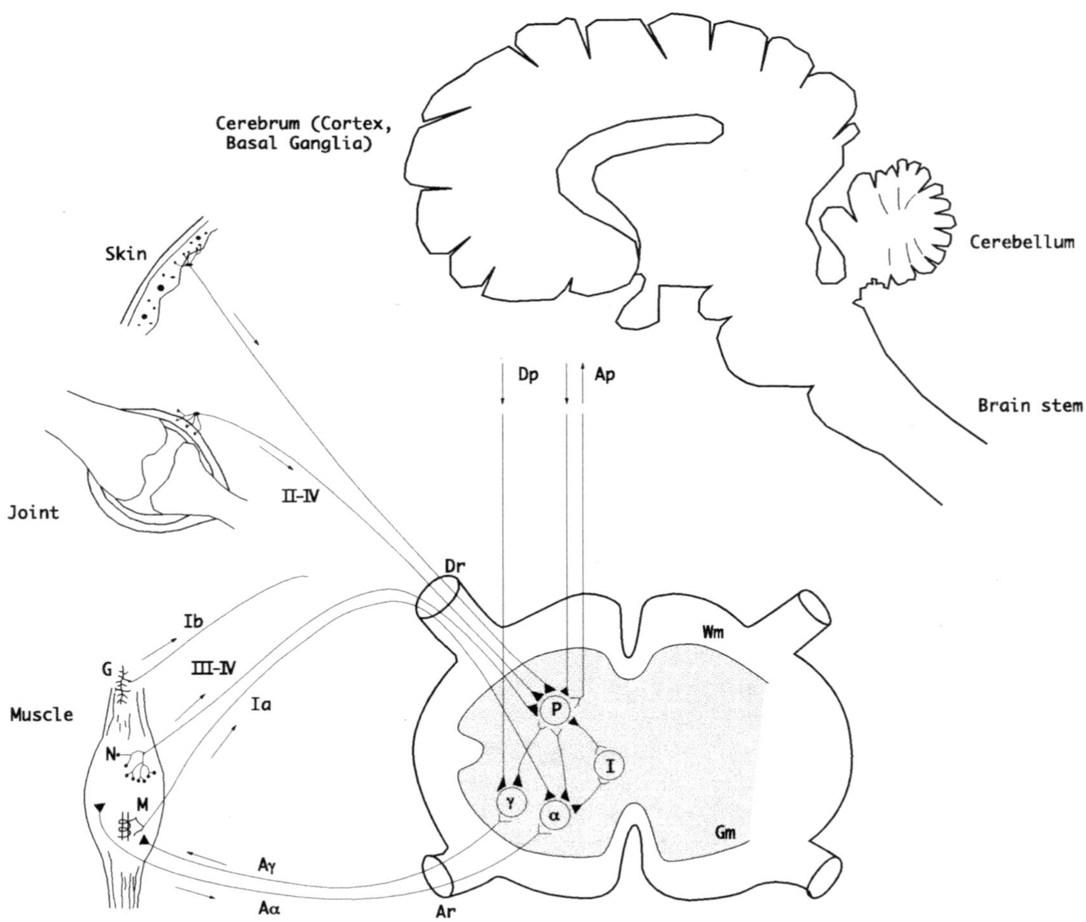

Figure 2.2 The spinal cord as integrative area for the cord reflexes and other motor functions.

fibers in a motor unit (gross control, not fine control). Both excite contraction of skeletal muscle fibers. Inhibitory presynaptic and postsynaptic neurons, together with a pool of interneurons, regulate the innervation of the alpha motor neurons.

Gamma motor neurons: The gamma motor neurons transmit impulses through the A gamma (Aγ) fibers to small special skeletal muscle fibers, that is, intrafusal fibers, in the muscle spindles. There are two classes of gamma motor neurons—one controlling the dynamic sensitivity of the muscle spindles (gamma-dynamic or gamma-d) and the other controlling the static sensitivity (gamma-static or gamma-s) (4).

The gamma motor neurons are constantly influenced by the mechanoreceptors of the joints and the descending motor neurons (pyramidal tract, reticulospinal fibers). With this mechanism, the muscle stiffness can be directly influenced by the CNS, which is important for voluntomotoricity. The whole gamma motor neuron loop (gamma motor neurons-muscle spindles-primary muscle spindle afferent pathways) may contribute to the preprogramming of the stiffness of muscles around the joint and thereby also to the regulation of joint stiffness and joint stability (4). The primary (more than the secondary) muscle spindle afferent pathways seem to have great importance in the regulation of muscle stiffness (4). The information from the muscle spindle is conveyed to the spinal cord via both primary and secondary afferent pathways.

Interneurons

Interneurons are present in all areas of the cord gray matter and are highly excitable. They have many interconnections and regulate the innervation of the anterior motor neurons. Most signals from the spinal nerves or from the brain stem are transmitted through interneurons, where they are processed. After this process, with control of muscle function and coordination of muscles, reflexes become possible.

Muscle Sensory Receptors

Qualitatively high control of muscle function requires not only excitation of the skeletal muscle by the anterior motor neurons but also continuous sensory feedback from the muscle to the spinal cord. The sensory feedback alerts the brain about the status of the muscle at the moment and also about length of the muscle and tension, and how they are changing. To provide this information, the muscles and their tendons are supplied with two special types of sensory receptors: muscle spindles in the belly of the muscle send information to the CNS about either muscle length or rate of change of its length, and Golgi tendon organs, which are located in the muscle tendons, transmit information about tension or its rate of change (3). Both types of receptors transmit vast amounts of information to the spinal cord, the cerebellum, and the cerebral cortex, helping these areas in their function for motor control.

Muscle Spindles: Dynamic and Static Stretch Reflex

Stretching a muscle causes excitation of the muscle spindles and consequently, reflex contraction of the skeletal muscle fibers of the same muscle (muscle stretch reflex). The stretch reflex can be divided into two components: dynamic stretch reflex, caused by rapid stretch of the muscle, and static stretch reflex, elicited by the continuous static receptor signals. This static reflex continues to cause muscle contraction as long as the muscle is maintained at excessive length.

The stretch reflex has also a dampening function. This ability to smooth muscle contractions prevents jerkiness of body movements.

Golgi Tendon Reflex: Dynamic and Static

The tendon organ has two different responses: dynamic, when the muscle tension suddenly increases, and static, when the muscle tension settles down to a lower level of steady-state firing (3). With these responses the tendon organs provide the nervous system with instantaneous information on the tension of each muscle.

The signals from increased muscle tension are transmitted to the spinal cord and cause reflex effects in the respective muscle. This inhibitory reflex provides a negative feedback mechanism that prevents muscle tension from becoming too high.

Muscle spindles and tendon organs also apprise the higher motor control centers of instantaneous changes in the muscles. Additional pathways transmit similar information into the brain stem and the motor areas of the cerebral cortex. The information transmitted to the brain stem and motor areas of the cerebral cortex is crucial for feedback control of motor signals that originate in these regions.

Voluntary Motor Activity

Signals transmitted from the motor cortex or other areas from the cerebrum stimulate in most instances not only the alpha motor neurons but also the gamma motor neurons at the same time. This so-called *coactivation* causes contraction of the extrafusal and the intrafusal muscle fibers at the same time.

Lower Brain

Several descending pathways are directly or indirectly under the control of the brain stem, the basal ganglia, and the cerebellum (see figure 2.3). Each hierarchical level receives information from the periphery so that the sensory input can modify the action of the descending commands. These different areas are also essential for normal motor function.

Brain Stem

The brain stem consists of midbrain, medulla oblongata, and pons; it is the stalk of the brain connecting the brain and the spinal cord. All sensory and motor nerves pass through the brain stem. It contains motor and sensory nuclei that perform motor and sensory functions. A specialized collection of neurons helps to coordinate skeletal muscle function. The brain stem serves as a way station for command signals from higher neural levels, which command the brain stem to modify specific control functions throughout the body (3). But the brain stem also plays an important role in controlling body movement and equilibrium. Especially important are the reticular and vestibular nuclei plus the vestibular apparatus that sends most of the equilibrium control signals. The brain stem contains the circuitry to stabilize posture.

Cerebellum

The cerebellum is crucial to the control of all rapid and complex muscular activities like running. It plays a major role in the timing of motor activities and in rapid progression from one movement to the next. It assists the functions of both the primary motor cortex and the basal ganglia. It controls movement patterns by smoothing out the movement that would otherwise be jerky and uncontrolled. Corrective adjustments are made in the body's motor activities so that they conform to the signals directed by the motor cortex and other levels. As it compares the intended program of muscle contractions from the specific motor areas with the continuously updated sensory information from the peripheral parts of the body, it acts as an integration system. The cerebellum transmits with this feedback system appropriate corrective signals into the motor system if necessary. All incoming information about the exact tension and position of the joints, muscles, and tendons and the body's position are noted relative to the environment, and then it determines the

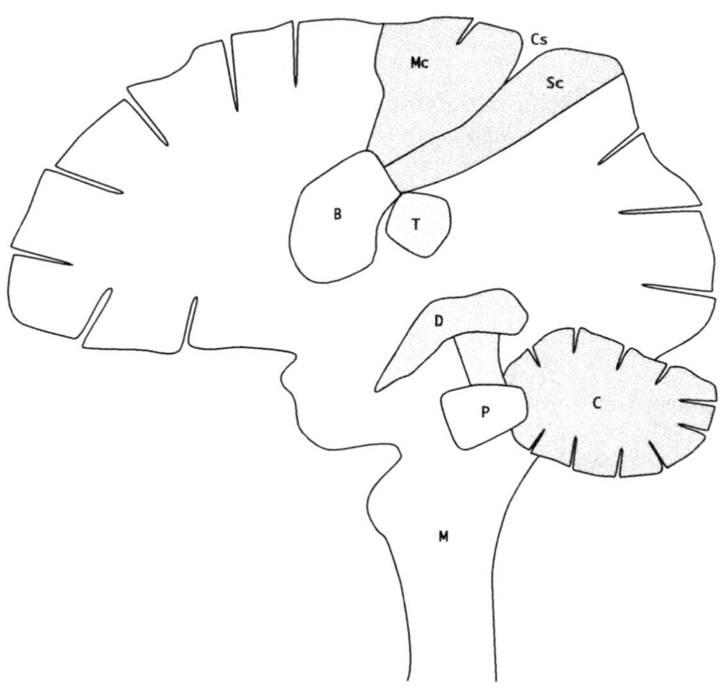

Figure 2.3 Different major regions of the brain.

correct plan of action to produce the desired movement (9).

The motor cortex makes the decision to perform a specific movement. This decision is relayed to the cerebellum. The cerebellum itself decides, based on the input from the periphery, what is the best plan of action to accomplish this movement.

Additionally, the cerebellum aids the cerebral cortex in planning the next step of movement in advance while the current movement is still performed, thus helping to progress smoothly from one movement to the next.

The cerebellum has also the ability to learn by its mistakes. The specific movements are made stronger or weaker after an error, adapting the excitability of the appropriate cerebellar neurons. Subsequent muscle contractions are brought into better correspondence with the planned movements.

Basal Ganglia

The basal ganglia are in the cerebral white matter, deep to the cortex. They consist of caudate nucleus, putamen, globus pallidus, substantia nigra, and subthalamic nucleus. Almost all of the motor and sensory nerve fibers connecting the cerebral cortex and spinal cord pass between the basal ganglia. Like the cerebellum they act as an accessory motor system that functions not by itself but in close association with the cerebral cortex and the corticospinal system.

One of the principal functions of the basal ganglia is the control of complex patterns of motor activity. Additionally, they initiate movements of sustained and repetitive nature (walking, running) and are therefore involved in maintaining posture and muscle tone.

Caudate Nucleus and Cognitive Control

Cognitive control of a motor activity means that the motor action occurs as a consequence of thoughts generated in the mind. The caudate nucleus plays an important role in this control system. The nucleus receives much of its input from the association areas of the cerebral cortex, the areas that integrate the specific sensory and motor information into usable thought patterns.

Cerebral Cortex

The cerebrum is composed of two hemispheres that are connected to each other by the corpus callosum. The cerebral cortex forms the outer portion of the cerebral hemispheres; it registers sensory stimuli and allows the voluntary control of specific movements. The cerebral cortex controls complex movement patterns. All voluntomotoricity involves conscious activity in the cerebral cortex. The control by the cortex involves simultaneous activation of different functions in the spinal cord, brain stem, basal ganglia, and cerebellum (3). These lower centers send their specific activating signals to the muscles.

The cerebral cortex has two functional areas: the motor cortex (anterior to the central sulcus) and the somatic sensory cortex (posterior).

Motor cortex

The motor cortex is divided into three different areas: the *primary motor cortex*, the *premotor area*, and the *supplementary motor area*. Each has its own topographical representation of muscle groups and specific motor functions.

Primary Motor Cortex

This area controls fine voluntary movements. Its left aspect controls the right side of the body, and its right aspect controls the left side. Its neurons (pyramidal cells) are responsible for consciously controlled movements of the skeletal muscles.

Premotor Area

Most nerve signals from the premotor area cause specific task movements. Together with the primary motor cortex, the basal ganglia, and the thalamus, the premotor cortex constitutes an overall system for coordinated muscle activity. It is involved in the development of motor skills.

Supplementary Area

This area functions together with the premotor area to provide attitudinal movements. It is concerned especially with bilateral synergic movement (8).

Corticospinal Tract

The signals from the motor cortex are transmitted directly to the spinal cord through the corticospinal tract (pyramidal tract) and indirectly through such accessory pathways as the basal ganglia, cerebellum, and nuclei of the brain stem.

The corticospinal tract is the most important pathway from the motor cortex. After leaving the cortex it forms the pyramids of the medulla. Most of the pyramidal fibers cross to the opposite side and descend in the lateral corticospinal tracts of the cord terminating on the interneurons in the intermediate regions of the cord gray matter. A few of the fibers do not cross and pass down the cord in the ventral corticospinal tract.

Corticospinal neurons of the motor cortex control the spinal reflexes. The axon of a single pyramidal neuron makes widespread connections within several motor neuron pools. In addition to making direct monosynaptic connections with individual motor neurons, they make connections with the same interneurons that also mediate spinal reflexes. This allows the motor cortex to govern complex patterns of muscle activation through the control of automatic reflex behaviors organized at lower levels (7).

Neurons of the motor cortex have peripheral receptive fields and are controlled by this somatic sensory system. Some neurons respond to tactile stimuli, others to joint rotation or compression, and others to stretch of muscles. This input-output association is responsible for the close relationship between the target muscle and the peripheral area that excites the neuron. The motor cortex is excited by sensory information; it reacts with the appropriate course of motor action.

Summary

Overall motor control of movements can be summarized according to the different levels as shown in figure 2.4.

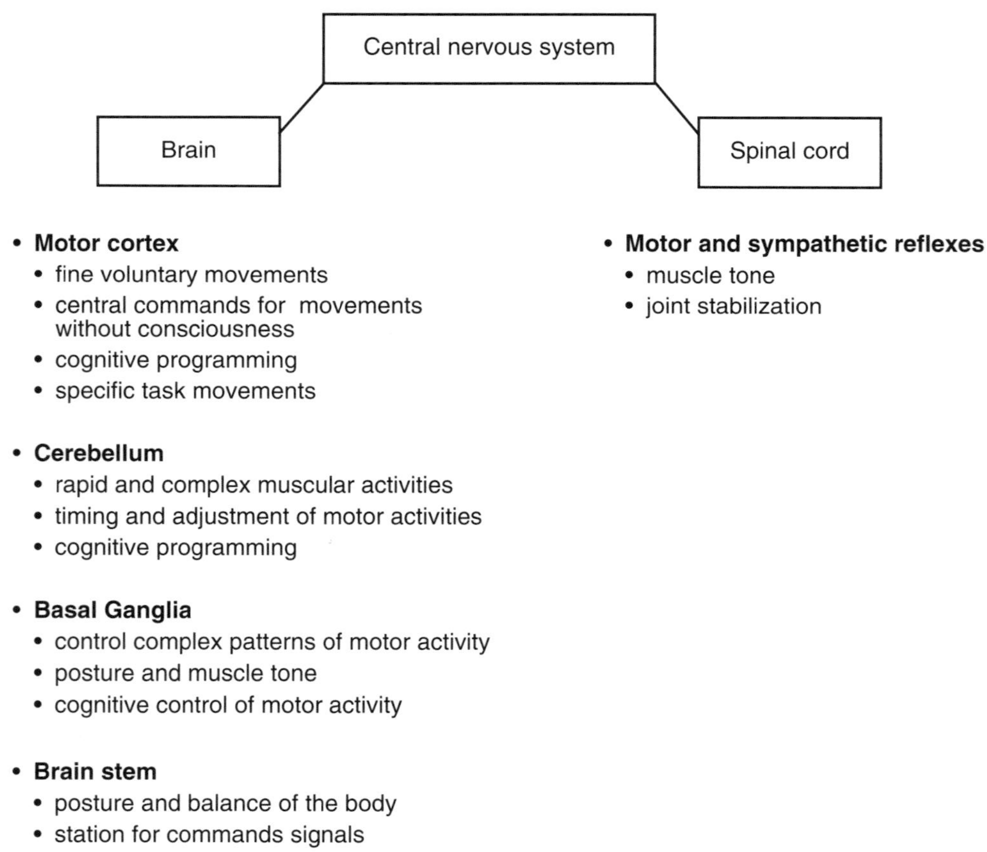

Figure 2.4 Main functions of the different levels of the nervous system motor control.

References

1. Biedert R, Stauffer E, Friederich N. (1992) Occurrence of free nerve endings in the soft tissue of the knee joint. *Am J Sports Med* 4: 430–33.
2. Biedert R, Meyer S. (1996) Propriozeptives Training bei Spitzensportlern. Neurophysiologische und klinische Aspekte. *Sportorthopädie—Sporttraumatologie* 12.2: 102–105.
3. Guyton A. (1996) *Textbook of medical physiology,* 9th ed. Philadelphia: Saunders.
4. Johansson H. (1991) Role of knee ligaments in proprioception and regulation of muscle stiffness. *J Electromyogr Kinesiol* 3: 158–79.
5. Lephart S, Giraldo J, Borsa P, Fu F. (1996) Knee joint proprioception: A comparison between female intercollegiate gymnasts and controls. *Knee Surg Sports Traumatol Arthroscopy* 4: 121–24.
6. Lephart S, Pincivero D, Giraldo J, Fu F. (1997) The role of proprioception in the management and rehabilitation of athletic injuries. *Am J Sports Med* 1: 130–37.
7. Lüscher H. (1988) The sensory motor systems: Reflex and voluntary control of movement. Johnstone concept in the treatment of stroke patients. Lecture handout for course taught in 1988 at Solothurn.
8. Schafer RC. (1987) *Clinical biomechanics: Musculoskeletal actions and reactions,* 2d ed. Baltimore: Williams & Wilkins.
9. Wilmore J, Costill D. (1994) *Physiology of sport and exercise.* Champaign, IL: Human Kinetics, p. 55.

CHAPTER 3

Functional Anatomy of the Cerebellum

Scott F. Dye, MD

Brushing one's teeth, smoothly descending stairs, jogging down the street, and hitting a baseball are activities that most people take for granted. Even to those who have had some medical training, performing such an activity would seem a fairly simple and straightforward process of proper activation, solely in the opposite motor cortex of the cerebrum, of different muscles under the direct control of neurological phenomena. This impression would, however, be wrong.(3, 7, 8) There exists a largely subconscious set of neurological mechanisms that constantly monitor, adjust, correctly sequence, and anticipate musculoskeletal actions, without which none of the complex or even many simple motor activities would be possible. The main components of this neurological complex are the cerebellum, basal ganglia, spinal cord, and an immense network of proprioceptive sensors supplying data to these central nervous system components.

The purpose of this work is to provide a brief overview of the functional neuroanatomy of one of the most intricate and intriguing elements of the central nervous system—the cerebellum. The complete neuroanatomy of this central nervous system component is vastly complex and beyond the scope of this presentation. Of necessity, some details will therefore be left uncovered. Even a summary exposure to the cerebellum, however, should prove of interest to the student of the musculoskeletal sciences. The cerebellum (L., little brain) may be the most important, yet underappreciated, component of normal musculoskeletal function. To perform its monitoring, adjustment, sequencing, and planning functions, this vital central nervous system element has evolved a unique neuroanatomy, containing more nerve cells than the *rest of the central nervous system combined*. (1) The cerebellum is located in the posterior fossa of the cranium and in sagittal section is composed of three lobes: the anterior, posterior, and flocculonodular lobes (see figure 3.1). (5, 9) The flocculonodular lobe is phylogenetically the most ancient component of the cerebellum, and its functions evolved in conjunction with the vestibular system to which it has direct connections in order to help maintain postural balance. The anterior and posterior lobes are functionally divided in coronal section into three zones: the axial vermis and the lateral hemispheres, which are further functionally divided into the intermediate and lateral zones (see figure 3.2). The vermis monitors and modifies movements of axial musculoskeletal components, including the neck, shoulders, and hips. The intermediate zone monitors and modifies motor activities of the distal portions of the extremities. The lateral zones, which in humans are proportionately the largest of any vertebrate, help planning of sequential movements before they occur.

The *afferent input* to the cerebellum from the periphery arrives primarily through dorsal and ventral spinocerebellar tracts (see figure 3.3), which contain the most rapidly conducting nerves in the entire human neurological system (approximately 100 m/s). The dorsal spinocerebellar tracts provide data from the proprioceptive system, including muscle spindles, somatic sensors, Golgi tendon organs, tactile receptors of the skin, and other joint receptors. The data provides information regarding position and rate of change of joint movements, tension of muscles, and forces acting on musculoskeletal components. The ventral spinocerebellar tracts provide nearly instantaneous information concerning the actual sequence of motor signals that have arrived at the anterior horn cell level within the spinal cord. (5, 9) The cerebellum thus constantly receives what is called an *efference* copy of the neurological signals that have already arrived at the spinal cord level, which initiate the dynamic sequencing of millions of motor unit contractions. The cerebellum also receives input from the cerebral cortex (2, 4, 12) via the cerebropontile tracts, which have their origin in the motor, premotor, and sensory cortices, from the vestibular apparatus through the short vestibulocerebellar tracts.

The *efferent output* of the cerebellum reaches the motor cortex primarily through connections between the deep nuclei (including dentate, vestigial, and interpositus), the red nucleus, and the thalamus (see figure 3.4). (5, 9) For example, a pathway that

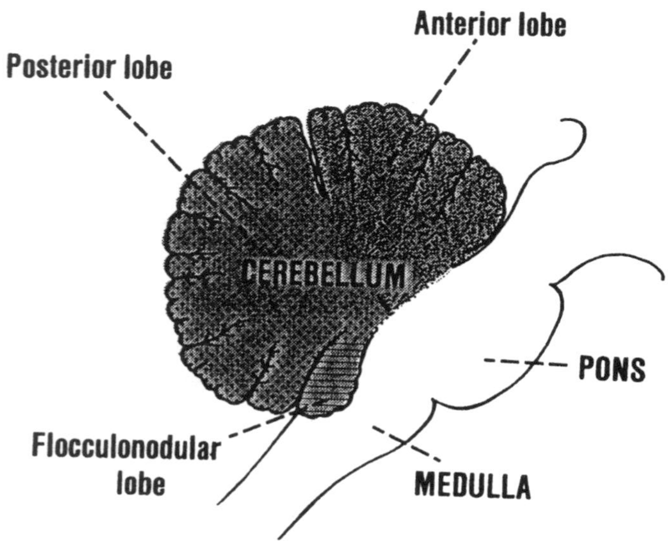

Figure 3.1 The anatomic lobes of the cerebellum as seen in sagittal view, showing the anterior lobe, the posterior lobe, and the flocculonodular lobe.
Reprinted with permission from Guyton AC: *Textbook of Medical Physiology.* Philadelphia: Saunders, 1986.

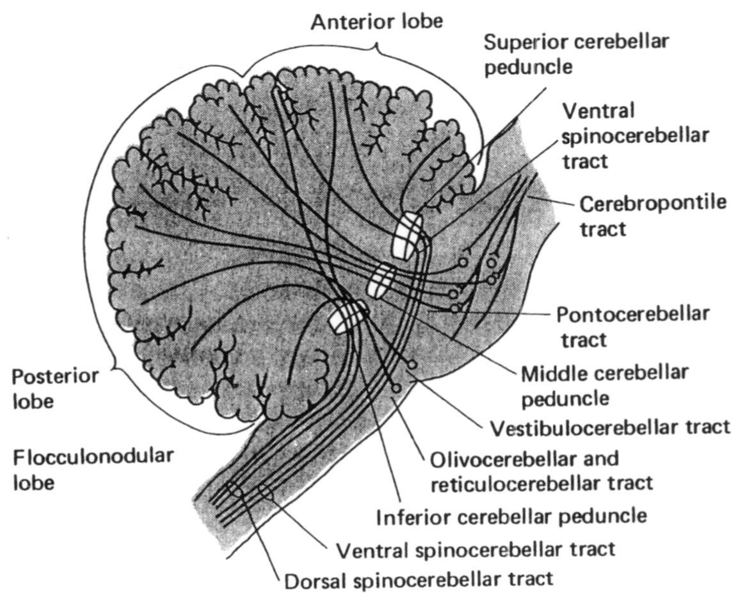

Figure 3.3 The principle afferent input tracts to the cerebellum.
Reprinted with permission from Guyton AC: *Textbook of Medical Physiology.* Philadelphia: Saunders, 1986.

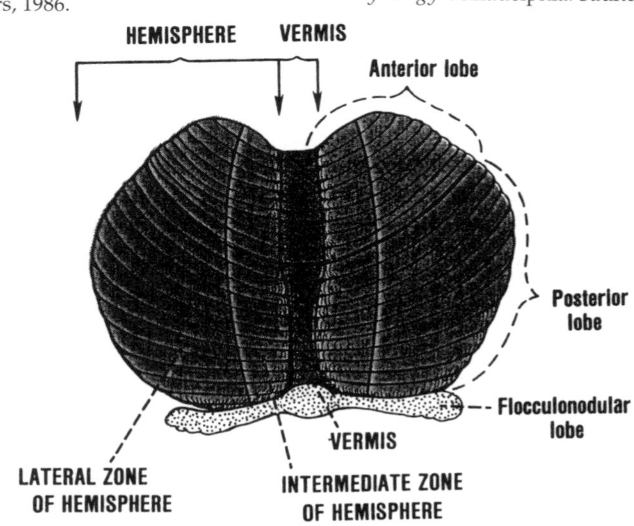

Figure 3.2 The functional parts of the cerebellum as seen in a coronal view, showing the midline vermis and the hemispheres with the intermediate and lateral zones.
Reprinted with permission from Guyton AC: *Textbook of Medical Physiology.* Philadelphia: Saunders, 1986.

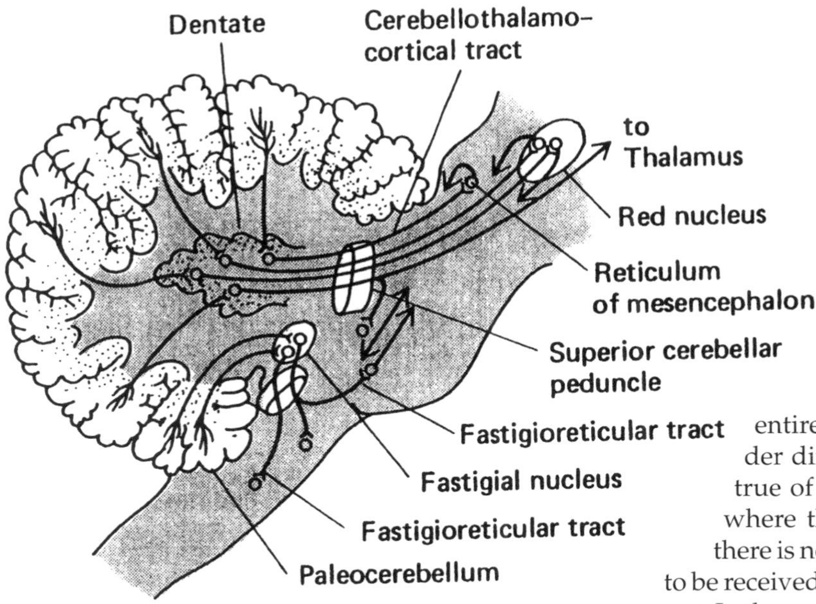

Figure 3.4 The principle efferent output tracts from the cerebellum.
Reprinted with permission from Guyton AC: *Textbook of Medical Physiology*. Philadelphia: Saunders, 1986.

originates in the intermediate zone travels through the nucleus interpositus to the thalamus, and then to the motor cortex to modify its output to the spinal cord, and then through peripheral motor nerves to the extremity muscles.

The main functional neural unit of the cerebellar cortex consists of a combination of various cell types and morphologies arranged in cortical layers, including what are termed Purkinje cells, climbing fibers, mossy fibers, and granular cells (see figure 3.5). The functional circuitry of these neuronal structures is designed to provide a type of "delayed-line" negative feedback output to the deep nuclear cells that effectively provides time-delayed dampening signals to the motor cortex. (9)

The cerebellum is particularly important in regulating the intensity and sequence of motor actions of agonist and antagonist muscle groups (see figure 3.6). A primary function of the cerebellum is to compare the intentions of the cerebral motor control system, which are supplied by the cerebropontile tracts, with the actual musculoskeletal movements, as supplied through the dorsal spinocerebellar tracts, and the efference copy of motor signals arriving at the anterior horn cells, as supplied through the ventral spinocerebellar tracts. During rapid movements, the motor cortex transmits more motor impulses to the agonist muscles than are needed. The cerebellum acts to inhibit the motor cortex controlling the agonist muscles and simultaneously excites the antagonist muscles at just the proper degree and in just the proper sequence (in milliseconds) to control a musculoskeletal movement. (5, 9) Such movements occur too rapidly for the motor cortex to reverse voluntarily, and it is clear that the excitation of an antagonist muscle towards the end of a movement is an entirely subconscious process and not under direct, willed control. This is especially true of ballistic movements, such as typing, where the movement occurs so rapidly that there is not enough time for proprioceptive data to be received to modify cerebellar and cerebral output. In these circumstances, the cerebellum, through the time-delay circuitry of the Purkinje system, automatically sends a delayed inhibitory signal to the motor cortex, stopping the agonist muscles and then concurrently activating the antagonist muscles, without proprioceptive data having arrived from the periphery.

The lateral zones of the cerebellum are most highly evolved in man, compared to other vertebrates. (9) Their primary input is from the premotor and somatosensory portions of the cerebrum, rather than from the peripheral proprioceptive system. These zones are involved with planning of the next set of movements, before they occur. The neurons in the dentate nucleus, though which the effective output of the lateral zones is channeled, manifest a copy of the next sequence of motor signals at a time when a current musculoskeletal movement is in progress. The motor control function of the lateral zones thus seems to be involved with what will be occurring during the next sequential movement.

Recent research using functional magnetic resonance imaging (1, 6) points to potentially extensive *nonmotor* operations of the lateral zones, including their function in diverse cognitive actions with information acquisition and analysis. (10, 11) Thus, it may be as important for someone like Gary Kasparov, a chess champion, to posses excellent cerebellar functioning in cognitive planning as it would be for a professional basketball player such as Michael Jordan to possess fine motor control skills. Different cerebellar components and functions would be involved, however, between these dissimilar activities.

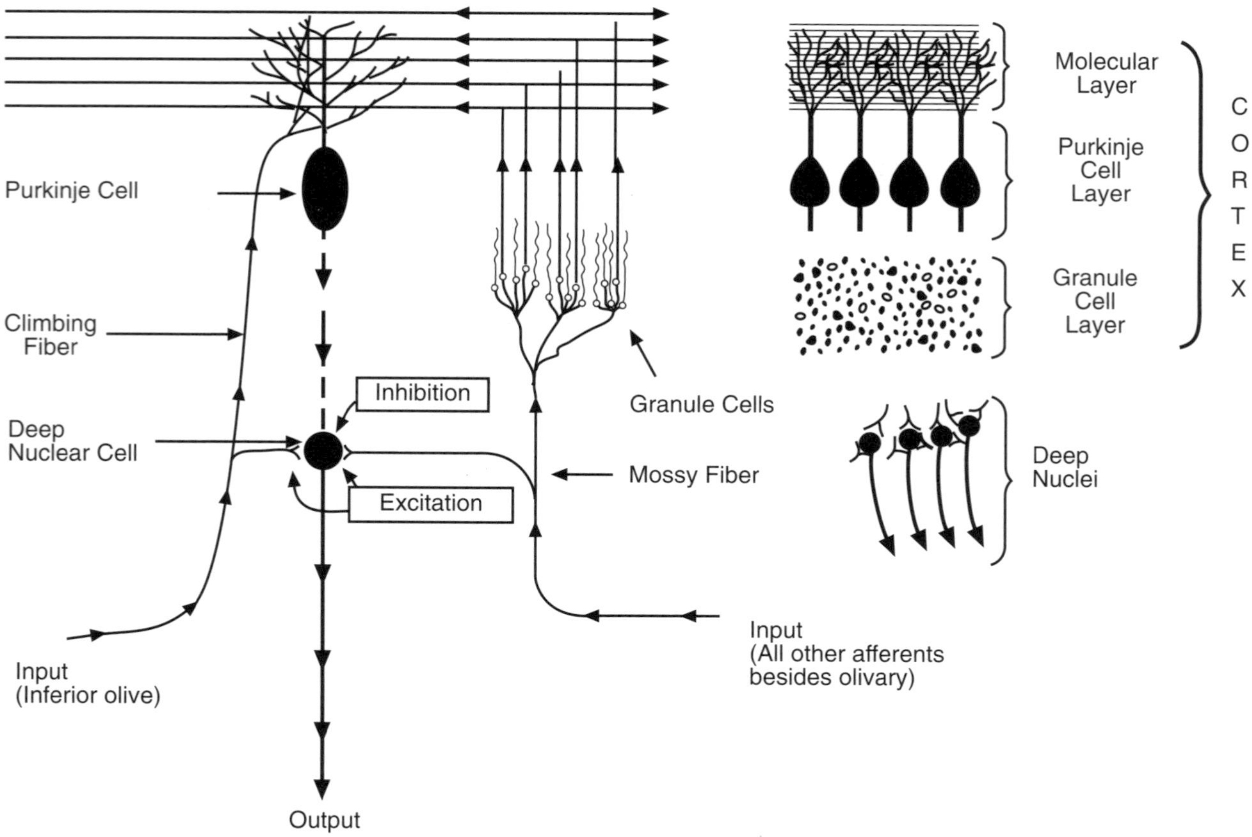

Figure 3.5 The basic neuronal time delay circuitry of the cerebellum, showing excitatory and inhibitory effects on the deep nuclear cell.
Reprinted with permission from Guyton AC: *Textbook of Medical Physiology.* Philadelphia: Saunders, 1986.

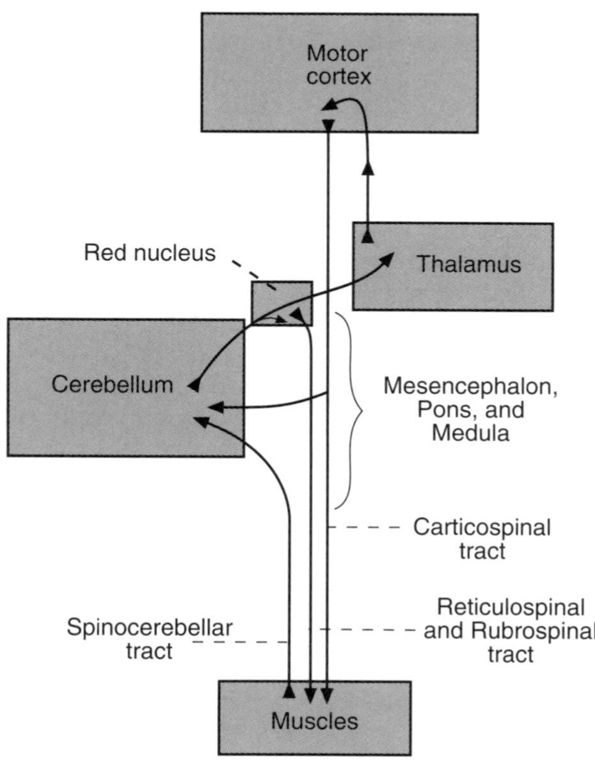

Figure 3.6 Simplified pathways for cerebellar control of voluntary movements.
Reprinted with permission from Guyton AC: *Textbook of Medical Physiology.* Philadelphia: Saunders, 1986.

Summary

In this brief overview of functional neural anatomy of the cerebellum, it can be understood that this unique central nervous system component is vital to the proper sequencing of motor activity and that, in addition, it performs a function as yet not fully clarified in cognitive analysis independent of motor control. It is expected that in the next century the detailed function of the cerebellar systems and neuronal connections will be better defined and perhaps even controlled, which will permit us to provide improved musculoskeletal function in patients.

References

1. Allen G, Buxton RB, Wong RC, Courchesne E. Attentional activation of the cerebellum independent of motor involvement. *Science* 275: 1940–942, 1997.
2. Allen GI, Tsukahara N. Cerebrocerebellar communication systems. *Physiol. Rev.* 54: 957, 1974.
3. Eccles JC. *The Understanding of the Brain.* New York: McGraw-Hill, 1973.
4. Evarts EV, Thatch WT. Motor mechanisms of the CNS: Cerebrocerebellar interrelations. *Annu. Rev. Physiol.* 31: 451, 1969.
5. Everett NB, Sundsten JW, Lund RD. *Functional Neuroanatomy.* Philadelphia: Lea & Febiger, 1971.
6. Gao JH, Parsons LM, Bauer JM, Xiong J, Li J, Fox PT. Cerebellum implicated in sensory acquisition and discrimination rather than motor control. *Science* 272: 545–47, 1996.
7. Granit R. *The Basis of Motor Control.* New York: Academic Press, 1970.
8. Grillner S. Locomotion invertebrates: Central mechanisms and reflex interaction. *Physiol. Rev.* 55: 247, 1975.
9. Guyton AC. *The Textbook of Medical Physiology,* 7th edition. Philadelphia: Saunders, 1986.
10. Sanes JS: A theory of cerebellar function. *Math. Biosci.* 10: 25–51, 1971.
11. Schmahmann, JD. An emerging concept: The cerebellar contribution to higher function. *Arch. Neurol.* 48: 1178–187, 1991.
12. Wiesendanger M, Miles TS. Ascending pathway of low-threshold muscle efference to the cerebral cortex and its possible role in motor control. *Physiol. Rev.* 62: 1234, 1982.

CHAPTER 4

Contribution of the Peripheral Somatosensory System to Balance and Postural Equilibrium

Bryan L. Riemann, MA, ATC
Kevin M. Guskiewicz, PhD, ATC

Introduction

Balance is the single most important factor underlying movement strategies within the closed kinetic chain. Acquisition of effective and efficient movement strategies is essential for athletic performance. Proper maintenance of balance and postural equilibrium is therefore a vital component in the rehabilitation of joint injuries and should not be overlooked. Traditionally, however, orthopedic rehabilitation has emphasized isolated joint mechanics, such as improving joint range of motion and increasing muscle strength and endurance, rather than afferent information obtained by the joint(s) to be processed by the postural control system.

The postural control system utilizes complex processes involving both sensory and motor components. Maintenance of postural equilibrium requires sensory detection of body motions, integration of sensorimotor information within the central nervous system (CNS), and execution of appropriate musculoskeletal responses (see figure 4.1). The position of the body in relation to gravity and its surroundings is determined by combining visual, vestibular, and somatosensory inputs. Balance movements involve controlled, coordinated actions along the kinetic chain (see figure 4.2). All of these processes are vital for producing fluid sport-related movements. The aim of this paper is to describe the *somatosensory* system's contribution to the maintenance of balance.

The relationship between *balance* and *postural equilibrium* should first be addressed, because the terms are often used interchangeably. Balance is the process of maintaining the center of gravity (COG) within the body's base of support (56). In contrast, postural equilibrium is a broader term that describes the balanced state of forces and moments acting on the body's center of mass. When postural equilibrium is achieved, the body's center of mass moves uniformly and minimally (postural sway) around the body's equilibrium point. From a clinical perspective, this involves the body maintaining the center of gravity within the minimal limit of stability (LOS) through equalization of forces and optimal alignment of the joint segments. The LOS is the maximum anterior-posterior (A-P) and medial-lateral (M-L) angles that keep the vertical projection of the COG within the area representing the base of support. When the COG sway angle exceeds the LOS the individual will fall unless effective postural adjustments are made through the use of ankle, hip, or "stepping" strategies (56, 57).

Control of Balance

The postural control system operates as a control circuit between the sensory sources, CNS, and the

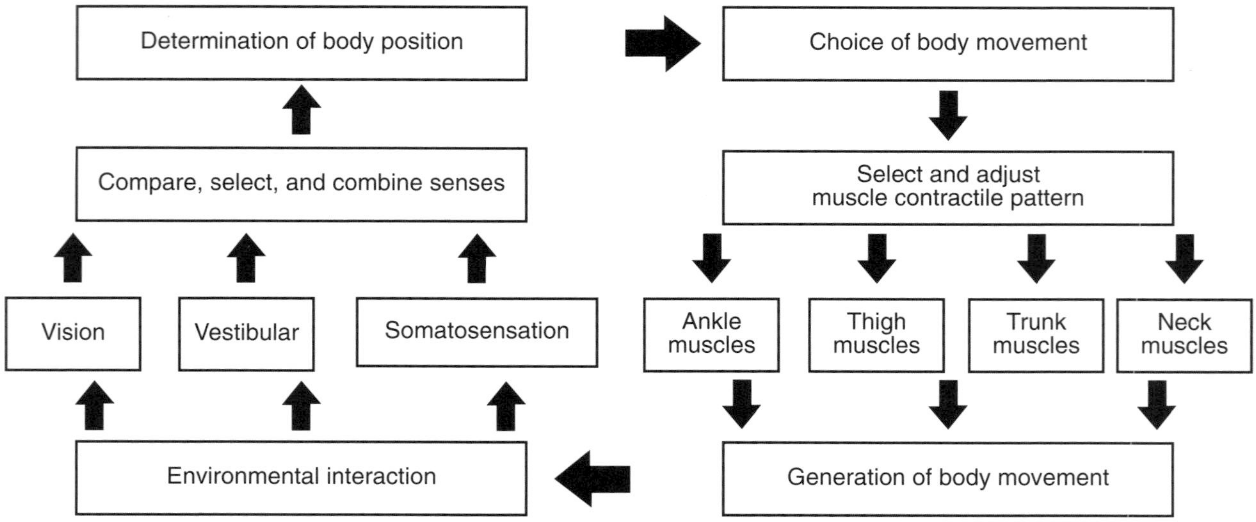

Figure 4.1 Dynamic equilibrium. (Adapted from Allison L, Fuller K, Hedenberg R, et al. Contemporary Management of Balance Deficits. Clackamas, OR, NeuroCom International, 1994; with permission.)

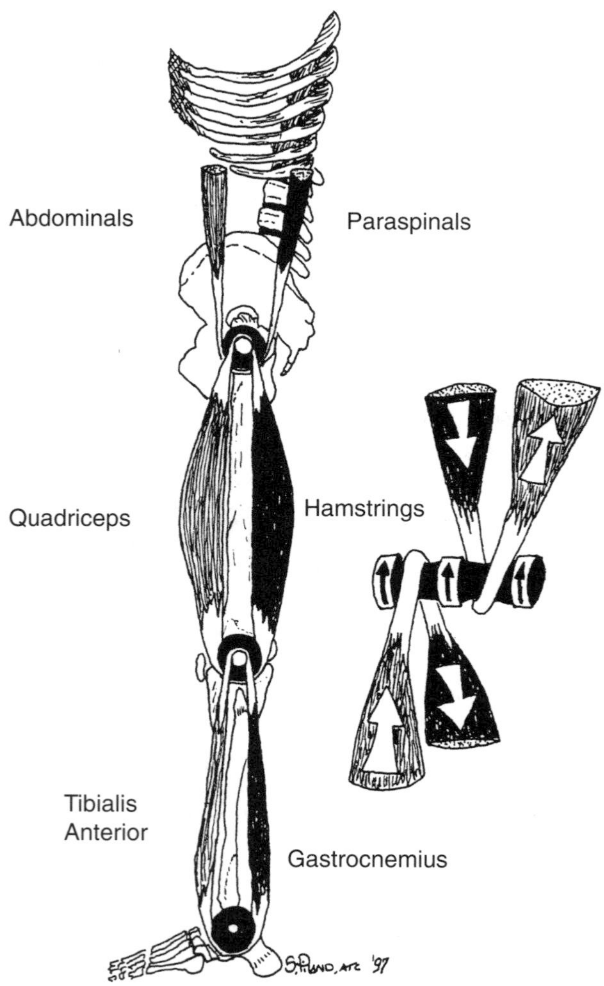

Figure 4.2 Paired relationships between major postural musculature, which executes coordinated actions along the kinetic chain to control the center of gravity.

musculoskeletal system. Afferent information supplied to the postural control system collectively comes from visual, vestibular, and somatosensory inputs. *Somatosensory* input provides information concerning the orientation of body parts to one another and to the support surface (22, 56). *Vision* plays an important role in maintaining balance, as it measures the orientation of the eyes and head in relation to surrounding objects. The *vestibular* apparatus supplies information that measures gravitational, linear, and angular accelerations of the head in relation to inertial space. It does not, however, provide orientation information in relation to external objects and therefore plays only a minor role in the maintenance of balance when the visual and somatosensory systems are providing accurate information (56).

The CNS's involvement in maintaining upright posture can be divided into two components. The first component, *sensory organization*, involves those processes that determine the timing, direction, and amplitude of corrective postural actions based upon afferent information (53). Despite the availability of multiple sensory input, the CNS generally relies on only one sense at a time for orientation information, and impairment or alteration of one of the sensory inputs can usually be compensated for by the remaining two. For example postural sway only increases slightly with eye closure in normal individuals. In this case, visual information becomes eliminated and the somatosensory and vestibular systems compensate. The second component, *muscle coordination*, describes the generation and execution of corrective motor responses with respect to temporal sequencing and distribution of contractile activity among the muscles of the body. Ineffective sequencing or improper coordination may result in disequilibrium (56).

Somatosensation as it Relates to Balance

The terms *somatosensation*, *proprioception*, *kinesthesia*, and *postural balance* are often used to describe similar concepts. Somatosensation, a more global term, is used to describe the peripheral afferent mechanisms related to postural control. Proprioception, therefore, is defined best as a specialized variation of the sensory modality of touch that encompasses the sensation of joint movement (kinesthesia) and joint position (joint position sense) (49). Somatosensation and postural balance work closely, as the postural control system utilizes sensory information related to movement and posture from peripheral sensory receptors (e.g., muscle, joint, and cutaneous receptors); the terms, however, are not synonymous. So the question remains: How does somatosensation influence postural equilibrium and balance?

The organs of the somatosensory system detect the sensations of touch, pressure, vibration, and tickle, all of which are commonly referred to as the tactile senses. The senses of position, velocity, and tension, which determine the relative positions and movement rates of the different body parts, are commonly referred to as proprioceptors (36, 71). These receptors are found abundantly throughout joint, muscle, connective, and ligamentous tissues. This section contains an overview of the somatosensory organs and the types of sensory information as related to the postural control system. The second half of this section presents an overview of the contribution and significance of somatosensory information for postural control.

Sources of Somatosensation

Each tactile and proprioceptive sense of the somatosensory system can be subdivided into two functional groups (slow adapting and fast adapting) with respect to the manner in which they respond to temporal (constant or enduring) characteristics of stimuli (51). Possessing both types of receptors is essential for the postural control system to operate during static, dynamic, and functional activities.

The sensations of touch, pressure, and vibration are conveyed to the CNS via the tactile sense organs. Each somatosensory organ is triggered by a unique stimulus. Hair follicle cells are the principal mechanoreceptors in areas of hairy skin, while glabrous (hairless) skin contains Meissner corpuscles (fast adapting) and Merkel receptors (slow adapting). Deep to both hairy and glabrous skin in the subcutaneous tissues are Ruffini corpuscles (slow adapting) and Pacinian corpuscles (fast adapting), each of which has a large receptor field. Based on their slow adaptation characteristic, Ruffini corpuscles can signal continuous states of deformation of the skin and deeper tissues. Pacinian corpuscles, the most widely studied tactile sensory organ, are stimulated by high frequency vibratory stimuli and very rapid movements of tissues, adapting within a few hundredths of a second. Acting simultaneously, the population of mechanoreceptors located in the plantar surface of the foot can detect the site, force, velocity, and acceleration of transient forces exerted during dynamic activity.

Proprioception is subdivided into two categories: sense of static position (position sense) and sense of movement (kinesthesia or dynamic proprioception). These senses are primarily attributable to joint and muscle mechanoreceptors, with the tactile senses playing contributory roles. Joint receptors include Pacinian corpuscles, Meissner corpuscles, Ruffini endings, and free nerve endings distributed throughout the articular structures (9, 26, 33, 64, 74). Similar to their cutaneous counterparts, the Pacinian corpuscles embedded within joint capsules are rapid adapting while the Ruffini endings are low-threshold, slow-adapting receptors (9, 33). Free nerve endings are found abundantly throughout many articular structures and are believed to become activated only during high degrees of mechanical deformation (33).

Mechanoreceptors located within musculotendinous tissue include the muscle spindles and Golgi tendon organs (GTOs). Both provide the CNS with continuous feedback as to the instantaneous status of each muscle (36, 49). The GTOs, located near their musculotendinous junction, are responsible for sending information to the motor control systems about muscle tension or changes in tension (36, 71). They also serve a protective function by inducing relaxation in a muscle that is being overstretched through polysynaptic inhibitory reflexes (71).

Muscle spindles are embedded in parallel within the contractile components (36, 71), while the GTOs are embedded in series with the musculotendinous fibers. Muscle spindles are considered most often for their role in activating fast monosynaptic reflexes in response to a muscle being stretched (71). They transmit information to the CNS about the rate and magnitude of muscle length change. Muscle spindles consist of specialized afferent nerve endings (primary and secondary) that are wrapped around several modified muscle fibers (intrafusal fibers), all of which is enclosed in a capsule of connective tissue. The intrafusal fibers function as the sensory organs of the apparatus, with only the peripheral areas possessing contractile abilities.

Muscle spindles are unique sensory organs containing both afferent and efferent innervation. The efferent motor neurons (gamma efferents) provide for a method of adjusting the muscle spindle sensitivity by regulating the level of contraction in the intrafusal fibers. This contraction pulls on the central regions of the intrafusal fibers, heightening their sensitivity to changes in muscle length (30). When gamma neuron stimulation accompanies alpha motor neuron activation by the CNS, the process is termed alpha-gamma coactivation. In addition, the levels of gamma activation can be adjusted independently of alpha activation. For example, joint and cutaneous mechanoreceptor stimulation has been reported to influence the muscle spindles via the gamma motoneurons (46). The significance of this aspect of neurophysiology on postural control remains unknown at the present time.

Significance of Somatosensation for Maintenance of Postural Equilibrium

The comprehensive purpose of the somatosensory system is to provide the postural control system with information concerning the orientation of body segments relative to one another as well as to the support surface (22, 56). Each somatosensory organ is triggered by a unique stimulus and thus has a particular role in postural equilibrium. More confidence surrounds the understanding of the role that the somatosensory system has on postural equilibrium as a whole than the individual contributions of each somatosensory component.

Researchers have identified various roles of the somatosensory system by using subjects who have deficient or absent peripheral sensory abilities, such as neuropathy patients (43), or by using methodological approaches that decrease afferent information through anesthesia, ischemia, and alterations in support surfaces (13, 14, 16, 18, 20, 41). Generally, these investigations have revealed that somatosensory input derived from the contact forces and motions between the feet and the support surface is the dominant sensory input to balance under normal (fixed) support surface conditions (41, 53). It has been suggested that somatosensory inputs compensate for both eye closure and vestibular deficit (6, 7, 13, 41, 58, 67) when maintaining balance.

Selective blocking of afferent information from the lower legs revealed that somatosensory information from pressure receptors in the foot and from muscle and joint receptors is important for postural stabilization during low frequencies of movement (13). During rapid displacements, somatosensory inputs from the legs provide the most sensitive means of perceiving postural sway, while at higher sway velocities, visual inputs provide similarly sensitive means of perceiving sway (20). Large disturbances of posture are required before vestibular mechanisms provide perceptual information about body sway (20).

In addition to the function of the somatosensory organs in detecting postural sway, researchers have suggested that they also trigger the selection and coordination of postural responses (13, 41). Feedback from the various somatosensory organs is required to adjust motor programs such as when encountering ground irregularities during walking (16). This is accomplished by incorporating feedback from both the tactile and proprioceptive organs. Horak and coworkers (41) reported that subjects deprived of somatosensory information from the foot through ischemia induced at the ankles responded to external perturbations with well-coordinated movements at normal latencies but that the postural movements were often either ineffective or inefficient for the environmental context in which they were used. In other words, somatosensory inputs distal to the ankle do not appear to be essential for the initiation of automatic postural responses but rather are essential for determining the availability of postural compensatory strategies.

Other studies (8, 41) have examined the role of somatosensory information by altering or limiting somatosensory input through the use of platform sway referencing or foam platforms. Similarly, these studies reported that subjects still responded with well-coordinated movements but the movements were often either ineffective or inefficient for the environmental context in which they were used.

Contributions of Individual Somatosensory Components

While debate has long existed as to whether cutaneous, joint, or muscle receptors are most important to the maintenance of balance, contemporary belief is that all contribute significantly. Several studies have been conducted considering the various functions of each component with the intent to identify the somatosensory source having the most substantial role in postural equilibrium (17, 41, 50, 62, 73). Many of these studies have reached contradictory conclusions, which could be due to several factors. For example, research has demonstrated compensatory mechanisms with each of the sensory modalities involved with balance. It is quite probable that the individual components of the somatosensory system have the ability to function in a similar manner. This section focuses on an overview of the research identifying the contributions of individual somatosensory components to postural equilibrium.

Cutaneous Receptors

Postural sway during static stance causes the location of the center of pressure (COP) to change relative to the support surface (10). Both the magnitude and distribution of these changes are detected by the plantar cutaneous receptors, as body sway increases significantly in their absence even when visual information is altered (17, 50). During static stance these receptors have been reported to transduce information concerning whether weight is distributed equally between the two feet and whether weight is more forward or backward on the feet (36).

In addition to reporting postural sway during static conditions, plantar cutaneous receptors appear to have significant roles during dynamic and functional movements. Both animal and human experiments have demonstrated that cutaneous afferent receptors influence segmental motor reflexes and modify voluntary motor commands (10). During upright stance, the stimulation of the plantar cutaneous receptors may provide additional muscular support by increasing the tone of intrinsic foot musculature. Stimulation of foot mechanoreceptors was demonstrated to have widespread reflex actions on multiple muscles throughout the lower extremity (10). Further, the reflex patterns of different muscles and within a single muscle have been reported to change according to the task undertaken. In other words, cutaneous reflex activity may affect both short-latency as well as long-latency pathways (10). Researchers think that, during walking, the plantar cutaneous receptors are contributing to muscle activation on an ongoing basis (73).

Muscle Receptors

In contrast, Fitzpatrick and others eliminated all cutaneous receptor (21) information from the feet and ankles and revealed that muscle mechanoreceptors in the leg muscles (gastrocnemius and tibialis anterior) were capable of providing sufficient somatosensory information for stable standing. They speculated that group I or group II muscle spindle afferents and group Ib afferents from GTOs were the probable sources of this somatosensory input. Similarly, no increases in postural sway were reported following ischemia induced at the level of the ankles, suggesting that proprioceptive inputs from the ankle musculature may have the dominant role in detecting postural sway (41). By selectively inhibiting the sensory information from muscle spindles in different muscle groups, Pyykko and coworkers (62) suggested that postural muscles vary in their predominate function. Based on the increases in postural sway associated with disruption to each muscle considered, several muscles appeared more essential for stabilization, while others appeared to serve more locomotive functions.

Support for the essential need for muscle mechanoreceptors has also followed investigations utilizing various platform perturbations (13, 16, 54). Traditionally, rotational and translational perturbations have been associated with eliciting postural reflexes by stretching opposing musculature, thereby stimulating reflexes via the muscle spindles. Although empirical observation might suggest that monosynaptic myotactic reflexes would have functional significance in the regulation of equilibrium, more contemporary views consider the stimulation of muscle spindles as being more significant in initiating complex, polysynaptic proprioceptive responses (15). Electromyographic (EMG) response latencies following platform perturbations have been reported to be longer than those normally associated with classical myotactic responses (13, 54).

Selection of Muscle Strategy

Three principal joint systems (ankles, knees, and hips) are located between the base of support and the COG. This allows for a wide variety of postures that can be assumed, while the COG is still positioned above the base of support. Motions about a given joint are controlled by the combined actions of at least one pair of muscles working in opposition. When forces exerted by pairs of opposing muscles about a joint (e.g., anterior tibialis and gastrocnemius-soleus) are combined, the effect is to resist rotation of the joint relative to a resting position. The degree to which the joint resists rotation is called joint stiffness. The resting position and the stiffness of the joint are each altered independently by changing the activation levels of one or both muscle groups (42, 56).

When a person's balance is disrupted by an external perturbation, movement strategies involving joints of the lower extremity coordinate movement of the COG back to a balanced position. In general, the relative effectiveness of *ankle, hip, and stepping strategies* in repositioning the COG over the base of support depends on the configuration of the base of support, the COG alignment in relation to the LOS, and the speed of the postural movement (40). The *ankle strategy* shifts the COG while maintaining the placement of the feet by rotating the body as a rigid mass about the ankle joints. This is achieved by contracting either the gastrocnemius or anterior tibialis muscles to generate torque about the ankle joints. The ankle strategy is most effective in executing relatively slow COG movements when the base of support is firm and the COG is well within the LOS perimeter. The ankle strategy is also believed to be effective in maintaining a static posture with the COG offset from the center. The thigh and lower trunk muscles contract and thereby resist the destabilization of these proximal joints due to the indirect effects of the ankle muscles on the proximal joints (see table 4.1). Under normal sensory conditions, activation of ankle musculature is almost exclusively selected to maintain equilibrium.

Persons with somatosensory loss, however, appear to rely on their hip musculature to retain their COG while experiencing forward or backward perturbation or with different support surface lengths (22). If the ankle strategy is not capable of controlling excessive sway, the *hip strategy* is available to help control motion of the COG through the initiation of large and rapid motions at the hip joints with antiphase rotation of the ankles. It is most effective when the COG is located near the LOS perimeter and when the LOS boundaries are contracted by a narrowed base of support. Finally, when the COG is displaced beyond the LOS, a step or stumble (*stepping strategy*) is the only strategy that can be used to prevent a fall (56, 57). It is proposed that LOS and COG alignment are altered in individuals exhibiting a musculoskeletal abnormality such as an ankle or knee sprain.

Balance Assessment

The complexity of the postural control system often makes identifying and isolating the source of balance problems difficult. A variety of approaches are available, ranging from evaluations of steadiness during static stance to stability during functional activity. Although static, dynamic, and functional assessments contain common underlying postural components, each of them appears to measure unique aspects of postural equilibrium (70). Measurements of performance during these various tasks are considered to have either a subjective or objective basis. Subjective tests involve an examiner judging balance performance based on qualitative criteria, whereas objective tests encompass the gathering and analysis of quantitative data from devices such as force platforms and motion analysis equipment. Several investigations have considered the relationships between qualitative assessment methods (using categorical scales) and quantitative force plate measures of postural sway. One investigation has reported a valid and reliable method of evaluating postural stability during three different stances on stable and unstable surfaces (see figure 4.3) (63).

Many of the various assessment methods have resulted from attempts to isolate and evaluate the

Table 4.1 Functional Anatomy of Muscles Involved in Balance Movements

	Extension		Flexion	
Joint	Anatomic	Functional	Anatomic	Functional
Hip	Paraspinals Hamstrings	Paraspinals Hamstrings Tibialis	Abdominals Quadriceps	Abdominals Quadriceps Gastrocnemius
Knee	Quadriceps	Paraspinals Quadriceps Gastrocnemius	Hamstrings Gastrocnemius	Abdominals Hamstrings Tibialis
Ankle	Gastrocnemius	Abdominals Quadriceps Gastrocnemius	Tibialis	Paraspinals Hamstrings Tibialis

(Adapted from Nashner, LM. Physiology of Balance. In *Handbook of Balance and Function Testing*, G Jacobson, C Newman, and J Kartush (eds.), St. Louis: Mosby Year Book, 1993, pp. 261-279.)

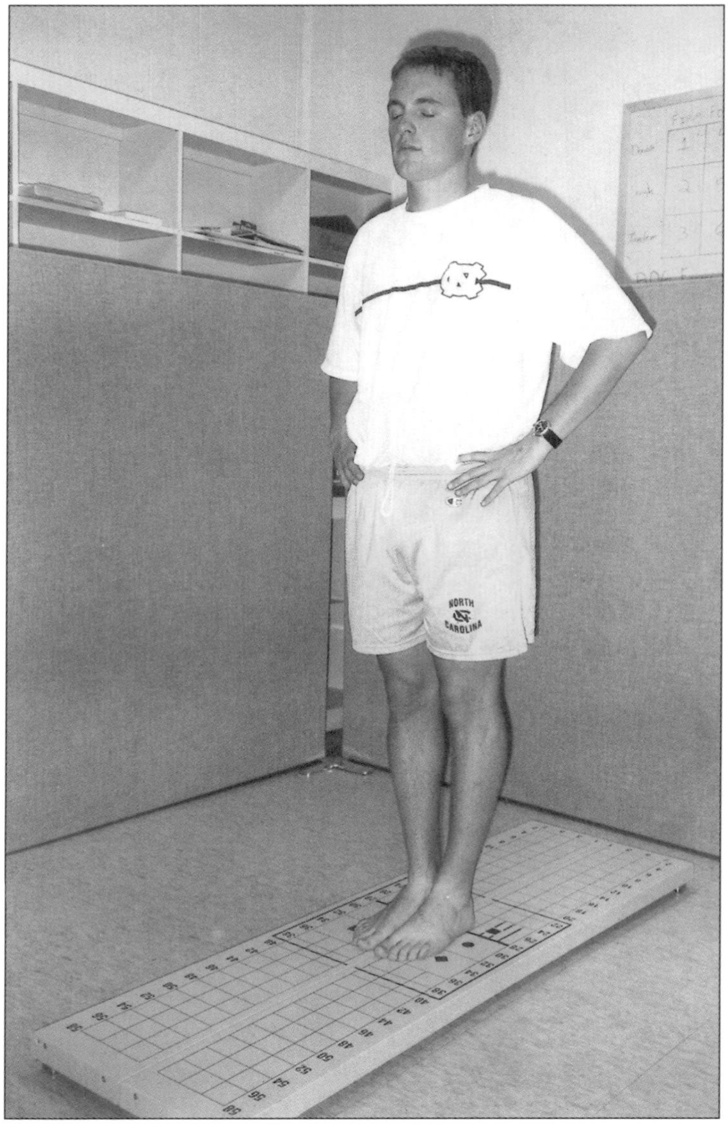

Figure 4.3 The testing position used by Riemann and Guskiewicz for the double-leg stance on a firm surface.

function of individual postural control system components (sensory, central integration, and motor). Force plate technology has allowed for quantitative evaluations of sensory inputs (visual, vestibular, somatosensory) through the Clinical Test of Sensory Interaction and Balance (CTSIB) and the Sensory Organization Test (SOT) (see figure 4.4). The CTSIB uses combinations of three visual and two support-surface conditions during assessment of postural sway (66). The technique to conflict sensory input involves alteration of somatosensation (foam surface vs. hard surface), vision (eyes closed vs. eyes open), and vestibular (conflict dome vs. normal vision) input. In a similar manner, the SOT evaluates the integrity of the three sensory modalities by selectively disrupting somatosensory or visual information or both regarding body COG orientation in relation to vertical and then measuring the patient's ability to maintain balance through a series of six conditions (55) (see figure 4.5). Sway referencing involves the tilting of the support surface, the visual surround (wall), or both, in an A-P direction according to the patient's COG sway. Under sway-referenced conditions, the orientation of the support surface and the visual surround remains constant in relation to the COG sway angle (55, 58). The theory behind sway referencing is similar to the theory behind the CTSIB, as healthy subjects should ignore functionally inaccurate sway-referenced sensory input(s) and maintain balance using other sensory inputs. Increased postural instability under selected conditions can identify sensory in-

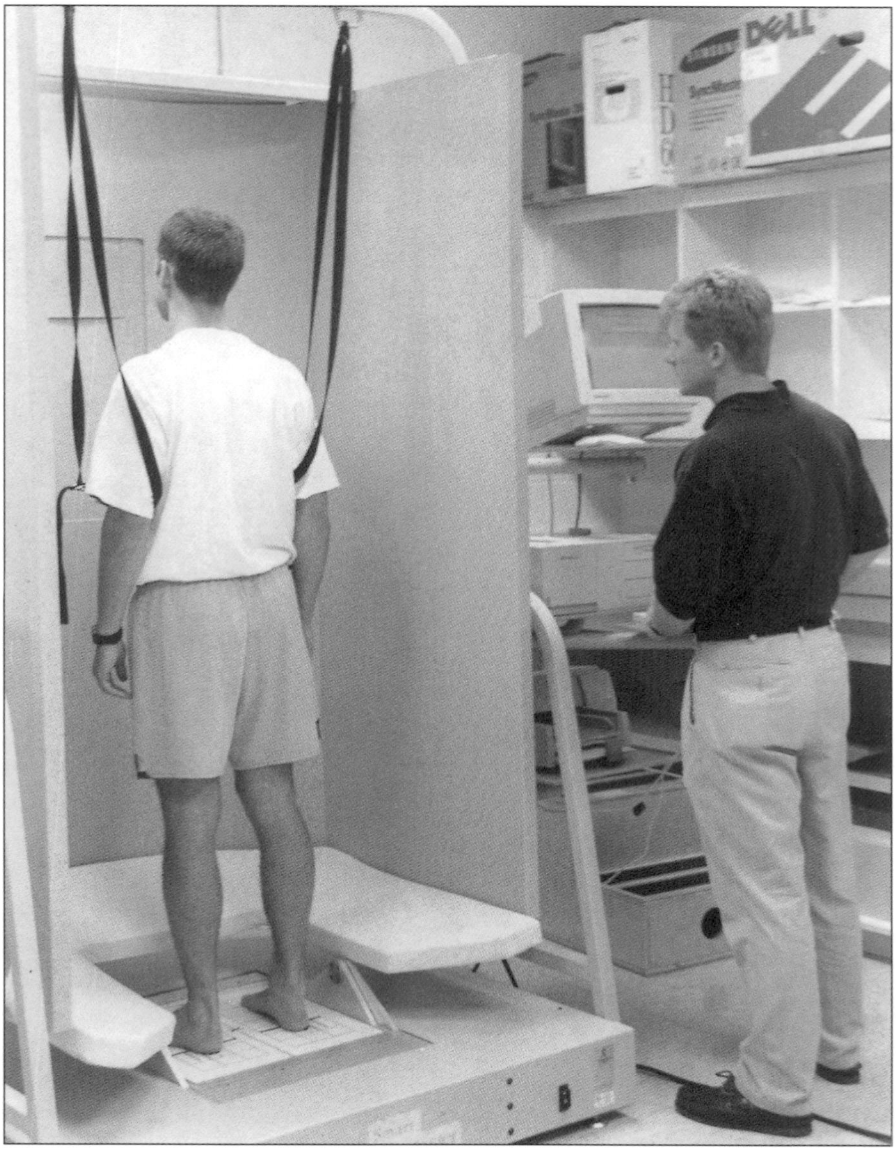

Figure 4.4 The NeuroCom Smart Balance Master (NeuroCom, Inc., Clackamas, OR) designed for computerized dynamic posturography testing protocols with moving visual surround and platform.

teraction problems such as a loss of somatosensory feedback.

In addition, accurate motor responses are important for the maintenance of balance and should be considered during balance assessments. Translational and rotational postural perturbations can be utilized to elicit discrete motor responses such as during the motor control test (MCT) and posture-evoked response test (PER) protocols on the NeuroCom EquiTest system (55). Automatic postural responses to the perturbations can be measured though electromyography or compensatory forces exerted against the support surface. Additionally, muscle strategy selections can be evaluated in response to various perturbations by measuring horizontal shear forces exerted against the support surface or through the use of accelerometers attached to the head, hip, and ankle.

Many of the assessment systems can also be used for balance training and rehabilitation (35) (see figures 4.6 and 4.7). As with assessment procedures, balance training should focus on location of the deficiency within the postural stability system. Balance training should require the person to keep or return the COG over the base of support during various environmental conditions and changes in body position. Eye closure will eliminate vision, as well as some vestibular information, thereby tax-

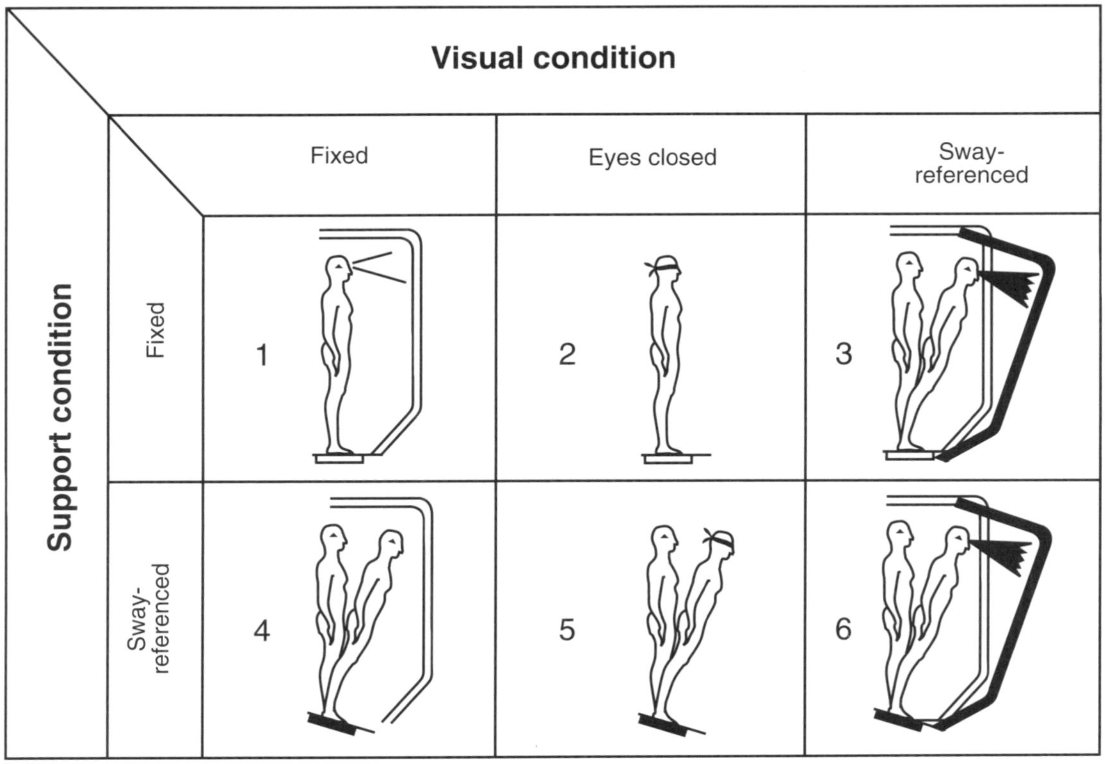

Figure 4.5 The six testing conditions used during the sensory organizational test. The first three involve a fixed platform across the three visual conditions (eyes open, eyes closed, sway referenced) and the last three involve a sway-referenced platform across the same three visual conditions.

ing the somatosensory system. During balance routines without the use of a balance system, exercises can include balancing on a rocker, wobble board, BAPS board, or multiaxial disk, which records change in deflection or postural sway. Other feasible routines, such as Thera-Band kicks, single-leg hop tests, and single-leg tests on foam, have been proposed and utilized by clinicians.

Injury and Balance

It has long been theorized that failure of stretched or damaged ligaments to provide adequate neural feedback in an injured extremity may contribute to decreased proprioceptive mechanisms necessary for maintenance of proper balance. Research has revealed these impairments in individuals with ankle injury (24, 34, 69) and anterior cruciate ligament (ACL) injury (4, 59). It has been suggested that the lack of proprioceptive feedback resulting from such injuries may allow excessive or inappropriate loading of a joint (11). Furthermore, Wilkerson and Nitz (72) state that although the presence of a capsular lesion may interfere with the transmission of afferent impulses from the joint, a more important effect may be alteration of the afferent neural code that is conveyed to the CNS. Decreased reflex excitation of motor neurons may result from either or both of the following events: (1) a decrease in proprioceptive input to the CNS, (2) an increase in the activation of inhibitory interneurons within the spinal cord. All of these factors may lead to progressive degeneration of the joint and continued deficits in joint dynamics, balance, and coordination.

Ankle Injuries

Joint proprioceptors are believed to be damaged during injury to the lateral ligaments of the ankle because joint receptor fibers possess less tensile strength than the ligament fibers. Damage to the joint receptors is believed to cause joint deafferentation, therefore diminishing the supply of messages from the injured joint up the afferent pathway, disrupting proprioceptive function (25). Freeman and coworkers (25) were the first to report a decrease in

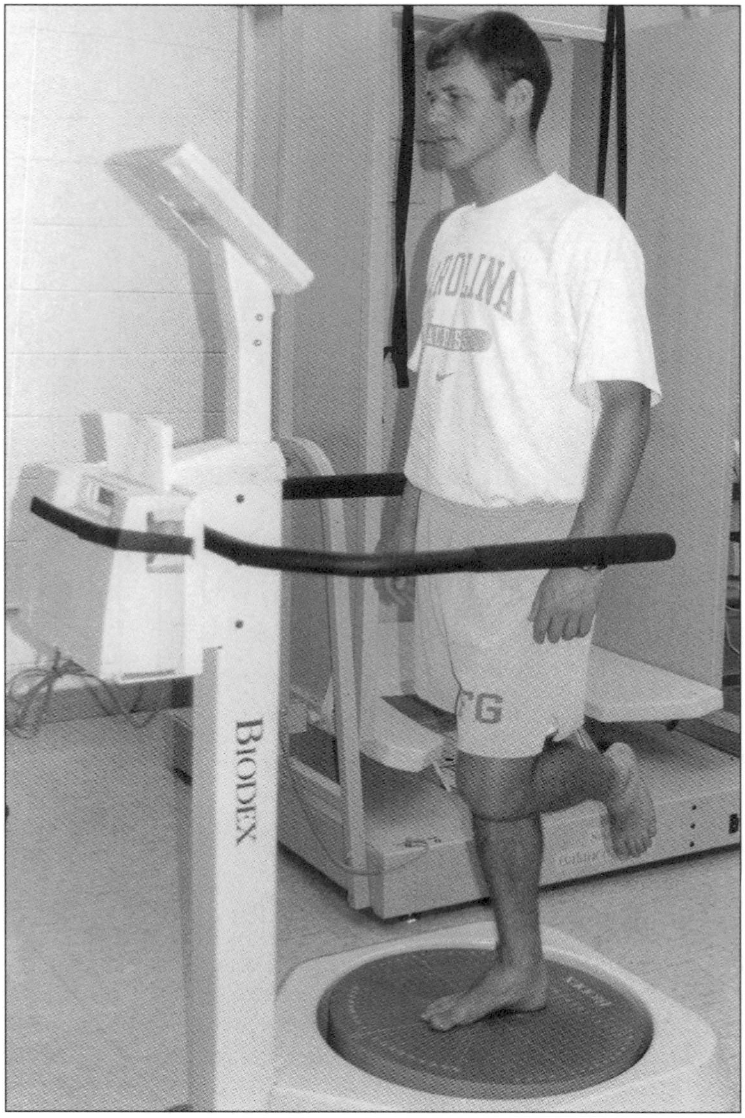

Figure 4.6 The Biodex Stability System. (Biodex Medical Systems, Shirely, NY)

the frequency of functional instability following ankle sprains when coordination exercises were performed as part of rehabilitation. Thus the term "articular deafferentation" was introduced to designate the mechanism that they thought to be the cause of functional instability of the ankle. This finding led to the inclusion of balance training in ankle rehabilitation programs.

Since 1965, Freeman (24) has theorized that if ankle injuries cause partial deafferentation and functional instability, a person's postural sway would be altered due to a proprioception deficit. While some studies (5, 44, 68, 69) have not supported Freeman's theory, other studies have revealed balance deficits in ankles following acute sprains (27, 29, 34, 47, 60) and in ankles with chronic instabilities (12, 23, 28).

Friden and others (27) identified differences between injured and uninjured ankles using a computerized strain gauge force plate. Four of five possible postural sway parameters (standard deviation of the mean COP dispersion, mean sway amplitude, average speed, and number of sway amplitudes exceeding 5 and 10 mm) taken in the frontal plane from a single-leg stance position were reported to discriminate between injured and noninjured ankles. The authors reported that the application of an ankle brace eliminated the differences between injury status when tested on each parameter, therefore improving balance performance. More importantly this

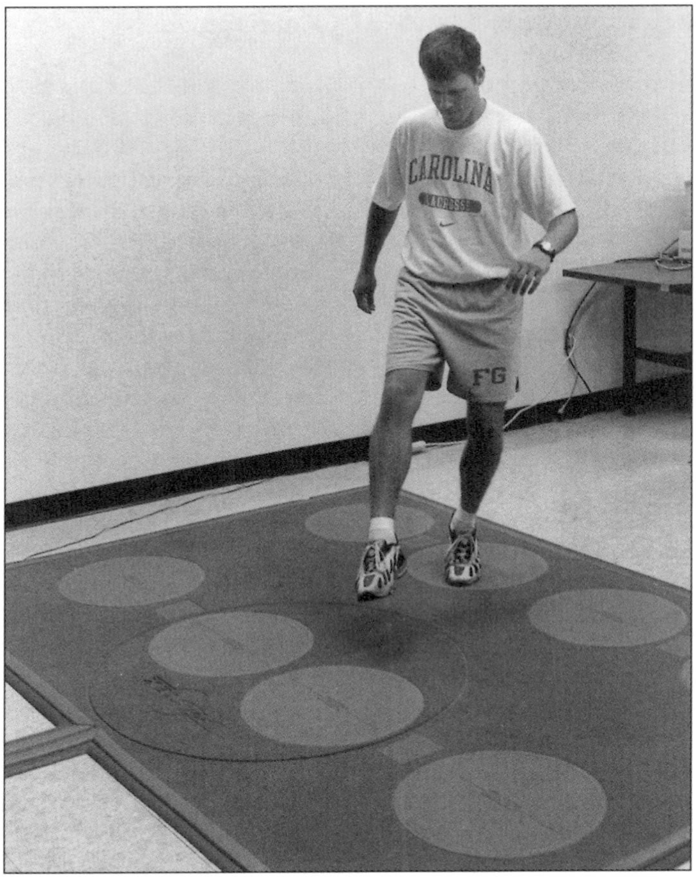

Figure 4.7 The Functional Activity System for Testing and Exercise (FASTEX). (Cybex Division of Lumex, Inc., Ronkonkoma, NY)

study suggests that the stabilometry technique of selectively analyzing postural sway movements in the frontal plane, where the diameter of the supporting area is smallest, leads to higher sensitivity. Because difficulties of maintaining balance after a ligament lesion involve the subtalar axis, it is proposed that increased sway movements of the different body segments would be found primarily in the frontal plane. The authors speculated that this could explain nonsignificant findings of earlier stabilometry studies (68, 69) involving injured ankles.

Interventions such as orthotics, taping, and rehabilitation have been shown to improve postural control in subjects with acutely injured ankles. Guskiewicz and Perrin (34) compared injured and uninjured subjects for postural sway under two treatment conditions (orthotic, nonorthotic) and four platform movements (stable, inversion-eversion, plantar flexion-dorsiflexion, medial-lateral perturbations). Results revealed that ankle-injured subjects swayed more than uninjured subjects when assessed in a single-leg stance. The analysis revealed that custom-made orthotics may restrict undesirable motion at the foot and ankle and enhance joint mechanoreceptors to detect perturbations and provide structural support for detecting and controlling postural sway in ankle-injured subjects. A similar study by Orteza and coworkers (61) reported improvements in static balance for injured subjects while wearing custom-made orthotics. Decreased postural control due to ankle sprains has also been shown to improve following taping of the ankle (47) and proprioceptive rehabilitation of the ankle (29, 47).

Studies involving subjects with chronic ankle instabilities (12, 23, 28, 61) indicate that individuals with a history of inversion ankle sprain are less stable in single-limb stance on the involved leg as compared to the uninvolved leg or noninjured subjects. Cornwall and Murrell (12) reported significant differences between injured and uninjured subjects for sway amplitude but not sway frequency using a standard force plate. Pintsaar and coworkers (61) studied the effect of stance perturbation on frontal plane postural control in three groups of subjects: (1) control (no previous ankle injury), (2) functional ankle instability and 8 wk training program, and (3) mechanical instability without functional instability (without shoe, with shoe, with brace and shoe). The authors reported a relative change from ankle to hip synergy at medially directed translations of the support surface on the NeuroCom EquiTest. The impairment was restored after 8 wks of ankle disk training and the effect of a shoe and brace did not exceed the effect of the shoe alone. Impaired ankle function was shown to be related to coordination, as subjects changed from ankle toward hip strategies for postural adjustments.

Similarly, Hertel and coworkers (38) reported that lateral ankle joint anesthesia did not alter postural sway or passive joint position sense but affected the center of balance position (similar to center of pressure) during both static and dynamic testing. This suggests the presence of an adaptive mechanism to compensate for the loss of afferent stimuli from the region of the lateral ankle ligaments (38). Subjects tended to shift the center of balance medially during dynamic balance testing and slightly laterally during static balance testing. The authors speculated that center of balance shifting may provide additional proprioceptive input from cutaneous receptors in the sole of the foot or stretch receptors in the peroneal muscle-tendon unit, which therefore prevents increased postural sway.

Increased postural sway frequency and latencies are parameters thought to be indicative of impaired ankle joint proprioception (13, 65). Cornwall and coworkers (12) and Pintsaar and others (61), however, found no differences between chronically injured subjects and control subjects on these measures. This raises the question as to whether postural sway was in fact caused by a proprioceptive deficit. Increased postural sway amplitudes in the absence of sway frequencies might suggest that chronically injured subjects recover their ankle joint proprioception over time (12).

In summary, results of studies involving both chronic and acute ankle sprains suggest that increased postural sway and balance instability may not be due to a single factor but to disruption of both neurological and biomechanical factors at the ankle joint. Loss of balance may result from abnormal or altered biomechanical alignment of the body, thus affecting the transmission of somatosensory information from the ankle joint. It is possible that observed increased postural sway amplitudes following injury result from joint instability along the kinetic chain rather than deafferentation.

Knee Injuries

Ligamentous injury to the knee has been proven to affect the ability of subjects to accurately detect position (2-4, 48, 49). The general consensus among numerous investigators performing proprioceptive testing is that a clinical proprioception deficit occurs in most patients after an ACL rupture causing functional instability and that this deficit seems to persist to some degree after an ACL reconstruction (2). Because of the relationship between proprioception (somatosensation) and balance, it would follow that a patient's ability to balance on the ACL-injured leg may also be decreased (4, 59).

Studies have evaluated the effects of ACL ruptures on standing balance using force plate technology and, while some studies have revealed balance deficits (27, 52), others have not (19, 37). Results from these studies appear to conflict, depending on which parameters are measured. Mizuta and others (52) found significant differences in postural stability when measuring COP and sway distance area between 11 functionally stable and 15 functionally unstable subjects who had unilateral ACL-deficient knees. In contrast, Faculjak and others (19) found no differences in postural stability between 8 ACL-deficient subjects and 10 normal subjects when measuring average latency and response strength on an EquiTest system.

Several potential reasons for these discrepancies exist. It has been suggested that there may be a link between static balance and isometric strength of the ankle and knee musculature (1). Isometric muscle strength may therefore compensate for any somatosensory deficits in the involved knee during a closed chain static balance test. Secondly, many studies fail to discriminate between *functionally unstable* ACL-deficient knees and those that were not *functionally unstable*. This presents a design flaw, especially considering that functionally stable knees would most likely provide adequate balance despite ligamentous pathology. Another suggested reason for failing to differentiate between injured knees and uninjured knees on static balance measures could be explained by the role that joint mechanoreceptors play. Neurophysiological studies (31, 32, 45, 49) have revealed that joint mechanoreceptors provide enhanced kinesthetic awareness in the near terminal range of motion or extremes of motion. It can be speculated, therefore, that if the maximum LOS is never reached during a static balance test, damaged mechanoreceptors (muscle or joint) may not even become a factor. Dynamic balance tests or functional hop tests that involve dynamic balance could challenge the postural control system (ankle strategies are taken over by hip or stepping strategies) requiring more mechanoreceptor input. These tests would most likely discriminate between functionally unstable ACL-deficient knees and normal knees.

Summary

Balance is a complex process involving the integration of neurological sensory afferent information, muscular coordination, and biomechanics. This chapter has attempted to present the physiological foundations of the postural control system with an emphasis on somatosensory input to central processing. Postural control requires input from all three sensory systems (vestibular, visual, and somatosensory); however, it is the somatosensory system that most healthy people rely on for maintaining postural equilibrium under most environmental conditions. The somatosensory system consists of both tactile and proprioceptive receptors that convey information to the CNS relative to body and limb positions. Information is then sent via motor pathways so that postural control adjustments can be made by the initiation of selected movement strategies (ankle, hip, stepping). The significance of individual somatosensory sources in postural equilibrium remains unknown, although it is apparent that all sources (muscle, joint, and cutaneous) play a major role. Several methods of postural stability assessment are available that allow for the isolation and evaluation of various postural system components as well as different aspects of postural control. Injury to the joints of the lower extremity appears to have an inhibitory effect on a person's proprioceptive ability, which could potentially affect his or her ability to maintain balance.

References

1. Balogun J, Adesinasi C, Marzouk D. The effects of a wobble board exercise training program on static balance performance and strength of lower extremity muscles. *Physiother Canada* 44: 23–30, 1992.
2. Barrack R, Lund P, Skinner H. Knee joint proprioception revisited. *J Sport Rehabil* 3: 18–42, 1994.
3. Barrack R, Skinner H, Buckley S. Proprioception in the anterior cruciate deficient knee. *Am J Sports Med* 17: 1–6, 1989.
4. Barret D. Proprioception and function after anterior cruciate reconstruction. *J Bone Joint Surg* (Britain) 73: 833–37, 1991.
5. Bernier J, Perrin DH, Rijke A. Effect of unilateral functional instability of the ankle on postural sway and inversion and eversion strength. *J Athl Train* 32: 226–32, 1997.
6. Black F, Nashner L. Postural control in four classes of vestibular abnormalities. In *Vestibular and Visual Control of Posture and Locomotor Equilibrium,* Igarshi M, Black F (Eds.), 271–81. Basel: Karger, 1985.
7. Black F, Nashner L. Vestibulospinal control differs in patients with reduced versus distorted vestibular function. *Acta Otolaryngol* 406: 110–14, 1984.
8. Black F, Wall C, Nashner L. Effect of visual and support surface orientations upon postural control in vestibular deficient subjects. *Acta Otolaryngol* 95: 199–210, 1983.
9. Boyd, IA. The histological structure of the receptors in the knee joint of the cat correlated with their physiological response. *J Physiol* (London) 124: 476–88, 1954.
10. Burke D, Dickson H, Skuse N. Task-dependent changes in the responses to low-threshold cutaneous afferent volleys in the human lower limb. *J Physiol* 432: 445–58, 1991.
11. Co F, Skinner H, Cannon W. Effect of reconstruction of the anterior cruciate ligament on proprioception of the knee and the heel strike transient. *J Orthop Res* 11: 696–704, 1993.
12. Cornwall M, Murrell P. Postural sway following inversion sprain of the ankle. *J Am Podiatric Med Assoc* 81: 243–47, 1991.
13. Diener H, Dichgans B, Guschlbauer b, Mau H. The significance of proprioception on postural stabilization as assessed by ischemia. *Brain Res.* 296: 103–109, 1984.
14. Diener H, Dichgans J, Guschlbauer B, et al. Role of visual and static vestibular influences on dynamic posture control. *Human Neurobiol* 5: 105–13, 1986.
15. Dietz V. Human neuronal control of automatic functional movements: Interaction between central programs and afferent input. *Physiol Rev* 72: 33–69, 1992.
16. Dietz V, Horstmann G, Berger W. Significance of proprioceptive mechanisms in the regulation of stance. *Prog Brain Res* 80: 419–23, 1989.
17. Do M, Bussel B, Breniere Y. Influence of plantar cutaneous afferent on early compensatory reactions to forward fall. *Exp Brain Res* 79: 319–24, 1990.

18. Dornan J, Fernie G, Holliday P. Visual input: Its significance in the control of postural sway. *Arch Phys Med Rehabil* 59: 586–91, 1978.
19. Faculjak P, Firoozbakshsh K, Wausher D, McGuire M. Balance characteristics of normal and anterior cruciate ligament deficient knees. *Phys Ther* 73: S22, 1993.
20. Fitzpatrick R, McCloskey D. Proprioceptive, visual, and vestibular thresholds for the perception of sway during standing in humans. *J Physiol* 478: 173–86, 1994.
21. Fitzpatrick R, Rogers D, McCloskey D. Stable human standing with lower limb muscle afferents providing the only sensory input. *J Physiol* 480: 395–402, 1994.
22. Flores A. Objective measures of standing balance. *Neurology Report-Am Phys Ther Assoc* 16: 17–21, 1992.
23. Forkin D, Koczur C, Battle R, Newton R. Evaluation of kinesthetic deficits indicative of balance control in gymnasts with unilateral chronic ankle sprains. *J Orthop Sports Phys Ther* 23: 245–50, 1996.
24. Freeman M. Instability of the foot after injuries to the lateral ligament of the ankle. *J Bone Joint Surg* 47B: 678–85, 1965.
25. Freeman M, Dean M, Hanham I. The etiology and prevention of functional instability of the foot. *J Bone Joint Surg* 47B: 669–77, 1965.
26. Freeman M, Wyke B. Articular reflexes at the ankle joint: An electromyographic study of normal and abnormal influences of ankle joint mechanoreceptors upon reflex activity in the leg muscles. *Br J Surg* 54: 990–92, 1967.
27. Friden T, Zatterstrom R, Lindstrand A, Moritz U. A stabilometric technique for evaluation of lower limb instabilities. *Am J Sports Med* 17: 118–22, 1989.
28. Garn S, Newton R. Kinesthetic awareness in subjects with multiple ankle sprains. *Phys Ther* 68: 1667–671, 1988.
29. Goldie P, Evans O, Bach T. Postural control following inversion injuries of the ankle. *Arch Phys Med Rehabil* 75: 969–75, 1994.
30. Gordon J, Ghez C. Muscle receptors and spinal reflexes: The stretch reflex. *Princ Neural Sci* 340–53, 1991.
31. Grigg P. Mechanical factors influencing response of joint afferent neurons from cat knee. *J Neurophysiol* 38: 1473–484, 1975.
32. Grigg P. Response of joint afferent neurons in cat medial articular nerve to active and passive movements of the knee. *Brain Res* 118: 482–85, 1976.
33. Grigg P, Hoffman A, Fogarty K. Properties of Golgi-Mazzoni afferents in cat knee joint capsule, as revealed by mechanical studies of isolated joint capsule. *J Neurophysiol* 47: 31–40, 1982.
34. Guskiewicz K, Perrin D. Effect of orthotics on postural sway following inversion ankle sprain. *J Orthop Sports Phys Ther* 23: 326–31, 1996.
35. Guskiewicz K, Perrin D. Research and clinical applications of assessing balance. *J Sport Rehabil* 5: 45–63, 1996.
36. Guyton A. *Textbook of Medical Physiology* (8th ed.). Philadelphia: Saunders, 1991.
37. Harrison E, Duenkel N, Dunlop R, Russell G. Evaluation of single-leg stance following anterior cruciate ligament surgery and rehabilitation. *Phys Ther* 74: 245–52, 1994.
38. Hertel J, Guskiewicz K, Kahler D, Perrin D. Effect of lateral ankle joint anesthesia on center of balance, postural sway, and joint position sense. *J Sport Rehabil* 5: 111–19, 1996.
39. Horak F. Clinical measurement of postural control in adults. *Phys Ther* 67: 1881–885, 1987.
40. Horak F, Nashner L. Central programming of postural movements: Adaptation to altered support surface configurations. *J Physiol* 55: 1369–381, 1986.
41. Horak F, Nashner L, Diener H. Postural strategies associated with somatosensory and vestibular loss. *Exp Brain Res* 82: 167–77, 1990.
42. Houk J. Regulation of stiffness by skeletomotor reflexes. *Ann Rev Physiol* 41: 99–114, 1979.
43. Inglis J, Horak F, Shupert C, Jones-Rycewicz C. The importance of somatosensory information in triggering and scaling automatic postural responses in humans. *Exp Brain Res* 101: 159–64, 1994.
44. Isakov E, Mizrahi J. Is balance impaired by recurrent sprained ankle? *Br J Sports Med* 31: 65–67, 1997.
45. Johansson H, Alexander I, Hayes K. Nerve supply of the human knee and its functional importance. *Am J Sports Med* 10: 329–35, 1982.
46. Johansson H, Sjölander P. Neurophysiology of joints. In *Mechanics of Human Joints*, Wright V, Radin EL (Eds.), 243–90. New York: Marcel Dekker, 1993.
47. Leanderson J, Eriksson E, Wilson C, Wykman A. Proprioception in classical ballet dancers. *Am J Sports Med* 24: 370–74, 1996.
48. Lephart S, Kocher M, Fu F. Proprioception following ACL reconstruction. *J Sport Rehabil* 1: 186–96, 1992.
49. Lephart S, Pincivero D, Giraldo J, Fu F. The role of proprioception in the management and rehabilitation of athletic injuries. *Am J Sports Med* 25: 130–37, 1997.
50. Magnusson M, Enbom H, Johansson R, Pyykko I. Significance of pressor input from the human

feet in anterior-posterior postural control. *Acta Otolaryngol* 110: 182–88, 1990.
51. Martin J, Jessel T. Modality coding in the somatic sensory system. *Princ Neural Sci* 340–52, 1991.
52. Mizuta H, Shirasishi M, Kubota K, Kai K, Takagi K. A stabilometric technique for evaluation of functional instability in the anterior cruciate ligament-deficient knee. *Clin J Sports Med* 2: 235–39, 1992.
53. Nashner L. Adaptation of human movement to altered environments. *Trends Neurosci* 5: 358–61, 1982.
54. Nashner L. Adapting reflexes controlling the human posture. *Exp Brain Res* 26: 59–72, 1976.
55. Nashner L. Computerized dynamic posturography. In *Handbook of Balance Function and Testing,* Jacobson G, Newman C, Kartush J (Eds.), 280–307. St. Louis: Mosby Year Book, 1993.
56. Nashner L. Practical biomechanics and physiology of balance. In *Handbook of Balance Function and Testing,* Jacobson G, Newman C, Kartush J (Eds.), 261–79. St. Louis: Mosby Year Book, 1993.
57. Nashner L. Sensory, neuromuscular, and biomechanical contributions to human balance. In *Balance: Proceedings of the APTA Forum*, Duncan P (Ed.), 5–12. June 13–15, 1989.
58. Nashner L, Black F, Wall C. Adaptation to altered support and visual conditions during stance: Patients with vestibular deficits. *J Neurosci* 2: 536–44, 1982.
59. Noyes F, Barber S, Mangine R. Abnormal lower-limb symmetry determined by function hop test after anterior cruciate ligament rupture. *Am J Sports Med* 19: 516–18, 1991.
60. Orteza L, Vogelbach W, Denegar C. The effect of molded and unmolded orthotics on balance and pain while jogging following inversion ankle sprain. *J Athl Train* 27: 80–84, 1992.
61. Pintsaar A, Brynhildsen J, Tropp H. Postural corrections after standardized perturbations of single-limb stance: Effect of training and orthotic devices in patients with ankle instability. *Br J Sports Med* 30: 151–55, 1996.
62. Pyykko I, Aalto H, Seidel H, Starck J. Hierarchy of different muscles in postural control. *Acta Otolaryngol* 468: 175–80, 1989.
63. Riemann B, Guskiewicz K. Relationship between clinical and force plate measures of postural stability. Manuscript submitted for publication.
64. Schultz R, Miller D, Kerr C, Micheli L. Mechanoreceptors in human cruciate ligament. *J Bone Joint Surg* 1072–76, 1984.
65. Shambers G. Influence of the fusimotor system on stance and volitional movement in normal man. *Am J Phys Med* 48: 225–27, 1969.
66. Shumway-Cook A, Horak F. Assessing the influence of sensory interaction on balance. *Phys Ther* 66: 1548–550, 1986.
67. Shupert C, Black F, Horak F, et al. Coordination of head and body in response to support surface translations in normals and patients with bilaterally reduced vestibular function. In *Posture and Gait: Development, Adaptation, and Modulation,* Amblard B, Berthoz A, Clarac F (Eds.), 281–89. New York: Elsevier Science, 1988.
68. Tropp J, Ekstrand J, Gillquist J. Factors affecting stabilometry recordings of single-limb stance. *Am J Sports Med* 12: 185–88, 1984.
69. Tropp J, Ekstrand J, Gillquist J. Stabilometry in functional instability of the ankle and its value in predicting injury. *Med Sci Sports Exerc* 16: 64–66, 1984.
70. Trulock S. A comparison of static, dynamic, and functional methods of objective balance assessment. Unpublished master's thesis, University of North Carolina at Chapel Hill, Chapel Hill, NC, 1996.
71. Vander A, Sherman J, Luciano D. *Human Physiology: The Mechanisms of Body Function* (5th ed.). New York: McGraw-Hill, 1990.
72. Wilkerson G, Nitz J. Dynamic ankle stability: Mechanical and neuromuscular interrelationships. *J Sports Rehab* 3: 43–57, 1994.
73. Yang J, Stein R, James K. Contribution of peripheral afferents to the activation of the soleus muscle during walking in humans. *Exp Brain Res* 87: 679–87, 1991.
74. Zimny M. Mechanoreceptors in articular tissues. *Am J Anat* 182: 16–32, 1988.

CHAPTER 5

Motor Learning, Motor Control, and Knee Injuries

William E. Garrett Jr., MD, PhD
Donald T. Kirkendall, PhD

Introduction

The concept of motor control actually encompasses two issues. The first is the control of the body with respect to stability (posture and balance). The second deals with movement of the body through space. To more completely understand motor control we need to understand the intimate relationship of action (control of musculoskeletal movements), perception (information about the interaction of the body in the environment), and cognition (e.g., attention, motivation, emotion). We realize that it is impossible to separate the individual from the task and the environment. These theoretical constructs will guide us in developing a paradigm for interpreting behavior, guide us in how we approach rehabilitation in the clinic, serve as a foundation for new ideas, and help us develop hypotheses directed at treatment.

Motor Control Theories

Before we discuss the most current theory, we describe briefly four examples of the many theories of motor control. These examples illustrate the complexities of the central nervous system and the difficulty of explaining a function about which we may *know* a great deal but, in reality, *understand* very little.

Reflex Theory

Sir Charles Sherrington (14) felt that reflexes served as the building blocks of more complex behaviors. A coordinated series of reflexes lead to the achievement of a common purpose. Reflexes were *chained together* to form complex behaviors. Limitations of reflex theory include the requirement of a sensory stimulus, the inability to explain rapid movements (movements that occur too fast for sensory input to trigger successive movements), and the fact that a single stimulus can result in many responses (16).

Hierarchical Theory

The brain is generally thought of as a "top down" organ, a divergent series of neural circuits originating from a higher center (5). Since the early 1920s, this notion has been modified to recognize that each neuronal level can impact on the others. Earlier work on the hierarchical model ignored the importance of reflexes in motor activity (e.g., the crossed extensor reflex—a lower motoneuron-dominated reflex). Reflexes are also considered as important modifiers of movement, not the sole determinants of motor behavior.

Motor Programming Theories

The more current theories of motor control view the central nervous system as a system that controls actions, not as a reactive system. In a reflex, if the motor pattern is separated from the stimulus a central motor pattern is described. This *motor program* (or central pattern generator) can be modified, not driven, by a stimulus, as we observe in the decerebrate cat, which can change its gait in the absence of inputs or descending patterns. Experiments like that on the cat identify a central pattern generator, a specific circuit to generate walking (7). This concept should not replace the idea of the importance of sensory input in controlling movement (6). Rather, the concept expands our understanding of the complexity of movement, especially when isolated from feedback (2).

Systems Theory

Perhaps movement should not be considered in terms of individual joints and limbs and instead should be considered as a major aspect of a whole system. Nicolai Bernstein (2) viewed the body as a whole—a mechanical system subject to internal and external forces. The same central command might lead to different movements (and different commands may result in similar movements) based on internal and external forces. Eventually, movement control was the result of many interacting systems. Bernstein reasoned that the higher levels in the nervous system simplified (minimized redundancies) control of movement.

Parallel Distributed Processing Theory

This theory is consistent with the current understanding of the central nervous system; the CNS processes information through both single (serial) pathways and parallel pathways (12). A "program" of planned activities is compared against the actual activity. If the two do not match, error has occurred. This error is used to change the activity to most closely approximate the original program. Such a concept can be used to predict how an injury will affect motor function. This theory also allows for redundant pathways to be used in the event that a major pathway is no longer functioning. Muscle reeducation is an example of this theory in practice.

The Forms of Learning

Following an injury, the rehabilitation process requires the reacquisition of extraordinarily complex tasks. One must be familiar with the basic process of learning to understand such complexities of learning skilled tasks.

Nonassociative Learning

Delivery of a repetitive stimulus results in nonassociative learning, leading the CNS to learn about the nature of the stimulus (9). If a person is exposed to a repetitive stimulus that gradually increases in intensity, which leads to a decrease in sensitivity to the stimulus, we say the person is habituated. Conversely, if stimulus intensity decreases, but the person is more responsive, then sensitization has occurred.

Associative Learning

When a patient with difficulty walking is instructed to shift his center of gravity by lifting his leg, he is associating two distinct movements into a single integrated movement (4). This style of learning helps one predict an outcome based on a single stimulus (classical conditioning) or associate the appropriate response (out of many) with a particular consequence (operant conditioning).

Classical conditioning can be demonstrated in the clinic by giving a visual cue to a patient before she makes some movement. With time, the patient may make the movement in response to the visual cue. The following statement best describes operant conditioning: rewarded behaviors are most likely to be repeated and nonrewarded behaviors are not repeated (4, 15).

Associative learning is sometimes classified by the type of acquired knowledge. Procedural learning refers to learned responses that are performed without conscious thought. Declarative learning is seen in gymnasts who mentally rehearse their routines just prior to performance (4, 15). In his mind, the gymnast is declaring, "I will do this, then this, then . . . ." Such types of declarative rehearsal have application in the clinic as patients attempt to relearn movements that have been altered due to injury.

Skilled Learning Theories

Four prominent theories of motor learning give us ideas about the nature of the acquisition of skills and the modification of learned pathways.

Closed-Loop Theory

This concept assumes that sensory feedback is used in the production and modification of movement (1). Feedback about the actual movement is compared with some stored pattern that was developed through practice. After some pattern stored in memory was activated, the sensory feedback would then modify movements as needed. A major limitation of this theory is that animals and humans can make and modify movements in the absence of sensory input (8).

Schema Theory

This theory emphasized open-loop control. Accordingly, specific movements are not stored. Rather, general patterns are stored and practice teaches one which general patterns are most effective (13). A schema is a psychological concept that suggests that we form an abstract concept in our minds. After multiple repetitions, we associate what we see or do with the abstract concept. For any movement, four things are stored: the initial movement conditions, parameters of the general motor pattern, movement outcome, and the consequences of the movement. For example, to learn to do a new movement, many repetitions are necessary. Inappropriate patterns are no longer called and the remaining rules of movement allow for the new pattern to be executed with a minimum of error.

Stages of Motor Learning

Three main stages of motor learning have been proposed (4). In the cognitive stage, the initial understanding of the task takes place. Strategies are devised and accepted or dropped during this phase where improvements are very rapid. The associative stage is for the refinement of the skill. Improvements are slow as variability in performance decreases. The autonomous stage is when the skill has become fairly automatic.

Learning as Exploration

The fundamental construct of this theory is the coordination between what was planned and what actually occurred within the constraints of the environment (10). During practice for an activity, performance is constrained by the environment. For example, learning to pick up a glass requires a planned motor pathway and sensory feedback about the environment—the weight of the glass, its texture, and how slippery it is are all environmental influences that must be accommodated.

There are many other factors about motor learning that have been explored: massed vs. distributed practice, whole vs. part training, transfer, guidance, and mental practice. These factors, among others, are beyond the scope of this discussion.

The Importance of the Motor Program

In our consideration of motor learning as applied to injury and rehabilitation, we must keep in mind the differences between an open-loop and a closed-loop system. The less flexible open-loop system has two components: the command and the effector components. This is not very flexible because changing situations can inappropriately modify the sequence of events. Closed-loop systems accept feedback and modify actions based on the feedback. This is flexible, but, as we shall see, problems can arise.

The delay in responding to an unanticipated stimulus is termed reaction time, which can range from 0.15 s (to kinesthetic stimuli) to 0.30 s (to visual and auditory stimuli). A human is sometimes considered to be a "single channel" organism. Let's say that the reaction time to a stimulus is 0.20 s. If there is a pause before a second stimulus, the reaction time will still be 0.20 s. If the second stimulus arrives during the reaction time for the first stimulus, however, the reaction time to the second stimulus is delayed (5). This suggests that we cannot process two overlapping stimuli at the same rate as we process the second stimulus after the completion of the reaction time to the first stimulus. This suggests that there is a reaction time delay, beyond the normal reaction time, to a second stimulus. This concept is critical when considering injuries that occur in reaction to an environmental stimulus.

A further consideration, especially when discussing athletes, is the time needed to alter movement. Many sporting activities include a reaction to the activities of an opponent. If the request to change a motor activity comes during the reaction time to the first stimulus, the pattern can be changed. However, if the second stimulus came after the reaction time was just completed, the activity would be carried out.

There are three elements to this discussion of reaction time (15). First, it takes 1 unit of reaction time for the athlete to process information presented while a movement is already in progress. Second, if the stimulus requires the athlete to change her movement, another unit of reaction time is necessary to begin to change the movement. Finally, the initial 0.20 to 0.30 s of any movement are preprogrammed and any change from the originally intended movement can't begin until the movement has been underway for about 0.30 to 0.50 s. And this is in an ideal setting. Given a sport setting such as skiing, ligament damage has been estimated to occur 79 ms after loading, and the muscle doesn't begin to contract until 213 ms after loading (11). This indicates that the ligament is already damaged before the body can respond to the load and compensate.

Anticipation can reduce some of these delays. For example, the batter needs to know how long it takes to swing the bat (from many practice sessions) so the time to initiate a swing is not solely in response to seeing the ball (called effector anticipation). The batter also needs to preview, or predict, where and when the ball will cross the plate so that initiation of the swing can begin at the correct time. This would all be delayed by at least one unit of reaction time (and when a pitch is only visible for 0.60 s, every unit of reaction time is precious) if the swing were purely in response to seeing the ball. In fact, the best performers in sports are ones who can anticipate what their opponents will do as well as disguising their movements to deprive their opponents of valuable clues, thus lengthening the opponents' reaction time.

The Motor Program

The length of reaction times indicates that motor activities can not be undertaken solely in response to environmental stimuli. Thus, we see the concept of the motor program, a stored set of muscle commands. Although research has not conclusively proven the existence of a "motor program," how could a person begin and stop a movement on a specified target in 0.10 s if a preprogrammed set of instructions had not been activated? If visual or kinesthetic information was needed to stop the movement, then the issuance of the command to stop the movement would have to have begun before the movement began. A motor program would have within it the commands to start, carry out, and stop the motion. In some movement patterns, this would argue against the closed-loop command discussed earlier.

Consider an activity that takes 0.60 s to complete. The activity might be underway for 0.30 s before the athlete must modify the movement. The new reaction time of about 0.20 s plus the first part of the movement means that at best the alteration would not occur for 0.50 s. Because the duration of sporting activities such as hitting and kicking is less than 0.50 s, the role of motor programs becomes more important in skill performance. Moving from a sensory based closed-loop system toward the open-loop system is the reason for practice. Given a new task (e.g., juggling), the subject will use sensory (e.g., visual) feedback to control the balls. With successful practice, a motor program will be developed for a more efficient motor pattern. In one sense, the motor program uses only those motor units appropriate for the movement by ruling out unnecessary pathways.

If we were to look at an athletic maneuver like cutting, we see further evidence that motor programs must be evident. An athlete runs and then, from some environmental influence (often an opponent), changes direction rapidly. Prior to planting the cutting foot, a series of events has already taken place that will influence the success of the cut. Immediately prior to ground impact of the plant foot, we see that the leg is flexed (an attempt to protect internal ligaments?) and the quadriceps muscle is also activated. At impact, the activation of the quadriceps increases in response to the eccentric load on the muscle. This activation at impact and during the milliseconds following is quite high, often larger than we would normally see during a maximal voluntary contraction. We have seen activation levels as high as 250% of NWC when the quadriceps contracts during the cutting motion. Such high activation levels suggest that there are incredibly high forces acting on the knee just from the contraction of the quadriceps.

This action, from heel strike to maximum quadriceps contraction takes only 0.12 s (unpublished observations). What would happen if, during the cut, the player was only slightly bumped immediately prior to heel strike. Based on the discussions above, the motor program for that step of the cut would be put into place, but any chance for a correction of the movement would likely begin well after heel strike. So the player initiated a pattern of muscle action, and he would be unable to change this pattern until after a ligament was torn.

Two more examples might be warranted. What about the player who plans to step on level ground but ends up stepping into a small hole in the grass? A pattern of events has begun, but the surface is not level, which means the program is no longer appropriate. When she steps into the hole, her proprioceptive response will likely be inappropriate—the response could well be a reactive contraction by the quadriceps causing excess tibial shear forces that tear the anterior cruciate ligament. Consider the volleyball player who goes up to hit a quick set at the net. She jumps and begins a series of preprogrammed events to perform the skill. If the set is a little high and behind, however, a midair correction must be made, which means the player will be landing differently than she had planned. Upon heel strike, the preplanned program can begin and the quadriceps could be performing normally. But with the knee and leg in an unfavorable position, tibial shear can result in tearing the ACL.

Now that the ligament has been injured, what might be some considerations with rehabilitation? Following such an injury, patients are known to be "weak." Hidden in this statement is the understanding that the muscle is not responding to central nervous system drive. We have asked postsurgical ACL patients to perform some muscular voluntary contractions (MVCs) periodically after surgery. As expected, the torque production by the surgical leg was below that of the nonsurgical leg. Of interest was the integrated EMG. If the IEMG of the surgical leg is indexed to that of the nonsurgical leg, the resulting ratio is very similar to a similar index of torque. This occurred across the range of MVC (25%, 50%, 75%, 100%) collected. This interesting finding suggests that the muscle is not responding adequately to the drive from the nervous system (unpublished observations). Whether this is due to some inhibition or through reduced central recruitment is unknown from this model.

What we are left with is the idea that the motor program is likely to be a real factor in athletic performance as well as a contributor to injury. Understanding the interaction of closed- and open-loop programs helps us in our understanding of performance and injury. In the future, such theories may better point us toward many mechanisms of injury that will suggest what measures must be taken to improve the safety of all sports.

References

1. Adams JA. A closed-loop theory of motor learning. *J Motor Behavior* 3: 111–50, 1971.
2. Bernstein N. *The coordination and regulation of movement.* London: Pergamon Press, 1967.
3. Dandel E, JH Schwartz, TM Jessel. *Principles of neuroscience,* 3d ed., 420–39. New York: Elsevier Science, 1991.
4. Fitts PM, MI Posner. *Human performance.* Pacific Grove, CA: Brooks/Cole, 1967.
5. Foerster O. The motor cortex in man in the light of Hughlings Jackson's doctrines. In *Scientific bases for neurophysiologic approaches to therapeutic exercise,* Payton OD, et al. (eds.), 13–18. Philadelphia: FA Davis, 1977.
6. Forssberg H, S Grillner, S Rossignol. Phase dependent reflex reversal during walking in chronic spinal cats. *Brain Res* 85: 103–107, 1975.
7. Grillner S. Control of locomotion in bipeds, tetrapods, and fish. In *Handbook of physiology,* vol. 2, Geiger SR (ed.), 1179–236. Bethesda, MD: American Physiological Society, 1981.
8. Ivry R. Representative issues in motor learning: Phenomena and theory. In *Handbook of perceptions and action: Motor skills,* Keel S (ed.). New York: Academic Press (referenced in Shumway-Cook and Woollacott, cited below).
9. Kupfermann I. Learning and memory. In *Principles of neuroscience,* 3d ed., Kandel ER, et al. (eds.), 997–1008. New York: Elsevier Science, 1991.
10. Newell KM. Motor skill acquisition. *Ann Rev Psychol* 42: 213–37, 1991.
11. Pope MH, RJ Johnson, DW Brown, C Tighe. The role of the musculature in injuries to the medial collateral ligament. *J Bone Joint Surg.* 61A: 398–402, 1979.
12. Rumelhart DE, JL McCelland. *Parallel distributed processing: Explorations in the microstructure of cognition,* vol. 1: *Foundations.* Cambridge, MA: MIT Press, 1986.
13. Schmidt RA. A schema theory of discrete motor skill learning. *Psychol Rev* 82: 225–60, 1975.
14. Sherrington, C. *The integrative action of the nervous system,* 2d ed. New Haven, CT: Yale University Press, 1947.
15. Shumway-Cook A, M Woollacott. *Motor control: Theory and practical applications.* Media, PA: Williams & Wilkins, 1995.
16. Taub E, AJ Berman. Movement and learning in the absence of sensory feedback. In *The neurophysiology of spatially oriented behavior,* Freedman SJ (ed.), 173–92. Belmont, CA: Dorsey Press, 1968.

CHAPTER 6

Functional Anatomy of the Knee: Bony Geometry, Static and Dynamic Restraints, Sensory and Motor Innervation

Scott F. Dye, MD
Geoffrey L. Vaupel, MD

Introduction

The human knee is one of the most complex systems in the biological realm. Composed of hundreds of billions of living cells, the knee acts as a type of biological transmission, whose purpose is to accept, transfer, and dissipate often high loads among the femur, tibia, patella, and fibula and still maintain tissue homeostasis over decades of use. (17, 20) The multiple asymmetric components of this joint, including a bicondylar femur, cruciate ligaments, and menisci, are extremely ancient in origin, with most having developed by 320 million years ago, soon after evolution of the earliest land vertebrates with limbs. (15) The ligaments can be conceptualized as sensate adaptive linkages within the biological transmission, with the menisci functioning as mobile sensate bearings. The muscles function in concentric contraction as cellular engines providing motive forces across the joint, and in eccentric contraction, they act as brakes and dampening systems, absorbing shock loads. The functional kinematics of the knee closely resembles a four-bar linkage mechanism, as described by Menschik and by Müller, with the point of femoral tibial contact moving posteriorly from extension to flexion (see figure 6.1, *a* and *b*). (47) Normal function of the living knee would be impossible without the complex neurological components providing sensory innervation, including proprioception, as well as active muscle control. This chapter provides an overview of the functions of the various anatomic components that comprise the knee (64) and a summary of its functional intraarticular sensory characteristics.

Femorotibial Joint

The knee is the articulation between the femur, tibia, and patella. This complex joint includes menisci and ligaments in a joint capsule. We discuss first the articulation between femur and tibia.

Osseous Anatomy

The medial knee compartment is more constrained and is therefore less tolerant of increases in femoral tibial translation and rotation than the lateral compartment, because of osseous, meniscal, and ligamentous morphology. This may explain the greater prevalence of medial meniscal injuries, as compared to the lateral meniscus. The medial femoral condyle is smaller in anterior-posterior diameter than the lateral femoral condyle, and the lateral condyle is broader in the transverse plane. The width of the medial femoral condyle is nearly constant, but the

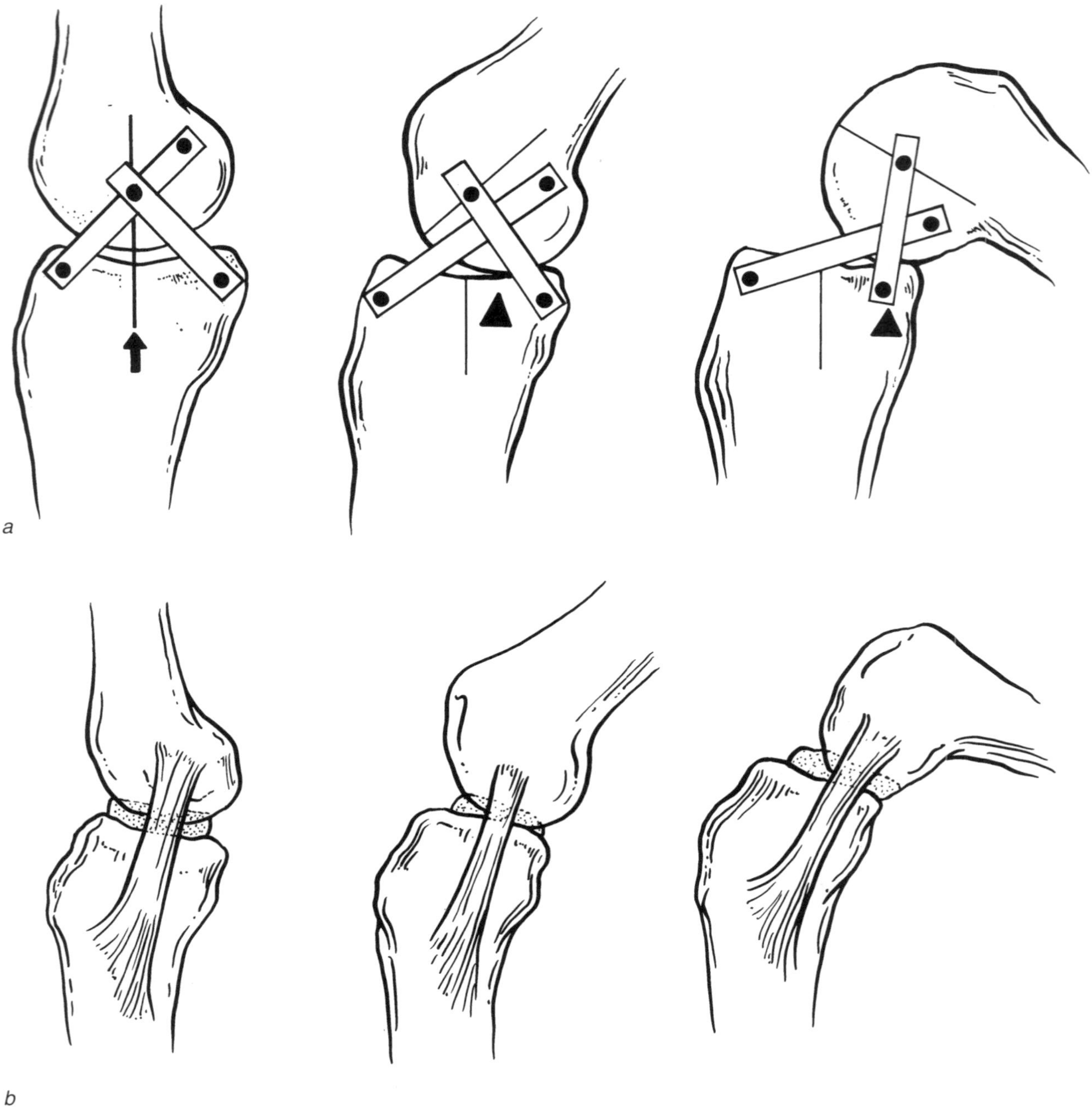

Figure 6.1 Functional kinematics of the human knee in sagittal projection showing the point of femoral tibial contact moving posteriorly in flexion. *(a)* Schematic of the four-bar linkage model. *(b)* Roll back of the femoral tibial contact point along with the medial meniscus. (Reprinted with permission from Dye SF: An evolutionary perspective of the knee. *J Bone Joint Surg* 7:976-983, 1987.)

lateral condyle is narrower on its posterior surface; the wider portion is in contact with the tibia during knee extension (see figure 6.2, *a-c*).

The medial tibial plateau is concave and, combined with the deepening of the medial meniscus, provides a more constrained articulation for the medial femoral condyle. The lateral tibial plateau is slightly convex, which appears to be incongruous with the shape of the femoral condyle, but this convex surface allows greater "rollback" of the lateral femoral condyle with flexion. (18) Both the convexity of the lateral tibial plateau and the larger surface area of the lateral femoral condyle contribute to the screw-home mechanism, that is, the internal rotation of the femur relative to a static tibia in terminal extension. In flexion this greater lateral compartment rollback, allowed by the posterior sloping lateral tibial plateau, results in functional

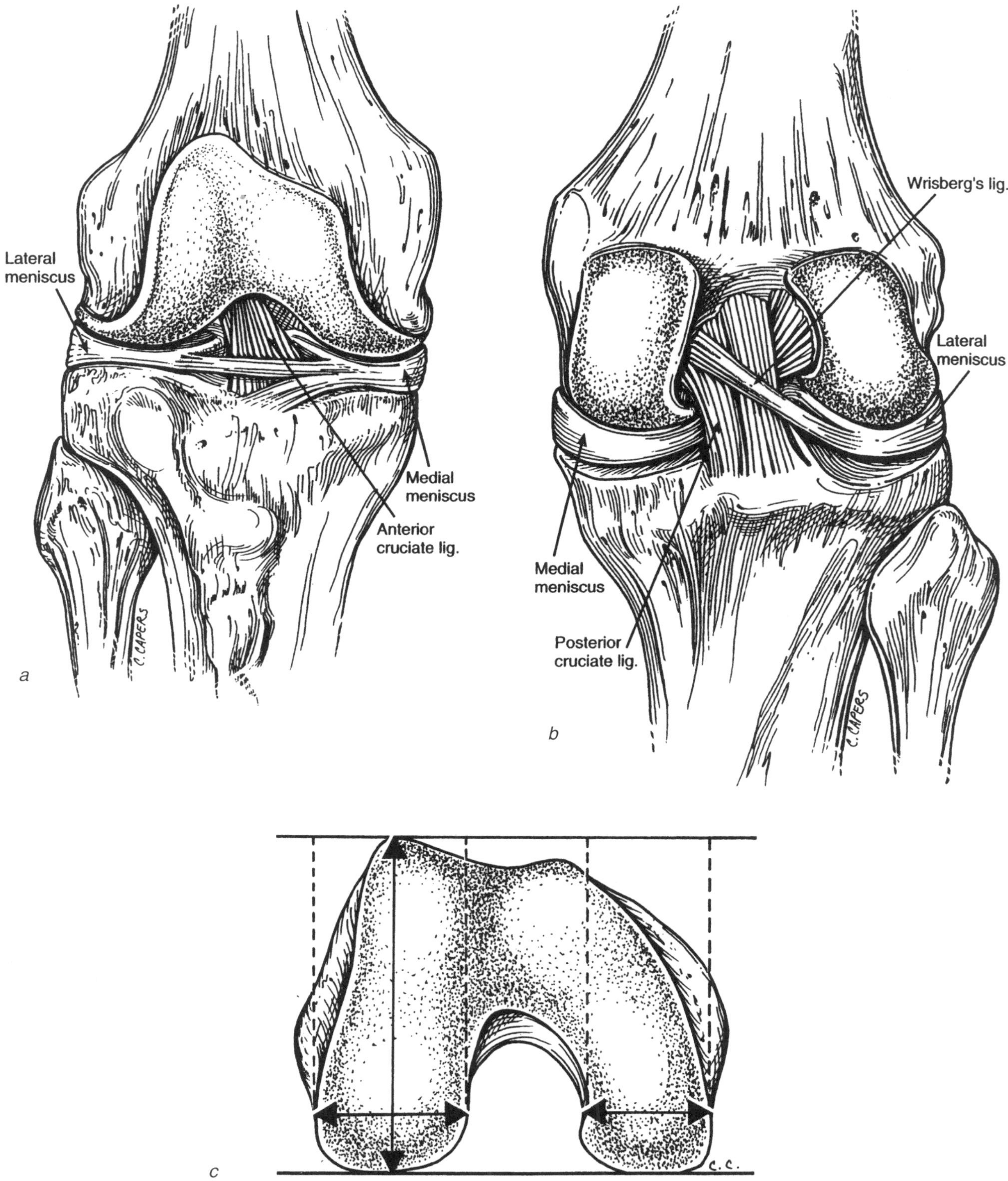

Figure 6.2 *(a)* Anterior view of the knee and *(b)* posterior view of the knee, showing osseous morphology, the menisci, and the orientation of the cruciate ligaments. *(c)* A comparison of the medial and lateral femoral condyles shows that the lateral condyle is broader in the transverse plane. (Reprinted with permission from Dye SF: An evolutionary perspective of the knee. *J Bone Joint Surg* 7:976-983, 1987.)

internal rotation of the tibia (and the attached foot) relative to a static femur.

The tibial surface slopes posteriorly about 10°. (33) Since the knee is flexed during running and cutting, this angulation brings the tibial plateau almost parallel with the weight-bearing surface. Without this natural posterior slope, the plateau would slope anteriorly in functional positions, which could compromise functional stability.

Menisci

The menisci are fibrocartilaginous wedges that lie between the femoral condyles and the tibial plateaus (see figure 6.3). The medial meniscus has been described as being more C-shaped than the nearly circular lateral meniscus. The lateral meniscus covers a larger surface area of the tibial plateau (approximately two-thirds) than the medial meniscus. The concave superior surface of each meniscus conforms to the shape of the femoral condyles, whereas the inferior surface is flat as it sits on the tibial plateau. The periphery of each meniscus is convex and thicker than the concave, thin inner margin. The menisci are divided into thirds for descriptive purposes: the anterior horn, the body, and the posterior horn. The posterior horn is usually thicker than the body and anterior horn. The anterior horn of each meniscus is connected to the other by the intermeniscal or transverse ligament.

The medial meniscus has a continuous and less mobile peripheral attachment than the lateral meniscus. There is an interruption in the peripheral attachment and blood supply (3) of the lateral meniscus where the popliteus tendon passes through a hiatus in the posterolateral aspect. The posterior horn of the lateral meniscus has attachments to the posterior cruciate ligament and medial femoral condyle through the ligaments of Wrisberg and Humphry. (8)

Both menisci passively follow the femur posteriorly with knee flexion. The lateral meniscus travels approximately twice as far posteriorly as the medial one (11 mm versus 5 mm, respectively) as documented by cine MRI. (62) The increased motion of the lateral meniscus necessitates a more compliant meniscotibial ligament attachment. The more adherent medial meniscus attachments predispose this structure to a greater incidence of tears, especially of the posterior horn. The contribution of the popliteus and the semimembranosus to active retraction, respectively, of the lateral and medial meniscus is unknown.

Many functions have been attributed to the menisci, including load transmission bearings, (17) shock absorbers, stress reducers, joint stabilizers limiting extremes of flexion and extension, and joint lubricators providing nourishment to articular cartilage. (55) The menisci also deepen the tibial plateaus, making the femoral articulation comparable to a shallow ball-and-socket arrangement. (32)

Intercondylar Region

The intercondylar region consists of the femoral intercondylar notch, the tibial intercondylar eminence or spine, both cruciate ligaments, and the anterior and posterior horn attachments of the menisci. This area, situated at the center of axial rotation in the

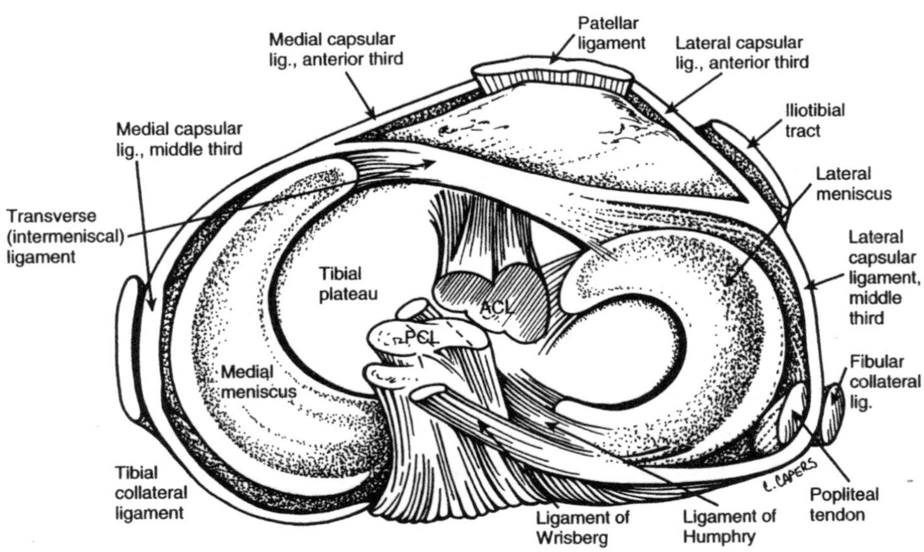

Figure 6.3 An overhead view of the menisci shows the ligamentous attachment by the transverse ligament and the ligaments of Humphry and Wrisberg. (Reprinted with permission from Vaupel GL, Dye SF: Anatomy of the knee. *The Hughston Clinic Sports Medicine Book*, ed. by C. Baker, Jr., Williams, and Wilkins, 1995, pp. 403-415.)

knee, is termed the *central pivot*. (47) The intercondylar eminence functions as the base of the central pivot. It helps guide and stabilize the femur through the flexion arc. This is accomplished in two ways: (1) the anterior and posterior horns of the menisci are anchored at the tibial eminence and thus serve as checkreins to rotation and translation of the femur, (2) the intercondylar articular surface of the femur articulates with the tibial eminence, sharing the compressive weight-bearing forces with the menisci and tibial plateau. Thus, the tibial eminence guides the femur, much as a monorail guides a train. This is especially significant in the middle range of flexion, when axial loads are great and the peripheral ligaments relatively lax. It also explains the typical position of osteochondritis dissecans on the lateral weight-bearing margin of the medial femoral condyle, which may be thought of more accurately as an osteochondral fracture rather than a pure vascular event.

Posterior Cruciate Ligament

Most authors feel the posterior cruciate ligament acts as the primary ligamentous contribution to the central pivot. (1, 33, 40, 47) Evidence to support this lies in its greater thickness (25) and strength as compared to the anterior cruciate ligament. (41) Furthermore, its position most closely approximates the axis of knee rotation. (65)

The posterior cruciate ligament is divided into the posteromedial and anterolateral bundles relative to the site of the femoral attachment (see figure 6.4, *a* and *b*.) Only the posteromedial fibers are taut in knee extension. During knee flexion, the anterolateral fibers become progressively tensed. At full knee flexion all fibers become equally taut. The posterior cruciate ligament assumes a nearly vertical orientation in full flexion and is more horizontal with knee extension. With full flexion, the posterior cruciate ligament is in contact with the roof of the posterior intercondylar notch. (51)

The tibial attachment of the posterior cruciate ligament is in the tibial fovea, just anterior to the posterior tibial condyles and extending 1 to 2 cm distal to the joint line. The femoral attachment, however, extends well anterior and ends just posterior to the articular surface of the intercondylar surface of the medial femoral condyle. The "tibial footprint" is almost square, whereas the femur is more oblong and rectangular because the posterior cruciate ligament fans out as it approaches the femur.

Simple point-to-point kinematics cannot explain the function of either the posterior or the anterior cruciate ligament. These structures must be thought of as a continuum of thousands of collagen fibers acting in concert through the flexion arc. Thinking in these terms, one can understand the frustration in trying to interpret isometric measurements.

Two meniscofemoral ligaments commonly are associated with the posterior cruciate ligament: the ligament of Humphry anteriorly and the ligament of Wrisberg posteriorly (see figure 6.3). They vary in size and are sometimes absent entirely. One or another of the two meniscofemoral ligaments is found in nearly every knee, but rarely are both found in the same knee, and even more rarely are both ligaments found in both knees. (63) The ligament of Wrisberg may be as large as half the diameter of the posterior cruciate ligament, whereas the ligament of Humphry is no larger than one-third the diameter of the posterior cruciate ligament. (29)

The ligament of Wrisberg is variably attached to the posterior lateral meniscus, the tibia, or the posterior capsule. It then runs proximally and obliquely across the posterior aspect of the posterior cruciate ligament and attaches to the medial femoral condyle at the posterior cruciate ligament attachment.

The ligament of Humphry arises from the posterior horn of lateral meniscus, runs anterior to the posterior cruciate ligament, and attaches to the medial femoral condyle with the anterolateral bundle.

The ligament of Humphry is taut in flexion, and the ligament of Wrisberg is taut in extension. Both ligaments tighten with internal rotation of the tibia and can confound the posterior drawer test. Thus, the posterior drawer test must also be done with the tibia in neutral position and in external rotation. (10)

Anterior Cruciate Ligament

The anterior cruciate ligament, like the posterior cruciate ligament, is an intracapsular but usually extrasynovial structure. It is usually covered by a synovial sheath, which protects it from the synovial fluid. The anterior cruciate ligament, like the posterior cruciate ligament, has been divided into bundles, but, instead of two bundles defined by femoral attachments, the anterior cruciate ligament has three bundles defined by the tibial attachments. (48) In many knees these bundles are difficult to discern on gross inspection. The purpose in describing them is to help readers conceptualize the different behavior displayed by the anterior and posterior fibers throughout the flexion arc.

In terminal knee extension all fibers of the anterior cruciate ligament are taut. The anterior fibers abut the intercondylar roof, though with progressive knee flexion the posterior fibers loosen and the

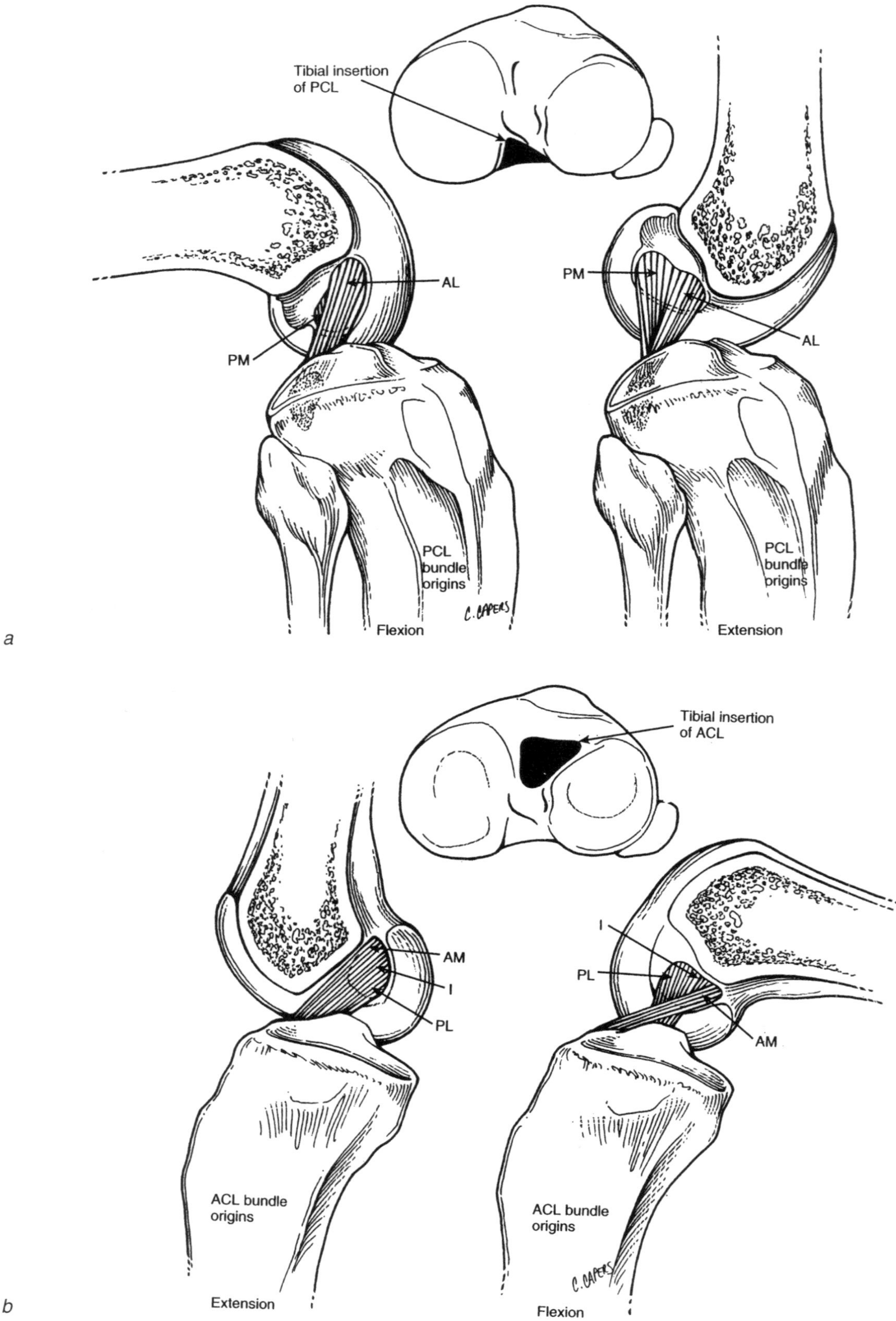

Figure 6.4 *(a)* Attachment sites of the posterior medial (PM) and anterior lateral (AL) bundles of the posterior cruciate ligament (PCL). During knee flexion the anterior lateral fibers are progressively tensed. *(b)* The anterior cruciate ligament is divided into three bundles based on the tibial attachment: the anterior medial (AM), the intermediate (I), and the posterior lateral (PL). With knee flexion the posterior fibers loosen and the anterior medial fibers coil around the posterior lateral fibers. (Reprinted with permission from Vaupel GL, Dye SF: Anatomy of the knee. *The Hughston Clinic Sports Medicine Book*, ed. by C. Baker, Jr., Williams, and Wilkins, 1995, pp. 403-415.)

anteromedial fibers coil around the posterolateral fibers. The anterior fibers remain taut throughout the flexion arc and are the most isometric. Therefore, the anterior edge of the anterior cruciate ligament serves as the rotational axis of the ligament during knee motion. (51) The anterior cruciate ligament is the principal restraint to anterior tibial translation and is a secondary restraint to varus and valgus forces.

Patellofemoral Joint

The patella acts as a large slide bearing within the biological transmission of the knee. (17) It increases the force of the quadriceps pull by increasing the lever arm of the extensor mechanism. The thickness of the patella displaces the patellar tendon away from the femorotibial contact point. (2) The patella has three facets, medial, lateral, and odd. The medial and lateral facets are separated by a longitudinal ridge called the median ridge. The odd facet is smaller in area than the medial and lateral facets and lies at the extreme medial border of the patellar articular surface. The articular cartilage on the undersurface of the patella is the thickest of any of the human diarthrodial joints. It is thickest in cross section at its midportion and relatively thinner near the proximal and distal poles. (23)

The trochlea (L., pulley) is that portion of the anterior femur that articulates with the patella. Its two facets, medial and lateral, unite in the midline to form a groove. The median ridge of the patella rides in this groove, whereas the medial and lateral facets of the patella contact the corresponding trochlear facets. The lateral facet projects farther anterior and proximal than the medial facet, adding to patellar stability.

The area of contact between the patella and femur varies with the position of the knee (see figure 6.5). (37) With the knee in full extension the patella lies superior and lateral to the trochlea and rests in the supratrochlear pulvinar (L., a cushioned seat) or fat pad. (16) The distal patellar surface contacts the proximal trochlea in 20° of flexion. As the knee flexes the patella becomes centralized within the femoral trochlea and by 30° of flexion the patella sits farthest anterior, giving the extensor mechanism its greatest lever arm. By 45 to 60° of flexion the midportion of the patella articulates with the midportion of the trochlea. Further flexion creates maximum centralization of the patella at 80°, which

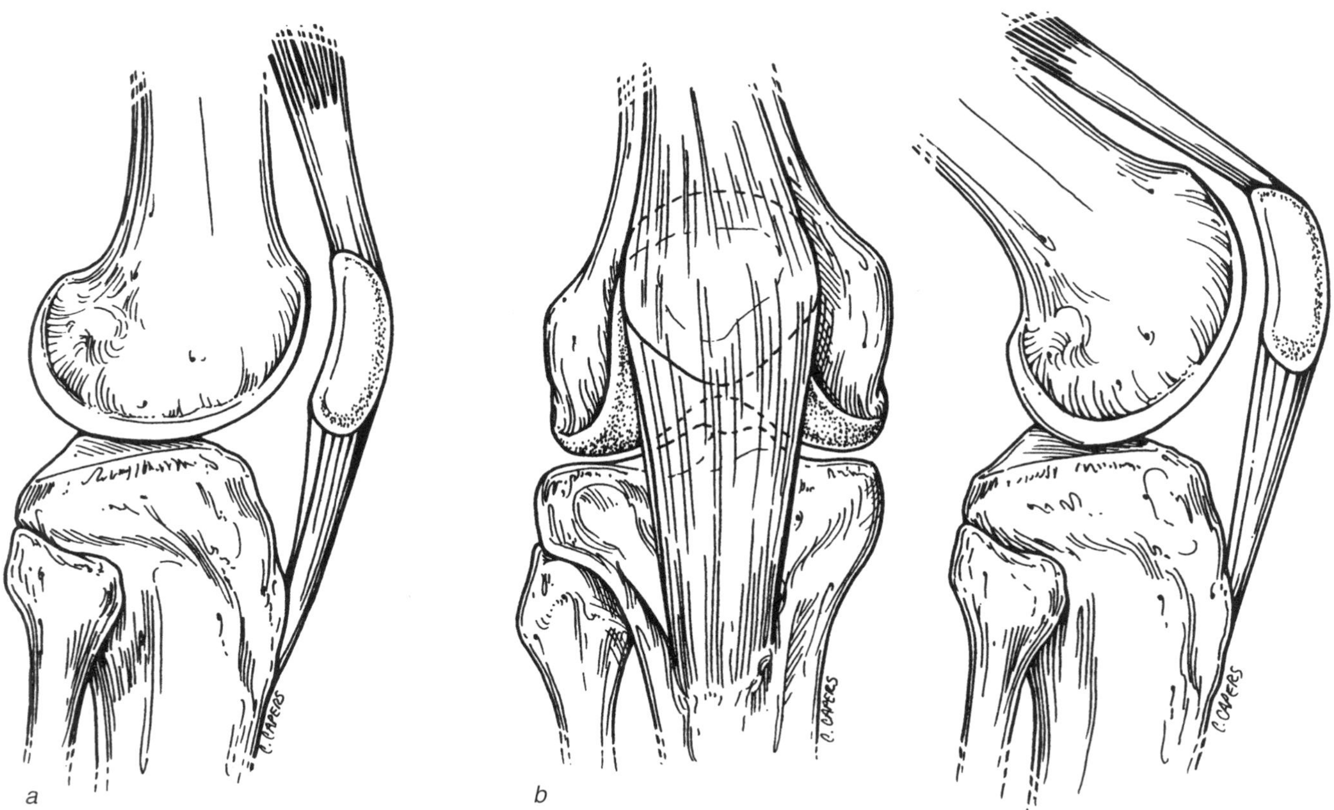

a b

Figure 6.5 *(a)* With the knee in extension the patella is superior and lateral to the trochlea. *(b)* At 30° of flexion the patella sits anteriorly, giving the extensor mechanism its greatest lever arm. (Reprinted with permission from Vaupel GL, Dye SF: Anatomy of the knee. *The Hughston Clinic Sports Medicine Book*, ed. by C. Baker, Jr., Williams, and Wilkins, 1995, pp. 403-415.)

is maintained throughout the remainder of flexion. At 90° of flexion the proximal patella contacts the distal trochlea, and at full flexion (at least 135°) only the supralateral patella and the odd facet articulate with the femur distal to the trochlea on the lateral femoral condyle and lateral surface of the medial femoral condyle. (23)

The Q angle is the angle between the quadriceps mechanism and the patellar tendon. It is measured with the knee in full extension and quadriceps contracted or with the patient seated and the knee in 90° of flexion. Normal values for these two measurements are 10° or less with the knee in extension and 0° with the knee in flexion. (35)

The screw-home mechanism has a profound influence on patellofemoral kinematics. As the knee extends the tibia rotates externally, causing an increase in the Q angle. This creates a lateral, or valgus, vector on the patella, which is resisted principally by the vastus medialis obliquus and the medial retinaculum. (23)

The infrapatellar fat pad rests in the cavity posterior to the patellar tendon and sends a frenulum, called the *infrapatellar plica* or *ligamentum mucosum* to the roof of the anterior intercondylar notch. The fat pad is well innervated (19) and well vascularized and may be an important nociceptive source for many patients' anterior knee pain. Injury to the fat pad may result in a hematoma with subsequent fibrosis, scar contracture, and possible development of patella baja. (32)

Knee Capsule

The knee capsule, which is also well innervated, (19) extends proximally from the femoral trochlea, on average 4 to 5 cm, and is termed the *suprapatellar pouch.* (23) This rather voluminous cavity is commonly interrupted by a transverse fibrous band called the *suprapatellar plica,* a vestigial rest that once divided the embryonic knee into two cavities. (69) The adult expression of this structure is variable, in that it may be a complete septum separating the knee joint cavity from the suprapatellar bursa or several variations of an incomplete septum. (12)

The superomedial portion of the suprapatellar plica blends with the medial patellar plica, which runs distally in the medial gutter and attaches to the infrapatellar fat pad. The medial patellar plica occasionally becomes inflamed when it is pinched between the medial facet of the patella and medial femoral condyle or when it snaps over that condyle. Because of the horseshoe shape of this interrelated complex, and the close association with the articularis genus muscle, it is felt that the plica constitutes a "synovial type of tendon aponeurosis of the articularis genus muscle" (see figure 6.6). (32)

Extraarticular Ligaments

Anterior

The patellar tendon is the terminal extension of the extensor mechanism. Some authors refer to this as the *patellar ligament,* since its fibers run from patella to tibia, as any ligament runs from bone to bone. However, tendinous fibers from the vastus medialis, vastus lateralis, and rectus femoris form an intermediate layer within the quadriceps tendon, which attaches to the superior pole of the patella. These fibers continue over the anterior patella and

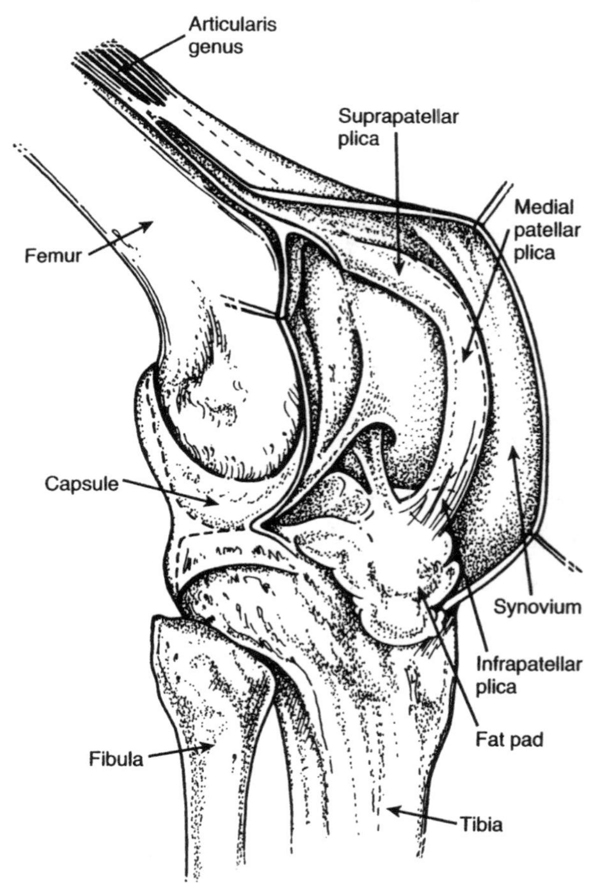

Figure 6.6 The plica is thought to act as a synovial-type tendon aponeurosis for the articularis genus muscle. (Reprinted with permission from Vaupel GL, Dye SF: Anatomy of the knee. *The Hughston Clinic Sports Medicine Book,* ed. by C. Baker, Jr., Williams, and Wilkins, 1995, pp. 403-415.)

then distally, as the patellar tendon, to the insertion at the tibial tuberosity. In this sense, the patellar tendon behaves as a direct extension of the quadriceps muscle group and its function is thus more consistent with a tendon.

The anterior capsule lies medial and lateral to the patellar tendon. This is a relatively weak tissue, except where its fibers form the medial and lateral patellofemoral and patellotibial ligaments. (61)

Medial

The medial collateral ligament (or as Hughston prefers, the tibial collateral ligament) (32) is a long, well-defined structure that lies superficial to the medial capsule and capsular ligaments. Its origin is the medial femoral epicondyle, and it inserts 6 to 9 cm distal to the joint line on the posterior half of the tibial metaphysis, deep to the pes anserinus tendons. The medial collateral ligament is the principal restraint to valgus force. (66)

Deep to the medial collateral ligament are the capsular or coronary ligaments, which have been divided into the anterior, middle, and posterior thirds (see figure 6.7, *a* and *b*). A small bursa separates the medial collateral ligament from the capsular ligaments. (7) The middle third medial capsular ligament is sometimes termed the *deep medial collateral ligament,* because it acts as a strong secondary restraint to valgus force. These capsular ligaments, both medially and laterally, are also referred to as *meniscofemoral* and *meniscotibial ligaments,* because they act as peripheral attachments for the menisci to the femur and tibia. They also

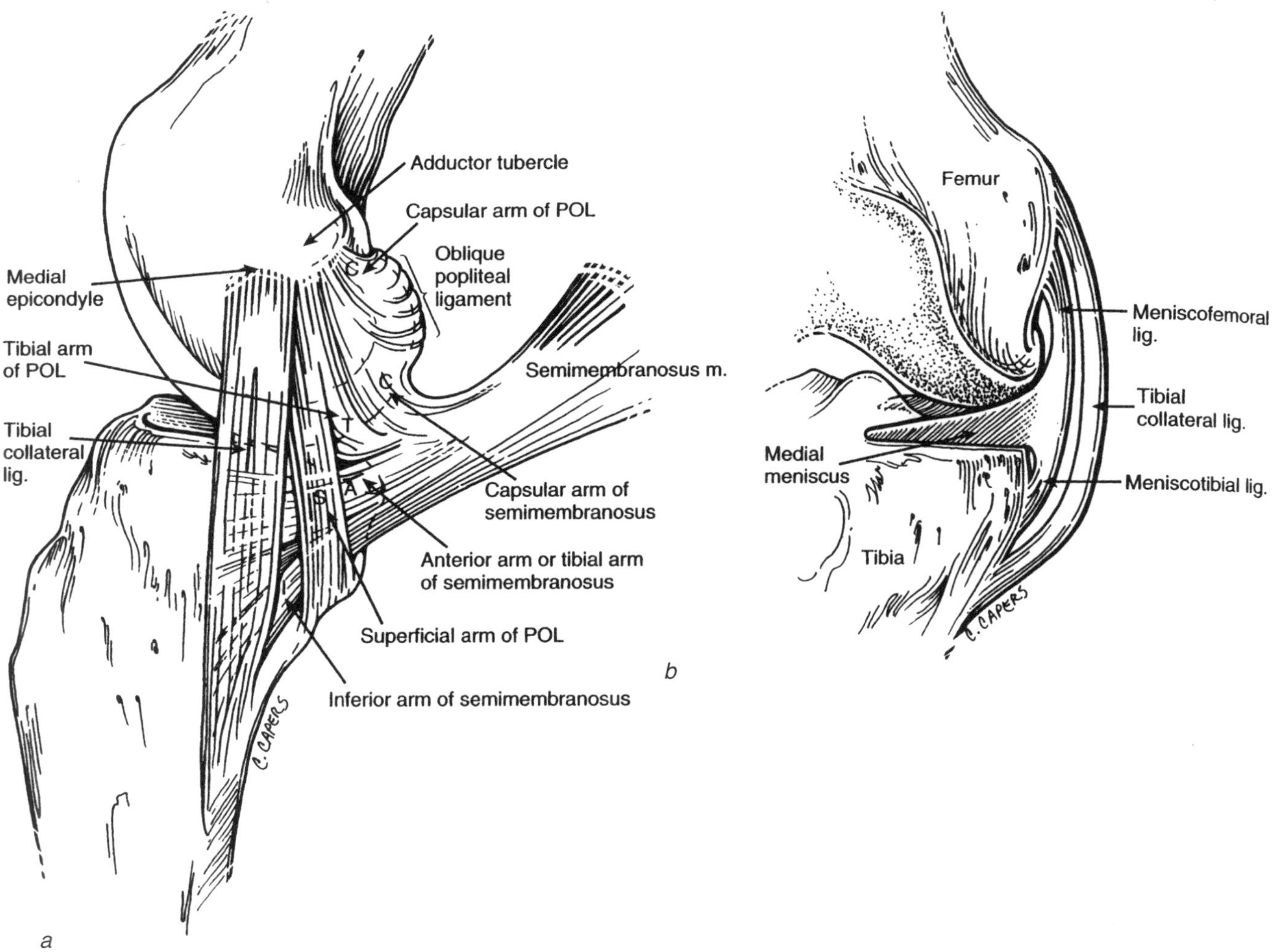

Figure 6.7 The medial ligaments of the knee: *(a)* medial view, *(b)* anterior posterior view. (Reprinted with permission from Vaupel GL, Dye SF: Anatomy of the knee. *The Hughston Clinic Sports Medicine Book,* ed. by C. Baker, Jr., Williams, and Wilkins, 1995, pp. 403-415.)

act as secondary restraints to valgus and varus forces. (49)

Directly posterior to the medial collateral ligament is the posterior oblique ligament (POL), which has its femoral attachment at the adductor tubercle. The POL has been described as having three arms, the superficial, tibial, and capsular arms. The POL contributes to dynamic stability of the knee in flexion through its capsular arm by confluence of its fibers with the semimembranosus. (34)

Lateral

The static structures of the lateral knee are lax in flexion. Only when the dynamic lateral muscle groups contract will these ligaments become taut in flexion. The iliotibial band (ITB) is the distal extension of the tensor fascia lata. The posterior half of the ITB is called the iliotibial tract. The ITB sends an attachment (the iliopatellar ligament) obliquely toward the patella. The ITB inserts at the anterior half of the lateral tibial tubercle, and the iliotibial tract inserts at the posterior half of the lateral tibial tubercle (see figure 6.8). (32) The ITB acts as a knee extensor in 0 to 30° of flexion and a flexor in 40 to 145° of flexion. (47) It also acts as a static stabilizer of the knee through its attachment to the intermuscular septum and the iliopatellar ligament. The iliopatellar ligament provides further stability by its condensation with the lateral patellotibial and patellofemoral ligaments.

The fibular collateral ligament has been described as a "cordlike" ligament attaching on the lateral epicondyle of the femur and distally on the tip of the

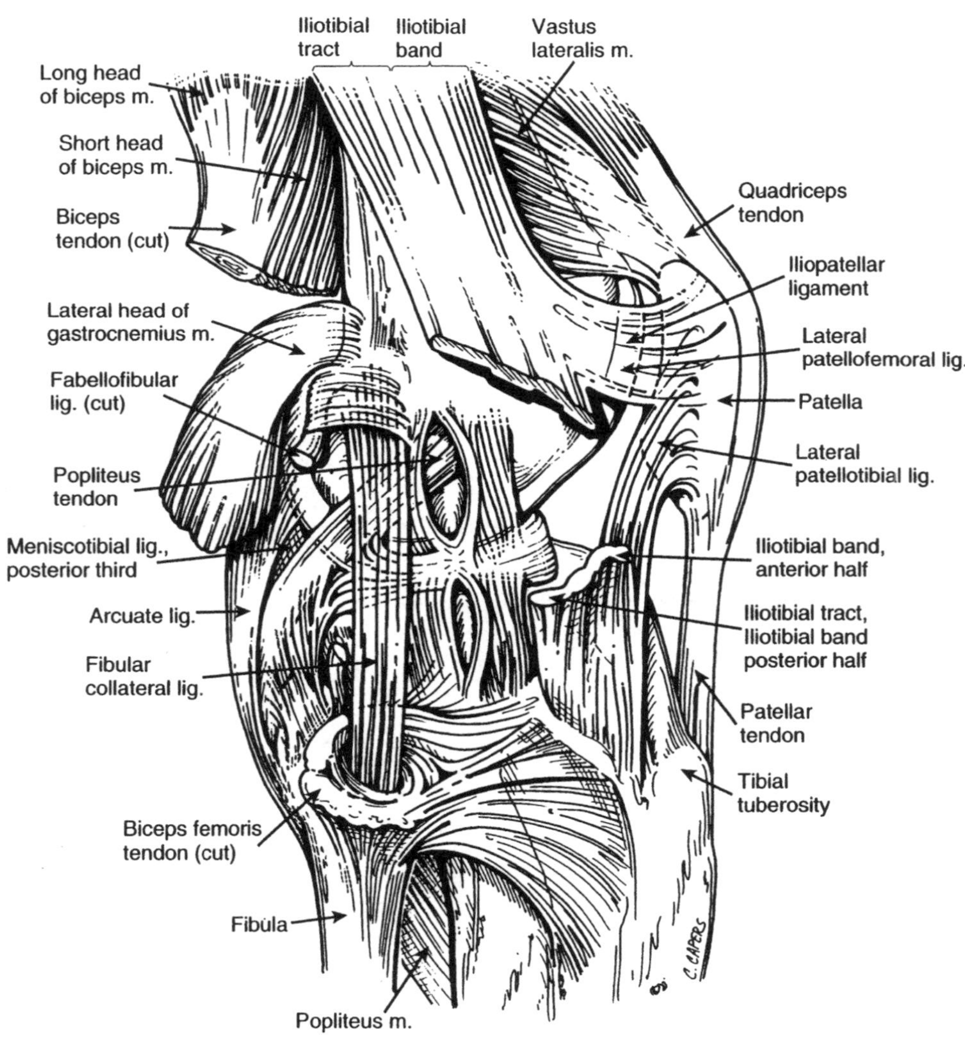

Figure 6.8 The lateral ligaments of the knee. (Reprinted with permission from Vaupel GL, Dye SF: Anatomy of the knee. *The Hughston Clinic Sports Medicine Book*, ed. by C. Baker, Jr., Williams, and Wilkins, 1995, pp. 403-415.)

fibular head. These descriptions have been proven misleading by dissection in vivo: fibers from the arcuate ligament and the fascia of the lateral head gastrocnemius envelop the fibular collateral ligament. Furthermore, distal expansions of the fibular collateral ligament envelop the fibular head, blending with the biceps femoris and sending fibers to the fascia overlying the anterior muscle compartment of the leg. Regardless, the fibular collateral ligament functions principally as a static restraint against varus force. (49)

Posterior

The arcuate ligament is a condensation of the posterolateral capsule that covers the posterolateral femoral condyle. Its proximal attachment is just beneath the origin of the lateral head of the gastrocnemius where its fibers are enmeshed with the gastrocnemius tendon. The distal expansion of the arcuate ligament becomes the posterior third of the meniscotibial ligament where it blends with the popliteus. This is the immediate area of attachment for the capsular arm of popliteus to the posterior horn lateral meniscus. The arcuate also sends an attachment to the posterior fibular head. The arcuate acts as a restraint to posterior and posterolateral forces.

The oblique popliteal ligament is an expansion of the semimembranosus, running from the semimembranosus insertion at the posteromedial tibia obliquely, proximally, and laterally toward the origin of the lateral head of the gastrocnemius on the posterolateral femur. The oblique popliteal ligament acts as a secondary restraint to posterior instability.

Muscle Anatomy

The quadriceps comprises four separate muscles: the rectus femoris, the vastus intermedius, the vastus lateralis, and the vastus medialis. These four muscles condense in the quadriceps tendon to a common attachment on the superior pole of the patella (see figure 6.9). The vastus lateralis and vastus medialis have oblique arms that insert into the patella as well. The angles of insertion in the sagittal plane vary between each of these arms: 15 to 18° for the vastus medialis, 50 to 55° for the vastus medialis obliquus, 12 to 15° for the vastus lateralis, and 38 to 48° for the vastus lateralis obliquus. (28, 61)

These muscles act in concert to extend the knee with concentric contraction. Eccentric contraction of the quadriceps acts as a decelerator and important shock absorber of the knee. (36) During knee extension and deceleration, a balance must be attained between these muscles in order to stabilize dynamically the patella. If there is an imbalance between the vastus lateralis and vastus medialis, the result is a tendency for subluxation of the patella to the "stronger" side. Of course, the static restraints also play an important role in stabilizing the patella.

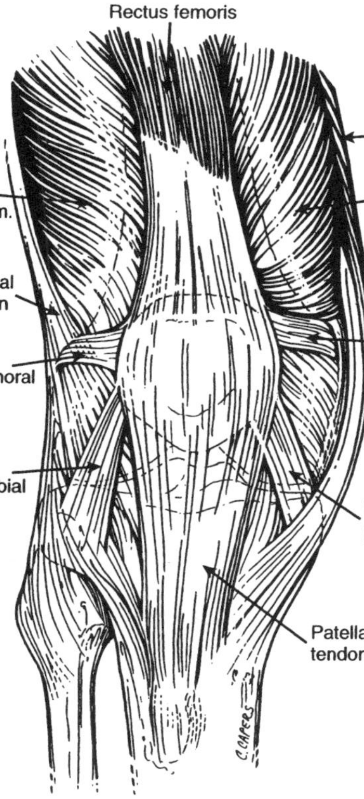

Figure 6.9 Muscular anatomy of the anterior aspect of the knee. (Reprinted with permission from Vaupel GL, Dye SF: Anatomy of the knee. *The Hughston Clinic Sports Medicine Book*, ed. by C. Baker, Jr., Williams, and Wilkins, 1995, pp. 403-415.)

The articularis genus muscle (the "fifth quadriceps muscle") is a small muscle deep to the vastus intermedius. Its origin is on the anterior surface of the distal femur, and its insertion is into the proximal knee joint capsule. Its function is felt to be proximal retraction of the suprapatellar pouch with quadriceps contraction. (32)

The quadriceps acts synergistically with the posterior cruciate ligament to stabilize the knee against posterior subluxation. Conversely, the hamstrings (specifically semimembranosus and biceps femoris) act in concert with the anterior cruciate ligament to prevent anterior subluxation. (46)

The hamstrings act as knee flexors and comprise the semitendinosus, semimembranosus, and biceps femoris. The pes anserinus is the combined insertion of the tendinous expansion of the sartorius, gracilis, and semitendinosus (see figure 6.10). The pes is thought to act as an internal rotator and flexor

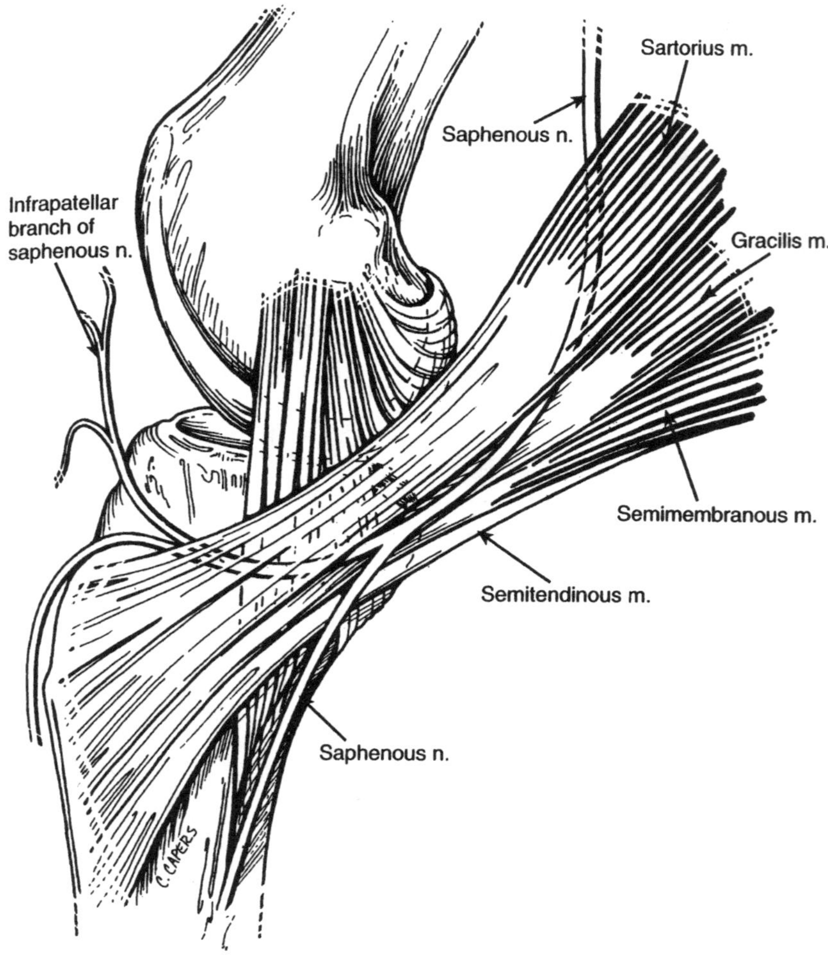

Figure 6.10 The pes anserinus is the insertion of the tendinous expansions of the sartorius, the gracilis, and the semimembranosis muscles. (Reprinted with permission from Vaupel GL, Dye SF: Anatomy of the knee. *The Hughston Clinic Sports Medicine Book*, ed. by C. Baker, Jr., Williams, and Wilkins, 1995, pp. 403-415.)

of the tibia; thus it stabilizes the knee against anteromedial rotatory instability. (32)

The semimembranosus typically has five insertions into the posteromedial aspect of the knee: (1) the oblique popliteal ligament, (2) the posterior capsule and posterior horn medial meniscus, (3) the anterior or deep arm, (4) the direct arm, and (5) the inferior arm. This complex insertion pattern serves several functions, including tightening the posterior oblique ligament and oblique popliteal ligament and thereby dynamically stabilizing the knee in flexion. It also retracts the posterior horn of the medial meniscus posteriorly in flexion, preventing a compression injury to the meniscus between the posterior femoral condyle and tibial plateau. (32)

The biceps femoris has a long and short head of insertion. The long head is more superficial, attaching to the fibular head as well as sending investing fibers around the fibular head and extending distally to the proximal tibia. The deeper fibers also coalesce with the fibular collateral ligament. The short head of the biceps femoris arises from the lateral and medial linea aspera on the posterior femur and inserts into the long head of the biceps femoris, as well as into the posterolateral capsule.

The function of the biceps femoris is to actively flex the knee and to retract the posterior horn of the lateral meniscus posteriorly with knee flexion, similar to the semimembranosus medially.

The popliteus muscle has a tripartite attachment proximally and extends obliquely, distally, and medially to originate on the posterior tibia. The tripartite attachment is divided between the lateral femoral condyle, the posterior horn lateral meniscus, and the fibular head. The fascicular attachments from the popliteus tendon have been demonstrated in detail by Stäubli and Birrer. (60) Through this complex scheme of bony anchors, the popliteus is felt to act both dynamically and statically. The dynamic function is to produce internal rotation of the tibia and retraction of the posterior horn of the lateral meniscus. Its static function is as a secondary restraint to posterolateral rotation, varus, and hyperextension forces. It also maintains hoop tension in the lateral meniscus.

The gastrocnemius muscle has a medial and a lateral head, which originate from the popliteal surface of the femur above the medial femoral condyle and the lateral aspect of the lateral femoral condyle, respectively. The two heads join in the posterior aspect of the Achilles tendon to insert on the posterior calcaneus. The gastrocnemius, because of its origin proximal to the knee, assists in knee flexion, though its primary function is plantar flexion of the foot.

The soleus muscle originates from the soleal line on the posterior proximal tibia and fibula. It then joins with the gastrocnemius on the anterior surface of the Achilles tendon. The plantaris muscle is a feeble plantar flexor of the foot and an accessory knee flexor as it accompanies the gastrocnemius. Its origin is the lateral supercondylar ridge of the femur, and it extends obliquely to its insertion on the medial border of the Achilles tendon.

Vasculature

The popliteal artery is the primary blood supply to the knee. It is commonly injured with knee dislocation and fractures because it is securely fixed proximally at the adductor hiatus and distally under the soleus muscle. Damage is usually incurred by stretching of the vessel away from the point of firm attachment with a knee dislocation or by direct puncture from a bony fragment.

The medial and lateral superior genicular arteries branch off the popliteal artery proximal to the posterior joint space. The medial and lateral inferior genicular arteries branch off the popliteal artery distal to the joint space. The lateral inferior genicular artery runs along the lateral joint line, making it susceptible to injury with lateral meniscal surgery. All four vessels pass forward to form an anastomosis called the rete articulare genus. (47)

The middle genicular artery arises directly from the anterior aspect of the popliteal artery and pierces the posterior capsule, supplying the cruciate ligaments and the posterior capsule. It has two branches that run anteriorly along the periphery of the medial and lateral menisci to anastomose at the anterior meniscal horns. The anterior tibial recurrent artery arises from the anterior tibial artery and exits the anterior muscle compartment laterally to anastomose with the medial inferior genicular artery anteriorly.

Two areas of the knee deserve special mention with regard to vascular supply, the patella and the menisci. There has been increasing concern about patellar avascular necrosis secondary to iatrogenic injury. The principal patellar blood supply is from an anterior anastomotic ring supplied by the medial and lateral superior genicular arteries and the medial and lateral inferior genicular arteries. There is also a small contribution from an infrapatellar anastomosis in the fat pad. (56) If medial and lateral capsular incisions are made (as is common for total knee arthroplasty), the patella is at great risk of developing avascular necrosis. (45)

The meniscal blood supply has been well documented. A perimeniscal capsular plexus within the synovium and capsule supplies blood to the peripheral 10 to 30% of the menisci, except for the area immediately adjacent to the popliteus tendon, which is completely avascular. (3) This suggests that meniscal healing is more predictable in the peripheral vascular zones. The inner portions of the menisci depend upon diffusion for their nutrition.

Neuroanatomy

Motor Innervation

The femoral nerve, tibial nerve, and common peroneal nerve are the primary nerves that innervate muscles about the knee. The femoral nerve divides into anterior and posterior divisions approximately 4 cm distal to the inguinal ligament. The anterior division gives off two cutaneous branches (medial femoral cutaneous nerve and intermediate femoral cutaneous nerve) and two muscular branches (sartorius and pectineus). The posterior division gives off one cutaneous branch (saphenous nerve) and all of the muscular branches to the quadriceps muscles.

The tibial nerve arises in the lower one-third of the posterior thigh, passes through the popliteal fossa, and enters the posterior compartment beneath the soleus muscle. It supplies the gastrocnemius, soleus, popliteus, semimembranosus, semitendinosus, and long head of the biceps femoris.

The common peroneal nerve enters the popliteal fossa on the lateral side of the tibial nerve and follows closely the medial border of the biceps femoris muscle. It then leaves the fossa by crossing superficially the lateral head of the gastrocnemius, passes behind the head of the fibula, and then crosses the fibular neck before piercing the peroneus longus muscle. The muscle branch to the short head of biceps femoris is given off proximally in the popliteal fossa. The peroneal nerve is vulnerable to injury because it lies just under the skin at the fibular neck.

Sensory Innervation

The femoral nerve supplies sensory innervation to the proximal medial quadrant of the knee. The medial femoral cutaneous branches descend with the vastus medialis muscle and then pass laterally across the midline above the joint space.

The saphenous nerve provides sensation along the medial aspect of the leg (see figure 6.10). The infrapatellar branch of the saphenous nerve may be injured with medial meniscal repair or with harvesting of the hamstring tendons because it emerges between the tendons of the sartorius and gracilis muscles. The infrapatellar branch crosses the midline to supply the skin, subcutis, knee capsule, infrapatellar fat pad, and iliotibial tract. An anterior longitudinal skin incision, utilized to harvest the patellar tendon before placement of total knee components, thus invariably results in decreased cutaneous sensation lateral to the wound. The lateral aspect of the knee has a cutaneous nerve supply, from the lateral femoral cutaneous nerve proximally and the lateral sural cutaneous branch distally.

The knee joint itself has sensory contributions from the obturator nerve with its terminal branches, the tibial, peroneal, and saphenous nerves, and branches from the vastus lateralis, vastus intermedius, and vastus medialis muscles.

The medial articular nerve should be identified and protected when dissecting near the proximal medial collateral ligament. (47) This nerve descends across the adductor tubercle close to the femoral attachment of the medial collateral ligament. It then passes into the joint capsule, to the fat pad, and below the patellar tendon to the lateral knee. Multiple different end organ sensors have been documented histologically in and about the knee, including free nerve endings, (6, 44) Golgi-like tension receptors, (39, 50) and mechanoreceptors of the cruciate ligaments, (13, 38, 43, 57, 58) as well as the meniscus (71) and other knee tissues. (70)

Functional Intraarticular Sensation of the Knee

Much evidence indirectly indicates that various intraarticular components of the knee are sensate, that is, they generate neurosensory signals that reach the spinal, cerebellar, and higher central nervous system levels. These neurosensory signals can ultimately result in conscious perception. The main research supporting this belief has been indirect and based on histological evidence of neurostructures within intraarticular components, (6, 13, 22, 24, 26, 27, 31, 38, 43, 57, 58, 70, 71) the documentation of sensory evoked potentials, (53) or on proprioceptive characteristics of the human knee. (4, 5, 11, 54, 59, 67) It should be noted, however, that proprioceptive studies have been primarily designed to elicit conscious detection of small movements of the knee. Such data summarize neurosensory output from the entire joint and limb, including the extraarticular structures, and thus do not isolate possible intraarticular sensory signals. Documentation of sensory evoked potentials with electrical stimulation of intraarticular structures of anesthetized patients at surgery does not answer the questions of whether and to what extent a person would consciously experience palpation of those components.

We (SFD and GLV) concluded that a simple method to directly document possible conscious neurosensory perception of the intraarticular components of the knee would be to arthroscopically palpate the components without intraarticular anesthesia and record the subjective experience. The senior one of us (SFD) had both knees inspected arthroscopically (by GLV) without intraarticular anesthesia. The various structures were palpated by an instrumented probe. The sensation was recorded from 0—no perception, to 4—severe pain, as well as whether the sensations could be accurately localized (A) or not (B). The results of this study are represented in figure 6.11. (19)

This study, by probing the human knee without intraarticular anesthesia, provides direct evidence of the conscious perception of neurosensory output of internal structures. The anterior synovial tissues, fat pad, and capsule were exquisitely sensitive to the mechanical stimulus of the probe, whereas the sensation experienced with similar probing of the cruciate ligaments and menisci did not result in accurate spatial localization. This observation can provide an explanation for the often poor localization of structural damage that many

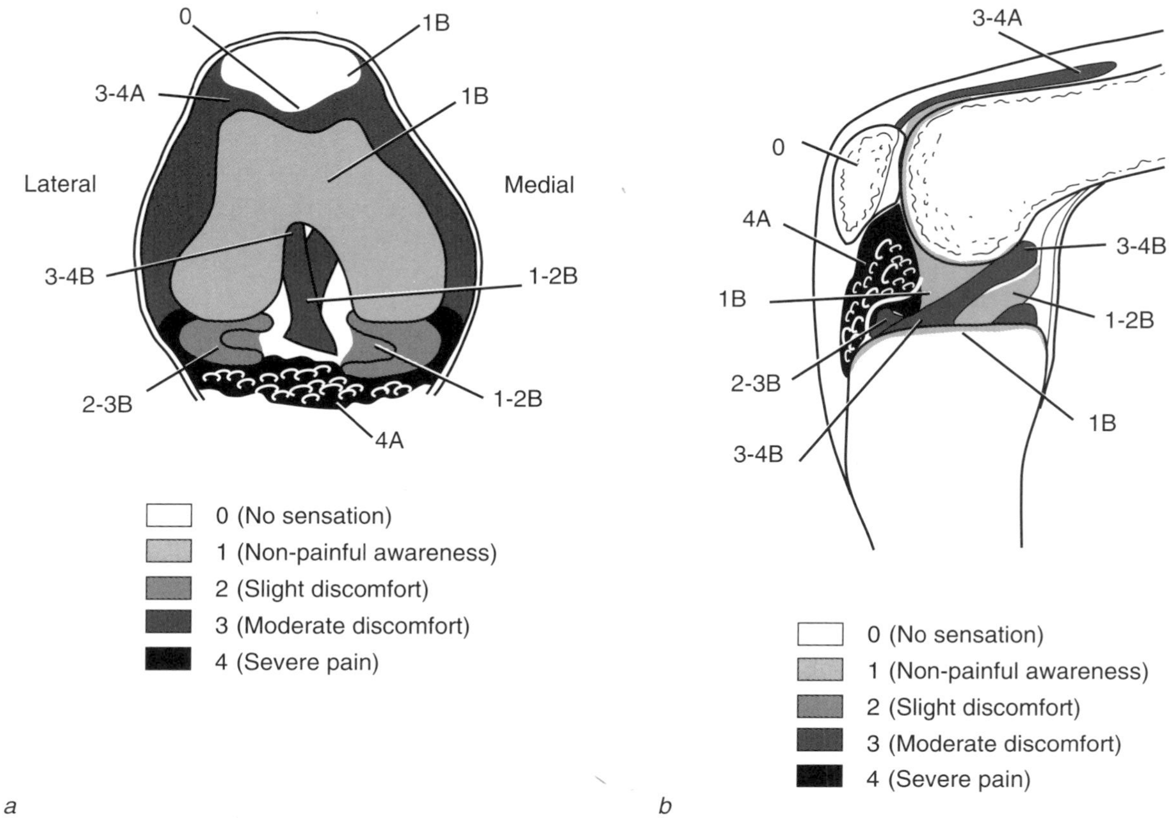

Figure 6.11 *(a)* Coronal and *(b)* sagittal schematic representations of the conscious neurosensory findings of the intraarticular structures of the knee. The right knee is illustrated. (A) Accurate spatial localization and (B) poorly localized sensation. (Reprinted with permission from Dye SF, Vaupel GL, Dye CC: Conscious neurosensory mapping of the internal structures of the human knee without intraarticular anesthesia. *Am J SportsMed* 1998; 26:773-777.)

patients experience with a cruciate ligament or meniscal injury. The painful synovitis and capsular information frequently associated with a meniscal injury may be a more important factor in the subjective localization of the site of possible cartilage damage than sensation arising solely from the damaged meniscus.

Of interest, we noted that the patellae of both knees have grade III chondromalacia, and yet they were totally asensate, even to deep probing. This finding may enhance the opinion of those who dispute a direct causal connection between the presence of chondromalacia of the patella and anterior knee pain.

It is well documented that the absence of joint sensation can lead to eventual destruction due to a variety of diseases, (9, 21, 42, 52, 68) as is seen in patients with Charcot joints and those born with congenital insensitivity to pain. (14, 30) We, therefore, believe that sensation of most intraarticular structures of the knee is crucial for long-term joint function and maintenance of tissue homeostasis. The failure of certain intraarticular reconstructions and tissue transplants may be due, in part, to absence of restoration of neurosensory characteristics. Future research, which is designed to delineate factors that determine, maintain, and restore normal neurosensory characteristics of intraarticular structures, may ultimately lead to the development of techniques that result in true restoration of joint homeostasis and function.

References

1. Abbott LC, Saunders JB, Bost FC, Anderson CF. Injuries to the ligaments of the knee joint. *J Bone Joint Surg* 26A: 503, 1944.
2. Aglietti P, Buzzi R, Insall JN. Disorders of the patellofemoral joint. In *Surgery of the Knee*, 2d ed. JN Insall et al., eds. New York: Churchill Livingstone, 1993.
3. Arnoczky SP, Warren F. Microvasculature of the human meniscus. *Am J Sports Med* 10: 90, 1982.
4. Barrack R, Lund P, Munn B, et al. Evidence of reinnervation of free patellar tendon autograft

used for anterior cruciate ligament reconstruction. *Am J Sports Med* 25: 196–202, 1997.
5. Barrett D, Cobb A, Bentley G. Joint proprioception in normal, osteoarthritic, and replaced knees. *J Bone Joint Surg.* 73B: 53–56, 1991.
6. Biedert R, Stauffer E, Friederich N. Occurrence of free nerve endings in the soft tissue of the knee joint: A histological investigation. *Am J Sports Med* 20: 430–33, 1992.
7. Brantigan OC, Voshell AF. The tibial collateral ligament: Its function, its bursae, and its relation to the medial meniscus. *J Bone Joint Surg* 25A: 121, 1943.
8. Brantigan OC, Voshell AF. Ligaments of the knee joints: The relationship of the ligament of Humphry to the ligament of Wrisberg. *J Bone Joint Surg* 28: 66, 1946.
9. Chong A, Bruce W, Goldberg J. Treatment of the neuropathic knee by arthroplasty. [Australia, NZ] *J Surg* 65: 370–71, 1995.
10. Clancy WG Jr, et al. Treatment of knee joint instability secondary to rupture of the posterior cruciate ligament: Report of a new procedure. *J Bone Joint Surg* 65A: 310, 1983.
11. Clark F, Horch K, Bach S, Larson G. Contributions of cutaneous and joint receptors to static knee position sense in man. *J Neurophysiol* 42(3): 877–88, 1979.
12. Dandy DJ. Anatomy of the medial suprapatellar plica and medial synovial shelf. *Arthroscopy* 6: 79, 1990.
13. Denti M, Monteleone M, Berardi A, Panni A. Anterior cruciate ligament mechanoreceptors: Histological studies on lesions and reconstruction. *Clin Orth Rel Res* 308: 29–32, 1994.
14. Derwin K, Glover R, Wojtys E. Nociceptive role of substance-P in the knee joint of a patient with congenital insensitivity to pain. *J Pediatr Orthop* 14: 258–62, 1994.
15. Dye SF. An evolutionary perspective of the knee. *J Bone Joint Surg* 7: 976-83, 1987.
16. Dye SF. Patellofemoral anatomy. In *The Patellofemoral Joint,* JM Fox, W Del Pizzo, eds. New York: McGraw-Hill, 1993.
17. Dye SF. The knee as a biological transmission with an envelope of function. *Clin Orth Rel Res* 325: 10–18, 1996.
18. Dye SF, Shapeero L, Lipton MJ, et al. Quantitative assessment of functional knee morphology by means of cine computed tomography. *Am J Sports Med* 15: 387, 1987.
19. Dye SF, Vaupel GL, Dye CC. Conscious neurosensory mapping of the internal structures of the human knee without intraarticular anesthesia. *Am J Sports Med* 26: 773–77, 1998.
20. Dye SF, Wojtys EM, Fu FH, Fithian DC, Gillquist J. Factors contributing to function of the knee joint after injury or reconstruction of the anterior cruciate ligament. *J Bone Joint Surg* 80A: 1380–393, 1998.
21. Farsetti P, Caterini R. Idiopathic Charcot's arthropathy. *Arch Orthop Trauma Surg* 111: 282–83, 1992.
22. Freeman M, Wyke B. The innervation of the knee joint: An anatomical and histological study in the cat. *J Anat* 101:505–32, 1967.
23. Fulkerson JP, Hungerford DS. Normal anatomy. In *Disorders of the Patellofemoral Joint,* 2d ed. Baltimore: Williams & Wilkins, 1990.
24. Gardner E. The innervation of the knee joint. *Anatom Rec* 95: 109–30, 1948.
25. Girgis FG, Marshall JL, Al-Monajem ARS. The cruciate ligaments of the knee joint: Anatomical, functional, and experimental analysis. *Clin Orthop* 106: 216, 1975.
26. Grabiner M, Koh T, Draganich L. Neuromechanics of the patellofemoral joint. *Med Sports Exerc* 26: 10–21, 1994.
27. Greep R, Weiss L. *Histology,* 3d ed. New York: McGraw-Hill, 1973.
28. Hallisey MJ, Doherty N, Bennett WF, Fulkerson JP. Anatomy of the junction of the vastus lateralis tendon and the patella. *J Bone Joint Surg* 69A: 545, 1987.
29. Heller L, Langmen J. The meniscofemoral ligaments of the human knee. *J Bone Joint Surg* 46B: 307, 1964.
30. Hirsch E, Moye D, Dimon J 3d. Congenital indifference to pain: Long term follow-up of two cases. *South Med J* 88: 851–57, 1995.
31. Horner G, Dellon A. Innervation of the human knee joint and implications for surgery. *Clin Orth* 301: 221–26, 1994.
32. Hughston JC. *Knee Ligaments: Injury and Repair.* St. Louis: Mosby Year Book, 1993.
33. Hughston JC, Andrews JR, Cross MJ, Moschi A. Classification of knee ligament instabilities: Part I. The medial compartment and cruciate ligaments. *J Bone Joint Surg* 58A: 159, 1976.
34. Hughston JC, Eilers AF. The role of the posterior oblique ligament in repairs of acute medial (collateral) ligament tears of the knee. *J Bone Joint Surg* 55A: 923, 1973.
35. Hughston JC, Walsh WM, Puddu G. Diagnosis. In *Patellar Subluxation and Dislocation.* Philadelphia: Saunders, 1984.
36. Hughston JC, Walsh WM, Puddu G. Functional anatomy of the extensor (decelerator) mechanism. In *Patellar Subluxation and Dislocation.* Philadelphia: Saunders, 1984.

37. Hungerford DS, Barry M. Biomechanics of the patellofemoral joint. *Clin Orthop* 144: 9, 1979.
38. Johansson H, Sjölander P, Sojka P. A sensory role for the cruciate ligaments. *Clin Orthop* 268: 161–78, 1991.
39. Kennedy JC, Alexander IJ, Hayes KC. Nerve supply of the human knee and its functional importance. *Am J Sports Med* 10: 329–35, 1982.
40. Kennedy JC, Grainger RW. The posterior cruciate ligament. *J Trauma* 7: 367, 1967.
41. Kennedy JC, Hawkins RJ, Willis RB, Danvlchuk KD. Tension study of the human knee ligaments: Yield point, ultimate failure, and disruption of the cruciate and tibial collateral ligaments. *J Bone Joint Surg* 58A: 350, 1976.
42. Koshino T. Stage classifications, types of bone destruction, and bone scintigraphy in Charcot joint disease. *Bull Hosp Joint Dis Orthop Inst* 51: 205–17, 1991.
43. Krauspe R, Schmidt M, Schaible H. Sensory innervation of the anterior cruciate ligament. *J Bone Joint Surg* 74A: 390–97, 1992.
44. Lobenhoffer P, Biebert R, Stauffer E, et al. Occurrence and distribution of free nerve endings in the distal iliotibial tract system of the knee. *Knee Surg Sports Traumatol Arthroscopy* 4: 111–15, 1996.
45. McMahon MS, et al. Scintigraphic determination of patellar viability after excision of infrapatellar fat pad or lateral retinacular release in total knee arthroplasty. *Clin Orthop* 260: 10, 1990.
46. More RC, et al. Hamstrings—an anterior cruciate ligament protagonist: An in vitro study. *Am J Sports Med* 21: 231, 1993.
47. Müller W. *The Knee: Form, Function, and Ligament Reconstruction.* New York: Springer-Verlag, 1983.
48. Norwood LA, Cross MJ. Anterior cruciate ligament: Functional anatomy of its bundles in rotatory instability. *Am J Sports Med* 7: 23, 1979.
49. Noyes FR, Grood ES, Butler DL, Paulos LE. Clinical biomechanics of the knee ligament restraints and functional stability. In *American Academy of Orthopaedic Surgeons Symposium on the Athlete's Knee: Surgical Repair and Reconstruction.* St. Louis: Mosby, 1980.
50. Nyland J, Brosky T, Currier D, et al. Review of the afferent neural system of the knee and its contribution to motor learning. *J Sports Phys Therapy* 19: 2–11, 1994.
51. O'Brien WR, Friederich NF, Müller W, et al. Functional anatomy of the cruciate ligaments. American Academy of Orthopaedic Surgeons Instructional Videotape. Park Ridge, IL. AAOS, 1991.
52. O'Connor B, Visco D, Brandt K, et al. Neurogenic acceleration of osteoarthrosis: The effects of previous neurectomy of the articular nerves on the development of osteoarthrosis after transection of the anterior cruciate ligament in dogs. *J Bone Joint Surg* 74: 367–76, 1992.
53. Pitman M, Nainzadeh N, Menche D, et al. The intraoperative evaluation of the neurosensory function of the anterior cruciate ligament in humans using somatosensory evoked potentials. *Arthroscopy* 8(4): 442–47, 1992.
54. Proske U, Schaible H, Schmidt R. Joint receptors and kinesthesia. *Exp Brain Res* 72: 219–24, 1988.
55. Renström P, Johnson RJ. Anatomy and biomechanics of the menisci. *Clin Sports Med* 9: 523, 1990.
56. Scapinelli R. Blood supply of the human patella: Its relation to ischemic necrosis after fracture. *J Bone Joint Surg* 49B: 563, 1967.
57. Schultz R, Miller D, Kerr C, Micheli L. Mechanoreceptors in human cruciate ligaments. *J Bone Joint Surg* 66A: 1072–1076, 1984.
58. Schutte M, Dabezies EJ, Zimny M, et al. Neural anatomy of the human anterior cruciate ligament. *J Bone Joint Surg* 69A: 243–47, 1987.
59. Skinner H, Barrack R. Joint position sense in the normal and pathologic knee joint. *J Electromyogr Kinesiol* 1: 180–90, 1991.
60. Stäubli HU, Birrer S. The popliteus tendon and its fascicles at the popliteal hiatus: Gross anatomy and functional arthroscopic evaluation with and without anterior cruciate ligament deficiency. *Arthroscopy* 6: 209, 1990.
61. Terry GC. The anatomy of the extensor mechanism. *Clin Sports Med* 8: 163, 1989.
62. Thompson WO, Theate FL, Fu FH, Dye SF. Tibial meniscal dynamics using three-dimensional reconstruction of magnetic resonance images. *Am J Sports Med* 19: 210, 1991.
63. Van Dommelen BA, Fowler PJ. Anatomy of the posterior cruciate ligament: A review. *Am J Sports Med* 17: 24, 1989.
64. Vaupel GL, Dye SF. Anatomy of the Knee. In *The Hughston Clinic Sports Medicine Book,* C Baker Jr, ed. 403–15. Baltimore: Williams & Wilkins, 1995.
65. Wang CJ, Walker PS. Rotatory laxity of the human knee joint. *J Bone Joint Surg* 56A: 161, 1974.
66. Warren LA, Marshall JL, Girgis F. The prime static stabilizer of the medial side of the knee. *J Bone Joint Surg* 56A: 665, 1974.

67. Warren P, Olanlokun T, Cobb A, Bentley G. Proprioception after arthroplasty: The influence of prosthetic design. *Clin Orth* 297: 182–87, 1993.
68. Yoshino S, Fujimori J, Kajino A, et al. Total knee arthroplasty in Charcot's joint. *J Arthroplasty* 8: 335–40, 1993.
69. Zidorn T. Classification of the suprapatellar septum considering ontogenetic development. *Arthroscopy* 8: 459, 1992.
70. Zimny M. Mechanoreceptors in articular tissues. *Am J Anat* 182: 16–32, 1988.
71. Zimny M, Albright D, Dabezies E. Mechanoreceptors in the human medial meniscus. *Acta Anat* (Basel) 133: 35–40, 1988.

CHAPTER 7

Neuromuscular Contributions to Knee Kinematics and Kinetics: Normal Versus Pathological State

Timothy E. Hewett, PhD
Mark V. Paterno, MS, PT
Frank R. Noyes, MD

Sagittal Plane Flexion-Extension Motion and Moments

Normal Flexion-Extension Kinematics and Kinetics at the Knee

To best appreciate the dynamic neuromuscular contributions to knee joint stability and the specifics of its kinematics and kinetics, it becomes necessary to break these complicated motions and forces down into manageable phases. A simple and clinically significant means to accomplish this is to examine the separate phases of gait. Through this breakdown, the muscular contributions to knee joint stability become evident.

Muscular Control in the Sagittal Plane

Most normal motion at the knee joint occurs in the sagittal plane. This motion represents a biphasic pattern of flexion and extension (21, 36). By using gait analysis, it becomes clear how sagittal motion, combined with smaller motions in the coronal and transverse planes, creates a synchronous, stable motion at the knee. Through EMG analysis during gait, trends in muscle firing patterns have been determined with respect to magnitude and timing of the necessary activity to produce not only flexion and extension but also coronal and transverse motion (36).

Knee extension is accomplished through the firing of several muscles. Four heads of the quadriceps muscle, including the vastus intermedius, vastus lateralis, vastus medialis longus, and vastus medialis obliquus, contribute to knee extension exclusively because they cross only the knee joint. The rectus femoris represents a two-joint muscle, crossing both the knee and the hip and contributing to extension of the knee while also flexing the hip. Finally, the upper gluteus maximus acts as a knee extensor as it tensions the iliotibial band, which attaches at the anterolateral rim of the tibia, thus producing knee extension (17, 36).

During normal gait, the knee reaches a maximum of approximately 60° of flexion during swing phase and 20° of flexion during stance phase. The exact amount of flexion varies with the speed of motion, specific subject, and method of measurement; however, most authors agree that maximum flexion is between 60° and 70° (9, 13, 17, 21, 24, 36). The magnitude and pattern of sagittal knee motion has been well documented (see figure 7.1).

Knee flexion is achieved through the coordination of eight muscles. The popliteus and the short head of the biceps femoris represent single-joint knee flexors acting only to produce knee flexion.

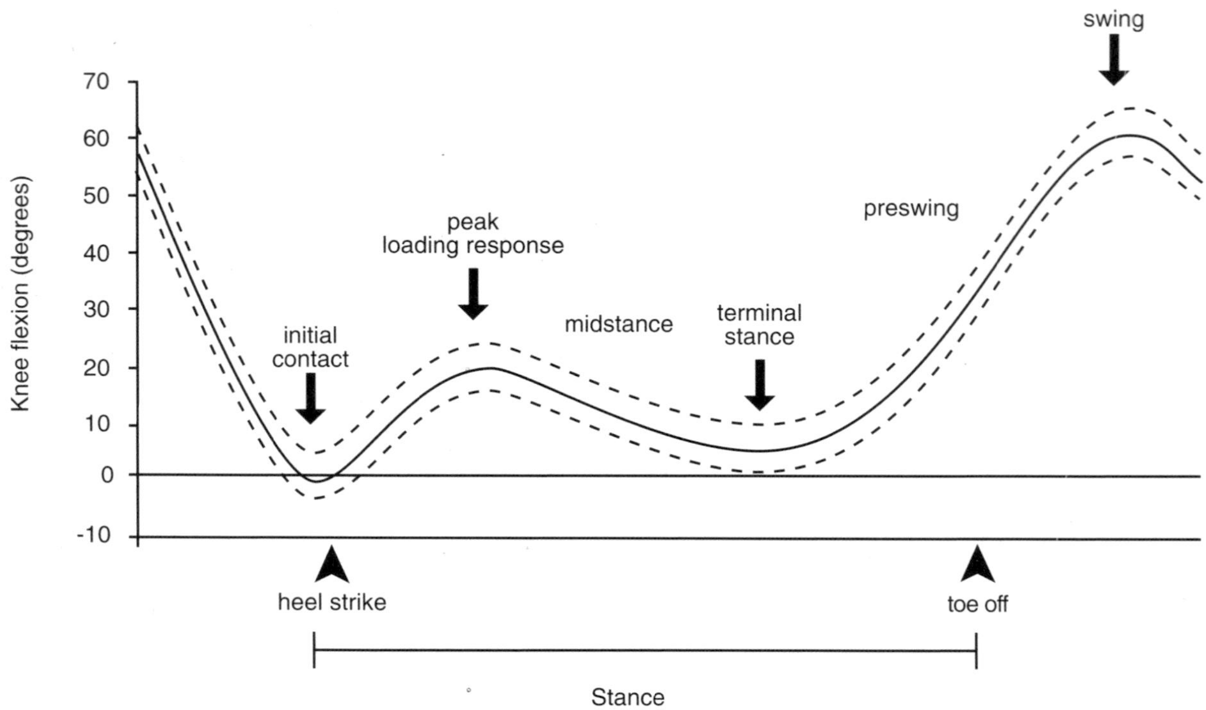

Figure 7.1 The pattern of sagittal knee motion during the normal gait cycle. (Adapted with permission from Noyes FR, Dunworth LA, Andriacchi TP, Andrews M, Hewett TE. Knee hyperextension gait abnormalities in unstable knees. Recognition and preoperative gait retraining. *Am J Sports Med* 24(1): 35-45, 1996).

Additionally, flexion is attained through the action of the semimembranosus, semitendinosus, and the long head of the biceps femoris. Muscular contraction of the gastrocnemius plays a role in knee flexion, as do contractions of the gracilis and sartorius (17, 36).

Neuromuscular Contributions to Stance Phase of Gait

Coordinated muscle activity around the knee joint during the stance phase of gait is reflected by the external flexion-extension moment at the knee. During normal stance phase the external flexion-extension moment shows a biphasic pattern (see figure 7.2). After a short extension peak at heel strike, the flexion moment increases during loading response and peaks at early midstance. The external flexion moment is the external torque that tends to flex the knee and is dependent on the limb inertia, limb weight, and the resultant ground reaction force, which is passing posterior to the flexed knee joint. Mechanical equilibrium dictates that this external flexion moment be balanced by an "internal" extension moment during gait in order to prevent the subject from collapsing to the ground. This internal extension moment is assumed to be derived predominantly from the quadriceps muscle. Nissan (25) showed this to be a valid assumption. Once the body center of gravity passes forward of the knee joint during midstance, then the extension moment predominates. The external extension moment is balanced primarily by the hamstrings and then the gastrocnemius as the limb passes through midstance and terminal stance (40).

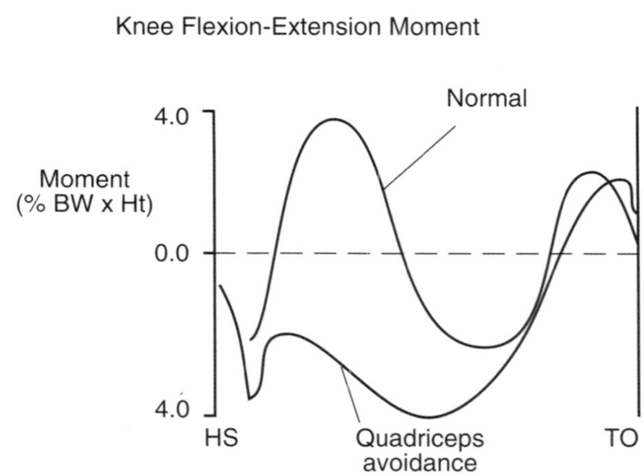

Figure 7.2 The normal pattern of the flexion-extension moment at the knee during stance phase of gait and the pattern of "quadriceps avoidance" observed in some ACL-deficient subjects.

Initial contact

As the foot hits the ground at initial contact, the knee is near full extension in a stabilized position (17, 36). Alignment of the ground reaction force lies anterior to the knee joint resulting in an external extension moment (3, 10, 28). This extended position at the knee is maintained by eccentric contraction of the knee extensor musculature, primarily the vastus group. Contraction of the upper gluteus maximus also contributes to extension via the iliotibial band. In addition, low levels of hamstring activity are present to serve as a protective counterbalancing flexion force (10, 36).

Loading response

As the lower extremity progresses through stance phase, the knee continues to flex until it reaches its maximum stance phase flexion near 20° at loading response (17, 28). During this phase the lower extremity must work to absorb the shock of the transfer of body weight onto the limb. The limb achieves stability through knee flexion. The onset of flexion is encouraged as the ground reaction force moves posterior to the knee, creating an external flexion moment (3, 36). Residual swing phase hamstrings activity terminates early in loading response and yields to strong eccentric contraction of the vastus muscles, which prevents greater than 20° of flexion and provides stability and shock absorption (17, 36). Quadriceps firing is crucial at this stage. Deficits in quadriceps strength lead to gait abnormalities. These abnormalities result from attempts to maintain stability in a weakened knee joint (6).

Midstance

During midstance phase the knee progresses again towards extension. This motion, however, is not dominated by neuromuscular control of the vastus alone. In the initial portion of midstance the vastus muscles are active to bring the knee toward extension and maintain the knee at the slightly flexed position (17). As midstance progresses vastus activity is decreased as the tibia becomes stabilized through the contraction of the soleus. Tibial stability allows femoral advancement over the knee due to the momentum generated from the swing limb. This passive mechanism of knee extension decreases demands on the quadriceps muscles until they cease contracting at peak midstance (36).

At this point of midstance, the body vector passes through the knee from posterior to anterior, resulting in a passive extension force (3). Stability during the remainder of midstance is dependent on this passive knee extension (10).

Terminal stance

As midstance progresses knee flexion decreases until terminal stance phase, when it reaches near full extension. Knee extension occurs in an attempt to maintain stability and increase stride, prior to an initiation of flexion to prepare for swing. This is accomplished through minimal neuromuscular control at the knee joint. Rather, momentum and a coordination of actions at the ankle and foot allow for this extension at the knee to be maintained (10, 36).

Contraction of ankle plantar flexors maintains the previously attained tibial stability. This action is coupled with maintenance of momentum generated from the swing limb, which causes most of the force necessary for extension. Finally, the forefoot acts as a rocker to aid in the advancement of the body vector beyond the leg. The tensor fascia lata contracts to prevent hip hyperextension, which tenses the iliotibial band. This tension assists in the maintenance of knee extension.

The sum of the extensor forces adequately provides the necessary force to accomplish the goals of terminal stance. To ensure maintenance of the proper position of the knee in slight flexion at the midpoint of this phase, the gastrocnemius and popliteus fire. This activity continues through the end stage of terminal stance, resulting in an increase in knee flexion. Additionally, tibial stability is lost when the body vector is too far anterior and forward rotation occurs at the foot, encouraging knee flexion. Five degrees of flexion is attained prior to the end of terminal stance (10, 36).

Preswing

The second period of flexion follows at the initiation of preswing (36). At this point, the rate of flexion increases dramatically, as the leg must now prepare for limb advancement. Flexion increases to 40° at the end of preswing and peaks at 60° during initial swing. At 60°, the knee has attained adequate flexion to accomplish limb advancement, a critical event in gait (10, 36). Neuromuscular contributions at this time relate to preparation for swing. This is attained through three mechanisms. The first is tibial advancement, which progresses secondary to the position of the base of the ground reaction force vector anterior to the metatarsals. This facilitates a flexed knee posture. In addition, the tibia is further advanced secondary to residual gastrocnemius activity causing heel off. Finally, knee flexion increases as a result of the direct action of the gastrocnemius and popliteus (36).

Neuromuscular Contributions to Swing Phase of Gait

During the swing phase of gait, the lower extremity has progressed from a closed kinetic chain to an open kinetic chain. No longer is the function of the knee to act as a shock absorber and stabilizer; rather it functions to aid the lower extremity in limb advancement. This is accomplished through both neuromuscular contributions and momentum.

During initial swing the 60° of knee flexion necessary for foot clearance and limb advancement are achieved through several means. The forward progress of the limb is primarily due to the momentum generated by rapid hip flexion. Active knee flexion occurs as a result of contraction of the short head of the biceps femoris in conjunction with low-level activity from the sartorius and gracilis to allow foot clearance (17). Throughout midswing knee extension occurs as the limb advances. This action occurs completely through passive means at the knee. All motion at the knee is secondary to momentum (10).

The limb completes advancement and prepares for stance during the final phase of the gait cycle, terminal swing. At this point passive momentum continues to progress the tibia; however, this force alone is inadequate. Therefore, the vastus musculature acts to extend the knee toward full extension (21, 36). Antagonistic activity of the hamstrings acts eccentrically to decelerate the limb at the end of terminal swing. The knee then begins to flex slightly in preparation for initial contact and another stride in the gait cycle (10).

An Example of the Pathologic State: The ACL-Deficient Knee

Pain plays an important role in the development of gait pathology at the knee. Kinematic pathologies resulting from knee pain occur most commonly in the sagittal plane, usually involving inadequate flexion or extension. An inappropriate relative balance of quadriceps and hamstrings activity during stance phase is often associated with these changes in knee kinematics.

A percentage of patients with knee pathology develop functional gait adaptations in an attempt to modify their symptoms. These functional gait adaptations have been well documented in patients with advanced degenerative joint disease of the knee (14, 32). In addition, functional gait adaptations in anterior cruciate ligament- (ACL-) deficient knees have been documented (6, 42). These gait changes may be an attempt by the patient to modify symptoms of pain and instability. Noyes and coworkers (26, 30) reported on a young active ACL-deficient population at an average of 5.5 yrs postinjury. They found that with a course of rehabilitation, one-third of their patients improved enough to participate in recreational activities, another third could perform activities of daily living but had to discontinue strenuous activity, and one-third of these patients had difficulties with activities of daily living. What accounts for this difference between the fully functional third and the essentially nonfunctional third of these patients? We hypothesize that the functional third adapt their musculature in a way to stabilize the knee joint and decrease pain symptoms. It was noted, however, that a 44% incidence of degenerative changes on radiographs of the knee occurred in this active "functionally adapted" group of patients. Therefore, it remains in question whether these "functional adaptations" protect the knee joint from degenerative changes.

Factors that have been shown to be related to outcome in ACL-deficient patients include the degree of instability (20), associated ligament injury (1), meniscal pathology (1, 5, 26), expectations about returning to strenuous activity (5, 8, 26, 30), activity modification (5, 30), rehabilitation program (30), occupation (8, 20), and age (8). Each of these factors must be considered in order to predict a patient's functional outcome. We hypothesize that differences in neuromuscular adaptation levels are also involved. These adaptations may help to explain why some ACL-deficient patients demonstrate a higher functional level than others do.

Berchuck and others (6) showed that a majority of ACL-deficient patients possessed no measurable external knee flexion moment during the stance phase of gait (see figure 7.2). Tibone and others (42) demonstrated using electromyography (EMG) that quadriceps activity does indeed decrease with ACL deficiency. Hence, if the measurable external knee flexion moment is decreased, then it is assumed that the need for a "balancing" internal extension moment (primarily quadriceps derived) is likewise decreased. Therefore, Berchuck and coworkers (6) termed this observed decrease in the external flexion moment at the knee the "quadriceps avoidance gait". They reported that 75% of ACL-deficient patients (12 of 16) they tested demonstrated this adaptation. Please refer to Dr. Andriacchi's discussion in this text of "Functional Adaptations in Patients With ACL-Deficient Knees" for a more in-depth discussion of this topic.

It is unclear if this described functional gait change (the so-called "quadriceps avoidance gait") protects the knee joint. If one examines the forces about the knee, one could make an argument that quadriceps avoidance does protect the joint. A number of studies have shown that there is increasing strain in the ACL as quadriceps contractions are performed at angles less than 45° of knee flexion (4, 7, 12, 16, 23). In an ACL-deficient knee, this force would tend to displace the tibia anteriorly. This "quadriceps avoidance gait" appears to be an adaptive change that decreases this anteriorly directed force. Data from other analyzed activities (i.e., jogging and stair climbing) is also consistent with the hypothesis that "quadriceps avoidance" is an adaptive response to increased anterior tibial subluxation and ACL strain. At angles greater than 45° there is decreasing strain in the ACL with quadriceps contraction. Therefore, with activities performed at higher knee flexion angles (jogging: 40°, stair climbing: 60°) one would expect the flexion moment to be present in these "gait adapted" individuals. Berchuck and others (6) demonstrated that the flexion moment was indeed present in ACL-deficient knees during jogging and stair climbing.

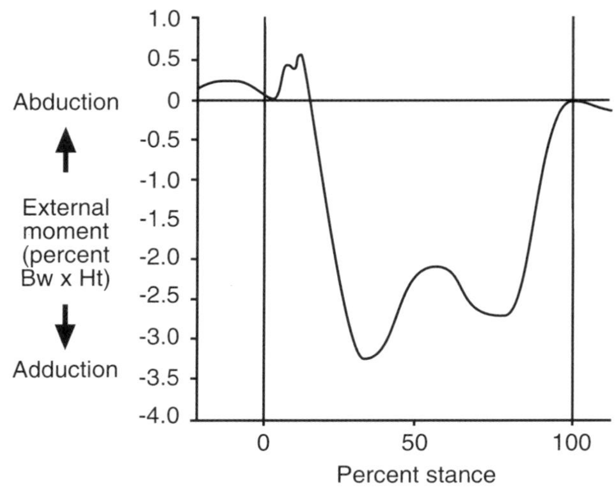

Figure 7.3 The abduction-adduction moment pattern of gait during stance phase in a normal subject. (Adapted with permission from Andrews M, Noyes FR, Hewett TE, Andriacchi TP. Lower limb alignment and foot angle are related to stance phase knee adduction in normal subjects: A critical analysis of the reliability of gait analysis data. *Journal of Orthopaedic Research* 14(2): 289-295, 1996.)

Coronal Plane: Abduction and Adduction Motion and Moments

Normal Abduction-Adduction Kinematics and Kinetics at the Knee

The magnitude of motion in the coronal plane is significantly less than that which occurs in the sagittal plane during gait: 8° to 12° of normal motion occurs in the coronal plane in comparison to 60° to 70° in the sagittal plane (9, 17, 21, 36). The function of this motion at the knee joint is to aid in the maintenance of vertical balance over the lower extremity, which is accomplished through movement into abduction and adduction during periods of stress, especially during single-limb support (36). Kettelkamp and others (21) reported that maximum knee abduction occurs during stance, either at initial contact or in the loading response phase (21). The knee returns toward a more neutral position during the swing phase of gait.

During the normal stance phase, the external adduction moment dominates (as the ground reaction force passes medially to the knee joint). This moment is double peaked, with a peak at loading response and another peak in terminal stance (see figure 7.3). Dynamic control of coronal plane motion is necessary during periods of stress to prevent excessive motion and undue strain on static stabilizers. During loading response, as the body experiences an unloading of the swing limb, the knee attains an abducted position of approximately 8° to 12° and a peak adduction moment (17, 36). As a result, lateral stability is necessary. The neuromuscular contributions to this stability include contraction of the long head of the biceps femoris and the upper gluteus maximus acting to tension the iliotibial band (36). Contraction of the sagittal plane musculature, namely quadriceps and hamstrings, acts to compress both the lateral and medial compartment of the knee joint. This contraction serves to resist the dominating adduction moment in the coronal plane (40). Additionally, contraction of the tensor fascia lata may provide support in some instances (3, 36). As the body progresses toward midstance, the center of gravity migrates laterally, thus decreasing the adduction moment. As a result, dynamic stability is no longer necessary to control movement. The exception remains a slight contraction of the iliotibial band, serving as a hip abductor, offering some dynamic control (36).

The Pathological State: The ACL-Deficient Varus Knee

Pain also plays a role in gait pathologies in the coronal plane. The ACL-deficient knee can progress into varus alignment postinjury (26, 32). Medial meniscal damage may accompany injury. These factors lead to increased loads in the medial compartment, medial compartment osteoarthritis, and increased tensile forces in the lateral ligaments. Patients with pain due to medial arthrosis or lateral joint opening may demonstrate neuromusculature adaptations to decrease symptoms of pain and functional instability.

The Varus Knee

Prodromos and others (38) analyzed the adduction moment at the knee pre- and postoperative high tibial osteotomy (HTO) in varus knees. They demonstrated that patients with low preoperative knee adduction moments showed significantly better objective and subjective results than those patients with high preoperative knee adduction moments. Wang and coworkers (43) followed this cohort of patients over three to nine years and found that patients with low adduction moments continued to report higher subjective outcome scores than individuals with high preoperative adduction moments. These authors suggested that those patients with varus knees and low adduction moments adapt their gait to decrease this external torque. An increased adduction moment tends to increase medial compartment loads and lateral tensile forces, resulting in a more painful knee. They postulated that one possible mechanism of adaptation was an increased toe-out gait in these subjects.

The ACL-Deficient Varus Knee

Noyes and coworkers (32) demonstrated that a varus angulated ACL-deficient knee shows significant alterations in gait from normal. These knees show decreased external knee flexion moments ("quadriceps reduction gait") and increased external knee extension moments (or a "hamstrings overuse pattern"). The external knee flexion moment was approximately one-third lower in ACL-deficient varus knees than in normal knees. Therefore, there is a tendency toward the quadriceps avoidance phenomenon reported by Berchuck and coworkers (6); however, the adaptation in these knees was much less pronounced. Only 40% of these patients demonstrated external flexion moments that were decreased to more than one standard deviation below control value (see figure 7.4). None of the 32 subjects was a true quadriceps avoider (they did not demonstrate a complete absence of an external flexion moment during midstance). The absence of a true quadriceps avoidance pattern in this population could be related to the pronounced varus angulation of these knees. As the degree of varus alignment worsens there is increased tension in the lateral soft tissues and a tendency for lateral liftoff (32, 40). The ACL is a secondary stabilizer to lateral joint opening. The ACL-deficient varus knee has significantly less static stabilization (11, 29, 32, 40), and patients may recruit additional sagittal (quadriceps and hamstring) muscle force to avoid lateral joint liftoff (23, 32, 35). The external extension moment (and balancing hamstrings contraction) was significantly higher than control in 50% of the involved knees. This increased hamstrings contraction may indicate a neuromuscular adaptation to decrease anterior tibial subluxation and to close down the lateral compartment of the joint. These increased moments may arise from an attempt to dynamically stabilize the knee; however, these increased sagittal plane moments lead to increased medial compartment loads.

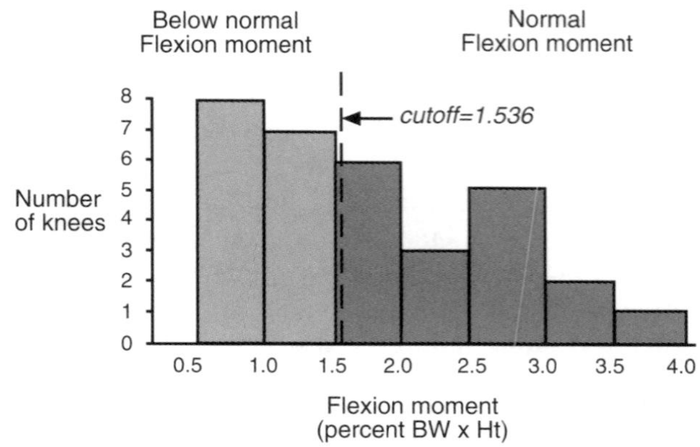

Figure 7.4 Bar graph of flexion moment distribution in ACL-deficient varus population. (Adapted with permission from Noyes FR, Schipplein OD, Andriacchi TP, Saddemi SR, Weise M. The anterior cruciate ligament deficient knee with varus alignment. An analysis of gait adaptations and dynamic joint loadings. *Am J Sports Med* 20(6): 707-716, 1992.)

Noyes and coworkers (32) also showed that a majority (20 of 32) of the ACL-deficient varus knees had a high external adduction moment. However, approximately 40% of this population showed normal adduction moments despite severe varus alignment. We conducted a study to determine if normal gait parameters were restored following HTO in a population of ACL-deficient varus knees (15). Another objective was to determine if a predictive relationship existed between the alteration in alignment and the change in dynamic loads at the knee. Gait analyses were performed pre- and post-HTO on 34 ACL-deficient varus patients. Patients were subdivided into normal and high adduction moment groups. Preoperatively, these two groups demonstrated equal magnitudes of varus alignment. However, the normal adduction moment group showed significantly lower adduction moments. The high adduction group demonstrated a significant preoperative correlation between mechanical alignment and adduction moment, whereas the low adduction group did not. We postulate that the normal adduction group employs a neuromuscular adaptation to decrease the loads in the medial compartment of the knee in response to pain originating in this compartment.

Correction of the Pathological State to Normal: High Tibial Osteotomy

Andrews and others (2) showed that in normal knees the mechanical axis correlates with the adduction moment. This is further evidence that patients with painful knees adopt functional adaptations in an attempt to lower the knee moments to effectively lower compartment loads. Normal knees and postoperative knees (with decreased pain levels) do not appear to require these functional adaptations.

We demonstrated that following HTO and ACL reconstruction in ACL-deficient varus knees the adduction moment and medial compartment load at the knee were significantly diminished postoperatively (15). There was a statistically significant correlation between the postoperative lower-limb alignment and the adduction moment during gait in both high and normal preoperative adduction moment subgroups. Previous studies showing a lack of correlation between lower-limb alignment and the knee adduction moment or force distribution in the joint confined their observations to preoperative knees with established arthrosis (14, 19, 32, 34). The possibility exists that pain and neuromuscular adaptations (body sway, stance phase time, foot progression angle, hip and ankle moments) provide additional variables that can mask the effect of lower-limb alignment. It is likely that gait adaptations play a role in the preoperative moment values of the normal adduction moment group. The high adduction group may demonstrate a relatively lower adaptative response to high medial compartment loads. Assuming that HTO relieves or diminishes pain symptoms, preoperative gait adaptations from arthrosis may diminish or normalize, and the correlation between limb alignment and adduction moment becomes apparent postoperatively.

The Transverse Plane

Normal Internal-External Rotation Kinematics at the Knee

The quantity of transverse motion relative to sagittal motion is minimal. The knee utilizes between 8° and 13° of transverse rotation to accommodate the body's change in alignment during gait (9, 21, 22, 36). Most motion occurs during stance when the transfer of body mass occurs over the knee from posterior to anterior, resulting in a rotational demand on the knee. Minor variations exist as to the magnitude and timing of transverse motion in the gait cycle; however, these are minimal (21, 22).

At initial contact the knee is affixed in a locked position with the femur in external rotation with respect to an internally rotated tibia (21, 22). As the body progresses through loading response, the tibia progresses further into internal rotation, reaching its peak at the end of loading response. Through the remainder of stance, the tibia externally rotates and resumes a position of maximum external rotation at the conclusion of preswing (17). The transverse rotation of the knee joint during the swing phase of gait represents a progressive internal rotation that peaks at terminal swing (22).

Dynamic control of transverse motion at the knee is minimal. Most transverse stability is provided through static ligamentous constraints while motion is dictated by rotational moments occurring at the ankle-foot complex (36). The primary transverse neuromuscular contribution at the knee occurs during loading response. At the initiation of stance, as the foot pronates, an internal rotation force is placed on the tibia that is translated to the knee. The pronation allows for increased shock absorption; however, it also results in a more unstable weight-bearing position. External tibial rotation is produced at the knee joint by contraction of the tensor fascia lata and biceps femoris muscles during the loading response phase. The contraction of these muscles acts to oppose excessive internal rotation motion, providing enhanced stability (36).

The Pathological State: The Triple Varus Knee

Excessive knee hyperextension during stance phase is common in patients with combined ACL or PCL and posterolateral ligamentous deficiencies. In a prior study (28) we described the abnormal hyperextension gait pattern in these patients. The loss of the normal knee flexion and extension pattern holds functional significance throughout the stance phase of the gait cycle: initial contact, loading response, midstance, terminal stance, and preswing (6, 28, 38). During the loading response phase, normal levels of knee flexion are needed for the knee joint to absorb shock (37, 39). A limb that is hyperextended during this phase transfers body weight directly from the tibia to the femur without the usual muscle energy absorption and cushioning that a flexed knee provides. The knee hyperextension pattern frequently causes pain in the medial tibiofemoral joint and posterolateral ligamentous structures.

Different types of abnormal knee motions and thrusts in the transverse plane occur during the stance phase of gait with hyperextension gait abnormalities (28). The abnormal varus recurvatum position of the knee due to ligamentous injury is markedly worse (e.g., symptoms, function, degree of malalignment) if there is associated tibiofemoral varus alignment. The "triple varus knee" syndrome (27, 31, 32) refers to the following combination of conditions: (1) varus tibiofemoral osseous alignment, (2) lateral tibiofemoral compartment separation due to lateral collateral ligament deficiency, and (3) knee hyperextension with involvement of the entire posterolateral ligament complex. A varus thrust is decreased with increasing external tibial rotation, while it is increased with internal rotation. With a valgus thrust, which occurs at loading response of stance phase, internal tibial rotation tends to decrease thrust, while external tibial rotation tends to increase it. In addition, there may be a tibiofemoral compartment rotational subluxation with a valgus thrust. Increases in this thrust occur with medial-posteromedial ligament injury. Increased external tibial rotation may occur with lateral-posterolateral ligament injury with posterior subluxation of the lateral plateau. It is important to note that abnormalities in tibiofemoral alignment markedly affect knee thrusting motions in the coronal, sagittal, and transverse plane and complicate treatment in that abnormal osseous alignment may require correction before soft tissue reconstructive procedures. This has been discussed in greater detail elsewhere (18, 27, 28, 32, 33, 43).

Because of the hyperextension gait pattern, the quadriceps muscles become relatively inactive during the stance phase whether or not quadriceps muscle weakness is the initial cause of the hyperextension. This results in marked quadriceps muscle atrophy, which further compounds the patient's subjective descriptions of knee instability and giving way. Awareness and correction of this gait pattern before surgery facilitates the postoperative rehabilitation program in restoring quadriceps muscle tone and strength (see figure 7.5).

Correction of Gait in the Pathological Triple Varus Knee: Gait Retraining

A comprehensive rehabilitation program is used to increase muscle strength and endurance of all of the muscle groups of the lower extremity in patients with

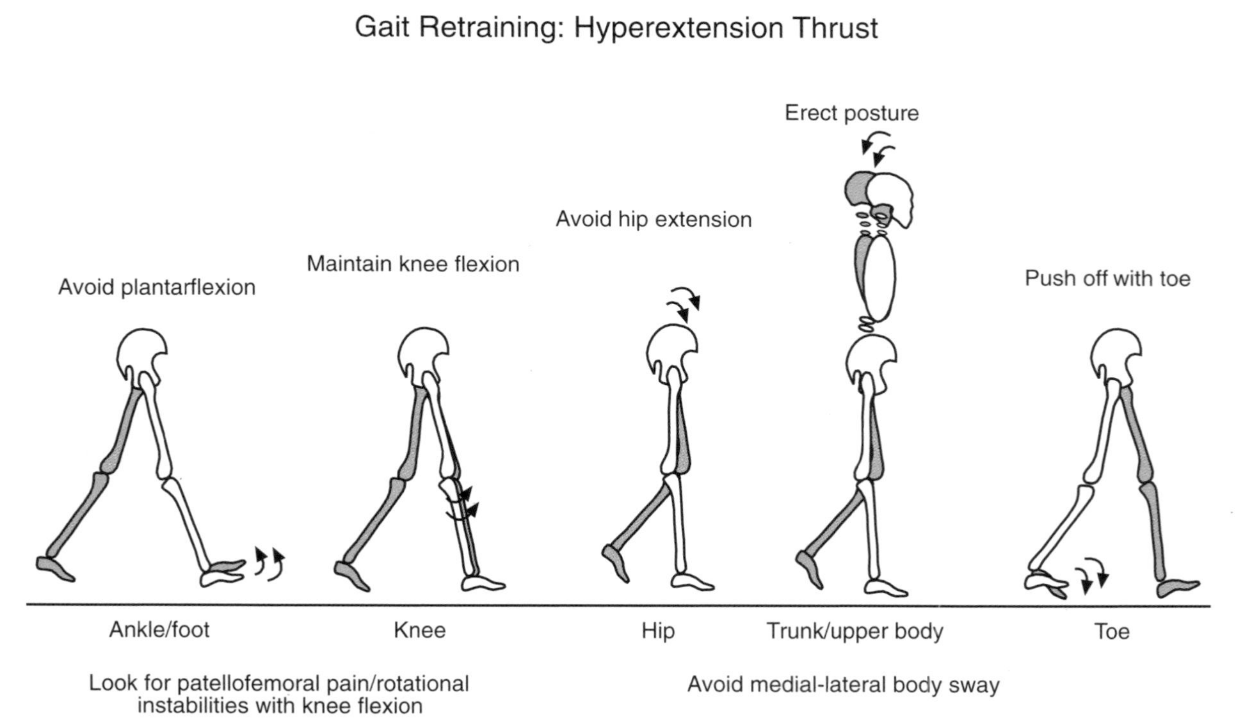

Figure 7.5 Graphic representation of gait abnormalities observed in patients before retraining. Filled gray anatomic structures represent the correct, retrained positions at the trunk and upper body, hip, knee, foot and ankle, and toes. (Adapted with permission from Noyes FR, Dunworth LA, Andriacchi TP, Andrews M, Hewett TE. Knee hyperextension gait abnormalities in unstable knees. Recognition and preoperative gait retraining. *Am J Sports Med* 24(1): 35-45, 1996.)

a triple varus knee and a hyperextension gait pattern (28). A flexed knee gait is introduced to strengthen the quadriceps muscle and contributes to the rehabilitation process. A flexed knee stance at approximately 5° at heel strike and 20° at loading response increases the moment arm of the quadriceps tendon and thus increases the mechanical advantage to the quadriceps muscle (37). A gait retraining program provides increased strength and endurance of the lower-extremity muscles and prevents abnormal loading of ligaments and soft tissue during knee hyperextension. Snyder-Mackler and coworkers (41) have noted an improvement in functional gait, knee flexion in particular, with improvement of quadriceps muscle strength.

Thrusting hyperextension motion at the knee is associated with an abnormally high adduction moment, which tends to increase medial compartment compression forces and lateral distraction forces. This moment may place ACL and posterolateral reconstructions at risk for stretching out posteriorly. The failure to recognize a hyperextension gait pattern and to institute gait retraining preoperatively may lead to failure of reconstructed ligaments if the abnormal gait pattern is resumed postoperatively.

The characteristics of the hyperextension gait pattern appear to be important factors in how the gait retraining affects the final outcome of the mechanics of the walking pattern. Patients with a type II pattern (knee hyperextension throughout the stance phase) (28) appear to be better suited for gait retraining (see figure 7.6). Patients with a type I pattern (early and midstance hyperexten-

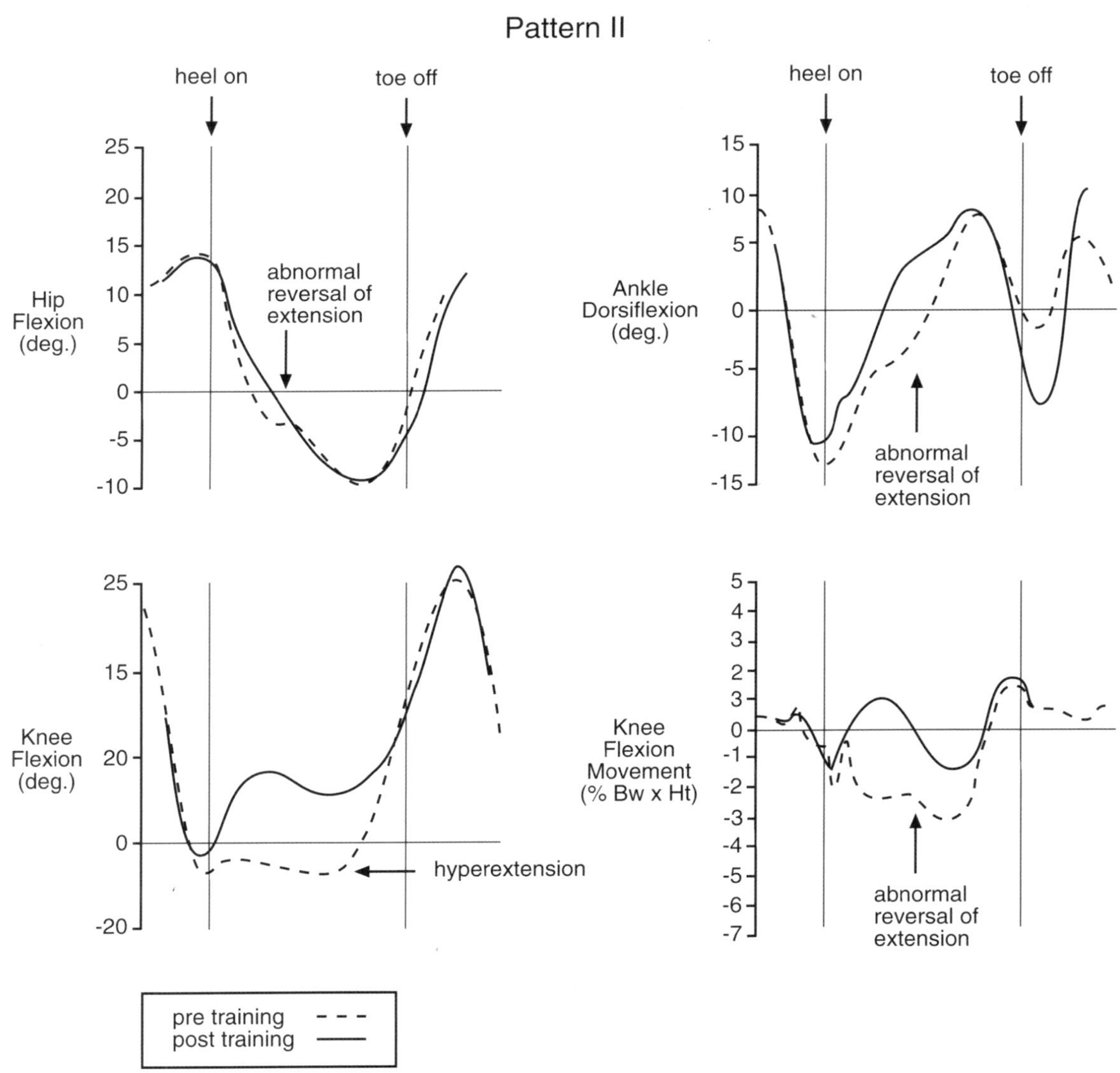

Figure 7.6 Abnormal flexion-extension moment in triple varus knees: pattern II. (Adapted with permission from Noyes FR, Dunworth, LA, Andriacchi TP, Andrews M, Hewett TE. Knee hyperextension gait abnormalities in unstable knees. Recognition and preoperative gait retraining. *Am J Sports Med* 24(1): 35-45, 1996.)

sion with knee flexion in between) have more difficulty in retraining as they must control a rapid "back and forth" hyperextension-flexion-hyperextension pattern (see figure 7.7). These patients may have severe ambulatory problems, often requiring a crutch support or a knee brace, and require more intensive retraining to regain a normal flexion-extension gait pattern. Retraining of neuromuscular patterning at the lower extremity can lead to the correction of abnormal transverse plane motions and moments in even the most recalcitrant patient.

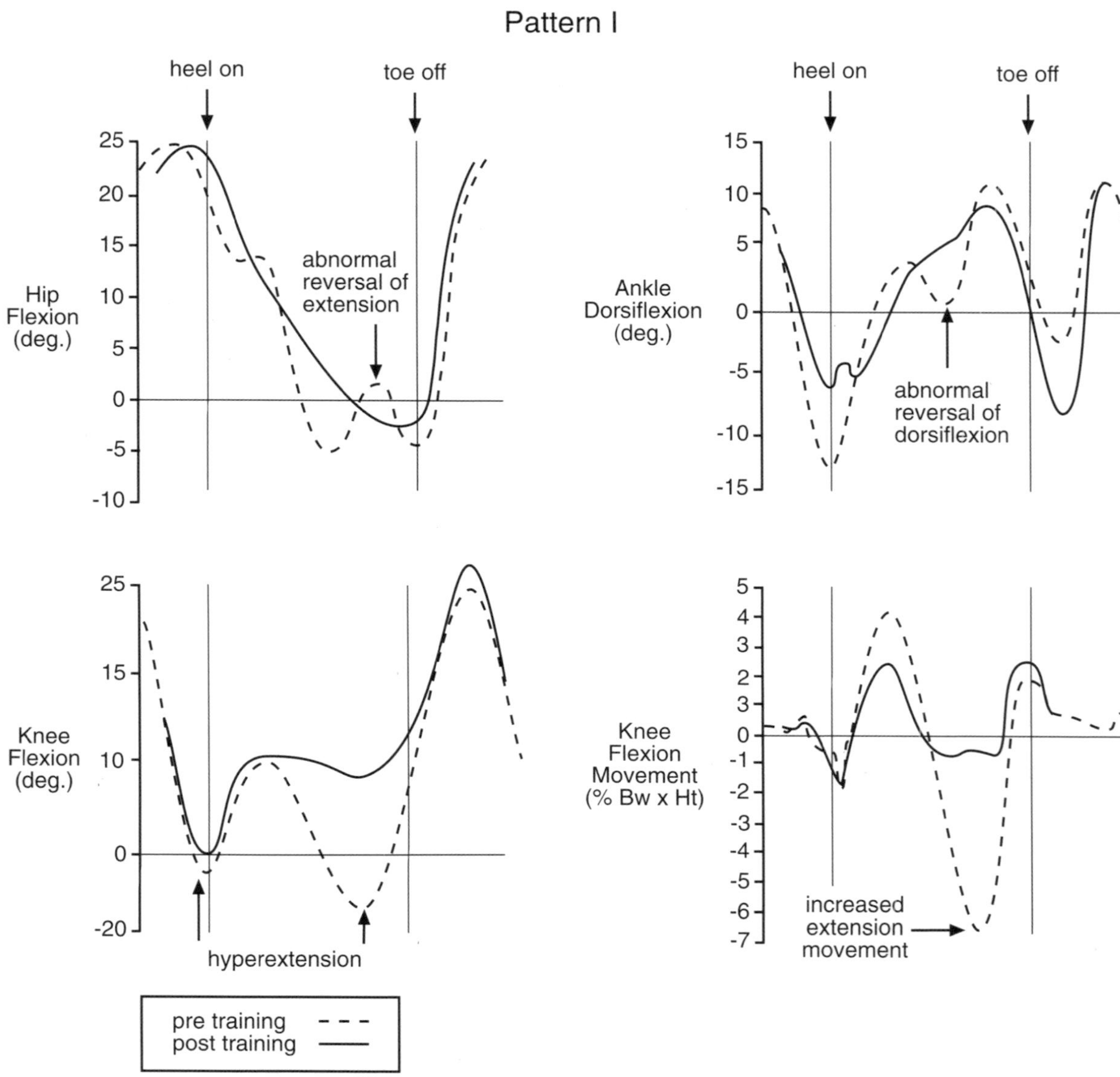

Figure 7.7 Abnormal flexion-extension moment in subject with hyperextension gait: pattern I. (Adapted with permission from Noyes FR, Dunworth LA, Andriacchi TP, Andrews M, Hewett TE. Knee hyperextension gait abnormalities in unstable knees. Recognition and preoperative gait retraining. *Am J Sports Med* 24(1): 35-45, 1996.)

References

1. Andersson C, Odensten M, Good L, Gillquist J. Surgical or nonsurgical treatment of acute rupture of the ACL: A randomized study with long-term follow-up. *J Bone Joint Surg* 71A(7): 965–74, 1989.
2. Andrews M, Noyes FR, Hewett TE, Andriacchi TP. Lower-limb alignment and foot angle are related to stance phase knee adduction in normal subjects: A critical analysis of the reliability of gait analysis data. *J Orthop Res* 14(2): 289–95, 1996.
3. Andriacchi TP, Galante JO, Draganich LF. Relationship between knee extensor mechanics and function following total knee replacement. In *Proceedings of the 1st Annual Meeting of the Knee Society,* 83–94. Baltimore: University Park Press, 1985.
4. Arms SW, Pope MH, Johnson RJ, Fischer RA, Arvidsson I, Eriksson E. The biomechanics of anterior cruciate ligament rehabilitation and reconstruction. *Am J Sports Med* 12(1): 8–18, 1984.
5. Barrack RL, Bruckner JD, Kniesl J, Inman WS, Alexander AH. The outcome of nonoperatively treated complete tears of the anterior cruciate ligament in active young patients. *Clin Orthop Rel Res* 259: 192–99, 1990.
6. Berchuck M, Andriacchi TP, Bach BR, Reider B. Gait adaptations by patients who have a deficient anterior cruciate ligament. *J Bone Joint Surg* 72A(6): 871–77, 1990.
7. Beynnon BD, Fleming BC, Johnson RJ, Nichols CE, Renstrom PA, Pope MH. Anterior cruciate ligament strain behavior during rehabilitation exercises in vivo. *Am J Sports Med* 23(1): 24–34, 1995.
8. Buss DD, Min R, Skyhar M, Galinat B, Warren RF, Wickiewicz TL. Nonoperative treatment of acute anterior cruciate ligament injuries in a selected group of patients. *Am J Sports Med* 23(2): 160–65, 1995.
9. Eberhart HD, Inman VT, Saunders JB, Levens AS, Bresler B, McCowan TD. Fundamental studies of human locomotion and other information relating to the design of artificial limbs. In *National Research Council Committee on Artificial Limbs*: University of California at Berkeley, 1947.
10. Gage JR. An overview of normal walking. Instructional Course Lectures XXXIX: 291–303, 1990.
11. Grood ES, Noyes FR. Diagnosis of knee ligament injuries: Biomechanics precepts. In *The Crucial Ligaments,* Feagin J, (ed), New York: Churchill Livingstone, 1988.
12. Grood ES, Suntay WJ, Noyes FR, Butler DL. Biomechanics of the knee extension exercise: Effect of cutting the anterior cruciate ligament. *J Bone Joint Surg* 66A(5): 725–34, 1984.
13. Gyory AN, Chao EYS, Stauffer RN. Functional evaluation of normal and pathologic knees during gait. *Arch Phys Med Rehab* 57(12): 571–77, 1976.
14. Harrington IJ. Static and dynamic loading patterns in knee joints with deformities. *J Bone Joint Surg* 64A(2): 247–59, 1983.
15. Hewett TE, Noyes FR, Weise MW, Andriacchi TP. A relationship between joint loads and alignment in ACL-deficient knees following high tibial osteotomy. *Orthop Trans,* in press.
16. Howell SM. Anterior tibial translation during a maximum quadriceps contraction: Is it clinically significant? *Am J Sports Med* 18(6): 573–78, 1990.
17. Inman VT, Ralston HJ, Todd F. Human walking. Baltimore: Williams & Wilkins, 1981.
18. Ivarsson I, Larsson LE. Gait analysis in patients with gonarthrosis treated by high tibial osteotomy. *Clin Orthop Rel Res* 239: 185–90, 1989.
19. Johnson F, Leitl S, Waugh W. The distribution of load across the knee: A comparison of static and dynamic measurements. *J Bone Joint Surg* 62B: 346–49, 1980.
20. Kannus P, Jarvinen M. Conservatively treated tears of the anterior cruciate ligament: Long-term results. *J Bone Joint Surg* 69A(7): 1007–1012, 1987.
21. Kettelkamp DB, Johnson RJ, Smidt GL, Chao EYS, Walker M. An electrogoniometric study of knee motion in normal gait. *J Bone Joint Surg* 52A(4): 775–90, 1970.
22. Levens AS, Berkeley CE, Inman VT, Blosser JA. Transverse rotation of the segments of the lower extremity in locomotion. *J Bone Joint Surg* 30A(4): 859–72, 1948.
23. Markolf KL, Kochan A, Amstutz HC. Measurement of knee stiffness and laxity in patients with documented absence of the anterior cruciate ligament. *J Bone Joint Surg* 66A(2): 242–53, 1984.
24. Murray MP. Gait as a total pattern of movement: Including a bibliography on gait. *Am J Phys Med* 46: 290–333, 1967.
25. Nissan M. Review of some basic assumptions in knee biomechanics. *J Biomech* 13: 375–81, 1980.
26. Noyes FR, A. MP, Matthews DS, Butler DL. The symptomatic anterior cruciate deficient knee. Part I: The long-term functional disability in athletically active individuals. *J Bone Joint Surg* 65A(2): 154–62, 1983.
27. Noyes FR, Barber SD, Simon R. High tibial osteotomy and ligament reconstruction in varus angulated, anterior cruciate ligament deficient knees: A two- to seven-year follow-up study. *Am J Sports Med* 21(1): 2–12, 1993.
28. Noyes FR, Dunworth LA, Andriacchi TP, Andrews M, Hewett TE. Knee hyperextension

gait abnormalities in unstable knees: Recognition and preoperative gait retraining. *Am J Sports Med* 24(1): 35–45, 1996.
29. Noyes FR, Grood ES. Diagnosis of knee ligament injuries: Five concepts. In *The Crucial Ligaments,* Feagin J, (ed), New York: Churchill Livingstone, 1988.
30. Noyes FR, Matthews DS, Mooar PA, Grood ES. The symptomatic anterior cruciate-deficient knee. Part II: The results of rehabilitation, activity modification, and counseling on functional disability. *J Bone Joint Surg* 65A(2): 163–74, 1983.
31. Noyes FR, Munns SW, Andriacchi TP, Mayhall MT. The double varus and triple varus anterior cruciate-insufficient knee: Gait analysis and surgical correction. *Trans Am Orthop Soc Sports Med* 11: 41, 1985.
32. Noyes FR, Schipplein OD, Andriacchi TP, Saddemi SR, Weise M. The anterior cruciate ligament-deficient knee with varus alignment: An analysis of gait adaptations and dynamic joint loadings. *Am J Sports Med* 20(6): 707–16, 1992.
33. Noyes FR, Stowers SF, Grood ES, Cummings J, VanGinkel LA. Posterior subluxations of the medial and lateral tibiofemoral compartments: An in vitro ligament sectioning study in cadaveric knees. *Am J Sports Med* 21(3): 407–14, 1993.
34. Ogata K, Yoshii I, Kawamura H, Miura H, Arizono T, Sugioka Y. Standing radiographs cannot determine the correction in high tibial osteotomy. *J Bone Joint Surg* 73B(6): 927–31, 1991.
35. Olmstead TG, Wevers HW, Bryant JT, Gouw GJ. Effect of muscular activity on valgus-varus laxity and stiffness of the knee. *J Biomech* 19(8): 565–77, 1986.
36. Perry J. Gait Analysis: Normal and Pathological Function. In 49–281. Thorofare, NJ: Slack, 1992.
37. Perry J, Antonelli D, Ford W. Analysis of knee joint forces during flexed-knee stance. *J Bone Joint Surg* 57A: 961–67, 1975.
38. Prodromos CC, Andriacchi TP, Galante JO. A relationship between knee joint loads and clinical changes following high tibial osteotomy. *J Bone Joint Surg* 67A(8): 1188–194, 1985.
39. Saunders JB, Inman VT, Eberhart HD. The major determinants in normal and pathological gait. *J Bone Joint Surg* 35A: 543–58, 1953.
40. Schipplein OD, Andriacchi TP. Interaction between active and passive knee stabilizers during level walking. *J Orthop Res* 9(1): 113–19, 1991.
41. Snyder-Mackler L, Ladin Z, Schepsis AA, et al. Electrical stimulation of the thigh muscles after reconstruction of the ACL. *J Bone Joint Surg* 73A: 1025–1036, 1991.
42. Tibone JE, Antich TJ, Fanton GS, Moynes DR, Perry J. Functional analysis of anterior cruciate ligament instability. *Am J Sports Med* 14(4): 276–84, 1986.
43. Wang J, Kuo KN, Andriacchi TP, Galante JO. The influence of walking mechanics and time on the results of proximal tibial osteotomy. *J Bone Joint Surg* 72A(6): 905–909, 1990.

CHAPTER 8

Gross Anatomy of the Shoulder: Bony Geometry, Static and Dynamic Restraints, Sensory and Motor Innervation

Lucio S. Ernlund, MD
Jon J.P. Warner, MD

Neurosensory and Neuromuscular Contributions to Joint Stability

The shoulder is a complex that involves three separate bones (the clavicle, the scapula, and the humerus) and four joints (glenohumeral, acromioclavicular, sternoclavicular, and scapulothoracic). Characterized as a multiaxial, spheroidal, and diarthrodial joint, the glenohumeral joint, the principal articulation of the shoulder, allows for remarkable ranges of motion due to its minimal articular constraints. Its surrounding capsular structures, ligaments, and muscles afford poor stability. However, normal kinematics depends on balanced coordination with scapulothoracic motion. The dynamic balance is maintained through the collaborative effect of ligaments and muscles mediated through proprioceptive afferent feedback.

The glenohumeral joint anatomic stability is divided into static and dynamic. This chapter presents the anatomic basis for proprioception and neuromuscular control of the shoulder joint.

Bony Geometry of the Humeral Head and Glenoid Fossa

Two conflicting functions are required for joint motion: to facilitate the desired motion and to restrict undesirable motion. Therefore the stable joint is the result of the sum of static bony congruity and ligament and capsular restraints, and dynamic stability from surrounding muscles (1).

The humeral head and the glenoid fossa of the scapula form the glenohumeral joint. Even though it is classified as a spheroidal (ball-and-socket) joint, as opposed to the hip joint, it has a lack of intrinsic stability, which allows for the large range of motion normally accessible to the glenohumeral articulation. Both the articular surfaces of the humeral head and the glenoid are curved and ovoid in the cross section. Despite the mismatch in the bony congruency between the glenohumeral joint surfaces, stereophotogrammetric studies of the curvature of fresh frozen human cadaver shoulders have shown the deviation from sphericity of the cartilaginous surface to be less than 1% (2). This discrepancy between bony and articular cartilage congruency is due in part to differences in thickness of the layer of hyaline cartilage that covers the articular surfaces. Whereas this layer is thicker at the periphery and thinner centrally of the glenoid, the reverse occurs in the humeral head (3, 4). One-half of the total depth of the glenoid fossa is provided by the surrounding labrum and the other half by the bony configuration and articular cartilage (2).

The glenoid fossa of the scapula has a comma-shaped face measuring an average of 25 mm anteroposteriorly and 35 mm superoinferiorly. By contrast, the humeral head has dimensions of 45 mm anteroposteriorly and 48 mm superoinferiorly. Thus, only 30% of the humeral head surface articulates with the glenoid throughout shoulder ranges of motion (5). This relationship was described by Saha (6) as the glenohumeral index (GHI), which is the ratio of the maximum glenoid diameter to the maximum humeral head diameter. The GHI is calculated to be 0.75 in the sagittal plane and 0.76 in the transverse plane (6–8).

Saha (6) classified the glenohumeral joint into three types: type A, in which the glenoid fossa has a curvature greater than the humeral head; type B, found most frequently in normal individuals, in which the glenoid fossa and the humeral head have the same curvature; and type C, in which the glenoid fossa has a curvature smaller than the humeral head. Saha also studied the glenoid orientation relative to the axial plane of the scapula using axillary and anteroposterior plane radiographs. He observed that 73.5% of his cases had an average of 7.4° of retroversion and 26.5% had anteversion ranging from 2° to 10°. Yet, because the plane of the scapula faces 30° anteriorly on the chest wall, the glenoid is anteverted 23° to 40° with respect to the coronal plane of the body (see figure 8.1). The glenoid is superiorly tilted an average of 5° relative to the scapula plane (6, 9) (see figure 8.2). This superior inclination has been shown to be an important factor in the stability of the glenohumeral joint (2).

Hurley and associates (10) described a computed tomography study designed to evaluate those patients with recurrent posterior shoulder instability. Their results showed an increasing glenoid retroversion on this population, suggesting that variable degrees of glenoid version may be associated with unstable shoulders.

Radiographic studies performed by Saha (6) demonstrated that the neck-shaft angle averages 130° to 140° with a retroversion of 30°, on average, relative to the transepicondylar line (see figure 8.3). These studies confirmed previous descriptions of French anatomists almost a century ago (11, 12).

The lesser tuberosity lies on the anterior aspect of the proximal humerus opposite the greater tuberosity in relation to the bicipital groove. These two tubercles are the insertion sites of the muscles of the rotator cuff (subscapularis inserts in the lesser tuberosity and supraspinatus, infraspinatus, and teres minor insert in the greater tuberosity). These attachments contouring the humeral head control part of the dynamic stability of the glenohumeral joint by producing compression forces toward the center of the joint.

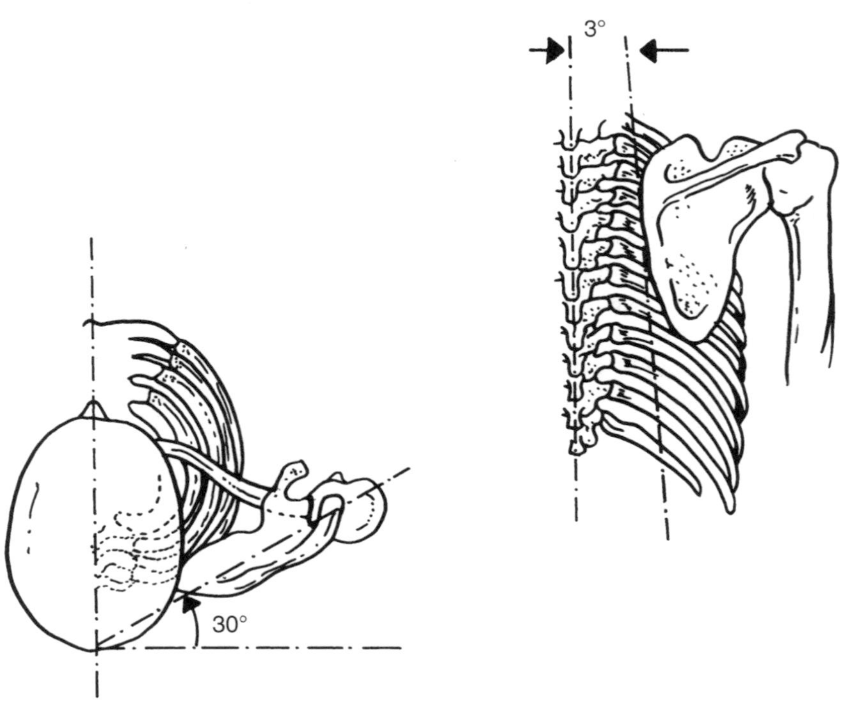

Figure 8.1 The scapular orientation on the chest wall: 30° anterior (left), 3° upward (right).

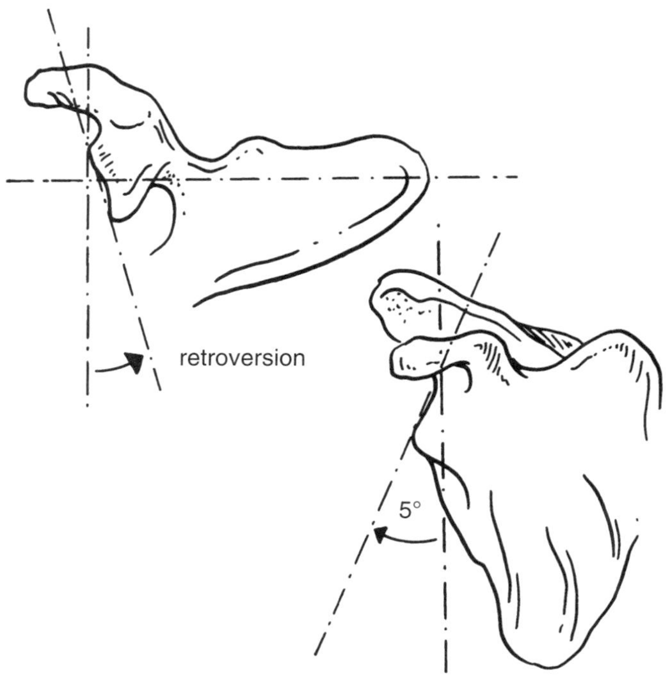

Figure 8.2 The scapular average 7° glenoid tilt (left) and 5° superior tilt (right).

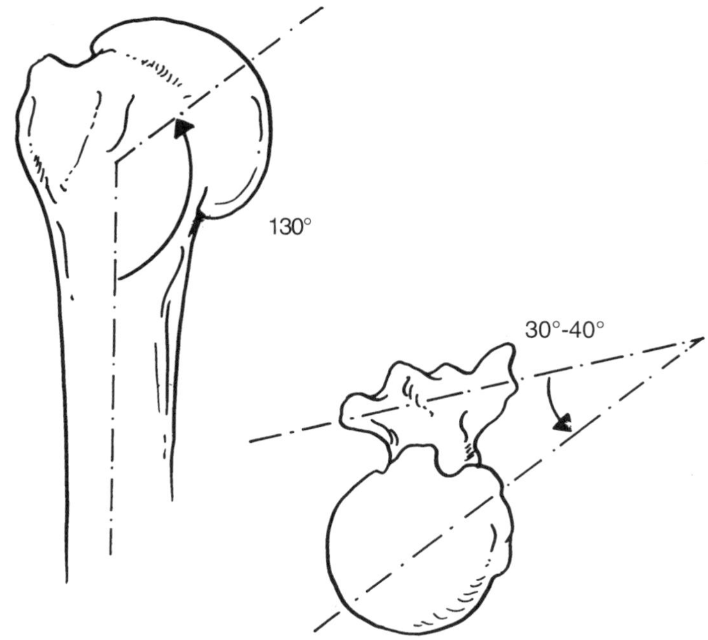

Figure 8.3 The scapular 130° neck-shaft angle (left) and the 30° to 40° retrotorsion relative to transepicondylar line (right).

Static Restraints

Articular Components

The scapulohumeral complex in humans has undergone a series of evolutionary stages that exchanged stability for mobility in order to promote the prehensile activity of the upper limb required by the erect position of the human being (8, 13). Normal bony geometry, as previously described in this chapter, as well as balanced muscular forces controlled by proprioceptive receptors (14) are critical components of a stable shoulder joint.

Glenoid Labrum

The labrum, as described by Perthes (15) and Bankart (16), is a fibrous triangular extension of the rim of the glenoid fossa. Its anatomy varies in size, thickness, presence, and attachment (17, 18). The most consistent finding is the anteroinferior attachment of the inferior glenohumeral ligament. In this region the labrum is consistently found to be firmly attached to the glenoid rim and is immobile. The anterosuperior labrum, above the equator of the glenoid, can be small or absent or even detached from the glenoid (7, 19). Recently, a unique variant of the normal capsulolabral anatomy, termed the Bufford complex, was described in 1.5% of 200 shoulder arthroscopies (20).

The glenoid labrum contributes to the control of glenohumeral joint stability by increasing the depth of the glenoid area, therefore increasing the humeral head fit to the glenoid. It may also act as a "chock block" to the translation of the humeral head out of the glenoid as well as forming the anchoring point for the glenohumeral ligaments and long head of the biceps tendon (7, 19, 21, 22) (see figure 8.4).

On the other hand, Townley (23) and Reeves (24) performed the removal of the anterior labrum through a posterior approach maintaining the integrity of the anterior capsular structures. They observed no anterior dislocation of the humeral head and concluded that secure attachments of the glenohumeral ligaments are more important than labrum integrity to prevent glenohumeral dislocations. Warner and coworkers, in their analyses of the results of arthroscopic Bankart lesion repair with a cannulated absorbable device, concluded that a complete healing of the Bankart repair does not seem to be a prerequisite for shoulder stability (25–27). Recent work by Lippitt and associates (28) demonstrated that the concavity-compression mechanism performed by the rotator cuff musculature represents an efficient glenohumeral stabilizer.

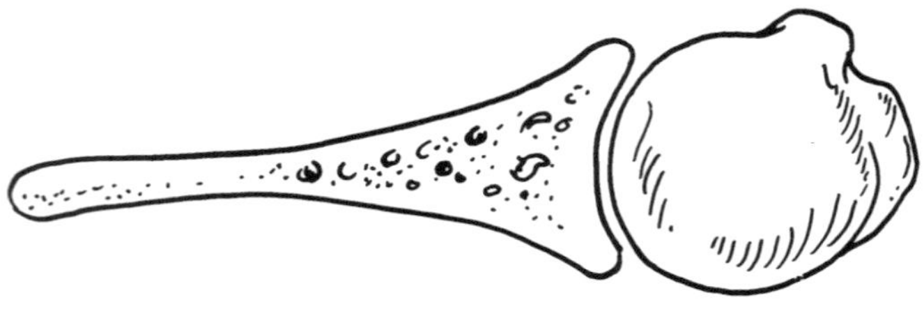

Figure 8.4 The glenoid concave shape and the chock effect of the labrum.

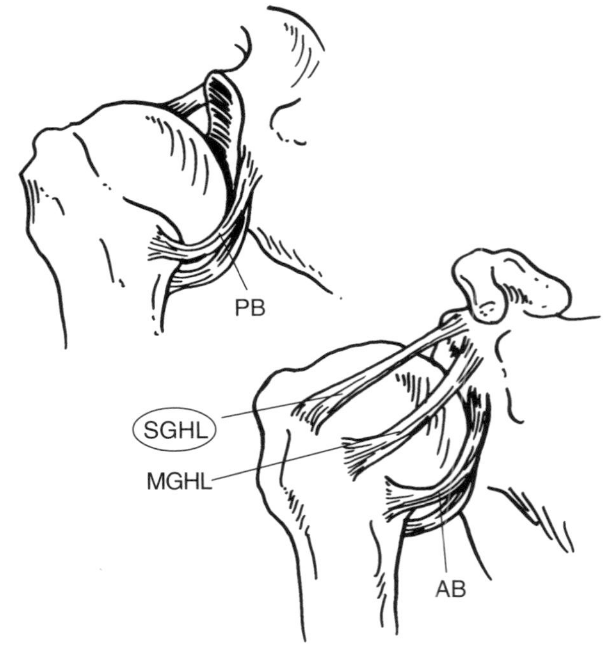

Figure 8.5 At 0° abduction the superior glenohumeral ligament (SGHL), and secondarily the middle glenohumeral ligament, is taut while the inferior glenohumeral complex (IGHLC) is lax.

Capsule and Ligaments

The glenohumeral ligaments are collagenous thickenings of the capsule of the shoulder joint (29, 30). They are best visualized arthroscopically without distention of the capsule (13, 17, 31), and their function is related to their integrity and attachment sites and to the position of the arm.

The anatomic gap between the anterior border of the supraspinatus tendon and the superior border of the subscapularis tendon is the triangularly shaped region known as the rotator interval. The superior glenohumeral ligament (SGHL) and the coracohumeral ligament (CHL) are the two ligamentous structures about the rotator interval, with the former bridging the interval and the latter attaching adjacent to the insertion of the long head of the biceps tendon (1, 8, 13, 32).

The CHL is a dense and fibrous structure with its origin in the lateral surface of the coracoid process and its insertion in the lesser and greater tuberosities adjacent to the bicipital groove, forming its roof (32, 33). Anatomic dissections carried out on 100 shoulders of fresh cadaver specimens demonstrated that the CHL is loose with internal rotation of the shoulder and taut as the shoulder is moved into external rotation below 60° of glenohumeral abduction, or extended and externally rotated below 60° of glenohumeral abduction, and when the arm is inferiorly pulled. Lesions of this ligament are seen in patients with rotator interval defects (7, 32).

The SGHL is a fairly constant structure that is present in more than 90% of the specimens (34). Recently, biomechanical studies showed that the SGHL has little effect on the static stabilization of the glenohumeral joint (35, 36) (see figure 8.5). Warner and associates (33) showed that the SGHL restrains inferior translation and that the sulcus sign reflects its integrity. Recent studies by Boardman and others (37), however, suggest that the CHL is far more important for shoulder stability.

The middle glenohumeral ligament (MGHL) is identified as the most variable of all glenohumeral ligaments (32, 38). It is not present in approximately 8% to 30% of shoulders (39). Its origin is located on the superior glenoid just below the insertion of the SGHL, medial to the glenoid labrum, and it inserts into the humerus just medial to the lesser tuberosity, under the tendon of the subscapularis (40). Two morphological variations are found for the MGHL: sheetlike and confluent with the anterior band of the inferior glenohumeral ligament (IGHL) or cordlike with a foraminal separation between it and the anterior band of the IGHL. It has been identified as a critical restrainer to external rotation of the glenohumeral joint between 60° and 90° of abduction (32).

The IGHL functions as a complex (IGHLC) consisting of an anterior band, an axillary pouch, and a posterior band arranged in such a way that simulates a hammock (39, 41). The IGHLC is the primary stabilizer for anterior, posterior, and inferior instability of the abducted glenohumeral joint (36, 42). It has its origin from the glenoid, labrum, or neck of the glenoid and labrum, and it inserts into the anatomic neck of the humerus (35, 39). At 45° of shoulder abduction the IGHLC develops, along with the MGHL, the most strain. At 90° of abduction the IGHLC plays an important role in anterior shoulder stability (42) (see figures 8.6 and 8.7).

Bigliani and associates (43) recently published their study on the tensile properties of the IGHLC.

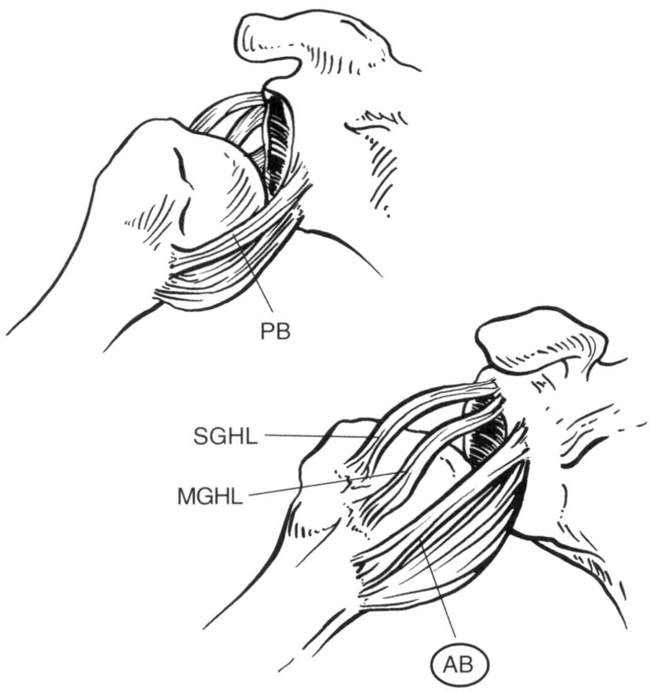

Figure 8.6 At 45° abduction all ligaments are lax.

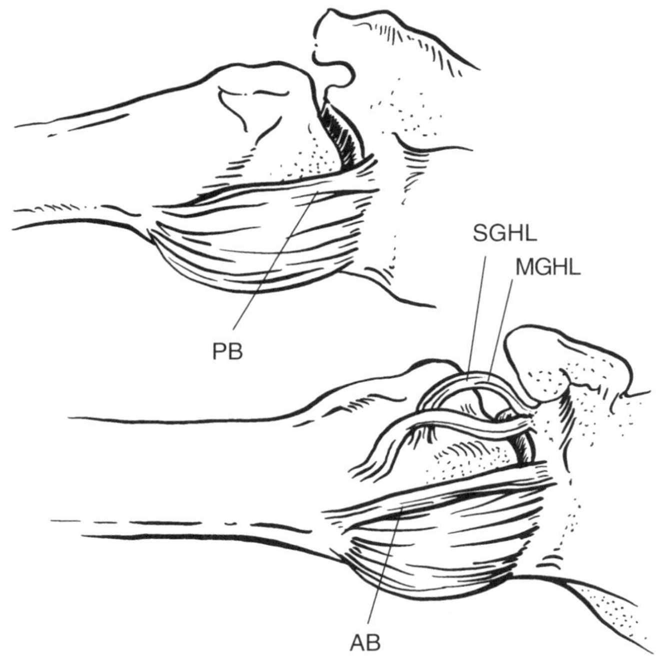

Figure 8.7 At 90° all of the superior ligaments are lax while the inferior ligaments are taut.

They concluded that the ligaments are not strong enough to statically resist shoulder dislocation, and they must work together with well-balanced muscles to prevent glenohumeral instability.

Negative Intraarticular Pressure

The glenohumeral joint has a normal negative intraarticular pressure relative to the atmospheric pressure. This factor is the consequence of the high osmotic pressure in the surrounding tissues, which acts to drain water from the joint. Although the glenohumeral joint can accommodate more than 30 cc of fluid, it normally contains less than 1 cc of fluid (2). Cadaveric studies have been carried out to investigate the role of the intraarticular negative pressure in shoulder stability. The researchers concluded that the negative intraarticular pressure is probably clinically important only in an adducted shoulder at rest. Arthroscopy and arthrography cause venting of the glenohumeral capsule and increased inferior laxity may occur (42, 44–46).

Dynamic Restraints

Rotator Cuff Muscles

This four-unit musculotendinous structure (subscapularis, supraspinatus, infraspinatus, and teres minor muscles) arises from the anterior and posterior aspects of the scapula and inserts in a hemispheric fashion about the lateral aspect of the proximal humerus (3, 11, 12). It represents the true dynamic stabilizer of the glenohumeral joint.

The subscapularis represents the anterior portion of the rotator cuff and arises from the subscapularis fossa on the anterior face of the scapula with insertion as a broad tendon on the lesser tuberosity. In shoulder arthroscopic procedures the subscapularis is distinct from the other muscles of the rotator cuff in its intraarticular appearance (17, 31). Its superior border is reinforced by the coracohumeral ligament, which creates, along with the supraspinatus tendon, the rotator interval (47).

The subscapularis muscle functions as an internal rotator, passive stabilizer to anterior subluxation, and humeral head depressor (48). The latter improves the efficiency of the moment arm of the deltoid in shoulder elevation.

The innervation of the subscapularis is accomplished by the upper and lower subscapular nerves, and their points of entry into the muscle have been studied by Checchia and associates (49). They concluded that the subscapular nerve entrance could be as close as 1 cm to the glenoid border, putting the nerve at risk when extensive release is performed.

The supraspinatus (SS) originates from the supraspinatus fossa and passes beneath the coracoacromial arch, inserting as a broad tendon on the greater tuberosity. The SS tendon is visualized easily arthroscopically with capsular distention (17).

The supraspinatus compresses the humeral head against the glenoid fossa and along with the deltoid muscle elevates the arm. Although both muscles are active during all ranges of motion, the deltoid becomes progressively more efficient with the improvement of its moment arm (2).

The suprascapular nerve, after emerging from the scapular notch beneath the transverse scapular ligament, is responsible for the innervation of the SS with two motor branches (3, 11, 12). Because of this unique anatomic characteristic this nerve could be entrapped at a number of locations along its course (50, 51).

The infraspinatus (IS) originates at the infraspinatus fossa of the scapula and inserts in a common tendon with the supraspinatus and teres minor at the greater tuberosity (3, 11, 12). It is primarily an external rotator and a humeral head depressor. According to Cain and associates (52), the IS, along with the teres minor muscle, is the most effective controller of strain of anterior structures of the shoulder due to its capacity to pull the humeral head posteriorly during external rotation of the shoulder.

The inferior branch of the suprascapular nerve divides into three to four motor branches after crossing the spinoglenoid notch innervating the IS muscle. This is also a site for nerve entrapment, which will lead to the differential diagnosis of rotator cuff tear (50).

The teres minor muscle has its origin from the middle portion of the lateral border of the scapula and the dense fascia of the infraspinatus. Its insertion site is the lower portion of the greater tuberosity. On its inferior border lies the triangular space medially and the quadrangular space laterally, which are crossed by the circumflex scapular artery in the former space and the axillary nerve and posterior humeral circumflex artery in the latter space.

The teres minor provides 45% of the shoulder external rotation force. Along with the IS muscle it also controls stability in the anterior direction (52). The teres minor is innervated by the posterior branch of the axillary nerve.

Biceps Tendon

The long head of the biceps brachii has its origin at the supraglenoid tubercle and the superior-most portion of the glenoid. The biceps brachii is innervated by branches of the musculocutaneous nerve. The biceps tendon is an intraarticular but extrasynovial structure (53), and it is the landmark that practitioners use to keep oriented during arthroscopic examination of the shoulder (31). After exiting the joint through a capsule defect the biceps tendon enters the bicipital groove where it is retained by the transverse humeral ligament. This is the portion of the tendon most often involved in pathologies.

Rodosky and associates (54) conducted a study to determine the role of the long head of the biceps in anterior stability of the shoulder. It was their conclusion that the biceps tendon helps to diminish the stress placed on the inferior glenohumeral ligament. The long head of the biceps is also considered an important humeral head depressor in the event of a rotator cuff tear (55). However, recent studies have suggested that its role may be minimal or nonexistent for superior stability of the joint during abduction in the plane of the scapula (56, 57).

Scapulothoracic Motion

Overhead activities require an optimal balance between mobility and stability of the shoulder joint, and a normal scapulothoracic muscle function is required for coordinated arm elevation. The serratus anterior and the trapezius are the most important muscles for scapula stabilization during arm elevation (48, 58–60), and they are more prone to fatigue during repetitive overhead activities such as swimming and throwing (61).

Warner and associates (58) designed a study using Moiré topographic analysis to evaluate the scapulothoracic motion. They demonstrated 36% scapular winging in patients with instability and a higher position of the scapula on the chest wall in the symptomatic shoulder as compared to the contralateral asymptomatic side in impingement patients. The serratus anterior protraction of the scapula, observed in the normal kinematics of the scapulothoracic motion, helps the trapezius rotate the scapula upward while keeping it stabilized against the chest wall. In both groups of the Warner study the fatigue and weakness of the serratus anterior, commonly seen in eccentric muscle contraction, permitted the coracoacromial arch to descend and impinge against the greater tuberosity during shoulder overhead elevation (58, 62).

This mechanism of injury is observed in the secondary impingement syndrome in throwing athletes, swimmers, golf players, and tennis players, as they all have the same pattern of overhead motion during their sport activities (63). A program of exercises directed to strengthen the scapular stabilizer muscles should be instituted among individuals with scapulothoracic disfunction (64).

Sensory and Motor Innervation

Both superficial and deep structures of the shoulder joint are innervated by the extensive network of nerves that cross this region. These nerves are derived from the C5, C6, and C7 nerve roots and in some individuals from the C4 root (3, 11–13, 36).

The ligaments, capsule, and synovial membrane of the shoulder are innervated by the axillary, suprascapular, subscapular, and musculocutaneous nerves, as they all cross the joint. The axillary and suprascapular nerves provide most of the nerve supply to the anterior capsule and glenohumeral joint (3, 11–13, 36, 49). The two branches of the suprascapular nerve are responsible for the innervation of the superior aspect of the shoulder (3, 11–13, 36, 51). Posteriorly, the main nerves are the suprascapular nerve in the upper region and the axillary nerve in the lower region. Inferiorly, the anterior portion is primarily supplied by the axillary nerve, and the posterior portion is supplied by a combination of the axillary nerve and lower ramifications of the suprascapular nerve.

The skin innervation over the shoulder is provided by the supraclavicular nerves, which come from the C3 and C4 nerve roots. The lateral brachial cutaneous nerve, which is a continuation of the axillary nerve, innervates the lower posterior and lateral aspects of the shoulder (3, 11–13).

Shoulder proprioception is mediated by peripheral receptors in articular, muscular, and cutaneous structures (14). The glenoid labrum and the glenohumeral ligaments have been found to contain nociceptive free nerve endings and mechanoreceptors such as Ruffini endings, Pacinian corpuscles and Golgi tendon organlike endings. Muscle and joint receptors are probably complementary to each other as they play a role in shoulder stability. Damage to this proprioceptor network will lead to shoulder joint instability (14).

References

1. Jobe CM: Gross anatomy of the shoulder. In Rockwood CA Jr, Matsen FA III (eds): *The Shoulder.* Philadelphia: Saunders, 1990, 34–97.
2. Simon SR (ed): *Orthopaedic Basic Science.* Rosemont, IL: American Academy of Orthopaedic Surgeons, 1994, 523–602.
3. Williams PL, Warwick R (eds): *Gray's Anatomy,* 36th ed. Philadelphia: Saunders, 1980.
4. Soslowsky LJ, Flatow EL, Bigliani LU, Mow VC: Articular geometry of the glenohumeral joint. *Clin Orthop Rel Res* 1992, 185: 181–90.
5. Boardman ND, Fu FH: Shoulder biomechanics. In McGinty JB, Caspari RB, Jackson RW, Poehling GG (eds): *Operative Arthroscopy.* Philadelphia: Lippincott-Raven, 1996, 625–33.
6. Saha AK: Dynamic stability of the glenohumeral joint. *Acta Orthop Scand* 1971, 42: 491–505.
7. Warner JP, Schulte KR, Imhoff AB: Current concepts in shoulder instability. *Advances Op Orthop* 1995, 3: 217–47.
8. Warner JP: The gross anatomy of the joint surfaces, ligaments, labrum, and capsule. In Matsen FA III, Fu FH, Hawkins RJ (eds): *The Shoulder: A Balance of Mobility and Stability.* Rosemont, IL: American Academy of Orthopaedic Surgeons, 1993, 7–27.
9. Basmajian JV, Bazant FJ: Factors preventing downward dislocation of the adducted shoulder joint in an electromyographic and morphological study. *J Bone Joint Surg* 1959, 41A: 1182–186.
10. Hurley JA, Anderson TE, Dear W, et al.: Posterior shoulder instability: Surgical versus conservative results with evaluation of glenoid version. *Am J Sports Med* 1992, 20: 396–400.
11. Testut L: *Traité d'anatomie humaine,* tome 1:*Osteologie, arthrologie, myologie,* ed 7. Paris: Doin, 1921.
12. Testut L, Jacob O: *Traité d'anatomie topographique avec applications medico-chirurgicales,* tome 2. Paris: Doin, 1909.
13. O'Brien SJ, Arnoczky SP, Warren RF, Rozbruch SR: Developmental anatomy of the shoulder and anatomy of the glenohumeral joint. In Rockwood CA Jr, Matsen FA III (eds): *The Shoulder.* Philadelphia: Saunders, 1990, 1–33.
14. Lephart SM, Warner JP, Borsa PA, Fu FH: Proprioception of the shoulder joint in healthy, unstable, and surgically repaired shoulders. *J Shoulder Elbow Surg* 1994, 3: 371–80.
15. Perthes G: Uber operationen bei habitueller Schulterluxation. *Deutsch Ztschr Chir* 1906, 85: 199–227.
16. Bankart ASB: Recurrent or habitual dislocation of the shoulder joint. *Br Med J* 1923, 2: 1132–133.
17. Hulstyn MJ, Fadale PD: Arthroscopic anatomy of the shoulder. *Orthop Clin North Am* 1995, 26: 597–612.

18. Detrisac DA, Johnson LL: *Arthroscopic Shoulder Anatomy: Pathologic and Surgical Implications.* Thorofare, NJ: Slack, 1996.
19. Cooper DE, Arnoczky SP, O'Brien SJ, et al.: Anatomy, histology, and vascularity of the glenoid labrum: An anatomic study. *J Bone Joint Surg* 1992, 74A: 46–52.
20. Williams MM, Snyder SJ, Bufford D Jr: The Bufford complex—the "cordlike" middle glenohumeral ligament and absent anterosuperior labrum complex: A normal anatomic capsulolabral variant. *Arthroscopy* 1994, 10: 241–47.
21. Howell SM, Galinat BJ: The glenoid-labral socket: A constraint articular surface. *Clin Orthop* 1989, 243: 122–25.
22. Lippitt SB, Vanderhooft JE, Harris SL, et al.: Glenohumeral stability from concavity-compression: A quantitative analysis. *J Shoulder Elbow Surg* 1993, 2: 27–35.
23. Townley CO: The capsular mechanism in recurrent dislocation of the shoulder. *J Bone Joint Surg* 1950, 32A: 370–80.
24. Reeves B: Arthrography in acute dislocation of the shoulder. *J Bone Joint Surg* 1968, 48B: 182.
25. Warner JP, Kann S, Marks P: Arthroscopic repair of combined Bankart and superior labral detachment anterior and posterior lesions: Technique and preliminary results. *Arthroscopy* 1994, 10: 383–91.
26. Warner JP, Miller MD, Marks P, Fu FH: Arthroscopic Bankart repair with the Suretac device. Part I: Clinical observations. *Arthroscopy* 1995, 11: 2–13.
27. Warner JP, Miller MD, Marks P: Arthroscopic Bankart repair with the Suretac device. Part II: Experimental observations. *Arthroscopy* 1995, 11: 14–20.
28. Lippitt SB, Vanderhooft JE, Harris SL, et al.: Glenohumeral stability from concavity compression: A quantitative analysis. *J Shoulder Elbow Surg* 1993, 2: 27–34.
29. Bowen MK, Deng XH, Warner JP, et al.: The effect of joint compression on stability of the glenohumeral joint. *Trans Orthop Res Soc* 1992, 17: 289.
30. Flood V: Discovery of a new ligament. *Lancet* 1829, 671–72.
31. Andrews JR, Carson WG: Shoulder joint arthroscopy. *Orthopedics* 1983, 6: 1157–162.
32. Ferrari DA: Capsular ligaments of the shoulder: Anatomical and functional study of the anterior superior capsule. *Am J Sports Med* 1990, 18: 20–24.
33. Warner JP, Deng X, Warren RF, Torzilli PA: Static capsuloligamentous restraints to superior-inferior translation of the glenohumeral joint. *Am J Sports Med* 1992, 20: 675–85.
34. Harryman DT II, Sidles JA, Clarke JM, et al.: Translation of the humeral head on the glenoid with passive glenohumeral motion. *J Bone Joint Surg* 1990, 72A: 1334–343.
35. Schwartz RE, O'Brien SJ, Warren RF, Torzilli PA: Capsular restraints to anteroposterior motion of the abducted shoulder: A biomechanical study. *Orthop Trans* 1988, 12: 727.
36. Arnoczky SP, Soslowsky LJ: Anatomy of the shoulder: Form reflecting function. In McGinty JB, Caspari RB, Jackson RW, Poehling GG (eds): *Operative Arthroscopy.* Philadelphia: Lippincott-Raven, 1996, 603–24.
37. Boardman ND, III, Debski RE, Warner JP, et al.: Tensile properties of the superior glenohumeral and coracohumeral ligaments. *J Shoulder Elbow Surg* 1996, 4: 249–54.
38. Caborn DNM, Warner JP, Berger R, et al.: Dynamic capsuloligamentous anatomy of the glenohumeral joint. *Trans Orthop Res Soc* 1992, 17: 498.
39. O'Brien SJ, Neves MC, Arnoczky SP, et al.: The anatomy and histology of the inferior glenohumeral ligament complex of the shoulder. *Am J Sports Med* 1990, 18: 449–56.
40. Turkel SJ, Panio MW, Marshall JL, Girgis FG: Stabilizing mechanisms preventing anterior dislocation of the glenohumeral joint. *J Bone Joint Surg* 1981, 63A: 1208–217.
41. O'Connel PW, Nuber GW, Mileski RA, Lautenschlager E: The contribution of the glenohumeral ligaments to anterior stability of the shoulder joint. *Am J Sports Med* 1990, 18: 579–84.
42. Miller MD, Cooper DE, Warner JP: *Review of Sports Medicine and Arthroscopy.* Philadelphia: Saunders, 1995, 113–64.
43. Bigliani LU, Pollock RG, Soslowsky LJ, et al.: Tensile properties of the inferior glenohumeral ligament. *J Orthop Res* 1992, 10: 187–97.
44. Warner JP, Deng X, Warren RF, Torzilli PA, O'Brien SJ: Superoinferior translation in the intact and vented glenohumeral joint. *J Shoulder Elbow Surg* 1993, 2: 99–105.
45. Kumar VP, Balasubramaniam P: The role of atmospheric pressure in stabilizing the shoulder. *J Bone Joint Surg* 1985, 67B: 719–21.
46. Gibb TD, Sidles JA, Harryman DT II, et al.: The effect of capsular venting on glenohumeral laxity. *Clin Orthop* 1991, 268: 120–27.
47. Clark J, Sidles JA, Matsen FA: The relationship

of the glenohumeral joint capsule to the rotator cuff. *Clin Orthop* 1990, 254: 29–34.
48. Inman VT, Saunders JB, Abbott LC: Observations on the function of the shoulder joint. *J Bone Joint Surg* 1944, 26A: 1–30.
49. Checchia SL, Doneux PS, Martins MG, Meireles FS: Subscapularis muscle enervation: The effect of arm position. *J Shoulder Elbow Surg* 1996, 5: 214–18.
50. Moore TP, Hunter RE: Suprascapular nerve entrapment. *Op Tech Sports Med* 1996, 4: 8–14.
51. Warner JP, Krushell RJ, Masquelet, et al.: Anatomy and relationships of the suprascapular nerve: Anatomical constraints to mobilization of the supraspinatus and infraspinatus muscles in the management of massive rotator cuff tears. *J Bone Joint Surg* 1992, 74A: 36–45.
52. Cain PR, Mutschler TA, Fu FH, Lee SK: Anterior stability of the glenohumeral joint: A dynamic model. *Am J Sports Med* 1987, 15: 144–48.
53. Burkhead WZ Jr: The biceps tendon. In Rockwood CA Jr, Matsen FA III (eds): *The Shoulder.* Philadelphia: Saunders, 1990, 791–836.
54. Rodosky MW, Harner CD, Fu FH: The role of the long head of the biceps muscle and superior glenoid labrum in anterior stability of the shoulder. *Am J Sports Med* 1994, 22: 121–30.
55. Perry J: Biomechanics of the shoulder. In Rowe CR (ed): *The Shoulder*. New York: Churchill Livingstone, 1988.
56. Warner JP, McMahon PJ: The role of the long head of the biceps brachii in superior stability of the glenohumeral joint. *J Bone Joint Surg* 1995, 77A: 366–72.
57. Speer JL. Anterior stability of the glenohumeral joint: A dynamic model. *Am J Sports Med* 1987, 15: 144–48
58. Warner JP, Micheli LJ, Arslanian LE, et al.: Scapulothoracic motion in normal shoulders and shoulders with glenohumeral instability and impingement syndrome. *Clin Orthop* 1992, 285: 191–99.
59. Freedman L, Munro R: Abduction of the arm in the scapular plane: Scapular and glenohumeral movements. *J Bone Joint Surg* 1966, 48A: 1503.
60. Saha AK: Mechanics of elevation of the glenohumeral joint. *Acta Orthop Scand* 1973, 44: 668.
61. Glousmann R, Jobe FW, Tibone J, Moynes MS, et al.: Dynamic EMG analysis of the throwing shoulder with glenohumeral instability. *J Bone Joint Surg* 1988, 70A: 220.
62. Perry J: Muscle control of the shoulder. In Rowe CR (ed): *The Shoulder*. New York: Churchill Livingstone, 1988.
63. Ticker JB, Fealy S, Fu FH: Instability and impingement in the athlete's shoulder. *Sports Med* 1995, 19: 418–26.
64. Burkhead WZ Jr, Rockwood CA Jr: Treatment of instability of the shoulder with an exercise program. *J Bone Joint Surg* 1992, 74A: 890–96.

CHAPTER 9

Peripheral Afferents of the Shoulder: Relationship Between Active and Passive Restraints Regulating Muscle Activation

Carlos A. Guanche, MD
Moshe Solomonow, PhD
Robert D. D'Ambrosia, MD

Introduction

The complexity of integrating the bony, muscular, ligamentous, and neural elements in the glenohumeral joint and understanding their interactions is daunting. The obvious components that lend both stability and mobility to the shoulder are the bony, muscular, and, to a certain extent, the ligamentous elements (4). The interaction of all these components is somehow mediated by the nerves supplying the joint. The extent to which the neural elements, especially the afferent portions, are utilized and how proprioceptive information is integrated by higher centers is unknown, except in very broad terms.

One aspect in delineating the workings of the shoulder complex has been the concept of reflexes. These neural influences may mediate or perhaps prevent abnormal joint excursions that result in injuries or progressive pathology of the shoulder (32). Ascertaining whether these reflexes effect immediate changes, which could prevent excessive translations or rotations within the glenohumeral complex, is a difficult project.

Actions about the joint, which we refer to in laymen's terms as reflexes, are not as expedient as the true reflex. In order to allow modification of joint position quickly enough to either avoid or produce motion, the speed of these reflexes needs to be significantly greater (1, 37).

Reflex, then, in the true sense of the word, may not be the proper terminology. The neural interconnections that serve to alter motions about joints should more properly be termed modulators. Their action would be a modifying one, rather than a reaction in an all-or-none pattern (5, 19).

Multilegged organisms display an example of this concept. If the swing phase of one leg is prolonged, the swing phase of the leg in front is blocked. This is an immediate afferent effect (from the blocked limb) unto the central pattern generator, which subsequently slows the swing phase of the next extremity (6). Proprioceptive (afferent) signals may help select the appropriate "synergy" of response from the rest of the body. If we think of these reflexive actions as modulators, then we can begin to incorporate them into treatment algorithms.

Capsular Neuroanatomy

The presence of neural elements within articular tissues would provide an anatomical basis for proprioception and joint position sense within the glenohumeral joint; these elements have been confirmed in essentially all joints of the human body (42). In an early study 120 normal feline knee joints were studied and compared to 18 that had undergone a surgical sympathectomy (33). Microscopy revealed a minority of nerves entering the capsule, independent of vessels. In cats that had undergone complete sympathectomy, the nervous distribution was still present in the capsule and synovium. This study disputed the previously held idea that all capsular fibers were autonomic since they appeared to travel exclusively with blood vessels.

Four general types of neuroreceptors have been identified and analyzed (9). These are Ruffini receptors, Pacinian receptors, Golgi tendon organs, and free nerve endings (see Table 9.1). The specific functions of each of these microanatomic organs have not been fully delineated, but some general comments with respect to their actions and their functions can be made (1, 9).

Ruffini receptors are thinly encapsulated end organs. The receptors are found usually in clusters of three to six corpuscles leading from the parent fiber. These structures vary in size and encapsulation. The nerve fibers that feed them may pass in and out of the corpuscle and are usually continuous with the connective tissue. The morphological variability of these receptors depends on the texture of the surrounding connective tissue (9).

Ruffini receptors are slow adapting, signaling speed and direction of movement. They exhibit a low threshold with a constant base impulse with continued stimulation. They function at the extremes of joint motion and signal impending injury (1).

Pacinian receptors are formed by a myelinated axon entering the base of a multilaminated corpuscle (9). The myelinated axon that enters the base of the corpuscle loses its sheath and continues through the end organ, subsequently terminating near the tip in a bulbous expansion. These receptors generate rapid bursts of impulses, followed by a rapid decline (quick adapting). They are sensitive to acceleration, vibration, or any deformation (1). They are best activated by local compression stimuli and are also responsive to tensile loading of the capsule (14).

These organs are distributed in the fibrous capsule and sometimes intermingled with Ruffini receptors; they are more prevalent in the deeper capsular tissue and especially in the subsynovial fibroadipose tissue.

The Golgi tendon apparatus is identical to that in the musculotendinous junction. It is enclosed within a fine connective tissue capsule and is innervated by a large myelinated parent axon. The nerve loses its sheath and breaks into several diverging branches that end in densely arborizing filaments. The terminal expansions of these fibers encircle small, compact fascicles of collagen from the capsule (9). These receptors are very slow adapting, high threshold organs that register direction of movement and exact joint position (9, 14).

Free nerve endings are present within the capsular tissue and are noncorpuscular, unmyelinated structures. Their size ranges from 0.5 to 1.5 μ and they usually arise from thinly myelinated parents that are anywhere from 1 to 4 μ in size. These fibers are high threshold, nonadaptive receptors that are primarily responsible for nociception. Free nerve endings exist throughout the capsular tissue (9, 14).

Table 9.1 Mechanoreceptor Types, Distributions, and Actions

Receptor type	Average size (microns)	Distribution	Action(s)
Ruffini ending	100 × 4	Interspersed between collagen fibrils	Responds to tissue stress (loads) Limit detectors Slow adapting, low threshold
Pacinian corpuscle	280 × 120	Fibrous capsule and subsynovial fibroadipose tissues	Fast adapting Responds to compression and tensile loading
Golgi tendon organ	600 × 100	Partially encircle collagen fascicles from capsule	Slow adapting, high threshold Registers direction of movement and joint position
Free nerve ending	0.5 to 1.5	Throughout capsular tissues	High threshold, nonadapting Primarily nociceptor

There are also a considerable number of proprioceptive fibers within the skin, muscle, and connective tissue of any particular joint (26, 29). Spindle receptors within muscle, called intrafusal fibers, are attached to sensory nerves. The gamma motor neurons that are attached to these receptors allow for the readjustment of muscle tension and hence, joint position, at all times (26, 34). In fact, it is possible to predict a joint's position using a model based solely on muscle spindle output (34).

More modern microscopic techniques have established the presence of neural elements in the feline shoulder (38). The entire capsular tissue from six shoulder capsules was analyzed using a modified gold chloride method. In all of the sections evaluated, free nerve endings, Golgi tendon organs, Ruffini endings, and Pacinian corpuscles were observed, with free nerve endings being the most numerous (38).

Attempts have been made to quantify the types and distribution of receptors within the glenohumeral joint. In one study, 15 human shoulders were analyzed and found to contain multiple serpentine axons (23). Theoretically, this configuration allows for stretching and motion about the capsule without significant tension on the nervous tissue. Type II (Pacinian) receptors were also identified. All of these were present beneath the synovial membrane and close to the humeral insertions of the joints (21).

Vangsness and others sampled multiple areas about the glenohumeral capsules of human cadavers (40). They identified neuroreceptors in all sections sampled. Pacinian corpuscles, two types of Ruffinis, and free nerve endings were all found. Most abundant were Ruffinis, with Pacinian corpuscles seen in lesser concentration.

Another study sampled three human cadaveric shoulders, with specimens obtained from the superior, middle, and inferior middle glenohumeral ligaments as well as the superior capsule (18). All sections contained neural elements. Within the superior glenohumeral ligament, 51% of the sections contained primarily Ruffini and Golgi receptors. Of the middle glenohumeral ligament specimens, 42% contained primarily Golgi and Ruffini types, while in the inferior glenohumeral ligaments, 48% of the sections contained Ruffini, Pacinian, or Golgi tendon organs (18).

Ide and coworkers have identified neural elements within the more peripheral structures about the glenohumeral joint (20). Three subacromial bursas were harvested and treated with antisera to substance P. Free nerve endings, Pacinian and Ruffini corpuscles, and two unclassified receptors were observed.

Finally, Gohlke and others have further delineated the three-dimensional neuroanatomy of the shoulder (13). Entire joint capsules, including the rotator cuff and coracoacromial ligaments were harvested. The morphology and distribution of mechanoreceptors was analyzed with monoclonal antibodies directed against the 68 kDa subunit of neurofilaments and to the basal lamina protein, laminin. The ligamentous tissue was aneuronal, whereas the periligamentous fatty or loose connective tissue contained a significant amount of nerve fibers. Pacinian corpuscles were found predominantly in the rotator cuff and along the anterior and inferior parts of the capsule. Golgi tendon organs were found only in the musculotendinous junction of the cuff. The receptors that were present within the capsular tissue were found in gaps between the collagen fiber bundles of the middle and outer layers of the capsule (13).

In summary, neural elements are present throughout the glenohumeral articulation in specific patterns. They are concentrated in the areas about the glenohumeral ligaments and accordingly are positioned for the registration of any stress that the joint capsule experiences. Additionally, the neural elements present within the extracapsular tissues must also play some role in registering joint motions. The specific type of receptors found within any given tissue does not appear to be random. Instead, a pattern that would maximize the information being sensed by each joint appears to be present.

Joint Innervation

The macroanatomic makeup of the shoulder joint also has been well evaluated. Gardner's serial sections of seven adult shoulders revealed a rich nerve distribution, with the axillary, anterior thoracic, posterior cord, and suprascapular nerve each found to provide capsular branches (10).

From the axillary nerve, twigs penetrate into the inferior capsule and track superiorly along both the anterior and posterior capsule (10). They penetrate the fibrous capsular layer and the synovial layer.

Posterior cord branches arise just proximal to its termination and traverse the ventral surface of the subscapularis, while others anastomose with articular branches from the axillary nerve. Some also pierce the subscapularis tendon to enter the capsule.

The suprascapular nerve branches into the capsule both before and after its main trunk to the supraspinatus. Both branches ramify adjacent to the capsule and overlap with the axillary nerve distribution.

The anterior inferior, and anterior superior, capsule are most replete with neural elements. Additionally, some sympathetic fibers are seen to track from the stellate ganglion into the capsule along all of the nerves (10).

An additional study evaluated fetal and cadaveric sections for nervous distribution (43). A similar pattern was documented, with the exception that the musculocutaneous nerve was also included as a contributor to the capsule.

In the feline shoulder, the neuroanatomy has been evaluated and follows a pattern similar to that of the human (17, 25, 38). The axillary nerve followed a consistent pattern in six adult cats, forming three consistent branches, which were labeled the anterior axillary articular nerve (AAAN), the inferior axillary articular nerve (IAAN), and the posterior axillary articular nerve (PAAN). These branches distribute themselves along the anterior, inferior, and posterior aspects of the capsule, respectively (17) (see figure 9.1). Additionally, the musculocutaneous nerve was seen to give off a consistent branch immediately prior to its insertion into the biceps muscle. This twig travels in a retrograde fashion along the biceps tendon and inserts into the more lateral aspects of the capsule (25). The suprascapular nerve also supplies the capsule both before and after branching to the supraspinatus (38).

Reflexive Activity About the Joint

Having documented a rich afferent supply to the glenohumeral joint, the next step is to delineate its integration with other structures about the joint. Intuitively, these elements provide sensations from the specific joints (23). Whether these are pain, position, or other sensations is not known. Additionally, the situations in which each of these sensations is registered by an individual have not been fully determined.

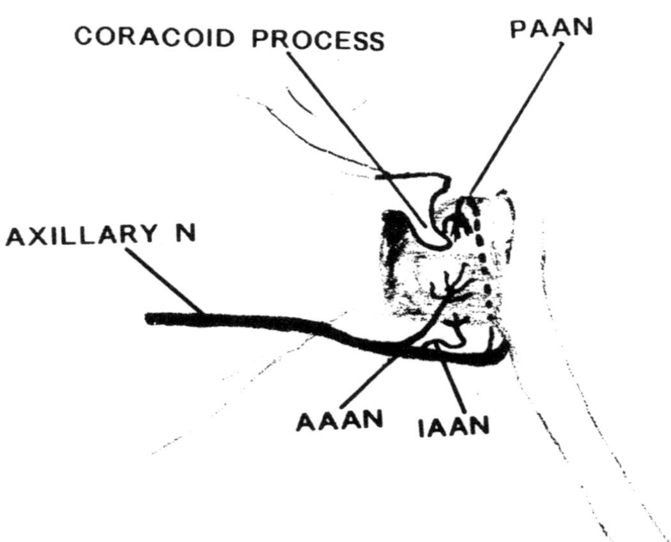

Figure 9.1 Diagrammatic representations of the feline glenohumeral capsule with its axillary nerve branch distribution. Key: AAAN—anterior axillary articular nerve, IAAN—inferior axillary articular nerve, PAAN—posterior axillary articular nerve.

The documentation of any glenohumeral reflexive activity would begin to integrate the neural elements with the muscular and passive elements about the joint. If the neural elements identified in the capsular tissues are afferent in nature, their stimulation should lead to some direct reaction by the musculature about the joint. Despite the fact that reflex activity may not be quick enough to control rapid movements, their possible integration into preprogrammed muscular activity may play a role in control of specific motions (39).

Studies about the knee have shown that there is a reflex that is activated by stress to either the capsular or ligamentous tissue (36). In one study, the feline anterior cruciate ligament (ACL) was stimulated and found to generate a reflexive hamstring contraction (36). A subsequent analysis has also delineated multiple routes of afferent activity emanating from the ACL of the adult feline (28). Subsequent authors have also evaluated this reflex and have found that the reflex occurs primarily after significant deformation of tissue (30).

The first glenohumeral reflexes documented were also in the feline model (17, 25, 38). In these studies, the glenohumeral joint of the adult cat was dissected in a live preparation. Branches of the axillary, subscapular, suprascapular, and musculocutaneous nerves were seen to have variable reflexive activity about the glenohumeral joint. The time from application of the stimuli to the generation of reflexive activity varied from 2.7 to 3.2 ms. Upon transection of these branches immediately distal to the main nerve trunk, reflexive activity was abolished. This lack of activity following transection confirmed the afferent nature of the branches.

The patterns generated by the nerves correlated, at least theoretically, with their presumed function about the joint. Specifically, the axillary nerve reflexive activity elicited was specific for each of three branches, with most of the activity localizing itself to the rotator cuff muscles (17) (see figure 9.2). Additionally, the musculocutaneous nerve reflex initiated a contraction in the biceps muscle (25). Finally, the suprascapular and the subscapular nerves had similar characteristic patterns of contractions with stimulation of their capsular branches, some of which were not muscles innervated by those nerves (38).

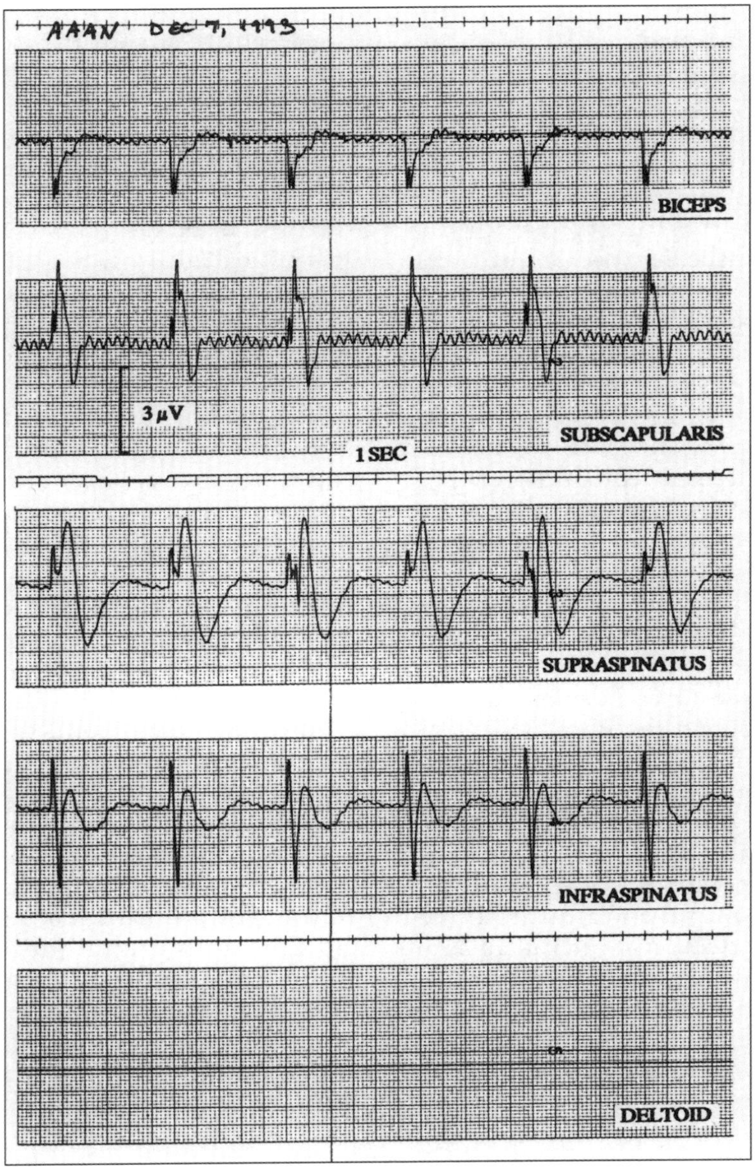

Figure 9.2 Reflexive EMG pattern obtained from stimulation of the anterior axillary articular nerve (AAAN) in the feline shoulder.

In a human study, Jerosch and coworkers confirmed the presence of reflexive activity while patients underwent arthroscopy of their glenohumeral joints (24). Using a bipolar electrode, they were able to establish reflexive activity between the capsule and the deltoid, trapezius, pectoralis, and rotator cuff muscles in 10 patients. The response time varied between 100 and 516 ms (24). This latency period was thought to be too long to be interpreted as a direct reflex.

With the existence of these reflexes, another piece of the puzzle with respect to the connection between the passive (ligamentous) and active (muscular) restraints about the glenohumeral joint has been confirmed. The overall importance of these reflexes, and any other feedback that may occur with activation of these receptors and how they interact, however, remains to be elucidated.

The obvious concern with these reflexive actions is whether or not their latency prevents them from being useful. If they are seen as simple reflexes, then the answer would be no (1). However, if they are seen as part of a network of interactions, which may immediately serve to modify a preprogrammed action at the spinal cord level, then they can be effective in altering motions (39).

Studies of Normal and Abnormal Proprioception

In order to position an extremity in space, a mechanism must exist to coordinate the transition from one alignment to another. The term proprioception has been used to describe this mechanism. Using this mechanism it should be possible to establish what limits the normal joint can achieve with respect to aligning a limb in the same position reproducibly. This concept has been termed the threshold to detection of passive motion (TTDPM) (3, 22, 23, 27).

A similar concept, termed reproduction of passive positioning (RPP), has been used to establish the reproduction of a specific angular position after the subject is removed from that position. Whereas TTDPM is thought to assess proprioception, RPP is thought to correlate to joint position sense (27).

Blasier and coworkers (3) and Lephart and others (27) have determined the normal TTDPM. Blasier found that an absolute angular proprioception of a "best" of 0.78° to a "worst" of 1.08° was reproducible in a normal population. Individuals with clinically determined generalized joint laxity, however, were found to be significantly less sensitive in their ability to detect motion (3). Finally, the detection of external rotation was significantly more sensitive than internal rotation, with this ability being more acute as the limit of external rotation was approached (3).

Lephart and coworkers determined that TTDPM ranged from 1.43° to 2.20° in a normal population (27). In a group of patients with surgically confirmed chronic, recurrent traumatic shoulder dislocations, a significantly higher TTDPM was found. The unstable shoulders also demonstrated significantly less accurate RPP values. When the normal values were compared to values for a group of patients having undergone repair of their instability, no significant mean difference was found for either TTDPM or RPP (27).

In a similar study, 30 patients undergoing anterior capsular repair were tested before and after surgery. At 12 mo follow-up, there was no significant difference between the surgical and uninvolved sides (10). These studies indicate that clinical stability may be established, to some extent, by the "retensioning" of the neural elements, which occurs with capsular reconstruction procedures (27).

The effects of muscular fatigue about the glenohumeral complex have also been documented (41). Employing a technique of RPP, it was found that following a fatigue protocol for the muscles, a significant difference was detected between prefatigue and postfatigue scores. This study underscores the necessity of increasing muscular endurance in shoulder rehabilitation (41). Interestingly, in comparing the available data in the shoulder with respect to that in the knee (35), fatigue does not appear to play a role in the proprioceptive ability of the knee. This may be a reflection of the inherent instability present in the shoulder as compared to the knee.

In a further confirmation of the presence of proprioceptive ability directly attributable to the joint innervation, a group of 60 normal volunteers underwent, while awake, ultrasonographic examination of their glenohumeral joints in order to determine the normal passive range of motion. Following this, each joint was infiltrated with local anesthetic and passive motion was again quantified. With the anesthetic, a significant increase in anterior, posterior, and inferior translation was found (21). The effect of the anesthetic indicates the presence of some physiological feedback mechanism that has some control in the limits of passive motion.

The available data on proprioception in joint position sense indicate that a significant amount of information is transmitted from a joint to a subject's central processing center, which alters joint position determinations. The ability to integrate this feedback into useful information that can be modified to improve either position sense or proprioception, or both, remains a challenge for both clinicians and basic scientists.

Coordination Between Passive and Active Restraints

The interactions of the afferent supply to the glenohumeral joint with the other structures about the joint are important to understand in order to develop treatment algorithms that would alter these interactions. If joint afferents somehow "sculpt" the central nervous system output to the musculature about the shoulder, then proprioceptive elements that respond to mechanical variables associated with muscles and joints would allow the central nervous system to make the available mechanical structures do its bidding for specific motion patterns (19). It appears that afferents play a crucial role in modulating the broad features of motor output. Through central pattern generators, which are constantly at work, afferent inflow is somehow able to mediate a movement or motion, thus altering the ultimate position of the joint. This immediate input and alteration of specific motions and positions is occurring on a constant basis (19).

During muscular action, there is tremendous activity not only in the agonist musculature but also in the antagonist (8). This high level of interaction is necessary for the fluidity of motion of human movement, which is much unlike the stilted movements of robots. More importantly, it is possible that this constant interaction between agonist and antagonist is what controls motions on a moment to moment basis. Moreover, it has been proposed that a direct selective cerebral control over single anterior horn cells exists (2). This concept would make possible a highly interrelated system that allows for the control of any motion and any required alteration on a short notice of less than a few milliseconds. While this may not be expedient enough to prevent injury from a sudden traumatic event, it would certainly augment motions that are under a person's control, such as pitching.

It may be possible to alter some of this interaction between the agonists and antagonists at any point. With muscular training, the control strategy that is employed by a certain muscle does not appear to change. However, the interaction of the muscle being trained with its antagonists is influenced. In other words, a diminution in antagonist activity is seen with periods of training (7, 39). Therefore, with specific training protocols, it may be possible to either decrease or increase the agonist or antagonist activity to effect a desired alteration in a motion.

The afferent activity from mechanoreceptors positioned in strategic locations about the glenohumeral articulation would be an important element of this concept. The question remains, however, whether this feedback can be modified by varying the muscular activation patterns that either develop abnormally or as a result of a remote traumatic event. Whether afferent input can alter the specific motion or a pattern would be one way to determine if these afferent inputs can be usefully altered. To this end, research in this field has revealed that motoneuron afferent input can induce recruitment order changes (5). In monkeys that were taught a specific reaching pattern, there was a constant afferent input to the muscles that was present for any specific motion. Subsequent to a partial deafferentation of the monkeys, the specific muscle firing patterns that were created were altered (5). Therefore, there is an integration of the afferent input into the muscle firing pattern, such that if an alteration occurs and afferent input is subsequently altered, the firing pattern for a specific motion changes.

Not only does afferent input allow alteration in motions, the initiation of voluntary activity may also play a role in muscle recruitment patterns (16). The order of the units has been shown to differ depending on the velocity of the initiation of motion. The varying order of recruitment can be changed when the state of facilitation of one of the units is altered (16). Also, a muscle that in a given situation is favored by rapid initiation of contraction, in another situation, may be favored by slow initiation. Hence it seems as though the varying recruitment order is governed not only by the inherent properties of the units but also by their state of facilitation (16). Finally, contraction of agonist musculature will recruit varying muscular contraction patterns, which are different from the normally established pattern (16). This may establish a format for the employment of varying muscle recruitment order in an attempt to effect changes in joint position leading to pathological motions.

It is possible to develop a model that would incorporate all of the afferent information coming into a person's central processor. During the course of movements, feedforward commands based on a proprioceptively updated internal model of the limb could allow the precise coordination between muscle action and interaction torques about a limb (32). This model would incorporate not only specific joint afferent information but that information emanating from all other sources (see figure 9.3).

The effect of such a model would be to control motions on an immediate basis. The alterations necessary to cause a change in a motion pattern can then be altered by either increasing or decreasing input from any of a number of sources. This rich availability of afferent information in a joint may be one reason why glenohumeral pathologies have been so difficult to treat and diagnose. This wealth, however, may also serve as a basis for treatment.

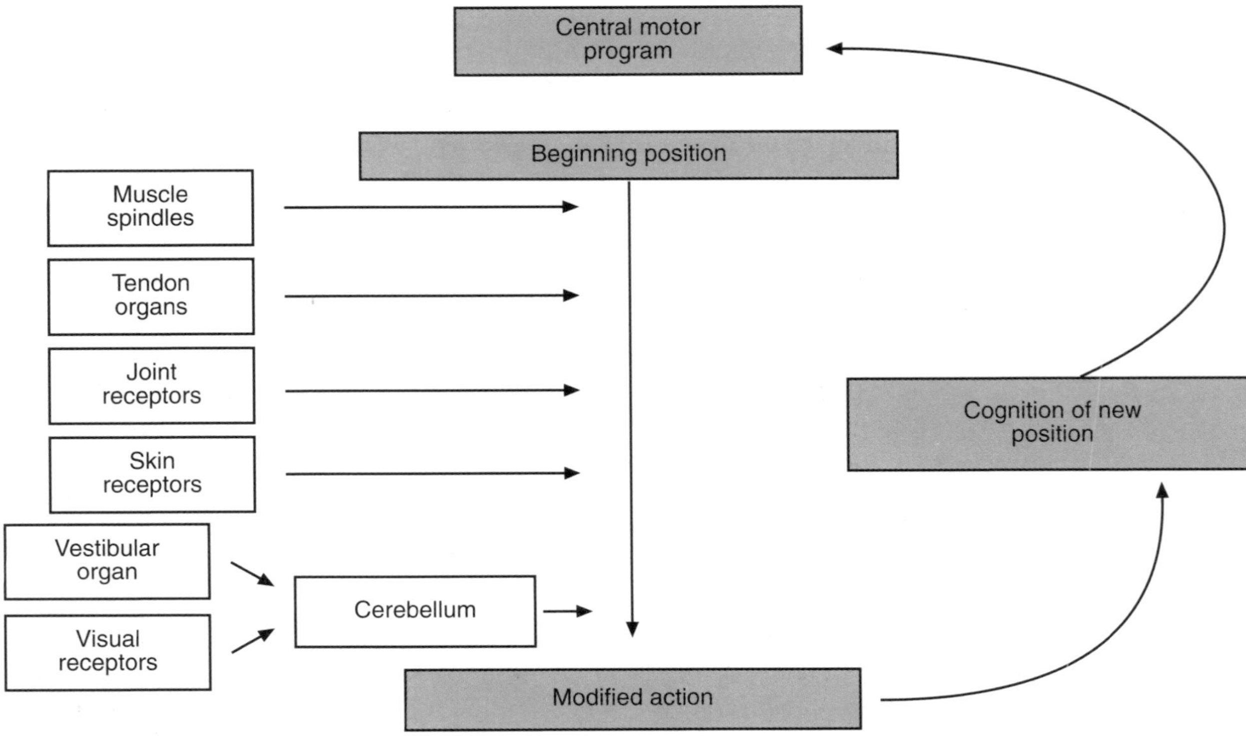

Figure 9.3 Diagram depicting the integration of the passive and active elements within the glenohumeral joint. (Adapted from Jerosch J, Prymka M. Proprioception and joint stability. *Knee Surg Sports Traumat* 4: 171-179, 1996.)

References

1. Barrack RL, Lund P, Skinner HB: Knee joint proprioception revisited. *J Sport Rehab,* 3: 18–42, 1994.
2. Basmajian JV: Control and training of individual motor units. *Science,* 141: 440–41, 1963.
3. Blasier RB, Carpenter JE, Huston LJ: Shoulder proprioception: Effect of joint laxity, joint position, and direction of motion. *Othop Rev,* 23: 45–50, 1994.
4. Borsa PA, Lephart SM, Kocher MS, Lephart SP: Functional assessment and rehabilitation of shoulder proprioception for glenohumeral instability. *J Sport Rehab,* 3: 84–104, 1994.
5. Clamman HP, Ngai AC, Kukulka CG, Goldberg SJ: Motor pool organization in monosynaptic reflexes: Responses in three different muscles. *J Neurophysiol,* 50: 725–42, 1983.
6. Dean J, Wendler G: Stick insects walking on a wheel: Perturbations induced by obstruction of leg protraction. *J Comp Physiol,* 148: 195–207, 1982.
7. Deluca CJ, LeFever RS, McCue MP, et al: Behavior of human motor units in different muscle during linearly varying contractions. *J Physiol* (London), 329: 113–28, 1982.
8. Flanders M: Shoulder muscle activity during natural arm movements: What is optimized? In Matsen FA, Fu FH, Hawkins RJ (eds): *The Shoulder: A Balance of Mobility and Stability.* Chicago: American Academy of Orthopaedic Surgeons, 1993, 635–45.
9. Freeman MAR, Wyke B: The innervation of the knee joint: An anatomical and histological study in the cat. *J Anat,* 101: 505–32, 1967.
10. Gallagher MA, Zuckerman JD, Cuomo F, Rokito A: The effect of instability and subsequent anterior shoulder repair on proprioceptive ability. *Orthop Trans,* 20(1): 274, 1996.
11. Gardner E: The innervation of the shoulder joint. *Anat Rec,* 102: 1–18, 1948.
12. Glousman R, Jobe F, Tibone J, Moynes D, Antonelli D, Perry J: Dynamic electromyographic analysis of the throwing shoulder with glenohumeral instability. *J Bone Joint Surg,* 70A: j220–26, 1988.
13. Gohlke F, Müller T, Sökeland T, Schmitz F, Messlinger K: Distribution and morphology of mechanoreceptors in the rotator cuff. *J Should Elb Surg,* 5(supp): S72, 1996.
14. Grigg P: Peripheral neural mechanisms in proprioception. *J Sport Rehab,* 3: 2–17, 1994.
15. Grigg P: The role of capsular feedback and pattern generators in shoulder kinematics. In

Matsen FA, Fu FH, Hawkins RJ (eds): *The Shoulder: A Balance of Mobility and Stability*. Chicago, American Academy of Orthopaedic Surgeons, 1993, 173–83.
16. Grimby L, Hannerz J: Recruitment order of motor units on voluntary contraction: Changes induced by proprioceptive afferent activity. *J Neurol Neurosurg Psych,* 31: 565–73, 1968.
17. Guanche CA, Knatt T, Solomonow M, Baratta RV, Lu Y: The synergistic action of the capsule and the shoulder muscles. *Am J Sports Med,* 23: 301–306, 1995.
18. Guanche CA, Noble J, Wink C: Periarticular neural elements in the human shoulder. Sixth International Congress on Surgery of the Shoulder, Helsinki, June 27–July 1, 1995.
19. Hasan Z, Stuart DG: Animal solutions to problems of movement control: The role of proprioceptors. *Ann Rev Neurosci,* 11: 199–223, 1988.
20. Ide K, Yasumasa S, Hiromoto I, Hironobu I: Sensory nerve supply in the human subacromial bursa. *J Should Elb Surg,* 5: 371–82, 1996.
21. Jerosch J, Castro WH, Halm H, Drescher H: Does the glenohumeral joint capsule have proprioceptive capability? *Knee Surg Sports Traumat,* 1: 80–84, 1993.
22. Jerosch J, Steinbeck J, Clahsen H, Schmitz-Nahrath M, Grosse-Hackman A: Function of the glenohumeral ligaments in active stabilization of the shoulder joint. *Knee Surg Sport Traumat,* 1: 152–58, 1993.
23. Jerosch J, Prymka M: Proprioception and joint stability. *Knee Surg Sports Traumat,* 4: 171–79, 1996.
24. Jerosch J, Steinbeck J, Schrode M, Westhues M: Intraoperative EMG-Ableitung bein Reizug der glenohumeralen Gelenkkapsel. *Unfallchir,* 98: 580–85, 1995.
25. Knatt T, Guanche CA, Solomonow M, Baratta RM, Lu Y: The glenohumeral-biceps reflex. *Clin Orthop Rel Res,* 314: 247–52, 1995.
26. Lephart SM, Pincivero DM, Giraldo JL, Fu FH: The role of proprioception in the management and rehabilitation of athletic injuries. *Am J Sports Med,* 25: 130–37, 1997.
27. Lephart SM, Warner JP, Borsa PA, Fu FH: Proprioception of the shoulder joint in healthy, unstable, and surgically repaired shoulders. *J Should Elb Surg,* 3: 371–80, 1994.
28. Miyatsu M, Atsuta Y, Takemitsu U: Afferent routes of mechanoreceptors in the anterior cruciate ligament. *Orthop Trans,* 18(2): 574, 1996.
29. Perlau R, Frank C, Fick G: The effect of elastic bandages on human knee proprioception in the uninjured population. *Am J Sports Med,* 23: 251–55, 1995.
30. Pope MH, Johnson RJ, Brown DW, Tigue C: The role of the musculature in injuries to the medial collateral ligament. *J Bone Joint Surg,* 61A: 398–402, 1979.
31. Safran MR, Caldwell GL, Fu FH: Proprioception considerations in surgery. *J Sport Rehab,* 3: 105–15, 1994.
32. Sainburg RL, Ghilardi F, Poizner H, Ghez C: Control of limb dynamics in normal subjects and patients without proprioception. *J Neurophys,* 73: 820–35, 1995.
33. Samuel EP: The autonomic and somatic innervation of the articular capsule. *Acta Anat,* 113: 53–70, 1952.
34. Scott SH, Loeb GE: The computation of position sense from spindles in monoarticular and multiarticular muscles. *J Neurosci,* 14: 7529–540, 1994.
35. Skinner HB, Wyatt MP, Hodgdon JA, Conrad DW, Barrack RL: Effect of fatigue on joint position sense of the knee. *J Orthop Res,* 4: 112–18, 1986.
36. Solomonow M, Baratta R, Zhou B, Shoji H, Bose W, Beck C, D'Ambrosia R: The synergistic action of the anterior cruciate ligament and thigh muscles in maintaining joint stability. *Am J Sports Med,* 15: 207–13, 1987.
37. Solomonow M, D'Ambrosia RD: Neural reflex arcs and muscle control of knee stability and motion. In Scott WN (ed): *Ligament and Extensor Mechanism Injuries of the Knee.* St. Louis: Mosby, 1991, 389–99.
38. Solomonow M, Guanche CA, Wink CA, Knatt T, Baratta RM, Lu Y: Shoulder capsule reflex arc in the feline shoulder. *J Should Elb Surg,* 5: 139–46, 1996.
39. Speer KP, Garrett WE: Muscular control of motion and stability about the pectoral girdle. In Matsen FA, Fu FH, Hawkins RJ (eds): *The Shoulder: A Balance of Mobility and Stability*. Chicago: American Academy of Orthopaedic Surgeons, 1993, 159–72.
40. Vangsness CT, Ennis M, Taylor JG, Atkinson R: Neural anatomy of the glenohumeral ligaments, labrum, and subacromial bursa. *Arthroscopy,* 11: 180–84, 1995.
41. Voight ML, Hardin JA, Blackburn TA, Tippett S, Canner GC: The effects of muscle fatigue on and the relationship of arm dominance to shoulder proprioception. *J Orthop Sports Phys Ther,* 23: 348–52, 1996.
42. Warner JP, Lephart S, Fu FH: Role of proprioception in pathoetiology of shoulder instability. *Clin Orthop Rel Res,* 330: 35–39, 1996.
43. Wrete M: The innervation of the shoulder-joint in man. *Acta Anat,* 7: 173–90, 1949.

CHAPTER 10

Neuromuscular Contributions to Normal Shoulder Joint Kinematics

Answorth A. Allen, MD

Introduction

The kinematics of the normal shoulder joint is dependent on the shoulder muscles and the capsuloligamentous structures. The rotator cuff and biceps tendon are the dynamic stabilizers of the glenohumeral joint and are responsible for coordinating normal shoulder motion. The capsuloligamentous structures are the primary static restraints and prevent excessive translation and rotation of the glenohumeral joint (1–3). Because they function at the extremes of motion, the static restraints may provide important feedback information that is used to orchestrate joint position sense and provide reflex muscle stabilization around the joint (4). It has been suggested that there are sensory afferent feedback systems, through which information from receptors in the skin, joints, and muscles is sent to the brain and spinal pathways, to produce motion that is appropriate for a given situation (5, 6). Proprioception is a specialized variation of the sensory modality of touch that includes the sensation of joint motion (kinesthesia) and joint position (joint position sense). There is relatively little published information on proprioception in the glenohumeral joint. Most of the information available has been extrapolated from the basic science and clinical studies done in other joints such as the knee (6). This chapter summarizes the basic science and clinical information available on shoulder proprioception.

Background

The primary function of the shoulder is to place the upper extremity in space so that the hand can perform its function. Proprioceptive feedback is essential for normal shoulder function (7). It has been hypothesized that peripheral afferents in the skin, muscle, and joint send information to the central nervous system, where it is integrated with visual and vestibular information to generate the appropriate motor response. The categories of motor response include cognitive programming, brain stem activity, and spinal reflexes (8). Cognitive programming involves the highest level of central nervous system function (motor, cortex, basal ganglia, and the cerebellum); it represents the appropriate voluntary response for a given situation and is stored as a central command (9). Afferent input to the brain stem from the eyes, ears, and joint proprioceptors is processed by the cerebellum and is used to maintain posture and balance of the body. The combination of cognitive programming and brain stem activity facilitates a constant awareness of body position and movement and allows performance of various activities without continual reference to consciousness. Spinal reflex refers to the reflex muscular activation when the joint is placed under a mechanical load (10–13).

It has been hypothesized that there is a neurological feedback mechanism that coordinates the actions of the shoulder muscles and protects the capsuloligamentous structures from excessive strain(4). Presumably, if there is a proprioceptive deficit this feedback mechanism is disrupted and the capsuloligamentous structures may become susceptible to excessive strain, thus increasing the risk for joint damage. Others have suggested that intramuscular receptors are the primary determinants of shoulder proprioception but little evidence is available to support this concept (14).

In a recent study Guanche and his coworkers demonstrated a reflex arc between the capsule and the muscles crossing the shoulder joint in a cat model (10). They identified three articular branches of the axillary nerve that innervate different regions of the capsule. The inferior axillary articular nerve innervates the inferior aspect of the capsule and when stimulated causes a reflex activation of the biceps, subscapularis, supraspinatus, and infraspinatus muscles. These muscles stabilize the glenohumeral joint with the arm abducted and externally rotated. The anterior axillary articular nerve innervates the superior quadrant of the anterior capsule and presumably the superior glenohumeral ligaments. Stimulation of this nerve also causes a reflex activation of the biceps subscapularis, supraspinatus, and infraspinatus muscles. These muscles also stabilize the joint during inferior and posterior displacement of the humerus, when the superior ligaments are stressed. The posterior articular axillary nerve innervates the posterior-superior aspect of the capsule, and when stimulated it causes a reflex contraction of the acromiodeltoid muscle, which resists inferior translation of the humeral head. This study demonstrated the presence of a reflex arc between the glenohumeral capsuloligamentous structures and the muscles crossing the joint and suggests that there is synergism between the static and dynamic stabilizers of the glenohumeral joint.

Receptors in the articular structures include the nociceptive free nerve endings, Pacinian corpuscles, Ruffini endings and corpuscles, and Golgi tendon organs. Peripheral receptors have been identified in the joint capsule that may be responsible for joint proprioception (15). Muscle spindle receptors and Golgi tendon organs are found in skeletal muscles. These mechanical receptors represent specialized neurons that have the ability to transduce mechanical deformation into electrical impulses and send information back to the central nervous system about joint position and motion. The Ruffini endings and Golgi tendon organs are relatively slow-adapting mechanoreceptors and appear to be responsible for providing information about joint position or change in joint position. The Pacinian corpuscles are quick-adapting mechanoreceptors and appear to detect rapid movements of acceleration or deceleration. They are probably the receptors responsible for reflex muscle contraction around the joint. The unmyelinated free nerve endings tend to respond to joint pain. In general the muscle and tendon receptors are relatively slow adapting.

These peripheral afferents that provide the anatomic basis of glenohumeral joint proprioception have been identified in the glenoid labrum and glenohumeral joints (16–19). Mechanoreceptors were initially identified in the shoulder joint of the cat by Shimamura and others (16). Subsequently, Murakami and his coworkers identified mechanoreceptors in the shoulder capsule of monkeys (17). These receptors were identified in the transitional zone between the labrum and the capsule. Vangsness and Ennis (18) observed neural structures and mechanoreceptors in the capsuloligamentous tissue of the human glenohumeral joint. Jerosch and associates (19) performed a histological study of 13 fresh human cadaveric shoulder capsules and demonstrated a diffuse pattern of neuroaxons of varying diameters, which appeared to have no specific relationship to the blood vessels or vessel walls. They concluded that these neuroreceptors were involved in shoulder proprioception. Although additional work needs to be done, these studies mentioned provide at least some evidence that mechanoreceptors are present in the human glenohumeral joint, and it can be extrapolated that these receptors may have a role in shoulder proprioception. Normal joint proprioception presumably would have a protective role by increasing neuromuscular control and stabilization of the glenohumeral joint. In the model proposed by Lephart and Henry (7) proprioceptive deficits from ligamentous injury will lead to decreased neuromuscular control and functional instability. The lack of appropriate proprioceptive feedback causes repetitive joint injury (see figure 10.1).

Clinical Relevance

Clinically, proprioception is assessed by measuring the threshold to detection of passive motion (kinesthesia) and joint position sense (reproduction of passive positioning and reproduction of active positioning). According to Lephart and coworkers (8), at slow angular velocities (0.5 to 2°/s) the threshold to detection of passive motion, as well as the reproduction of passive positioning, is thought to selectively stimulate Ruffini or Golgi-type mechanoreceptors in the articular structures. Reproduction of active positioning is thought to involve the stimulation of both joint and muscle receptors and provides a more functional assessment of the afferent pathways (8). There are relatively few clinical studies on shoulder proprioception. The data obtained from studying proprioception in other joints is often extrapolated to the shoulder. At times this may not be appropriate. The results from clinical studies must be interpreted in the context of the parameters being tested and the testing methods used.

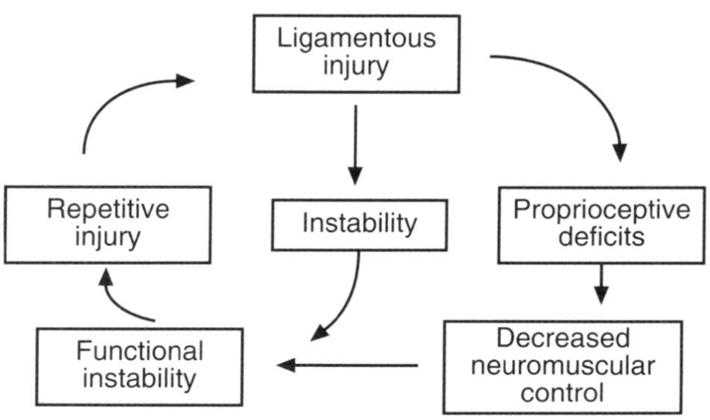

Figure 10.1 Functional stability paradigm depicting the progression of functional instability of the shoulder joint due to the interaction between mechanical instability and decreased neuromuscular control.

One of the first clinical studies demonstrating shoulder proprioception was performed by Hall and McCloskey in 1983 (14). They studied the detection of angular motion of the shoulder, elbow, and distal interphalangeal joint of the middle finger. These tests were performed in the mid ranges of motion of each joint but over a wide range of angular velocities. It was their conclusion that intermuscular receptors were the primary determinants of shoulder proprioception. In 1989, Smith and Brunolli (20) examined shoulder kinesthesia after anterior glenohumeral joint dislocation. They tested eight patients with anterior instability with a control group, measuring the accuracy of reproduction of a given angle and the detection for threshold of motion. They demonstrated a proprioceptive deficit in the patients with shoulder instability.

A number of shoulder proprioception studies have been performed at the University of Pittsburgh using a proprioception testing device that they developed. Fu and coworkers initially studied shoulder proprioception in college-age individuals without any history of shoulder injury (21). They found that there was minimal variation in proprioception and noted no differences between dominant and nondominant shoulders. Joint laxity or direction of rotation of the shoulder did not appear to affect proprioceptive sensitivity.

Blasier and others (22) subsequently tested 29 patients with clinically normal shoulders, in the age range from 20 to 42 years. Using a different test,

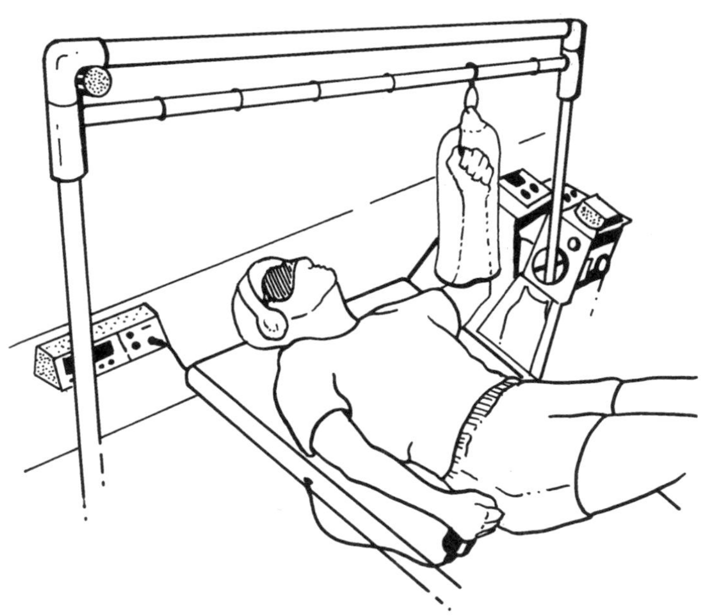

Figure 10.2 Shoulder proprioception testing device used at the University of Pittsburgh.

they measured the ability of the patients to detect passive shoulder rotation in the abducted shoulder (see figure 10.2). They determined that patients with generalized joint laxity had a higher threshold for detection of proprioception. Detection of external rotation was more sensitive than detection of internal rotation. The patient's ability to detect external rotation was found to be more sensitive as the capsule was tightened and a limit of external rotation was approached. They also determined that the absolute angle for proprioception for rotation of the abducted shoulder ranges from a best of 0.78° to a worst of 1.08°. They hypothesized that capsular tightening may play a role in the mechanism of shoulder proprioception.

Lephart and his coworkers subsequently measured shoulder proprioception in 90 subjects (4). They divided the subjects into three groups: group I, healthy college-age subjects who served as the control group; group II, patients with anterior instability and chronic recurrent traumatic anterior shoulder dislocation or subluxation who failed a rehabilitation program; group III, patients who had surgical stabilization of the shoulder with either an open or an arthroscopic technique. They measured kinesthesia and joint position sense with their proprioception testing device (see figure 10.3). They demonstrated that there was no significant difference in proprioception between the dominant and nondominant shoulder in group I for any test condition. There were significant differences between the unstable and involved shoulders for both kinesthesia and joint position sense in the patients in group II. In group III there were no significant differences between the surgically reconstructed and contralateral shoulders for any given test condition. They concluded that arm dominance does not affect proprioceptive sensibility. They also concluded that athletically active individuals with chronic traumatic anterior shoulder instability have significant proprioceptive deficits and that surgical reconstruction may normalize shoulder proprioceptive sensibility. It was not clear from their studies if there were any differences between patients who had an arthroscopic versus an open stabilization of the glenohumeral joint.

This study demonstrated that shoulder proprioception could be restored in patients with anterior shoulder instability by performing a capsulolabral reconstruction and retensioning the capsule. They suggested that by retensioning the capsuloligamentous structures that contain the mechanoreceptors, proprioceptive sensibility was restored (4). The finding of mechanoreceptors in the glenoid labrum and capsule and the presence of articular nerve branches and neuroaxons in the capsuloligamentous structures may be of significance when the type of capsulolabral reconstruction is contemplated. Guanche and his coworkers (10) have suggested that the capsule should be retensioned on the lateral side to decrease the risk of injury to the articular nerve branches and mechanoreceptors.

In spite of these studies, the role and relevance of shoulder proprioception is still not clearly defined. There does not appear to be any alteration in proprioception with open stabilization procedures, where the capsule is cut, and arthroscopic stabilization. Preliminary information suggests that glenohumeral arthroplasty does not affect shoulder proprioception. Some clinicians are still skeptical about the clinical significance of shoulder proprioception. Hopefully this skepticism will stimulate more discussions and investigations.

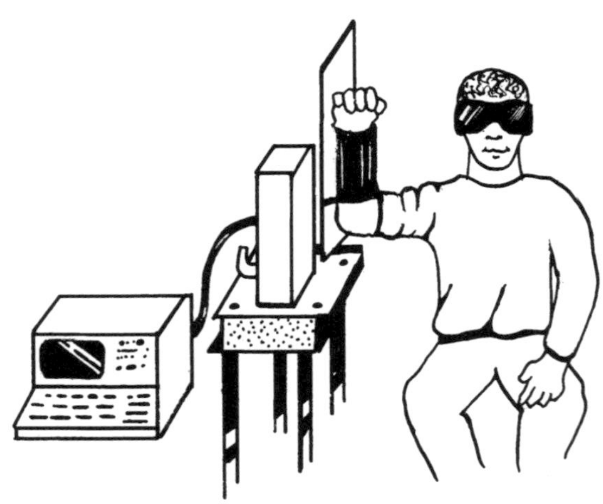

Figure 10.3 Shoulder proprioception testing device with a reclining adjustable seat. The height of the electrogoniometer and the seat position can be adjusted so that the arm is always in 90° elevation in the scapular plane.

Proprioception and Joint Kinematics

A number of biomechanical and electromyographic studies suggest that coordination and synergism of the rotator cuff and biceps muscles is required for normal shoulder function. According to Gowan and his associates (23), during the pitching motion in professional baseball pitchers, two groups of muscles control shoulder motion. The first group of muscles (the supraspinatus, trapezius, and biceps brachii) demonstrates increased electromyographic activity during the early and late cocking phase and decreased activity during the acceleration phase. This group of muscles positions the arm for the delivery of the pitch. The second group of muscles (the pectoralis major, serratus anterior, subscapularis, and latissimus dorsi) demonstrates increased electromyographic activity during the acceleration phase of the pitch. Subsequently, Glousman and coworkers (24), using the same measurement techniques, demonstrated changes in the electromyographic pattern in baseball pitchers with chronic anterior instability of the glenohumeral joint. Decreased electromyographic activity was demonstrated in the internal rotators of the arm (subscapularis, pectoralis major, latissimus dorsi, and the serratus anterior muscle), which contributed to anterior shoulder instability by allowing excessive external rotation during the late cocking and acceleration phases of pitching when the glenohumeral joint is susceptible to anterior subluxation. They also noted a compensatory increase in the activity of the biceps and supraspinatus muscles, which will enhance shoulder stability by directing the humeral head into the glenoid fossa. Alteration of the normal neuromuscular balance in patients with anterior instability can cause changes in the joint kinematics that can lead to repetitive microtrauma of the glenohumeral joint. Either way, this can lead to altered joint kinematics and repetitive microtrauma to the glenohumeral joint.

Conclusion

There is more evidence that there are proprioceptive receptors in both the static and dynamic stabilizers of the glenohumeral joint. Although it is difficult to assess the relative contributions from these structures there appears to be a synergistic relationship between receptors in the capsule and muscles surrounding the glenohumeral joint. The primary mechanism of shoulder proprioception appears to be capsular based, where stimulation of receptors in the capsuloligamentous structures by tension or mechanical deformation leads to the generation of electrical impulses that can cause a local or central response. Shoulder proprioception has been measured clinically with different testing devices. The parameters being measured are relatively subtle and can be influenced by a number of intrinsic and extrinsic variables. The proprioceptive deficit in patients with anterior glenohumeral instability appears to be improved with capsuloligamentous reconstruction.

Future Directions

The study of glenohumeral joint proprioception is in its relative infancy, and the role of shoulder proprioception is still not totally defined. More basic science research needs to be done to document the location and distribution of receptors in the capsuloligamentous structures and in the muscles around the glenohumeral joint. Further elucidation of local and central proprioceptive pathways is needed. The relationship between proprioceptive characteristics assessed in the laboratory and clinical function in both normal activities and in sports needs to be more clearly defined. The effect of upper extremity training on proprioception in normal and unstable shoulders needs further evaluation. The role of other shoulder pathology on proprioception such as glenohumeral joint arthritis, rotator cuff tears, and shoulder impingement needs further documentation.

References

1. Warner JJP. The gross anatomy of the joint surface, ligament, labrum, and capsule. In: Motsen FA III, Fu FH, Hawkins RJ, eds, *The shoulder: a balance of mobility and stability.* Rosemont, IL: American Academy of Orthopaedic Surgeons, 7–28, 1993.
2. O'Brien SJ, Neves MC, Arnoczky SP, et al. The anatomy and histology of the inferior glenohumeral ligament complex of the shoulder. *Am J Sports Med* 18: 449–56, 1990.
3. Warner JJP, Deng XH, Warren RF, Torzilli PA. Static capsuloligamentous restraints to superior-inferior translation of the glenohumeral joint. *Am J Sports Med* 20: 675–85, 1992.
4. Lephart SM, Warner JP, Borsa PA, et al. Proprioception of the shoulder in normal, unstable, and postsurgical individuals. *J Shoulder Elbow Surg* 3: 371–80, 1994.

5. Barrack RL, Skinner HB, Buckley SL. Proprioception in the anterior cruciate-deficient knee. *Am J Sports Med* 17: 1–6, 1989.
6. Grigg P. Peripheral neural mechanisms in proprioception. *J Sport Rehab* 3: 2–17, 1994.
7. Lephart SM, Henry TJ. The physiological basis for open and closed kinetic chain rehabilitation for the upper extremity. *J Sport Rehab* 5: 71–87, 1996.
8. Lephart SM, Pincivero DM, Giraldo JL, Fu FH. The role of proprioception in the management and rehabilitation of athletic injuries. *Am J Sports Med* 25: 130–37, 1997.
9. Tyldesling B, Greve JI. *Muscles, nerves and movement: Kinesiology in daily living.* Cambridge, MA: Blackwell Scientific, 268–84, 1989.
10. Guanche C, Knatt T, Solomonow M, et al. The synergistic action of the capsule and the shoulder muscles. *Am J Sports Med* 23: 301–306, 1995.
11. Barrett, DS, Cobb AG, Bentley G. Joint proprioception in normal, osteoarthritic, and replaced knees. *J Bone Joint Surg* (Britain) 73: 833–37, 1991.
12. Baxendale RA, Ferrell WR, Wood L. Responses of quadriceps motor units to mechanical stimulation of knee joint receptors in the decerebrate cat. *Brain Res* 453: 150–56, 1988.
13. Sojka P. Sjölander P, Johansson H, Djupsjöbacka M. Influence from stretch-sensitive receptors in the collateral ligament of the knee joint on the gamma-muscle spindle systems of flexor and extensor muscles. *Neurosci Res* 11: 55–62, 1991.
14. Hall AL, McCloskey DI. Detection of movement imposed on finger, elbow, and shoulder joints. *J Physiol* 335: 519–33, 1983.
15. Skoglund CT. Joint receptors and kinesthesia. In: *Handbook of sensory physiology.* Berlin: Springer-Verlag, 111–35, 1973.
16. Shimamura M, Kogure I, Fuwa T. Role of joint afferents in relation to the initiation of forelimb stepping in thalamic cats. *Brain Res* 297: 225–34, 1984.
17. Murakami M, Kojima Y, Maeda T, et al. Sensory nerve endings in the shoulder joint capsule of the monkey as sensors of dynamic stabilizing system. *Transactions of Combined Meeting of the ORS of USA, Japan, and Canada,* 315, 1991.
18. Vangsness CT, Ennis M. Neural anatomy of the human glenoid and shoulder ligaments. In: *Proceedings of the 59th annual meeting of the American Academy of Orthopedic Surgeons,* Washington, DC, February 20–25, 1992. Washington, DC: American Academy of Orthopaedic Surgeons, 205, 1992.
19. Jerosch J, Clahsen H, et al. Effects of proprioceptive fibers in the capsule tissue stabilizing the glenohumeral joint. Paper presented before the American Shoulder and Elbow Surgeons, Eighth Open Meeting, Washington, DC, February 23, 1992.
20. Smith RL, Brunolli J. Shoulder kinesthesia after shoulder dislocation. *Phys Ther* 69: 106–12, 1989.
21. Blasier RB, Carpenter JE, Huston LJ. Shoulder proprioception: Effect of joint laxity, joint position, and direction of motion. *Orthop Rev* 45–50, January 1994.
22. Gowan JP, Jobe, Tibone JE, Perry J, Moynes DR. A complete electromyographic analysis of the shoulder during pitching. *Am J Sports Med* 15: 586–90, 1987.
23. Glousmann R, Jobe FW, Tibone, et al. Dynamic electromyographic analysis of the throwing shoulder with glenohumeral instability. *J Bone Joint Surg* 70: 220–26, 1988.

CHAPTER 11

Peripheral Afferent Nerve Regeneration

Kevin P. Black, MD
Michael H. Rieber, MD

Introduction

Peripheral nerve is a composite tissue consisting of a number of cellular and connective tissue elements. An understanding of afferent nerve regeneration is dependent upon familiarity with the relationship between complex nerve anatomy, physiology, biomechanics, and mechanisms of impulse conduction. Each of these topics, therefore, is reviewed prior to the discussion of regeneration.

Anatomy and Physiology

Nerve fibers, or axons, are the extended processes of proximally located cell bodies. For afferent neurons, the cell bodies lie in the dorsal root ganglia, while motor neuron cell bodies lie in the spinal cord and sympathetic cell bodies in the sympathetic ganglia. The relationship of the axon to the cell body is a highly unique one in that the axon extends over a distance corresponding to many thousands of times the cell body diameter and contains 90% of the cytoplasm. Injury to any one area of the axon can result in serious deleterious effects to the entire neuron, including the nerve cell body (3, 12, 16, 30).

A second cellular element of the peripheral nerve is the Schwann cell. While both myelinated and nonmyelinated nerve fibers (53) are surrounded by a chain of Schwann cells, the relationship of the Schwann cell to the axon differs between the two. In myelinated nerve fibers there is a one-to-one relationship at any single level between the axon and Schwann cell. The myelin sheath is the membrane of the Schwann cell wrapped spirally around the axon in a multilayer sleeve of proteins and lipids. The Schwann cells are arranged linearly along the course of the axon and interdigitate with each other via fingerlike processes at the nodes of Ranvier, where the exchange of ions occurs between the axon and extracellular fluid. This results in rapid saltatory conduction of nerve impulses from node to node in myelinated fibers. In nonmyelinated fibers, multiple nerve fibers are located in internal troughs of a single Schwann cell, and the axon is not insulated from the surrounding extracellular fluid. As a result, the exchange of ions between the axoplasm and connective tissue is continuous, resulting in a much lower conduction velocity.

The connective tissue layers provide nutrition and protection to the nerve fiber (see figure 11.1). Each fiber is embedded in loose endoneural connective tissue, and bundles of fibers are collected in fascicles, each of which is protected by a second connective tissue layer, the perineurium (27). The perineurium is a dense, mechanically strong, multilamellar membrane that is composed of flattened cells with a basement membrane on both inner and outer aspects, which possesses a diffusion barrier to a number of extrinsic macromolecules and maintains an optimal intrafascicular environment for the fiber. Thus, the perineurium plays a vital role in the regulation and maintenance

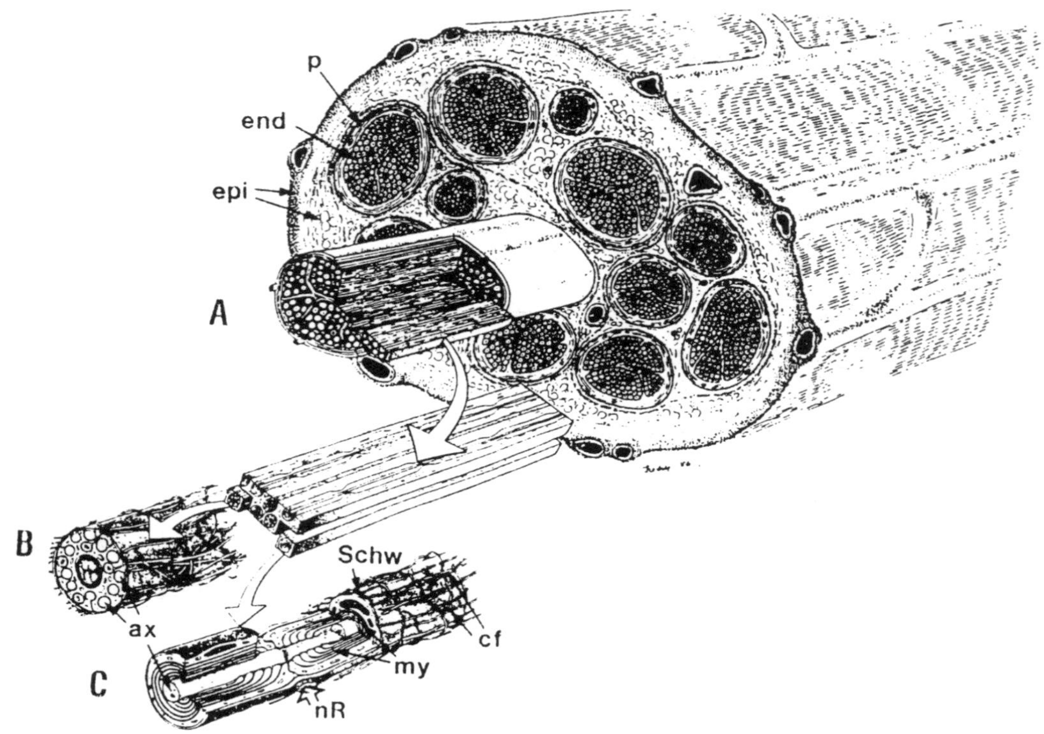

Figure 11.1 Schematic drawing of the microanatomy of the peripheral nerve trunk with all its components. (*a*) The fascicles of the peripheral nerve surrounded by the perineurium (p) and embedded in a loose connective tissue—the epineurium (epi). The intrafascicular tissue elements surrounding the nerve fibers are called endoneurium (end). (*b*) Nonmyelinated nerve fibers (ax) enclosed in troughs in one Schwann cell. (*c*) One axon around which one Schwann cell (Schw) is wrapped spirally. The place where two adjacent Schwann cells meet is called the node of Ranvier (nR). (Reprinted from Lundborg G. *Nerve injury and repair.* Edinburgh: Churchill-Livingstone, 1988, p. 33, with permission.)

of the endoneural space, which is of utmost importance for optimal nerve fiber function.

Nerve fascicles are embedded in the epineurium, a well-vascularized connective tissue membrane that protects the nerve cells from both compression and tensile injury. The amount of epineurium relative to the cross-sectional area of the nerve varies among nerves and nerve levels and is more abundant near joints, most likely to protect the nerve from friction and compression at these locations. The relationship of the epineurium to the extraneural connective tissue contributes greatly to the longitudinal movement of nerve trunks, which occurs with movement of the extremity. In addition, there is a deeper gliding layer of the epineurium that allows for sliding of the fascicles. Nerve gliding may be inhibited greatly by posttraumatic scarring.

Nerve function is dependent upon an energy supply delivered via an intraneural microvascular system, the main channels of which are located in the epineurium but that anastomoses throughout all the connective tissue layers. These anastomoses between vessels in different layers of nerve are very well developed and no single direction of blood flow is predominant in any segment of the nerve trunk. Although these anastomoses contribute to adequate blood flow when the nerve is transected or extrinsic vessels are damaged, low levels of strain interfere with intraneural microvascular circulation. Lundborg and Rydevik have demonstrated experimentally that a 15% strain results in a complete loss of intraneural circulation in the rabbit tibial nerve (35). The nerve regulates it own microcirculation via fine nerve endings from the sympathetic nervous system, which originate from fibers inside nerve trunks (2, 32). The Schwann cell membrane and retinacular and collagen fibrils of the endoneurium provide a framework of support for the nerve fiber known as the endoneural tube (38).

A slightly positive intrafascicular (endoneural) fluid pressure contributes to the stiffness of the nerve fascicles. If the perineural tube is transected, the endoneural contents herniate at the free ends, a process known as mushrooming. After ischemia or other nonpenetrating injuries there is a rapid increase in endoneural fluid pressure, resulting in a type of compartment syndrome that compromises the intrafascicular microvascular system.

Nerve fiber types are related to specific functions such as stretch, burning pain, temperature, and touch and have been classified into three types based on the relationship between fiber size and the shape of the compound axon potential. Myelinated somatic afferents and efferents comprise group A and are the largest and have the fastest conduction velocities. Group B consists of myelinated autonomic and preganglionic fibers, and group C fibers are thin, nonmyelinated slow-conducting visceral and somatic afferent fibers.

Within the axon there exists a continuous bidirectional transport system that allows for the transport of a wide variety of substances and organelles, including neurotransmitters, proteins, lipids, RNA, mitochondria, and membranous vesicles (17, 26). Transport from the nerve cell body down the axon is referred to as antegrade transport, while transport from the axon to the cell body is referred to as retrograde transport. Antegrade transport has been divided into five groups based upon the velocity of transport, and substances can be divided into these groups depending upon whether they are membrane-associated materials (fast) or cytoskeletal and associated proteins (slow). Antegrade transport is an energy-dependent process (6) in which intracellular microtubules (17) play a vital role.

Retrograde transport is, in general, slower than antegrade but plays an important role in recycling of materials already transported from the nerve cell body down the axon (4) and in the transfer of information regarding the status of the axon, its terminals, target cells, and environment (4, 54). That information is relayed to the cell body via neuronotropic factors, which are proteins supplied by the target territory, incorporated at the axon terminals, and transported to the cell body where their modulatory effects are exerted. These factors are essential for survival of the nerve and their absence after injury plays a major etiologic role for the functional and structural nerve cell body changes that take place after injury (5, 8, 16, 18).

Biomechanical Properties

Peripheral nerve has been demonstrated to have a very nonlinear stress-strain behavior (29). In the rabbit tibial nerve there is initially very little stress in the nerve with up to 15% strain. During this period much of the strain is due to the removal of slack in nerve fascicles and overall nerve. With strain exceeding 15%, lengthening of nerve fibers, endoneural tubes, and perineurium occurs. With strains exceeding 20%, endoneural tubes may rupture and ultimate strain approaches 40%. In situ strain of nerve varies with joint position. During typical physiological range of motion the nerve is under significant strain but well within the toe region of the stress-strain curve. Therefore, despite the fact that the nerve experiences a large amount of strain the stress within it remains small.

The perineurium, which is essential to maintain the environment of the endoneural space, has been demonstrated to be a major load carrying component of nerve (28). When loaded to failure, the perineural sheath will rupture at multiple sites along the specimen prior to injury to any other connective tissue components. Therefore, a peripheral nerve that appears to be grossly intact may have extensive structural and functional injury.

The specific effects of strain on the diffusion properties of the perineurium are not well understood. Significant differences in the sensitivity to strain have been reported by various investigators (11, 22, 39). Wall and coworkers (57) demonstrated a decrease in conduction velocity from as little as a 6% increase in strain beyond in situ levels and found these changes to be irreversible at 12% strain.

Impulse Conduction

A nerve cell consists of a cell body and numerous branches from it known as dendrites. As mentioned previously, in most neurons there is one dendritic process, the axon, which is longer and more uniform than the others are. Like all other types of cells, the nerve cell consists of a plasma membrane and cytoplasm (axoplasm). In contrast to the axoplasm, through which ions flow with relative ease, the plasma membrane acts as an ionic barrier between the cell interior and its surrounding environment, resulting in a much higher extracellular concentration of sodium and intracellular concentration of potassium. This membrane consists of a phospholipid bilayer with interspersed function-specific protein elements. As a result, the membrane is selectively permeable and can function as an insulator and also give rise to the nerve's excitable behavior (13, 24, 44).

At rest, the nerve membrane is more permeable to potassium than sodium while, as suggested by Hodgkin and Katz (23), the opposite is true at the peak of the action potential. They suggested that during nerve excitation, the nerve quickly becomes permeable to sodium, resulting in the flow of sodium ions down their concentration gradient and reversal of the resting membrane potential, and repolarization occurs as potassium ions move outward down their concentration gradient. In myelinated nerves, the myelin sheath functions as an insulator that results in the local axoplasmic currents flowing rapidly down the center of the nerve and exiting only at interruptions in the sheath, the nodes of Ranvier, a process known as saltatory conduction. The Schwann cells that synthesize the myelin are easily damaged by mechanical or ischemic injury.

Injury and Regeneration

Injury and regeneration of peripheral nerve is a highly complex process that must take into account not only the neuron but connective tissue components such as fibroblasts, macrophages, endothelial cells, and Schwann cells. Injury severity may be classified based upon functional deficit or pathoanatomy. Seddon (46–48) divided nerve injury into three groups based upon functional deficit. The earliest stage, neurapraxia, occurs after compression injury and corresponds to an acute local demyelinating block in which the continuity of the axon is preserved as well as the excitability of nerve structures distal to the lesion. Over weeks to months, myelin repair occurs in the injured segment, resulting in the restoration of axon excitability and conduction in the same area.

Seddon's next level of injury, axonotmesis, corresponds to a loss of axonal continuity at the site of injury in which the endoneural tubes remain intact to guide axonal regrowth. Wallerian degeneration of the axon occurs distal to the site of injury and functional recovery is dependent upon regeneration of the axon and the reinnervation of distal targets. However, irreversible damage may occur to target tissues during the time elapsed prior to reinnervation.

In Seddon's most severe injury, spontaneous regeneration does not occur and operative repair is required. Anatomically, this corresponds to total severance of the nerve or destruction of the perineurium and endoneural tube such that the interior anatomy of the nerve is grossly disrupted. Therefore, in contrast to axonotmesis, the endoneural tubes are not available to guide the regenerating axons to their target tissues.

Sunderland (51, 52) has introduced an alternate classification system, which is more detailed and based upon pathoanatomy of the nerve trunk components (see figure 11.2). Sunderland's first two groups correspond to neurapraxia and axonotmesis. In clinical practice, nerve injuries are often of a mixed nature and these two groups of injury may occur simultaneously. Groups three, four, and five correspond to a subdivision of neurotmesis based upon injury of individual connective tissue components. In third degree injury, the perineurium remains intact but axonal and endoneural tube continuity is lost. These injuries are typically accompanied by intrafascicular bleeding and edema, resulting in fibrosis. In fourth degree injury, the perineurium is disrupted but the epineurium remains intact, while in fifth degree injury the entire nerve trunk is severed.

Following axonal injury, regeneration can take place only if the nerve cell body has survived and if the growth terrain is acceptable for axon advancement. Markedly different responses occur in the proximal and distal nerve segments. Proximally, the nerve becomes dedicated to replacing the large volume of lost axoplasm (16, 18, 30, 31). Included among the changes are swelling of the cell body, a shift in protein synthesis toward components necessary for axon construction and decreased synthesis of synaptic transmission materials.

When injured, the axon degenerates proximally over a length corresponding to one or several internodal segments, leaving the endoneural tube an empty cylinder (52). Distally, fragmentation of the axon and myelin sheath occurs, a process known as wallerian degeneration. Distal Schwann cells and macrophages then proliferate and phagocytose debris. Axon sprouts, which have originated from the proximal stump, then spread distally, becoming embedded in the Schwann cell cytoplasm. In addition to serving as columns for axonal growth, the Schwann cells synthesize trophic factors for neuronal survival and growth. The most distal part of the sprouts develop growth cones, areas of swelling from which filipodia arise. These mobile, actin-containing microspikes play an essential role in determining the orientation and growth of the sprouts. The advancing sprouts that have originated from one myelinated axon are referred to as a regeneration unit (40, 41), and over time one of the axon sprouts usually matures and becomes myelinated while the others disappear. Regeneration units that make contact with their target organ mature and increase in diameter, probably as a result of trophic signals synthesized by the target, while those that do not, atrophy and disappear (1). The average rate of axon regrowth in adults is 1–2 mm/day; it varies with the magnitude and level of injury.

The survival of neurons and their regeneration following injury are also dependent on neurotrophic

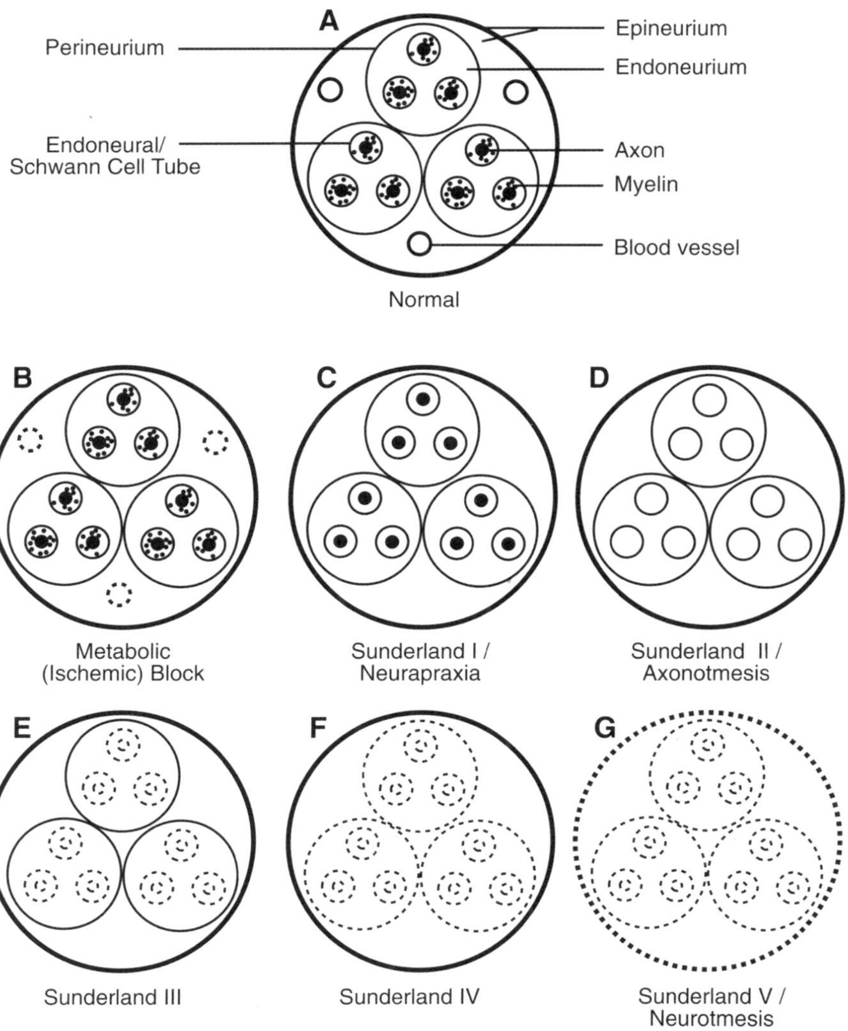

Figure 11.2 (A) Normal nerve with three fascicles and three vessels. (B) Metabolic (ischemic) block where vessels have been obliterated but remaining structures are intact. (C) Sunderland class I injury; Seddon, neurapraxia. Myelin is gone but fascicles are still present. (D) Sunderland class II injury; Sedon, axonotmesis. Axons and myelin are gone but endoneural tubes are preserved. (E) Sunderland class III injury. Endoneural tubes are gone but the perineurium is preserved (F) Sunderland class IV injury. Perineurium is gone but the epineurium remains. (G) Sunderland class V injury; Seddon, neurotmesis. All connective tissue coats of nerve, including epineurium, have been damaged.

and neurite promoting factors. Target tissues normally provide chemical signals to their innervating nerve cell, which are then transported back to the nerve cell body via retrograde transport and used to maintain essential cellular activities (54–56). The most studied of these chemicals is nerve growth factor (NGF), for which the necessary signal quantity is usually supplied by the target organ. When transected, however, this supply is lost and replaced by NGF synthesized by Schwann cells.

Although the process of chemotaxis is a well-accepted process in many biological systems, its existence in nerve regeneration has been somewhat controversial. Investigators have demonstrated preferential growth of a severed nerve toward a nerve graft or distal stump regardless of fiber alignment (14, 15, 42, 43). In addition, NGF has been observed to alter the direction of growth of axons from chick dorsal root ganglion neurons (19–21).

Many investigations have been done using biological chamber systems in which tubes of various materials have been utilized to bridge gaps between proximal and distal nerve stumps of transected nerves. In this manner the local environment can be manipulated to study its effects on regeneration. These studies have demonstrated that within a day of transection and implantation, a silicone chamber becomes filled with fluid containing both neurotrophic and neurite promoting factors. After between 3 and 7 days an acellular fibrin matrix, which connects the two stumps, forms, followed by both proximal and distal cellular invasion. The leading edge of the cells is composed of fibroblasts, followed by blood vessels, Schwann cells, and axons. Myelination is the last process to occur. Efforts to accelerate the formation of the fibrin matrix have stimulated the growth of all cellular elements (9, 10, 58). Similar studies using a silicone chamber model have demonstrated the importance of the distal nerve stump. Regeneration across gaps occurs only if the distal segment is nerve tissue and if the gap is 10 mm or less (33, 34, 45, 59).

Numerous techniques have been attempted and are still under investigation to modulate the regeneration process. These include utilization of a preceding conditioning lesion (36, 37), hormonal manipulation with substances such as triiodothyronine and growth hormone (7, 25), and electromagnetic fields (49, 50). Studies such as these hold promise for future methods to modulate the environment of the transected axon to promote its regeneration.

Models of nerve injury and regeneration described above have contributed tremendously to our understanding of peripheral nerve healing. Many questions remain, however, in regard to the clinical situation in which the injury occurs, not in the midaxon region, but rather in the region of the target organ and receptor. For example, when a shoulder dislocates anteriorly, significant strain occurs to both the target organ and receptor. How does this injury affect the neural receptor, what are its regenerative capabilities, and what effect does it have on the neurochemical signals that the target organ sends to it? What are the effects of prolonged strain injury (a shoulder that is dislocated for 4 h versus 20 min) or repeat injury (recurrent dislocater versus first time)? These same types of questions can certainly be applied to the knee and ankle joints and essentially throughout the entire musculoskeletal system. Further investigation of questions such as these will contribute greatly to our understanding of the effects of injury on proprioception.

References

1. Aitken TJ. The effect of peripheral connections on the maturation of regenerating nerve fibers. *J Anat* 83: 38–42, 1949.
2. Appenzeller O, Dithal KK, Cowen T, Burnstock G. The nerves to blood vessels supplying blood nerves: The innervation of vasa nervorum. *Brain Res* 304: 383–86, 1984.
3. Barron KD. Comparative observations on the cytologic reaction of central and peripheral nerve cells to axotomy. In: Kao CC, Bunge RP, Reier PJ, eds, *Spinal cord reconstruction.* New York: Raven Press, 7–40, 1983.
4. Bisby MA. Functions of retrograde axonal transport. *Fed Proc* 41: 2307–311, 1982.
5. Bisby MA. Retrograde axonal transport and nerve regeneration. In: Elam JS, Cancalon P, eds, *Axonal transport in neuronal growth and regeneration: Advances in neurochemistry,* vol 6. London: Pelham, 45–67, 1984.
6. Bray D. Fast axonal transport. *Nature* 315: 178–79, 1985.
7. Cockett SA, Kiernan JA. Acceleration of peripheral nervous regeneration in the rat by exogenous triiodothyronine. *Exp Neurol* 39: 389–94, 1973.
8. Cragg BH. What is the signal for chromatolysis? *Brain Res* 23: 1–21, 1970.
9. Danielsen N. Regeneration of the rat sciatic nerve in the silicone chamber model. *Restor Neurol Neurosci* 1: 253–59, 1990.
10. Danielsen N, Muller H, Pettman B, et al. Rat amnion membrane matrix as a substratum for regenerating axons from peripheral and central neurons: Effects in a silicone chamber model. *Dev Brain Res* 39: 39–50, 1988.
11. Denny-Brown D, Doherty MM. Effects of transient stretching of peripheral nerve. *Arch Neurol Psychiat* 54: 116–22, 1945.
12. Ducker TB. The central cell body and axonal regeneration. In: Gorio A, Millesi H, Mingrino S, eds, *Posttraumatic peripheral nerve regeneration: Experimental basis and clinical implications.* New York: Raven Press, 7–11, 1981.
13. Edidin M. Translational and rotational diffusion in membranes. *Ann Rev Biophys Bioeng* 3: 179–201, 1974.
14. Forssman J. Über die Ursachen, welche die Wachsthumsrichtung der peripheren Nervenfasern bei der Regeneration bestimmen. *Beitr Z Pathol Anat* 24: 56–100, 1998.
15. Forssman J. Zur Kenntnis des Neurotropismus. Weiter Beitrage. *Beitr Z Pathol Anat* 27: 407–30, 1900.
16. Grafstein B. The nerve cell body response to axotomy. *Exp Neurol* 48: 32–51, 1975.
17. Grafstein B, Forman DS. Intracellular transport in neurons. *Phys Rev* 60: 1167–283, 1980.
18. Grafstein B, McQuarrie IG. Role of the nerve cell body in axonal regeneration. In: Cotman CW, ed, *Neuronal plasticity.* New York: Raven Press, 155–95, 1978.
19. Gundersen RW. Sensory neurite growth cone guidance by substrate-absorbed nerve growth factor. *J Neurosci Res* 13: 199–212, 1985.

20. Gundersen RW, Barrett JN. Neuronal chemotaxis: Chick dorsal root axons turn toward high concentrations of nerve growth factor. *Science* 206: 1079–1080, 1979.
21. Gundersen RW, Barrett JN. Characterization of the turning response of dorsal root neurites towards nerve growth factor. *J Cell Biol* 87: 546–54, 1980.
22. Highet WB, Sanders FK. The effects of stretching nerves after suture. *Br J Surg* 30: 355–71, 1943.
23. Hodgkin AL, Katz B. The effects of sodium ions on the electrical activity of the giant axon of the squid. *J Physiol* (London) 108: 37–77, 1949.
24. Jain MK. *Introduction to biological membranes.* New York: Wiley, 1988.
25. Kanje M, Skottner A, Lundborg G. Effects of growth hormone treatment on the regeneration of rat sciatic nerve. *Brain Res* 475: 254–58, 1988.
26. Karlsson JO. Axonal transport in retinal ganglion cells. In: Osborne NN, Chader GJ, eds, *Progress in retinal research,* vol 3. Elmsford, NY: Pergamon Press, 105–23, 1984.
27. Key A, Retzius G. *Studien in der Anatomie des Nervensystems und des Bindegewebes.* Stockholm: Samson & Wallin, 1876.
28. Kwan MK, Rydevik BL, Myers RR, et al. Stretch injury of rabbit peripheral nerve: A biomechanical and histological study. *Proc 35th Ann Mtg, Orth Res Soc* 13: 430, 1988.
29. Kwan MK, Wall EJ, Weiss JA, Rydevik BL, et al. Analysis of rabbit peripheral nerve: In situ stresses and strains. *Biomechanics Sym, Am Soc Mech Engineers/AMD* 98: 109–12, 1989.
30. Lieberman AR. The axon reaction: A review of the principal features of perikaryal responses to axon injury. *Int Rev Neurobiol* 14: 49–124, 1971.
31. Lieberman AR. Some factors affecting retrograde neuronal responses to axonal lesions. In: Bellairs R, Gray EG, eds, *Essays on the nervous system.* Oxford, UK: Clarendon Press, 71–105, 1974.
32. Lundborg G. Ischemic nerve injury: Experimental studies on intraneural microvascular pathophysiology and nerve function in a limb subjected to temporary circulatory arrest. *Scand J Plast Reconstr Surg* 6(suppl): 1–113, 1970.
33. Lundborg G, Dahlin LB, Danielsen N, et al. Nerve regeneration in silicone chambers: Influence of gap length and of distal stump components. *Exp Neurol* 76: 361–75, 1982.
34. Lundborg G, Gelberman RH, Longo FM, Powell HC, Varon S. In vivo regeneration of cut nerves encased in silicone tubes: Growth across a 6 mm gap. *J Neuropathol Exp Neurol* 42: 412–22, 1982.
35. Lundborg G, Rydevik B. Effects of stretching the tibial nerve of the rabbit: A preliminary study of the intraneural circulation and the barrier function of the perineurium. *J Bone Joint Surg* (Britain) 55: 390–401, 1973.
36. McQuarrie IG. Acceleration of axonal regeneration in rat somatic motoneurons by using a conditioning lesion. In: Gorio A, Millesi H, Migrino S, eds, *Posttraumatic nerve regeneration: Experimental basis and clinical implications.* New York: Raven Press, 49–58, 1981.
37. McQuarrie IG, Grafstein B. Axon outgrowth enhanced by a previous nerve injury. *Arch Neurol* 29: 53–55, 1973.
38. Millesi H, Terzis J. Nomenclature in peripheral nerve surgery: Committee report of the International Society of Reconstructive Microsurgery. *Clin Plast Surg* 11: 3–8, 1984.
39. Mitchell SW. *Injuries of nerves and their consequences.* Philadelphia: Lippincott, 1872.
40. Morris JH, Hudson AR, Weddell G. A study of degeneration and regeneration in the rat sciatic nerve using electron microscopy: I. Traumatic degeneration of myelin in the proximal stump of the divided nerve. *Z. Zellforsch* 124: 76–102, 1972.
41. Morris JH, Hudson AF, Weddell G. A study of degeneration and regeneration in the rat sciatic nerve based on electron microscopy: II. The development of the regenerating unit. *Z Zellforsch* 124: 103–30, 1972.
42. Ramón y Cajal S. *Studien über Nervenregeneration.* Leipzig: 1908. (Quoted by Weiss, 1941).
43. Ramón y Cajal S. *Degeneration and regeneration of the nervous system,* vol 1. London: Oxford University Press, 1928.
44. Rothman JE, Lenard J. Membrane asymmetry. *Science* 195: 743–53, 1977.
45. Scaravilli F. The influence of distal environment on peripheral nerve regeneration across a gap. *J Neurocytol* 13: 1027–1041, 1984.
46. Seddon H. Three types of nerve injury. *Brain* 66: 237–88, 1943.
47. Seddon HJ. Peripheral nerve injuries. *Med Res Council Special Rep Series 282.* London: Her Majesty's Stationery Office, 1954.
48. Seddon H. *Surgical disorders of the peripheral nerves.* Edinburgh: Churchill Livingstone, 1972.
49. Sisken BF, Barr E, Estes RS. Electrical effects on nerve ganglia in vitro. In: Hunt TK, Heppenstall RB, Pines E, Rovey D, eds, *Soft and hard tissue repair: Biological and clinical aspects.* New York: Praeger, 1984.
50. Sisken BF, Smith SD. The effects of minute direct electrical currents on cultured chick embryo trigeminal ganglia. *J Embryol Exp Morph* 33: 29–35, 1975.
51. Sunderland S. A classification of peripheral nerve injuries producing loss of function. *Brain* 74: 491–516, 1951.

52. Sunderland S. *Nerves and nerve injuries*, 2d ed. Edinburgh: Churchill Livingstone, 133–41, 1978.
53. Thomas PK, Ochoa J. Microscopic anatomy of peripheral nerve fibers. In: Dyck PF, Thomas PK, Lambert EH, Bunge MB, eds, *Peripheral neuropathy*. Philadelphia: Saunders, 39–96, 1984.
54. Varon S, Adler R. Nerve growth factors and control of nerve growth. *Curr Top Dev Biol* 16: 207–52, 1980.
55. Varon S, Adler R. Trophic and specifying factors directed to neuronal cells. *Adv Cell Neurobiol* 2: 115–63, 1981.
56. Varon S, Manthorpe M, Williams LR. Neuronotrophic and neurite promoting factors and their clinical potentials. *Dev Neurosci* 6: 73–100, 1984.
57. Wall EJ, Kwan MK, Garfin SR, Woo SL-Y. Stress relaxation of a peripheral nerve. *Proc 36th Ann Mtg, Ortho Res Soc* 15: 579, 1990.
58. Williams LR. Exogenous fibrin matrix precursors stimulate the temporal progress of nerve regeneration within a silicone chamber. *Neurochem Res* 12: 851–60, 1987.
59. Williams LR, Powell HC, Lundborg G, Varon S. Competence of nerve tissue as distal insert promoting nerve regeneration in a silicone chamber. *Brain Res* 293: 201–11, 1984.

SECTION 2

Effects of Ligament Injury on the Sensorimotor System

Section Leaders: Thomas P. Andriacchi, PhD, and Joerg G. Jerosch, MD

Section Participants: Lars Konradsen, MD, Laura Huston, MS, Christian Fink, MD, Ivan Vassilev, MD, Arthur Kleipool, MD, Christopher D. Harner, MD, Roger Pollock, MD, Thomas Bochdansky, MD, Bruce D. Beynnon, PhD, David Beard, PhD, PT, Jorge L. Giraldo, MD, Marc R. Safran, MD, Freddie H. Fu, MD

The purpose of this section is to review techniques available for measuring the respective variables within the sensorimotor system, to elucidate the role of the sensorimotor system in maintenance of normal homeostasis, and to present the effects of articular pathology on the system.

Beynnon and associates provide an assessment of current techniques for measuring the knee joint variables on both the afferent and efferent pathways of the sensorimotor system, while Konradsen and associates discuss testing techniques specific to the ankle. Bochdansky and associates next discuss the role of electromyography in the assessment of motor control, followed by a discussion by Albright's group of methods for analyzing balance and neuromuscular responses of the spine and lower extremity.

Huston, Andriacci, Fink and their coauthors present issues related to injury of the anterior cruciate ligament (ACL) and the resulting physiological adaptations that occur with the sensorimotor system that promote knee joint stability. The chapters by Barrack and Munn, and Beard and Refshauge discuss the effects of ACL reconstruction on proprioception and neuromuscular control. Safran and coworkers then address sensorimotor issues specific to posterior cruciate ligament injury of the knee and surgical reconstruction.

The final chapters contained within this section address issues of ankle and shoulder instability. Konradsen and associates address issues related to the unstable ankle, while Jerosch and Pollack present material associated with the effects of shoulder instability on proprioception and the role of surgical restoration of the shoulder on motor control and kinematics.

This group provides an assessment of the current research findings and measurement techniques available in the clinical research laboratory for quantification of sensorimotor variables. One of the severe limitations related to our understanding of the sensorimotor system stems from a lack of specific instrumentation to test the variables contributing to the system. The knowledge base, therefore, is incomplete due to limited systematic research demonstrating normal and pathological data that describes the functional mechanisms of the system. Based on the expertise of the participants, and the observations of the research limitations in this area, the following future directions were identified, relating to the effects of ligament injury on proprioception and neuromuscular control.

Directions for Future Research

1. Determine the relevance of joint position and motion sense testing, and determine whether these tests are related to motor control mechanisms responsible to dynamic joint stabilization.
2. Discriminate between the mechanisms responsible for force proprioception and joint motion/sense and the clinical significance of these characteristics.
3. Establish the relationship between the acquisition and transmission of proprioceptive information and EMG output, and determine the functional significance of EMG data as it relates to dynamic joint stabilization.
4. Determine if levels of muscle tone can be accurately assessed. Determine if measurements of muscle tone are related to or the same as assessments of muscle stiffness, and ascertain the relevance of these characteristics to functional muscle tension and joint stabilization.
5. Establish valid and reliable EMG measurement techniques for assessment of motor control and dynamic joint stabilization related to such factors as normalization and coactivation.
6. Determine the mechanism responsible for proprioceptive decline with age, and establish the influence this decline has on function.
7. Determine if the surgical restoration of proprioceptive sense is related to tissue retensioning, reinnervation, or compensatory mechanisms from surrounding structures.
8. Establish the contribution of meniscal tissue to joint afference.
9. Determine the relative contribution of graft selection on restoration of joint afference.
10. Determine to what extent general locomotor reprogramming is a conscious/unconscious or voluntary/involuntary process.
11. Determine to what extent the reprogramming of general locomotor function to normal is related to restoration of proprioception, joint laxity, influence of secondary restraints, and degenerative changes.
12. Establish the normal timeline for functional adaptations in the ACL-deficient knee.
13. Discover functionally significant criteria to determine the onset latency of muscle activation and the mechanism responsible for these delayed firing responses. Once these assessment tools are established, determine the influence and functional significance of re-

habilitation and surgical intervention on the onset times.

14. Determine if the PCL contributes significantly to knee joint afference and whether not ligament injury results in functional deficits related to decreased proprioception and quadriceps alteration.
15. Determine if measurements of proprioception in the ankle and knee that are performed in the unloaded condition represent functional mechanisms

CHAPTER 12

Validation of Techniques to Measure Knee Proprioception

Bruce D. Beynnon, PhD
Per A. Renström, MD, PhD
Lars Konradsen, MD
Lars-Gunnar Elmqvist, MD, PhD
Daniel Gottlieb, MS
Marco Dirks, MD

Abstract

Joint position sense and joint kinesthesia are two measurement techniques that are used to evaluate knee proprioception; however, there has been very little validation or comparison of these methods. We compared the accuracy, repeatability, and precision of seven joint position sense techniques and one joint kinesthesia measurement technique in normal subjects with no history of knee injury. The joint position sense techniques that were evaluated varied the method and direction of setting the index angle and were characterized by three different error terms: absolute error, real error, and error variation. Accuracy was assessed by comparing dominant and nondominant legs. Repeatability was evaluated by comparing repeated trials conducted on the same day and trials conducted on different days. Precision was described by the standard deviation between repeated trials.

Joint kinesthesia was found to be more repeatable and precise than each of the joint position sense techniques. Therefore, studies designed to evaluate knee proprioception should consider using kinesthesia; this should result in increased power and sensitivity to detect significant differences if they truly exist. The joint position sense technique most frequently used in the orthopedic literature, passive setting of the knee index angle with movement of the leg into extension followed by active reproduction of the index angle, was found to be accurate and repeatable when the absolute error was analyzed. Another technique that relies on active setting of the index angle and subsequent active reproduction also gave accurate and repeatable results, but with improved precision. Using accuracy and repeatability as criteria to choose a proprioception measurement technique, we recommend utilizing joint kinesthesia, passive positioning of the knee into flexion to establish an index angle with active reproduction, and active positioning of the knee into flexion to establish an index angle with active reproduction. We found that the use of a handheld analog to estimate joint position resulted in poor repeatability. The large variability inherent in evaluation of joint position sense necessitates large sample sizes to find significant differences, if in fact they truly exist, and may explain the lack of consistent findings within the scientific literature.

Introduction

Joint position sense and kinesthesia are the two primary methods of measuring knee proprioception, and large variations exist with each approach. In addition, there are differences in the methods used to perform data analysis. Previous studies have analyzed the real error, absolute error, and the error variation. As a result of these differences in experimental techniques and methods of data analysis, comparison of knee proprioception studies is difficult.

Measurements of joint position sense have relied upon the matching of defined index angles (i.e., the knee flexion angle that must be reproduced by the study subject). Definition of the index angle has typically been accomplished passively without muscle contraction by the subject (2, 6, 12, 16), although muscle contraction has also been used (11, 15). Several approaches have been used to match index angles. They have included use of a visual analog of the leg (5), actively matching with the opposite limb (9), actively matching with the same leg (12, 16), and passively setting the contralateral leg (13). For each of these methods, differences exist in terms of how knee flexion angle is measured, the duration that the index angle is maintained, and the angular velocity of the leg. Flexion angle has been measured by monitoring linear translation of the foot, attaching a goniometer to the leg, analyzing video film, and using electrolytic tilt sensors. Angular velocity of the knee has ranged from 2°/s to uncontrolled. It is unclear how sensitive the measurement of joint position sense is to these differences in technique.

Differences also exist in terms of data analysis. Investigators have compared real errors (7, 10), absolute errors (4, 14, 16), and the variation of the error terms (8). Real errors contain both magnitude and direction information and characterize how a subject systematically underestimates or overestimates the index angle. Absolute errors contain only magnitude information, as the absolute value of the real error term is used, and cannot be used to determine if a subject underestimates or overestimates knee position. This term represents the subject's overall ability to reproduce the index angle. The variations of the error terms represent the precision of a subject's estimates and can be described by the standard deviation of the real error terms for a single trial. Each of these error terms represents a unique means of describing joint position sense, although they are probably not independent since it is likely that correlation exists between the values.

The technique for measuring knee joint kinesthesia has been fairly consistent across studies. With this approach, the subject sits in a chair with the legs supported by an external device. Observation of the legs is eliminated, and one leg is slowly flexed (or extended) at a rate of approximately 0.5°/s. The outcome measure is the magnitude of flexion (or extension) that the leg has moved at the point the subject detects motion of the leg. Previous studies that have measured knee kinesthesia have combined the measurements for flexion and extension of the leg; however, it is unclear whether there is a directional dependence and, as such, whether combining the results is appropriate.

While the importance of proprioception as a clinical outcome measure is becoming well recognized (3), the best measurement techniques have yet to be defined. An ideal method should have high sensitivity and specificity while also exhibiting good repeatability, precision, and accuracy. Rigorous statistical analysis of methods to verify repeatability and accuracy, in most instances, has not been performed. A comparison of the available techniques and methods of data analysis could yield one or a combination that is more reliable than others, would allow interpretation of the existing literature, and may guide future investigators. While it is not feasible to compare all of the variations in every technique that has been reported in the literature, the results of an analysis that employs representative methods should be capable of being extrapolated to methods with similar protocols.

Methods

The objectives of this study were to compare several proprioception measurement techniques and provide a database of normal values. Specifically, we were interested in the repeatability and accuracy of the techniques and whether joint kinesthesia (JK) measurement was superior in terms of accuracy and repeatability in comparison to commonly used joint position sense (JPS) measurement techniques. Each method of proprioceptive measurement provides an evaluation that is specific to each leg.

Human Subjects

The study was approved by the Institutional Review Board, and all subjects gave their informed consent prior to participation. Four separate groups of volunteers were used to evaluate the JPS1, JPS2–JPS3, JPS4–JPS7, and JK techniques (see table 12.1).

Table 12.1 Clinical Demographics of Subject Groups

Technique	JK	JPS1	JPS2-JPS3	JPS4-JPS7
Sample size (n)	11	10	9	11
Age: mean (range)	30 (24-34)	27 (24-32)	25 (21-32)	23 (20-30)
Lysholm scores: range	95–100	95–100	95–100	95–100
KT-1000 (Δ between legs)	< 2 mm	< 2 mm	< 2 mm	< 2 mm
Lachman test	Stable	Stable	Stable	Stable
Pivot shift test	Negative	Negative	Negative	Negative

All subjects were athletically active, participated in sport at least three times per week, had no history of a traumatic injury to either leg, and a Lysholm score that ranged between 95 and 100 (17). Subjects were both male and female and ranged between 18 and 34 yrs of age. Clinical examinations were normal for all subjects, and none showed any ligamentous defects.

Experimental Procedures

A consistent nomenclature was used to describe each JPS measurement technique (see table 12.2 and figure 12.1). The first portion of the description referred to the method and direction that was used to set the index angle (i.e., the knee flexion angle that must be reproduced by the subject), and the second portion referred to the method that was used to produce the matching angle (i.e., reproduction of the knee flexion angle). A total of seven different JPS and one JK measurement technique were tested in four different groups of subjects. Each measurement technique was referred to by its assigned number (see table 12.2 and figure 12.1).

All subjects were taught the JPS technique and allowed to practice prior to data collection. Subjects were seated for the techniques that involved extension of the knee to set the index and matching flexion angles. Subjects stood on a raised platform supporting their full body weight on one leg for techniques that involved flexion of the knee to set the index and matching knee angles. For these trials, the leg under study hung freely off the raised platform, and the subject maintained his or her balance by holding onto an arm rail.

Several procedures were common for each method. A blindfold or curtain was used to prevent visualization of the legs. An air cuff was used to minimize tactile cues when passively moving the knee. For the JPS techniques a 6 in. long cuff inflated to 1 lb/in^2 was placed around the ankle proximal to the malleoli. For the JK technique, an air boot (Aircast, Inc., Summit, NJ) inflated to 0.5 lb/in^2 was utilized. Electrolytic tilt sensors (MicroStrain, Inc., Burlington, VT) were strapped to the subject's proximal thigh and distal aspect of the lower leg, the signal amplified, sampled at 20 Hz, and stored for future analysis. Knee flexion angle was determined by comparing the output of the tilt sensors, one attached to the thigh and the other attached to the lower leg. These sensors were not sensitive to off-axis rotations (< 1% change in output for 45° off-axis alignment) and had high precision, which makes these devices an appropriate choice for measuring changes in knee flexion angle (10). The sensors were initialized at 45° with a handheld goniometer.

The dependent outcomes were the mean changes of knee flexion angle for the JK technique and the mean errors in repositioning of the knee for the JPS techniques. The error in repositioning of the knee was calculated as the difference between the index angle and the matching angle. Three different methods were used: real error, absolute error, and error variation (see Statistical Analysis section). The error values were used for statistical analysis and represent each subject's JPS.

The JPS1 group included 10 subjects, including 5 males and 5 females. Subjects ranged in age between 24 and 32 yrs (mean: 27 yrs). Subjects were seated on a Cybex 6000 dynamometer. The seat back was reclined 15° from vertical and was adjusted relative to the seat bottom to allow a 5cm space between the seat and the popliteal fossa. Legs were tested one at a time. To test the leg it was attached to the machine's lever arm and adjusted so that the center of rotation of the dynamometer was aligned with the center of rotation of the knee. The leg was passively extended at a rate of 2°/s. When the index angle was reached, the subjects were instructed to approximate their knee flexion angle using a plastic, handheld, visual analog of a leg fitted with a goniometer. The analog was similar in design to that used by previous investigators (4, 5). Each trial consisted of six different index angles ranging between

Table 12.2 Methods of Positioning and Repositioning the Joint for the Seven Joint Position Sense (JPS) Measurement Techniques

Technique	Method and direction used to set index knee angle	Method used to produce the matching knee angle	Position of subject
JPS1	Passive positioning into extension	Analog representation	Seated
JPS2	Passive positioning into flexion	Active flexion	Standing
JPS3	Active positioning into flexion	Multiple active flexion	Standing
JPS4	Passive positioning into extension	Active extension	Seated
JPS5	Active positioning into extension	Active extension	Seated
JPS6	Passive positioning into flexion	Active flexion	Standing
JPS7	Active positioning into flexion	Active flexion	Standing

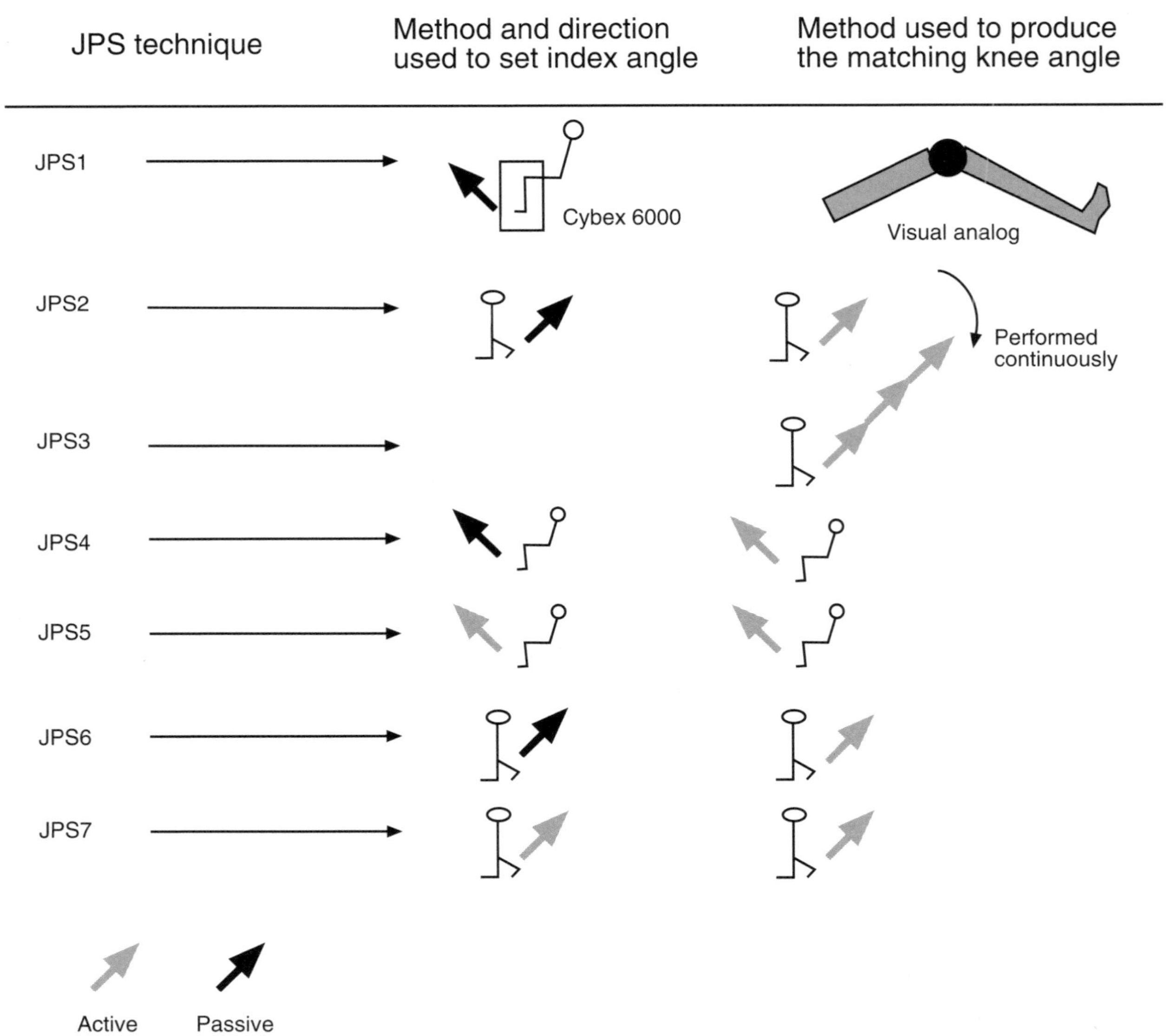

Figure 12.1 Pictorial description of the seven JPS techniques.

5° and 75°. The starting position of the leg was varied in a random sequence from one replicate to the next. There were two trials conducted on the first day and two trials on a subsequent day one week later. A rest period of approximately 1 h was given between trials conducted on the same day.

The JPS2 and JPS3 groups consisted of 9 healthy subjects, 1 male and 8 females, ranging in age between 21 and 32 yrs (mean: 25 yrs). The JPS2 and JPS3 measurements were performed concurrently with the subject in a standing posture. The limb under investigation was passively (no muscle activity) flexed by the examiner at a speed of 10°/s to an index angle between 10° and 80°. The index angle was maintained for 3 s and the leg was then passively returned to the initial, extended position. The subject then actively matched the index angle five times. Each trial consisted of five replicates. Two trials were conducted on the first day and one trial was conducted on a subsequent day one week later. The error for JPS2 was calculated as the difference between the passively set index angle and the first actively set matching angle. The error for JPS3 was calculated as the difference between the four successive matching angles (i.e., 2 – 3, 3 – 4, 4 – 5, 5 – 6). We used each successive angle for comparison rather than always comparing to the initial index angle because a pilot study found the former method produced the most precise results. For each replicate, four errors were calculated, and a complete trial had five replicates; the score was based on the mean of 20 individual error terms.

The JPS4, JPS5, JPS6, and JPS7 groups consisted of 11 healthy subjects including 5 males and 6 females ranging between 20 and 30 yrs of age (mean: 23 yrs). JPS4 and JPS5 were tested with the subjects in a seated position. A 1-liter intravenous bag was placed under the thigh to distribute the pressure at the seat-thigh interface. For JPS4 the examiner passively extended the leg at a rate of 10°/s, starting from 90°, to an index angle between 10° and 80° of flexion, this angle was maintained for 3 s, and the leg was then passively returned to the starting position at the same angular velocity. The subject then actively extended the leg to match the index angle. The procedure for JPS5 was identical to JPS4 except that the index angle was set by the subject actively extending the leg. In an attempt to prevent repeating the same index angle successively and to provide an equal distribution of index angles, instructions were given to select small (10°–30°), medium (30°–60°), or large (60°–80°) index angles. The JPS6 and JPS7 measurement techniques were performed during the same testing session and were identical to JPS2 and JPS3 with three exceptions: the two techniques were performed independently, index angles were repeated only once, and the number of replicates was increased to 25, in an attempt to improve precision. Thus, while performing JPS6 and JPS7, the subject only reproduced the index angle once. Twenty-five different index angles ranging between 10° and 80° were performed in a random order. Each technique was followed through to completion before beginning the next technique. Since the same group of subjects was used for JPS4–JPS7, the order of evaluating the four techniques was randomized. A 5 min rest was allowed between techniques. One week after completing the first trial, the subjects returned and completed another trial for each technique. Time constraints prevented these techniques from being repeated on the same day. Since there were 25 replicates per trial, repeatability within a day was evaluated by comparing replicates at the beginning versus the end of the trial.

The measurement of JK was performed in a manner similar to that used by others (2, 16), although small changes were instituted to reduce extraneous cues. The JK group consisted of 11 subjects including 8 males and 3 females ranging between 24 and 34 yrs of age (mean: 30 yrs). Subjects sat on a reclined chair, and the seat back was positioned such that the popliteal fossa did not touch the edge of the seat bottom when the leg was resting at 90° of flexion. Tests were initiated at 45° of flexion. After completing each motion the leg was returned to the 45° position only if the final position was greater than 48° or less than 42° of flexion. This effectively reduced the reinforcement that occurred when the leg was returned to its initial position after each replicate. Pilot tests indicated that some subjects could gain cutaneous cues from the cuff, so pressure was varied sinusoidally at 1 Hz between 0.4 to 0.6 lb/in^2 to eliminate this problem. Subjects were told that either leg could move in a flexed or extended direction beginning at a random time interval up to 45 s after the examiner signaled the start of the test. Once the subject detected motion of a leg, he or she pressed a button and confirmed the leg that moved and the direction of motion. Each trial consisted of three replicates for each of the four motions (flexion and extension of the right and left legs) performed in a random order, resulting in a total of 12 repetitions. In the event of incorrect identification of the motion, the repetition was returned to the randomization list so that three correct repetitions of each motion were completed for each trial. Data from incorrect responses were not analyzed.

Statistical Analysis

For each JPS technique, there were three scores calculated: the real error score (RES), the absolute error score (AES), and the error variation score (EVS). The RES was calculated as the true difference between the index and matching angles and was expressed in terms of degrees of rotation; this term contained both magnitude and direction information. The AES was calculated as the absolute value of the RES and contained only magnitude information. The EVS was used to describe the variability within a single trial and was calculated as the standard deviation across a single trial. Each score was evaluated independently. Thus, it was possible that within a single JPS technique, only certain types of scores produced accurate and repeatable results. For the JK technique, the threshold to detection of knee flexion angle rotation was used for statistical analysis.

For the JPS and JK measurement techniques, accuracy was evaluated by comparing error scores between dominant and nondominant legs. This comparison was based on the observations of Barrack and associates (3) and Corrigan and associates (6), who have also shown that symmetry exists between the legs of normal individuals for both JPS and JK. The error scores were compared with analysis of variance and correlation analysis for two reasons; correlation analysis provides no information on systematic differences between the variables, while with analysis of variance, differences become harder to detect (i.e., power drops) as the variability increases. A measurement technique and error score were considered accurate if there was a significant Pearson correlation coefficient (r) between dominant and nondominant legs and no significant difference between dominant and nondominant legs according to the analysis of variance.

Measurements of knee proprioception performed either on the same or different days should yield similar results that do not change in magnitude, and therefore we evaluated between- as well as within-day repeatability. Between-day repeatability was evaluated for all techniques, and within-day repeatability was evaluated for JPS1–JPS3 as well as JK. The error scores were compared with analysis of variance and correlation analysis. We used the intraclass correlation coefficient (R) to evaluate repeatability because it could be used to compare more than two repeated trials. Successive trials were not conducted on the same day for JPS4–JPS7, and therefore we could not formally evaluate within-day repeatability. There were, however, a large number of replicates within each trial (25), and therefore we tested for a systematic within-trial effect by comparing the first five replicates within each trial to the last five using a paired t test. A measurement technique and error score were considered repeatable within a day if there were no differences between successive trials conducted the same day as determined via analysis of variance. A measurement technique and error score were considered repeatable between days if there were no differences between trials conducted on different days and the interclass correlation coefficient was significant.

Standard deviations between legs and between repeated trials were included to provide a comparative measure of precision (variability). We calculated these values by using the square root of the mean square error taken from the analysis of variance. Since the experimental design involved repeated measures, the mean square error terms for each main effect were the effect by subject interaction. The large number of replicates employed for JPS4–JPS7 allowed us to test for flexion angle dependence. The mean real error score for index angles less than 45° were compared with those greater than 45° using a paired t test to determine if flexion angle affected the resultant error.

Since our previous work has determined that the absolute error score distributions did not consistently demonstrate a normal distribution (10), all data were plotted and checked for normality using the Shapiro-Wilk test. Distributions that were not normally distributed were normalized with an appropriate transformation before analysis. Comparisons were considered significant for $p < .05$.

Results

Many of the distributions violated the assumption of normality, and appropriate transformations (natural log and square root) were applied. Of the JPS techniques that utilized angle matching with the same leg (JPS2–JPS7), a consistent result was found: on average, all subjects overestimated the index angle (see table 12.3). This was evidenced by negative overall RES for JPS2, JPS3, JPS6, and JPS7.

Accuracy

Accuracy was evaluated by comparing differences and correlations between dominant and nondominant legs. Using this criteria the following techniques were found to be accurate: JPS1 (RES), JPS2 (RES and AES), JPS3 (RES and AES), JPS4 (RES and AES), JPS5 (AES and EVS), JPS6 (AES and EVS), JPS7 (RES, AES, and EVS), and JK (see tables 12.4 and 12.5).

Table 12.3 Average Results for Seven Joint Position Sense (JPS) Techniques, Each With Three Methods of Data Analysis, and the Joint Kinesthesia (JK) Technique, Mean (*SD*) in Degrees

Technique	RES	AES	EVS	JK
JPS1	−4.4 (7.9)	10.9 (4.5)	7.5 (2.7)	
JPS2	−5.6 (5.5)	7.0 (3.6)	3.4 (1.6)	
JPS3	−0.8 (1.0)	2.3 (0.8)	2.5 (0.8)	
JPS4	0.6 (2.6)	4.3 (1.2)	4.3 (1.2)	
JPS5	0.9 (1.7)	3.1 (0.9)	3.1 (0.9)	
JPS6	−3.7 (3.9)	5.8 (2.5)	5.8 (2.5)	
JPS7	−1.8 (1.7)	3.8 (1.0)	3.8 (1.1)	
JK				1.5 (1.0)

Table 12.4 Result of Analysis of Variance for the Eight Proprioception Measurement Techniques

Technique	Comparison	RES	AES	EVS	JK
JPS1	Between legs	.91	.9	.68	
	Between days	.19	.05*	.08^	
	Trials within a day	.03*	.98	.06^	
JPS2	Between legs	.74	.69	.7	
	Between days	.22	.37	.31	
	Trials within a day	.07^	.14	.29	
JPS3	Between legs	.67	.11	.024*	
	Between days	.53	.93	.19	
	Trials within a day	.90	.32	.54	
JPS4	Between legs	.22	.43	.96	
	Between days	.03*	.58	.53	
JPS5	Between legs	.07^	.25	.17	
	Between days	.98	.004*	.29	
JPS6	Between legs	.027*	.18	.24	
	Between days	.01*	.13	.74	
JPS7	Between legs	.14	.3	.26	
	Between days	.61	.43	.17	
JK	Between legs				.28
	Between days				.57
	Trials within a day				.06^

^.05 < p < .1; *p < .05

Table 12.5 Pearson Correlation (*r*) Coefficients Comparing Dominant and Nondominant Legs and Intraclass Correlation Coefficients (*R*) for Repeated Trials

Technique	Test	RES	AES	EVS	JK
JPS1	Between legs (*r*)	.53**	.28	.06	
	Repeated trials (*R*)	.62	.42	−.33	
JPS2	Between legs (*r*)	.72***	.51**	−.11	
	Repeated trials (*R*)	.77***	.26	−.46	
JPS3	Between legs (*r*)	.54**	.42**	.52**	
	Repeated trials (*R*)	.87***	.85***	.77***	
JPS4	Between legs (*r*)	.62**	.58*	.35 n.s.	
	Repeated trials (*R*)	.36	.8***	.56	
JPS5	Between legs (*r*)	.16	.6**	.59*	
	Repeated trials (*R*)	.55	.63**	.61*	
JPS6	Between legs (*r*)	.59*	.69**	.78**	
	Repeated trials (*R*)	.78***	.81***	.70*	
JPS7	Between legs (*r*)	.5*	.55*	.53*	
	Repeated trials (*R*)	.57	.32	.15	
JK	Between legs (*r*)				.86***
	Repeated trials (*R*)				.83**

*$p < .05$; **$p < .01$; ***$p < .001$

Measurements of knee proprioception performed either on the same or different days should yield similar results that do not change in magnitude, and therefore we evaluated between- as well as within-day repeatability. Between-day repeatability was evaluated for all techniques, and within-day repeatability was evaluated for JPS1–JPS3 as well as JK. The error scores were compared with analysis of variance and correlation analysis. We used the intraclass correlation coefficient (R) to evaluate repeatability because it could be used to compare more than two repeated trials. Successive trials were not conducted on the same day for JPS4–JPS7, and therefore we could not formally evaluate within-day repeatability. There were, however, a large number of replicates within each trial (25), and therefore we tested for a systematic within-trial effect by comparing the first five replicates within each trial to the last five using a paired *t* test (see table 12.6). A measurement technique and error score were considered repeatable within a day if there were no differences between successive trials conducted the same day as determined via analysis of variance. A measurement technique and error score were considered repeatable between days if there were no differences between trials conducted on different days and the interclass correlation coefficient was significant.

Standard deviations between legs and between repeated trials were included to provide a comparative measure of precision (variability). We calculated these values by using the square root of the mean square error taken from the analysis of variance. Since the experimental design involved repeated measures, the mean square error terms for each main effect were the effect by subject interaction. The large number of replicates employed for JPS4-JPS7 allowed us to test for flexion angle dependence. The mean real error score for index angles less than 45° were compared with those greater than 45° using a paired *t* test to determine if flexion angle affected the resultant error.

Repeatability Between Trials

A technique and analysis method were considered repeatable within a day if there were no differences between successive trials conducted the same day, as determined via analysis of variance. This analysis was not relevant for JPS4–JPS7 because these techniques were not repeated on the same day. Using these criteria the following techniques were repeatable: JPS1 (AES), JPS2 (RES, AES, and EVS, al-

Table 12.6 Comparison Between the RES of the First and Last Five Replicates for JPS4–JPS7 Techniques, Mean Value

Technique	Replicates 1–5	Replicates 21–25	*p* value
JPS4	0.1	0.5	n.s.
JPS5	1.0	0.3	.005
JPS6	–3.9	–3.9	n.s.
JPS7	–1.8	–2.1	n.s.

though $p = .07$ for the analysis of variance), JPS3 (RES, AES, and EVS), and JK (although $p = .06$ for the analysis of variance result).

Repeatability Between Days

A technique and analysis method were considered repeatable between days if there were no differences between trials conducted on different days and the intraclass correlation coefficient was significant. Using these criteria the following techniques were found to be repeatable: JPS2 (RES), JPS3 (RES, AES, and EVS), JPS4 (AES), JPS5 (EVS), JPS6 (AES and EVS), and JK.

Precision

Precision was described by the variation between repeated trials and between left and right legs (see table 12.7). The JPS technique with the least precision (greatest variation) was JPS1 while, in general, the most precise was JPS3. The JK technique had a precision similar to JPS3 (< 1).

Effect of Flexion Angle on the RES

For JPS4–JPS7, the RES was significantly more positive for replicates where the index angle was greater than 45° compared to those less than 45° (see table 12.8). For all techniques, the mean error was less than zero for the acute angles. The mean error was greater than zero for JPS4, JPS5, and JPS7.

Overall Results

The techniques and methods of data analysis that were both repeatable and accurate were JPS2 (RES), JPS3 (RES and AES), JPS4 (AES), JPS5 (EVS), JPS6 (AES and EVS), and JK. The protocol used for JPS2 and JPS6 was very similar, and therefore similar results were expected.

Discussion

The techniques utilized in this study do not represent all possible methods of measuring JPS and JK. The techniques not evaluated were omitted for one of two reasons: either they were considered not sensitive to within-subject differences, or the method would likely have large interobserver variation. The JPS techniques that have been used previously, but were not tested here, include matching with the opposite leg (either passively or actively) and passive matching with the same leg. When matching with the opposite leg the resulting error would be a combination of errors from each leg, and it would be impossible to determine which leg was the source. Our investigation focused on JPS techniques that could be used to detect problems produced by a knee injury; therefore, a specific test was necessary. Passive matching has the potential for large interobserver errors, and therefore this technique may not be repeatable when performed by other investigators. The results probably depend on the individual performing the test and the specific method used to zero in on the matching angle. We felt the techniques chosen, especially those where the subjects actively set both the index and matching angle, would lead to small interobserver errors, and therefore other investigators could replicate these methods and find similar results.

One can question how methods that are nearly identical (JPS2 and JPS6, and JPS3 and JPS7) yield somewhat different results. For JPS6 and JPS7 replicates were performed one at time, for a total of 25 replicates. The protocol for JPS2 and JPS3 differed in the number of replicates (5 for JPS2 versus 20 for JPS3). Another difference was the manner of testing: JPS2 and JPS3 were performed concurrently, while JPS6 and JPS7 were performed independently. Furthermore, for JPS3 the angle reproduction was repeated five times for each angle, while for JPS2 the index angle was only matched once. We would expect the increase in the number of replicates to improve the precision and thus the

Table 12.7 Standard Deviations (Precision) Between Legs and Between Repeated Trials for the Seven JPS Techniques, Each With Three Methods of Data Analysis, and the One JK Technique, in Units of Degrees

Technique	Comparison	RES	AES	EVS	JK
JPS1	Between legs	8.0	4.3	2.5	
	Between days	6.4	4.1	2.2	
	Trials within a day	5.9	4.8	2.8	
JPS2	Between legs	0.9	2.2	1.2	
	Between days	2.8	2.1	1.7	
	Trials within a day	3.3	3.7	2.2	
JPS3	Between legs	0.93	0.69	0.54	
	Between days	0.63	0.47	0.74	
	Trials within a day	0.46	0.41	0.51	
JPS4	Between legs	1.4	0.7	0.9	
	Between days	2.3	0.8	0.8	
JPS5	Between legs	1.6	0.6	0.7	
	Between days	1.23	0.88	0.55	
JPS6	Between legs	3.0	0.91	2.1	
	Between days	2.4	1.52	1.8	
JPS7	Between legs	1.3	0.75	0.63	
	Between days	1.6	1.73	1.1	
JK	Between legs				0.87
	Between days				0.64
	Trials within a day				0.89

Table 12.8 Comparison of Real Error Scores for Index Angles Less Than 45° With Those Greater Than 45° for Techniques 4–7

Technique	Mean (*SD*) for < 45°	Mean (*SD*) for > 45°	*p* value
JPS4	–2.0 (3.9)	2.8 (2.5)	<.001
JPS5	–0.8 (2.1)	3.0 (2.0)	<.001
JPS6	–6.2 (3.9)	–1.6 (4.5)	<.001
JPS7	–4.5 (3.2)	0.8 (2.6)	<.001

power of comparisons made with JPS6 and JPS7. We cannot discount the effect of different subject populations, testing conditions, and time required to complete each protocol. It took approximately 30 min to perform the measurements for JPS2 and JPS3, while it required about 2 h each day to complete the entire protocol for JPS4 through JPS7. The longer protocol may have increased the variability, thus reducing the repeatability and precision.

Prior to our investigation, we did not expect JPS to depend on the index angle. These findings have implications on the data analysis and may indicate something about the nature of joint position sense. Data should not be pooled if it is not homogeneous. Thus, we recommend that small and large index flexion angles be analyzed independently or that a smaller range of index angles be studied. The average RES were negative for index angles less than 45° and greater than zero for those larger than 45°; if these data were combined they would converge on an average near zero. This also has implications on the EVS. Because the errors occurring at each flexion angle may have little variability, and the mean error at each flexion may differ, the resulting standard deviation, and thus the EVS, may be inflated. However, this should not have affected the repeatability of the results since the distribution of flexion angles was the same for each trial.

It is not surprising that muscle activity affects the error associated with JPS measurements. JPS2–JPS3, JPS4–JPS5, and JPS6–JPS7 may be considered "matched" tests because the only difference was the active (with muscle contractions) or passive (without muscle contractions) setting of the index angle. For each of these pairs of tests, the absolute errors were consistently lower for the active test (JPS3, JPS5, and JPS7) compared to the corresponding passive test (JPS2, JPS4, and JPS6) (see table 12.3). The muscle force required to maintain the joint in a fixed position changed as the flexion angle was changed. Thus, subjects could utilize the sensation of muscle force in addition to the sense of position to replicate the index angle. Since the tests that required active setting of the index angle had consistently lower EVS than the passive tests, it appears that the senses of force and position produce more accurate results than the sense of position alone. This does, however, point out a potential limitation of the active tests: they may not be sensitive when evaluating subjects with intact force receptors but deficient position sensors.

We found that the passive tests also have limitations. Many subjects found it quite difficult or impossible to completely relax their lower leg musculature and remain passive as the leg was moved. This was particularly evident when performing the standing tests, where the leg under study was flexed. This effect can easily bias the results of a study, especially if different groups of subjects are compared, and one group finds it more difficult to remain passive than the other does. It is possible that biofeedback could be used to assist subjects in maintaining a relaxed state.

Four different groups of subjects were used for JPS1, JPS2–JPS3, JPS4–JPS7, and JK, and this may have confounded the comparisons. It would have been preferable to utilize a single group of subjects for all techniques, but this was not possible because many of the subjects were unable to make such a lengthy commitment to our investigation. However, all four groups were similar in terms of age, activity level, health, and knee status.

Comparison of the repeatability and accuracy data from the present study with those of previous investigations revealed contrasting results. Barrack and coworkers (3) reported a Pearson correlation coefficient of .94 between right and left legs of normal subjects for the JK technique. This value was comparable to the .86 found in our study. Barrett (5) evaluated the repeatability of the AES for a method similar to our JPS1 and reported a Pearson correlation coefficient of .82 for a group of 20 normal subjects tested two times. This is appreciably higher than the .42 and .62 we found for the AES and the RES. There are a few potential reasons for this discrepancy. First, Pearson's correlation coefficient tends to increase when the spread of the data is large. In Barrett's study (5) the highest values were approximately six times that of the lowest values; this was much larger than what we observed. Barrett also used more replicates per trial, which should reduce the variability and increase the correlation coefficient. The range of flexion angles utilized was much smaller in Barrett's study, which may have reduced the variability. Since we would expect the variability to decrease if the number of replicates increased and the range of angles tested was reduced, the differences found using analysis of variance could be expected to become more pronounced. Thus, it appears that even if we adjusted our technique by increasing the number of replicates and reducing the range of angles used, we would expect to find similar results.

The mean values that we found for JPS and JK were, in general, comparable to those of previous studies. Using methods analogous to our JPS4, other studies have reported mean AES for normal controls ranging between 2.6° and 5° (1, 6, 12, 16). We found a mean of 4.3°. We found an overall mean of 1.5° for the JK technique. Literature values for young subjects with normal knees range between 1.1° (6) and 3.9° (2). Using a method similar to our JPS1 technique, Barrett and coworkers (4) reported a mean AES of approximately 3°, which was substantially lower than the 10.9° we found. It may be that the difference is related to the larger range of flexion angles used in the current study and the subject's position during testing. We tested subjects in a seated position while Barrett and associates evaluated subjects in a prone position.

In the orthopedic literature, the AES has been used almost exclusively for JPS analysis. The reasons for this are unclear but may be related to the relative simplicity of interpretation and the possibility that the RES is not sensitive to differences in JPS. When using the RES, for instance, it may not be possible to say that one group has better or worse proprioception than another, even if the mean values are significantly different. This can easily occur if one group has a mean greater than zero and the other a mean of similar magnitude but negative. Barrack and coworkers (2) found that ballet dancers tended to overestimate the index angle more frequently than a group of normal controls, thus implying a difference in real error. In studies by Feuerbach and others (8) and Ferrell and associates (7) both the AES and RES were used for data analysis. Both studies reported significant differences when analyzing the AES but no differences when analyzing the RES. Our findings and these reports emphasize that use of the RES may provide precise and repeatable results, but use of this analysis technique may fail to find differences that exist when the AES is utilized instead.

Use of the EVS should not lead to the same difficulties in analysis and interpretation since a larger value is interpreted as poorer joint position sense. There are, however, several potential difficulties with the use of this value. First, the EVS will be increased by random errors in the measurement of flexion angle. Second, a subject will be classified as having excellent proprioception if he or she constantly errs to any degree, as long as the errors are consistent.

Conclusion

We have evaluated the repeatability and accuracy of several means of measuring knee proprioception and data analysis. We determined that JK was more repeatable and precise than each of the JPS techniques that were evaluated. While several techniques faired poorly, we found that the most common technique and method of data analysis (JPS4, AES) used in the literature were both accurate and repeatable. In addition to this technique, several "active" techniques were found to provide equally good results in terms of accuracy and repeatability. Researchers should either use the best techniques described here or validate a new technique before applying the method to answer research questions.

References

1. Barrack RL, Skinner HB, Cook SD: Effect of articular disease and total knee arthroplasty on knee joint-position sense. *J Neurophys* 1983; 50: 684–87.
2. Barrack RL, Skinner HB, Brunet ME, Cook SD: Proprioception of the knee joint: Paradoxical effect of training. *Amer J Phys Med* 1984; 63: 175–81.
3. Barrack RL, Skinner HB, Buckley SL: Proprioception in the anterior cruciate-deficient knee. *Amer J Sports Med* 1989; 17: 1–6.
4. Barrett DS, Cobb AG, Bentley G: Joint proprioception in normal, osteoarthritic, and replaced knees. *J Bone Joint Surg* 1991; 73B: 53–56.
5. Barrett DS: Proprioception and function after anterior cruciate reconstruction. *J Bone Joint Surg* 1991; 73B: 833–37.
6. Corrigan JP, Cashman WF, Brady MP: Proprioception in the cruciate deficient knee. *J Bone Joint Surg* 1992; 74B: 247–50.
7. Ferrell WR, Crighton A, Sturrock RD: Age-dependent changes in position sense in human proximal interphalangeal joints. *Neuroreport* 1992; 3: 259–61.
8. Feuerbach JW, Grabiner MD, Koh TJ, Weiker GG: Effect of an ankle orthosis and ankle ligament anesthesia on ankle joint proprioception. *Amer J Sports Med* 1994; 22: 223–29.
9. Goodwin GM, McCloskey DI, Matthews PBC: The contribution of muscle afferents to kinesthesia shown by vibration induced illusions of movement and by the effects of paralyzing joint affronts. *Brain* 1972; 95: 705–48.
10. Gottlieb DJ: An evaluation of joint position sense measurements: Accuracy, repeatability, and clinical potential. Master's thesis, University of Vermont, Burlington, 1993.
11. Gottlieb DJ, Beynnon BD, Dirks M, Renström PA: Is joint position sense clinically relevant? *Ortho Trans* 1994; 18(2): 394.
12. Harter RA, Osternig LR, Singer KM, James SL, Larson RL, Jones DC: Long-term evaluation of knee stability and function following surgical reconstruction for anterior cruciate ligament insufficiency. *Amer J Sports Med* 1988; 16: 434–43.
13. Horsch KW, Clark FJ, Burgess PR: Awareness of knee joint angle under static conditions. *J Neurophys* 1975; 38: 1436–447.
14. Klein BP, Blaha JD, Simons W: Anterior cruciate ligament deficient knees do not have altered proprioception. *Proc 38th Annual Ortho Res Soc* 1992.
15. Paillard J, Brouchon, M: Active and passive movements in the calibration of position sense. In: *The Neuropsychology of Spatially Oriented Behavior.* Belmont, CA: Dorsey Press, 37–55, 1968.
16. Skinner HB, Barrack RL, Cook SD: Age-related decline in proprioception. *Clin Ortho* 1984; 184: 208–11.
17. Tegner Y, Lysholm J: Rating systems in the evaluation of knee ligament injuries. *Clin Ortho* 1985; 198: 43–49.

CHAPTER 13

Techniques for Measuring Sensorimotor Control of the Ankle: Evaluation of Different Methods

Lars Konradsen, MD
Bruce D. Beynnon, PhD
Per A. Renström, MD, PhD

A number of methods seek to measure sensorimotor control of the ankle. The goal is usually to evaluate the afferent signal, but very often the methods include elements that require motor tasks and input from other sensory areas. The following chapter does not seek to judge whether or not measurements like movement threshold, reaction time, and the like have been validated, but whether or not the specific methods employed in ankle instability research can be considered to be well documented.

The methods that are in use in ankle sensorimotor control research have not been chosen from a cause and effect perspective in order to establish or verify a model that could connect a measured sensorimotor control deficit to the ability (or inability) to preserve functional ankle stability. Measuring the stability of single-limb stance evolved from clinical observations of the balance ability of functionally unstable subjects.[9] Kinesthesia and joint position sense were adopted from previous neurophysiological research on joint sensorimotor control. (2, 15) The idea of using functional jumping and running tests (4, 20) was duplicated from knee and foot reconstruction research, and peroneal nerve conduction velocity tests were employed to determine a neurophysiological explanation for a sensorimotor control deficit. (23) Only in the case of measuring peroneal reaction to sudden inversion does the connection between the measurement of sensorimotor control and the clinical significance of a deficiency seem clear. (30, 34)

The sensorimotor control measurement techniques can be organized into the following groups based on the neuromuscular pathways they measure:

- Measurements of general sensorimotor control functions involving a wide variety of motor skills
- Single-limb postural stability tests
- Single-limb agility tests
- Measurements primarily evaluating afferent information but also including efferent abilities to a varying degree
- Tests of kinesthesia (movement threshold)
- Tests of joint position assessment both as active and passive positioning
- Tests for the reaction of the peroneal muscles to sudden inversion
- Measurements evaluating neurophysiological afferent abilities
- Peroneal nerve conduction velocity measurements
- Measurement of H-reflex modulation and EMG response magnitude

Prior to discussing the background for some of the most widely used tests and the information available concerning their validity, we will review the approach used to perform validation.

Validation of a Method

To consider a method validated, information must first be available concerning its repeatability, accuracy, and precision. Repeatability is evaluated by comparing repeated trials that are performed either on the same day or on different days. Accuracy is the difference between an experimental measurement and a "gold standard." This is seldom available, and therefore reliability is usually evaluated through a comparison between dominant and nondominant legs. It is important to realize that this assumes bilateral symmetry. Precision is the variability, or experimental error, of a measurement technique and is often measured as the standard deviation between repeated trials performed on the same leg. Finally it is often of interest to know if the method demonstrates a learning effect, that is, a systematic change in the test results over repeated trials.

When these elements are accounted for, testing can proceed to the important question of whether or not the method is sensitive to the changes that are expected. Not many of the methods employed in research of sensorimotor control of the ankle have been validated, but for many of them, either repeatability or left-right comparisons have been performed.

Single-Limb Postural Stability Tests

Initially, the idea of a sensorimotor control deficit being responsible for functional ankle instability sprang from the observation that functionally unstable subjects had problems balancing on the affected foot. (9) The patients were asked to stand first on the uninjured and then on the injured side. The test was done with the eyes open as well as closed. The patient's stability when standing on the injured side was compared to stability when standing on the uninjured foot. When impaired stability was obvious to the examiner, the defect in sensorimotor control was described as "objective." In cases where the subject felt unstable when standing on the injured leg but no difference was obvious to the examiner, the defect was described as "subjective." The study showed a marked difference in objective and subjective test results between functionally stable and unstable subjects. However, a substantial number of tests were considered inconclusive, and they were excluded from the comparisons.

In 1985, Tropp and coworkers (36) generated an objective measurement of sway during single-limb stance. Tropp standardized the way subjects stood on a force platform (arms crossed, eyes open, contralateral leg flexed under the subject) and registered the location of the instantaneous center of pressure. The subjects were required to stand for 60 s. Based on the pressure location data, an ellipse was constructed to encompass 66% of the center of pressure points. The area of the ellipse was considered a measurement of the magnitude of sway during these 60 s. The coefficient of variation of repeated tests was found to be 8.3%. No difference was found between right and left limb tests in normal subjects. (36)

In the following studies this method was not adopted exactly as described in the thesis of Hans Tropp. (35) Instead, many factors were varied in the measurement of single-limb balance. The platform could be a stable force platform, (10, 35) an unstable instrumented wobble board, (6, 33) or programmed to do random perturbations. (7) Data collection required single-limb stance that ranged between 5 s (14) and 60 s; (35) and the data has been processed as the area of an ellipse, (12, 35) as a postural sway amplitude in medial-lateral or anterior-posterior direction, (7) as a lateral-medial and anterior-posterior sway variability, (17) as average speed, (10) or as a vertical force variation. (14) It is not possible to state that one approach is more "right" than another, as they all measure a variety of sensory input and motor outputs. Whether to decide on a short or a long period of data collection may depend on the group that is tested. Old people can't be expected to keep their balance for 60 s, while subtle changes seen in groups of soccer players might not manifest themselves in a 5 s observation period. It is thought that subtle changes in sensorimotor control become more detectable using an unstable support surface or a surface that can be programmed to make small perturbations.

To improve the sensitivity of one-leg stabilometry tests, Fridén and associates (10) chose to measure movement only in the frontal plane, where the support surface available to maintain upright posture is confined to the width of the foot. They studied the single-limb balance of 55 ankle-healthy volunteers on a static force plate with the following measurements: (a) mean value for the distance between the center of pressure and the reference line of the foot, (b) the standard deviation of this measurement, (c) average speed of frontal sway movements, (d) the mean sway amplitude, and (e) number of movements exceeding a certain amplitude of sway. Test-retest measurements showed that the best correlation was achieved for the average speed of frontal sway reflecting both amplitude and frequency ($R = .71$) with the other measurements producing correlation coefficients that ranged between .4 and .5.

Except for the first measurement, gender had no effect, and there was no right-left difference in any of the measurements. The latter four measurements were significantly different between functionally unstable and stable ankles.

Also using young healthy subjects, Goldie and coworkers (14) found that sway measurements collected over 5 s using the shear and vertical force output signals from the force platform showed more reliable results than measurements that were based on calculations of the movements of the center of pressure. The medial-lateral shear force was the best predictor for postural steadiness. In their study there was no difference in force balance measurements between preferred and nonpreferred balance leg.

Cornwall and Murrell (5) tested the postural sway of 30 healthy subjects on a force platform over 12.8 s and found no significant differences between dominant and nondominant legs using sway amplitude and mean power frequency. For both measurements they found a test-retest reliability of .73 to .78.

Right and left side comparisons on healthy control subjects have also been performed by Feuerbach and Grabiner (7) for medial-lateral postural sway amplitudes and sway frequency when small perturbations were added during single-limb stance; no significant differences were found.

Single-Limb Agility Test

The time it takes to complete a single-leg jumping course (20) is considered to be a measurement of sensorimotor control that is both objective and easy to perform in a clinical setting. A literature review has revealed no information regarding validation of the outcome measure.

Ankle Kinesthesia

Measurement of the threshold to detection of joint motion (ankle kinesthesia) requires slow, accurate movement of the joint under study. As the threshold levels are typically less than 2°, the methods require accurate sensors. External input to the neuromuscular system such as the pressure of the strapping system on cutaneous receptors should be excluded. In the knee and shoulder, kinesthesia has been employed frequently, using different methods for recording how and when a movement was perceived. With respect to the ankle, Garn and Newton (11) measured kinesthesia by moving the foot 5° in a plantar direction at a speed of 0.3°/s in only some of the situations of a total trial and then asking the subject whether he or she felt the foot move. The sensitivity for the "yes" and "no" signals was calculated as a measure of kinesthesia using Luce's choice theory. No validation data were given. Lentell and others (26) used the degree of inversion before detection of movement as the kinesthetic measurement. Intraclass correlation coefficient between three testing angles was found to be .78. Otherwise the method was not evaluated, and thus very little information is currently available regarding validation of kinesthesia tests for the ankle.

Joint Position Sense

Measuring joint position sense requires the subject to match a set of index angles set by the investigator. The differences that are typically found are small (< 2°), and this requires a precise method and accurate registration of limb motion. Methods have been used where the subject is required to match the index angles with a visual analog scale, (32) to replicate the index angle with the contralateral foot, (1) and to copy the index angle with the ipsilateral foot either actively (13, 16, 19, 25) or passively. (16, 25) The number of angles matched, the magnitude of the angles matched, and the direction of the angle matching vary from study to study, as does the investigational equipment. The results are typically expressed in terms of a mean absolute error value of joint position assessment, but the real errors with corresponding standard deviation about the mean have been used. (8)

There is currently very little information available regarding the measurement of ankle joint position sense. No left-right comparisons or test-retest measurements have been reported. In a recent study we have validated a method of measuring ankle inversion position sense. The technique required 10 repetitions of each of three inversion angles (10°, 15°, and 20°), which were initialized passively and matched actively with the same foot. Twenty ankle-healthy subjects were tested for accuracy, repeatability, and precision of the method. Absolute error, real error, and the standard deviation of the real error were calculated. We found the absolute error to be the most accurate, repeatable, and precise means of expressing ankle position sense in our setup (*accuracy* [dominant-nondominant comparison]: ANOVA: $p = .15$, correlation: $R = .70$, $p < .001$; *repeatability* [same day test-retest]: ANOVA: $p = .96$, correlation: $R = .92$, $p < .001$; *precision* [95% confidence limits for repeated trials]: 0.2°).

Peroneal Reaction Time to Sudden Ankle Inversion

Measurement of the time before a reactive peroneal muscle EMG signal is present after sudden ankle inversion is considered to be a measurement of the activation of a medium latency polysynaptic reflex arc under supraspinal control. With this method there are a number of methodological concerns. As the muscle reaction time appears to be dependent upon the speed of the ankle perturbation (28) it is necessary to try to reach speeds of inversion relevant to an injury condition, and these speeds may be as high as 1000°/s. The EMG signal should be isolated from cross talk. The lateral muscle group lies close to both the anterior and posterior compartment, and there has been concern that the short loop reflex measured in some cases in the peroneal muscles is a crossover signal from the triceps surae complex, where short loop reflexes are present. Finally, a definition of the onset of an EMG signal should be clear, automated, and not dependent on the interpretation of the observer. Most studies use a multiplum of the standard deviation of the baseline EMG activity before perturbation as the recognition level of a reflex signal. As a result, this level, and thus the latency measured, will depend on the magnitude of the baseline noise, which again is dependent on the equipment used, and on the number of standard deviations chosen to represent activity. The number of standard deviations that have been used in studies varies from 2 to 10. In a study by Moffroid and coworkers (29) 10 times the standard deviation was found to be most consistent with what a group of observers considered to be the onset of a signal.

Several researchers have compared muscle latencies in uninjured and injured ankles using a tilt platform setup. However, very little is reported on the reliability and repeatability of the muscle latency measurements.

Right-left comparisons in healthy subjects finding no significant differences between sides have been performed by Johnson and Johnson, (21) by Isakov and others, (18) and by Löfvenberg and associates. (27) Good test-retest reliability has been noted by a number of researchers, (3, 18, 21, 22, 25, 30) but extensive supportive data was not reported.

Lynch and coworkers (28) validated their sudden ankle inversion technique. The ankles of standing subjects were inverted at speeds up to 200°/s, and the threshold of the EMG signal was defined as a signal 10 times the standard deviation of the EMG signal prior to ankle perturbation. Reliability (left to right comparisons) was demonstrated for the peroneus brevis ($p = .38$) but not for the peroneus longus ($p = .03$). As mentioned, this has not been found in other reports. (18, 21, 27) The technique was repeatable (day-to-day testing) for both muscles (peroneus longus: $p = .48$; peroneus brevis: $p = .65$).

Neurophysiological Tests: Peroneal Nerve Conduction Velocity

It can be argued that testing nerve conduction velocity in the deep and the superficial peroneal nerve is not a measurement of a sensorimotor function. From a clinical perspective, however, the quality of the afferent information from the ankle area is interesting, particularly with respect to changes after ankle injury. Kleinrensink and coworkers (23, 24) have shown that the measurement is repeatable for ankle-healthy subjects.

Reflex EMG Amplitude and H-Reflex Modulation

Nishikawa and Grabiner (31) have studied the effect of ankle bracing on the peroneal muscles H-reflex amplitude and the magnitude of the integrated EMG of the short-medium latency reflex response to a sudden but slight inversion. The basic theory behind this approach is that even though changes in muscle latencies were not apparent in certain injury and bracing situations, changes in the facilitation of certain signals at a spinal level might be evident. Validity measurements of these methods were not given.

Conclusion

It can be concluded that most of the techniques measuring sensorimotor control in ankle research have been tested for right-left similarity and test-retest repeatability. However, only for a few tests of postural sway, ankle position assessment, and peroneal reaction time to sudden inversion can it be said that adequate validation has been performed. The testing procedures employed by different researchers within a single type of sensorimotor testing method are very different, and therefore validation of one procedure within a method can not lead to the conclusion that the other tests within the group are valid as well.

References

1. Berenberg RA, Shefner JM, Sabol JJ Jr. Quantitative assessment of position sense at the ankle:

A functional approach. *Neurology* 1987; 37(1): 89–93.
2. Browne K, Lee J, Ring PA. The sensation of passive movement at the metatarsophalangeal joint of the great toe in man. *J Physiol* 1954; 126: 448–58.
3. Brunt D, Andersen JC, Huntsman B, Reinhert LB, Thorell AC, Sterling JC. Postural responses to lateral perturbation in healthy subjects and ankle sprain patients. *Med Sci Sports Exer* 1992; 24(2): 171–76.
4. Chambers RB, Cook TM, Cowell HR. Surgical reconstruction for calcaneonavicular coalition. *J Bone Joint Surg* 1982; 66A: 829–36.
5. Cornwall MW, Murrell P. Postural sway following inversion sprain of the ankle. *J Am Podiatr Med Assoc* 1991; 81(5): 243–47.
6. DeCarlo MS, Talbot RW. Evaluation of ankle proprioception following injection of the anterior talofibular ligament. *J Sports Phys Ther* 1986; 8(2): 70–76.
7. Feuerbach JW, Grabiner MD. Effect of the aircast on unilateral postural control: Amplitude and frequency variables. *J Sports Phys Ther* 1993; 17(3): 149–54.
8. Feuerbach JW, Grabiner MD, Koh TJ, Weiker GG. Effect of an ankle orthosis and ankle ligament anesthesia on ankle joint proprioception. *Am J Sports Med* 1994; 22(2): 223–29.
9. Freeman MAR, Dean MRE, Hanham IWF. The etiology and prevention of functional instability of the foot. *J Bone Joint Surg* [British] 1965; 47B: 678–85.
10. Fridén T, Zätterström R, Lindstrand A, Moritz U. A stabilometric technique for evaluation of lower limb instabilities. *Am J Sports Med* 1989; 17(1): 118–22.
11. Garn SN, Newton RA. Kinesthetic awareness in subjects with multiple ankle sprains. *Phys Ther* 1988; 68(11): 1667–71.
12. Gauffin H, Tropp H, Odenrick P. Effect of ankle disk training on postural control in patients with functional instability of the ankle joint. *Int J Sports Med* 1988; 9(2): 141–44.
13. Glencross D, Thornton E. Position sense following joint injury. *J Sports Med Phys Fitness* 1981; 21: 23–27.
14. Goldie PA, Owen ME, Bach TM. Steadiness in one-legged stance: Development of a reliable force platform testing procedure. *Arch Phys Med Rehabil* 1992; 73: 348–54.
15. Goodwin GM, McCloskey DI, Matthews PBC. The persistence of appreciable kinesthesia after paralyzing joint afferents but preserving muscle afferents. *Brain Res* 1972; 38: 326–29.
16. Gross MT. Effects of recurrent lateral ankle sprains on active and passive judgment of joint position. *Phys Ther* 1987; 67: 1505–509.
17. Hoffman M, Payne VG. The effects of proprioceptive ankle disk training on healthy subjects. *J Sports Phys Ther* 1995; 21(2): 90–93.
18. Isakov E, Mizrahi J, Solzi P, Susak Z, Lotem M. Response of the peroneal muscles to sudden inversion of the ankle during standing. *Int J Sports Biomech* 1986; 2: 100–109.
19. Jerosch J, Bischof M. Proprioceptive capabilities of the ankle in stable and unstable joints. *Sports Exer Inj* 1996; 2: 167–71.
20. Jerosch J, Hoffstetter I, Bork H, Bischof M. The influence of orthoses on the proprioception of the ankle joint. *Knee Surg Sports Traumat Arthroscopy* 1995; 3(1): 39–46.
21. Johnson MB, Johnson CL. Electromyographic response of peroneal muscles in surgical and nonsurgical injured ankles during sudden inversion. *J Sports Phys Ther* 1993; 18: 497–501.
22. Karlsson J, Andreasson GO. The effect of external ankle support in chronic lateral ankle joint instability: An electromyographic study. *Am J Sports Med* 1992; 20(3): 257–61.
23. Kleinrensink GJ, Stoeckart R, Meulstee J, et al. Lowered motor conduction velocity of the peroneal nerve after inversion trauma. *Med Sci Sports Exer* 1994; 26(7): 877–83.
24. Kleinrensink G, Dijkstra P, Boerboom A, Stoeckart R. Reduced motor conduction velocity of the peroneal nerve caused by inversion damage: A prospective longitudinal study. *Acta Orthop Scand* 1996; 67(Suppl. 272): 83.
25. Konradsen L, Ravn JB, Sørensen AI. Proprioception at the ankle: The effect of anaesthetic blockade of ligament receptors. *J Bone Joint Surg* [British] 1993; 75(3): 433–36.
26. Lentell G, Baas B, Lopez D, McGuire L, Sarrels M, Snyder P. The contributions of proprioceptive deficits, muscle function, and anatomic laxity to functional instability of the ankle. *JOSPT* 1995; 21(4): 206–15.
27. Löfvenberg R, Kärrholm J, Sundelin G. Prolonged reaction time in patients with chronic lateral instability of the ankle. *Am J Sports Med* 1995; 23: 414–17.
28. Lynch SA, Eklund U, Gottlieb D, Renström PA, Beynnon B. Electromyographic latency changes in the ankle musculature during inversion moments. *Am J Sports Med* 1996; 24(3): 362–69.
29. Moffroid M, Tranowski J, Ricamato A, et al. Computer solutions to identify EMG latency of

automatic postural reactions. *IEEE Eng Med Biol* 1992; 11(4): 48–51.

30. Nawoczenski DA, Owen MG, Ecker ML, Altman B, Epler M. Objective evaluation of peroneal response to sudden inversion stress. *J Sports Phys Ther* 1985; 7(3): 107–109.
31. Nishikawa T, Grabiner MD. Ankle braces influence the reflex amplitude of muscle in response to stretch. 42nd Annual Meeting, Orthopaedic Research Society. *ORS Proceedings* 1996.
32. Robbins S, Waked E, Rappel R. Ankle taping improves proprioception before and after exercise in young men. *Br J Sports Med* 1995; 29: 242–47.
33. Soderberg GL, Cook TM, Rider SC, Stephenitch BL. Electromyographic activity of selected leg musculature in subjects with normal and chronically sprained ankles performing on a BAPS board. *Phys Ther* 1991; 71(7): 514-22.
34. Sprigings EJ, Pelton JD, Brandell BR. An EMG analysis of the effectiveness of external ankle support during sudden ankle inversion. *Canadian J Sports Sci* 1981; 6(2): 72–75.
35. Tropp H. Functional instability of the ankle joint. Master's thesis, Linköping University, Linköping, Sweden, 1985.
36. Tropp H, Ekstrand J, Gillquist J. Factors affecting stabilometry recordings of single-limb stance. *Am J Sports Med* 1984; 12(3): 185–88.

CHAPTER 14

The Role of Electromyography in the Assessment of Neuromuscular Control

Thomas Bochdansky, MD
Josef Kollmitzer, PhD
Gerold Ebinbechler, PhD

Introduction

It has been a long time in science since Swammerdam (1658) wrote one of the first books about electrophysiology and Luigi Galvani (1791) presented his famous work, *De viribus electricitatis in motu musculari commentarius* (18). More than a hundred years later it was Hans Piper (70) who first used the word "electromyogramm" (1909) and presented his work in a paper, "Elektrophysiologie menschlicher Muskeln" (1912). Since that time an immense number of publications have been presented on the use of the electromyographic method (EMG) in the various fields of both biomedical and clinical research and applications. Among these innumerable publications on this subject, textbooks like *Muscles Alive* (5), *Biomechanics and Motor Control of Human Movement* (88), and *Electrophysiological Kinesiology* (86, 2) have been published, which provide basic information. The aim of this article is to present a brief review on selected topics in the light of the results of our own experiments. References cannot be complete, and in most cases they are just examples.

Methodology

Units, terms, and standards in the reporting of EMG research have been defined by an ad hoc committee of the International Society of Electrophysiological Kinesiology chaired by D. Winter (members: G. Rau, R. Kadefors, H. Broman, and C. DeLuca) in August 1980. An update was published recently in the *Journal of Electromyography and Kinesiology* (vol. 6, no. 3, pp. iii–iv, 1996). The very latest review on this topic has been published by DeLuca (20).

Studies indicate that the influence of temperature (36, 66) and intracellular pH (62) on an EMG recording ought to be considered, although no influence of lactate accumulation could be demonstrated (46, 81, 14).

The reliability of average area measurement has been determined by Yang and Winter (92). The within-day coefficient of variation ranged between 8% and 10%. The range of between-days variability was 12% to 16%. Submaximal contractions are more reliable. In a more recent study Zakaria and coworkers (95) found an excellent test-retest reliability of integrated EMG within 2–8 days.

The information content of the surface EMG signal is band limited between 20 Hz and 500 Hz. The low frequency energy of the raw signal is mainly caused by movement artifacts such as movement of electrode, contact, or cable. There are also very low frequency shifts due to respiration or slow impedance changes of the electrode-skin interface. There is no EMG energy in frequencies higher than 500 Hz. There is, however, noise within the band limits, such as power line hum (50 Hz or 60 Hz according to location) and impact movement artifacts. Thus the signal filter is of complex structure. In general, it is a multiple band-pass and notch filter with fixed frequencies. The output results are amplitude- and frequency-related parameters, such as root mean square (*RMS*) or mean amplitude in the time domain and median frequency (MF) or centroid frequency in the frequency domain. Both types of parameters need to be investigated starting from the raw signal, to allow processing of power spectra or quality control of the many possible artifacts. The amplitude of the EMG signal roughly indicates the number of motor units that the nerve is recruiting in the pickup volume, whereas the frequency spectrum is chiefly a function of the ion flow dynamics within the muscle.

The processing of EMG data is done in digital form due to the flexibility and reliability of computer software. Thus the analog signal has to be sampled in digital representation without loss of information and without error propagation. As the frequency band may reach 500 Hz, the sampling frequency has to be at least 1000 Hz to avoid aliasing. This is necessary to prevent mirroring high-frequency components in the lower-frequency domain by the sampling procedure. As there is no way to identify and recalculate movement artifacts or hum in preprocessed data such as integrated EMG, the raw signal has to be stored for further processing. The best way of "recalculating" errors is not introducing errors. Therefore, the quality of the EMG signal starts with the reliability of the electrodes, the preprocessing of the skin to lower electrode impedance, and the cabling of the moving extremities. The connection of a freely moving subject to the measurement unit should preferably be telemetered.

Any force-producing task is a complex interaction of multiple muscle groups (agonists, antagonists, synergists, and fixation muscles as well as co-contractive contralateral groups). Therefore a functional (kinesiological) EMG has to be multichanneled. Thus, in addition to the quality of the EMG signal of each channel, the synchronization of the channels and the timing of repeated movements is crucial in order to calculate an "ensemble average" signal.

Thus the functional EMG needs additional sensor channels for event identification. These may be contact events or movement phases measured with appropriate sensors (pressure or acceleration sensors, goniometer, force transducer, strain gauges, etc.). The rapid change in measurement technology indicates the complexity of the functional EMG.

Neurophysiological Model

In order to allow a better understanding of the main principles of muscle function and the complex integrative synergies with other systems related to movement, we have created a model that is based on three spheres: information, structure, and energy.

We suggest that all three spheres interact and if one parameter of one sphere is changed, then the other two spheres also will be changed. This model takes into account the homeostatic (steady state) nature of such biological systems. Therefore, only a change of informational content—the change in structure and the turnover rate of metabolism being the major determinants, not only for muscle physiology—will be described.

For example, pain caused by tissue damage after trauma represents an influence on the informational sphere. This changes the central and peripheral sensomotoric loops, which thus may lead to a decreased muscular activity and maybe immobilization and associated adaptations of the metabolism of the muscle (energy sphere) as, for example, muscle atrophy (structure sphere). Or, for instance, in diabetic patients (energy sphere) muscle atrophy (structure sphere) may occur as the consequence of both a decrease in substrate supply due to microangiopathy (energy) and a decrease of information provided by the nervous system due to polyneuropathy (information). The EMG is generated at the interface between the information and the structural spheres and is affected by all three.

In view of the long history of EMG, the old fashioned "magic eye" in radio receivers in the pretransistor age of electric valve systems may serve as a symbol for the EMG signal. The information sphere is represented by the electromagnetic wave transmitted by the radio station. The structural sphere is represented by the modifying system, including antenna, detector, amplifier, and speaker. The energy sphere is represented by the power consumption of the total system. The kinematic or kinetic output (movement) is symbolized by the sound.

If the receiver is tuned well, the "magic eye" shows a visual reaction. The signal is pulsing according to the amplitude of the input. There is no way, however, to identify the radio station that is being received or even the content of the transmitted information. The signal is meant to support the tuning process and not to visualize the information output. This is also true for the EMG in a physiological context. It shows the activity of muscles without prediction of the resulting movement.

With this representation in mind, it is obvious that the neurophysiological and the kinesiological application of the EMG are basically different. Without information of any kinetic or kinematic output the neurophysiological application of the EMG can just tell us if the neuromuscular system is working (i.e., if the information reaches the muscle receiver). To get any further information a simultaneous kinematic and kinetic output representation is necessary. (A well-tuned radio also is useless without a speaker.) This additional information may be time events, angular position, torque across a joint, and all subsequently derived signals. The EMG is able to detect changes in the information and structural sphere but not in the energy sphere or in the kinematic and kinetic output.

A hi-fi receiver is a representation of intermuscular synchronized activity. In the hi-fi at least two totally different channels, and speakers with a defined phase shift and amplitude ratio, produce auditory output. Similar circumstances are required for smooth movement in the multimuscular system. Thus, any phase disharmony or unexpected change in amplitude relation leads to the loss of surround effect in auditory systems and the loss of smoothness in moving systems. Here the EMG is the only signal that is able to detect this unsynchronicity.

Thus there are two basically different applications of EMG: neurophysiological and kinesiological EMG (see figure 14.1). To discuss this connection we have developed another model composed of the following two domains:

1. A neurophysiological domain
2. A mechanical domain

Again it is not possible to separate one from the other.

The central element of the neurophysiological domain is the motoric pool according to Basmajian (5). In addition, we have several sensory inputs modulating the central drive to the alpha motor system and in parallel to the gamma motor system. These inputs arrive not only from proprioceptive sensors; there are also possible modulations coming from exteroceptors and from other afferent information. Therefore, we prefer to use the term "sensomotoric system."

To represent the mechanical domain we used a simple Hill-type model, which consists of contractile and elastic elements in parallel and in series and a pennation angle. The muscle-tendon system (MTS) has to perform two contradictory major functions. The first is to initiate movement, and the second is to inhibit movement. In other words, the MTS has to accelerate and decelerate the human body, and therefore it has to produce strain and resist strain. It can achieve this by two different forms of contractions: concentric contraction and eccentric contraction.

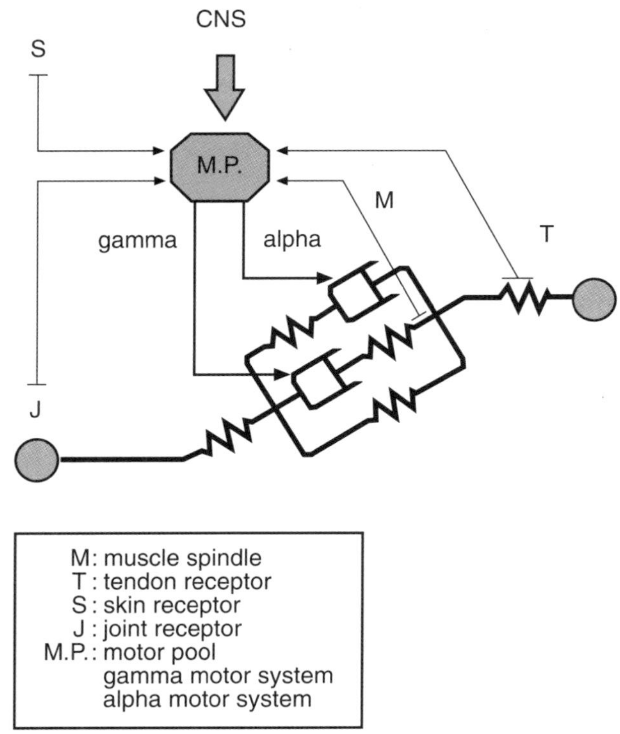

Figure 14.1 Neurophysiological muscle model.

With this very simple model it is easy to understand the different types of contraction. During concentric contraction there is an activation of the alpha motor system (together with the gamma system) and, subsequently, a contraction (shortening) of the contractile elements. If the strain in the whole mechanical system exceeds a certain limit the whole MTS shortens, and muscle-tendon length decreases. During eccentric contraction the alpha motor system again is activated to a certain extent, and therefore there is a shortening of the contractile elements. But in contrast to the concentric contraction, muscle-tendon length increases.

The EMG shows the activity of the efferent neuromotor system. The question is, in which way is there a connection between electrical activity (electrical input) and mechanical strain (mechanical output), and to what extent can strain in the MTS develop a movement?

We have four basic functional groups of muscles:

1. Agonists
2. Antagonists
3. Synergists
4. Fixation muscles

This requires that all of the different muscles (structure) work together in a well-coordinated way (information) in order to minimize the energy costs (energy) for a given movement.

During a single movement—like knee extension—we have different forms of contraction for the different muscle groups. We have concentric contraction for the agonists and synergists, eccentric contraction for the antagonists, and isometric contraction for the fixation muscles, which is an intermediate form between concentric and eccentric (shortening of the contractile elements and no change in muscle-tendon length).

Dynamometrical (Isokinetic) Tests

In order to investigate the relationship between electrical input and mechanical output we used a combination of a speed-controlled, hydraulically driven dynamometer for isokinetic knee extension and flexion (50) and a multichannel EMG system (Myo 2000, Noraxon). Torque was measured by a strain gauge system and the angular position was registered by a potentiometer. A convenient sample of 2 female (x: 30 a, 164 cm) and 8 male (x: 31 a, 187 cm) volunteers participated in our study. Before the test series started everybody had to perform a standardized warm-up program and several trials to become familiar with the unusual movement. The instruction was to extend the knee with "maximal voluntary contraction" throughout the whole test, no matter what happened with the lever arm. The knee extension test consisted of 4 periods. We started with an isometric contraction (Iso) lasting around 1.5 s, followed by a first concentric contraction (Con1) that was separated from a second concentric contraction (Con2) by a phase of eccentric contraction (Ecc), each of the contractions lasting 1 s. The 4 movement phases were identified by means of the angle position signal.

Test A was performed between 90° and 60° of knee flexion with an angular speed of 30°/s (0.57 rad/s). Test B had a range of motion from 60° to 30° with the same angular speed, and for test C we doubled the range of motion from 90° to 30° and the angular speed to 60°/s (1.05 rad/s). These angular speeds were chosen to keep contraction times constant for all tests because of the possible impact of fatigue (energy sphere). Each test was performed twice for both legs and the sequence of the tests was randomized.

EMG signals were recorded from the thigh muscles—vastus lateralis, vastus medialis, rectus femoris, and biceps femoris—using bipolar surface electrodes at an interelectrode distance of 2 cm (Medi-trace). The raw EMG signals were A/D converted with a sampling frequency of 1000 Hz (CMRR > 95 dB, input impedance > 10 Mohms, bandwidth 20–500 Hz antialiasing). Torque and angular position signals were stored in parallel with the EMG data (bandwidth 1.5–500Hz).

The unbiased raw EMG signal was full-wave rectified and linear envelopes were calculated by a low-pass filter (Butterworth 8th order, 5 Hz digital low pass, Matlab software). Each trial procedure was ensemble averaged separately. Artifact- or noise-affected signals were excluded from further processing when exhibiting a value of more than four standard deviations from the average signal (number of trials: 120; exclusion rate: vastus lateralis (1), vastus medialis (0), rectus femoris (2), biceps femoris (8))].

Results of the Kinematic Study

The total duration of each movement phase was found to be in the mean, t_m = 1100 ms (std < 10 ms). This is the high reproducibility that can be expected from automatically driven hydraulic machines (coefficient of variation < 1%) (see figure 14.2).

There was no detectable difference in the duration of eccentric and concentric trials. The hydraulic robotics mode of the machine was not accelerated or decelerated by the torque produced by subjects. No difference in the timing was found between tests A, B, and C. No correlation with subjects was detected.

To account for interindividual variability, torque was normalized to the preceding isometric contraction. Peak torque showed a modest decrease in Con1, a significant increase in Ecc ($p > .005$) and about the same level in Con2 (see table 14.1 and figure 14.3).

Results of the EMG

To analyze the time domain results, all EMG data are demonstrated as root mean square (RMS). In the first run we calculated RMS for all muscle groups during the whole period of each contraction type with normalization to the isometric phase. In contrast to the findings for torque, the differences between muscles and phases of contraction are not pronounced. Although the test has been performed in different angular positions and with different angular velocities, the electrical activity was the same during both the transition from concentric to eccentric contraction and during the transition from eccentric to concentric contraction. The normalization of RMS muscle activity to the isometric phase removes intermuscle effects. Thus in a second run,

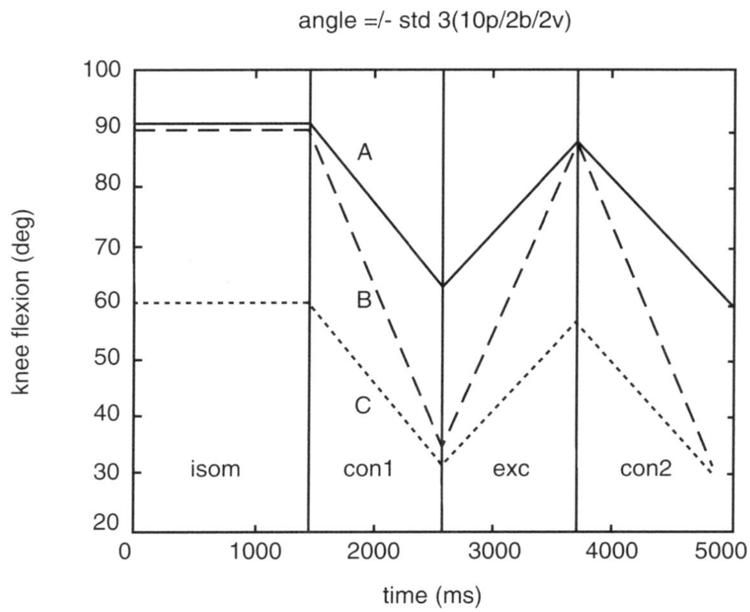

Figure 14.2 Mean angle position signals for trials A, B, and C calculated for 40 trials each ($SD = 2°$).

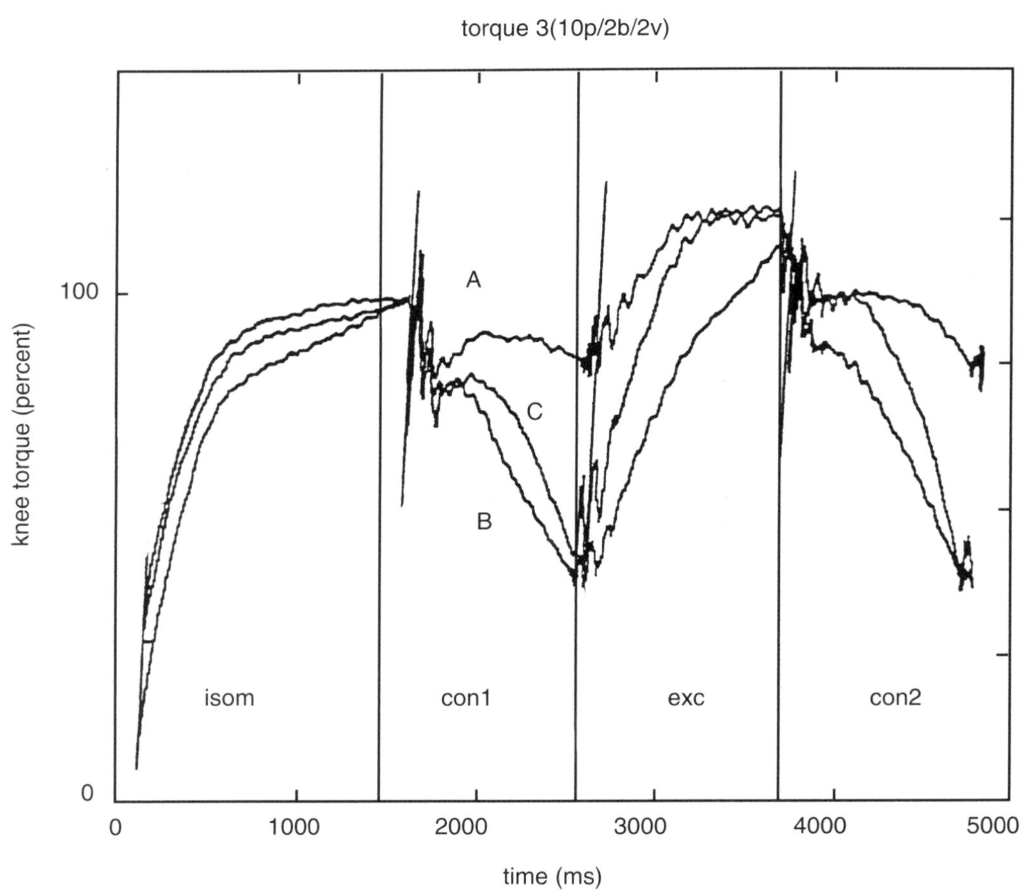

Figure 14.3 Mean torque (normalized) of the 3 different trials, each with 40 realizations.

in order to demonstrate the whole trend over time of the amplitude of the different muscles, we calculated the smoothed signal (linear envelope, 50 Hz high-pass filter, 10 Hz smoothing factor) averaged for each of the 3 different trial procedures as mentioned above. In all muscle groups EMG amplitude was highest in test C during the second concentric phase and lowest in test B. (See figures 14.4 and 14.5.)

Interestingly, there was a remarkable peak in amplitude about 50 ms after the beginning of the second concentric contraction phase in all muscle groups. Differences can be seen between the vastii as monoarticular muscles and the rectus femoris as biarticular muscle. The behavior of the biceps femoris as antagonistic muscle was low in absolute amplitude and showed an additional peak during the transition from first concentric to eccentric contraction. As co-contraction of antagonistic muscles does occur in a number of situations that require a high stability of the joint that the muscles are acting on, this additional peak can be interpreted as a stabilization activity rather than a stretch-reflex activity. The latter could be responsible for the peak in the agonistic muscles during the second concentric phase because of the time duration.

If one looks at the trend of the activity in the rectus femoris, an increase and decrease can be seen during each contraction phase. Although the standard deviation was high, one can speculate that these differences are due to a different central drive as described by Jacobs and Van Ingen Schenau (40).

The coefficient of correlation of the raw EMG signals during the same trial has been calculated. The results were averaged over subjects and trials. Highest signal correlation during dynamic "con-ex-con" trials was found between vastus lateralis and vastus medialis signals ($.5 \leq r \leq .6$). The lowest correlation could be detected between any correlation involving the rectus femoris muscle ($.13 \leq r \leq .15$). The correlation between both vastii and biceps femoris has been found to be also low ($.2 \leq r \leq .25$). (See figure 14.6.)

We found little cross correlation between rectus femoris and surrounding vastii. Thus we do not suppose that the high correlation between the vastii is due to volume conduction but can be interpreted as correlation of the central pattern. As the coefficient of correlation does not take into account phase shifts, it is not possible to estimate the amount of the cross talk between the correlated signals. Further investigation including phase shift influence is needed to explain this correlation. With that, one can decide if there is also a different role for monoarticular and biarticular muscles in multijoint movements with different types of contractions.

Frequency Domain Analysis

We calculated the median frequency during a window of 128 ms in the middle of the different phases for each test and for each muscle group (see table 14.2).

The energy of the hamstring was between 11 and 14% of that of rectus femoris, with about 70% of the noise. Therefore no further investigations were performed. A frequency shift to lower frequencies could not be found in any case during the "con-ex-con" trials, so it can be supposed that no fatigue occurred during the tests.

To summarize our results, we saw a very different behavior between torque and electrical activity during comparable movements. This is consistent with a study from Ghori and coworkers (28), who also found no fixed relationship between vastus lateralis activity and knee extension torque during maximum concentric and eccentric actions. The electromyographic activity differs with different angular sections but it does not appear that different angular velocities have an impact on the amplitude of EMG when maximal voluntary contraction is demanded.

The most important influence on the EMG activity derives from the contraction history. If a concentric contraction is preceded by an isometric contraction there is not as much electrical activity as when a concentric contraction is preceded by an eccentric contraction. This is in accordance with the well-known physiotherapeutic technique, "combination of isotonic," in the PNF (proprioceptive neuromuscular facilitation) concept developed by Kabat and Knott (41).

The question is What does the EMG signal have to do with muscular force output? What is the consistence of the association between EMG signal and muscular force output?

Force Production

Many papers have been published regarding the relationship between electrical activity and muscular force. In 1952, one of the first experiments was carried out by Lippold (53). He found a linear relation between integrated EMG activity and isometric force production on the calf muscles of humans. In 1954, Bigland and Lippold also demonstrated a linear relation between increasing velocity and muscle shortening (6). The electrical amplitude, however, remained almost independent of speed when the muscle was being lengthened. In a review

Table 14.1 Peak Torque in Percent of Each Individual's Value of Isometry (Standard Deviation)

	Test A [% Iso]	Test B [% Iso]	Test C [% Iso]
Concentric 1	93.3 (4.6)	93.0 (8.2)	90.5 (6.6)
Eccentric	110.5 (5.8)	114.5 (9.7)	113.9 (9.4)
Concentric 2	99.1 (8.6)	102.0 (9.3)	100.0 (8.5)

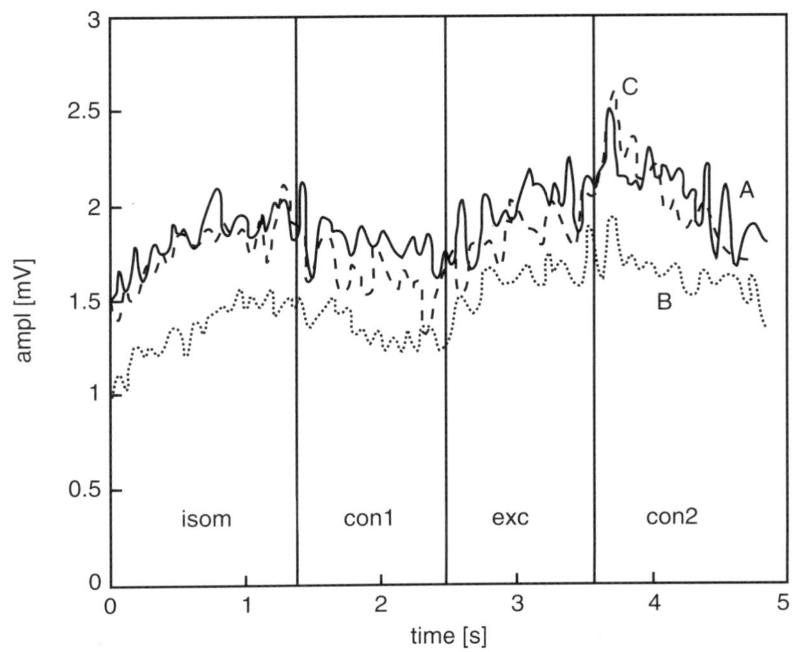

Figure 14.4 Amplitude (filtered and smoothed) of EMG signal of the vastus medialis during test A (–), test B (– ·), and test C (- -).

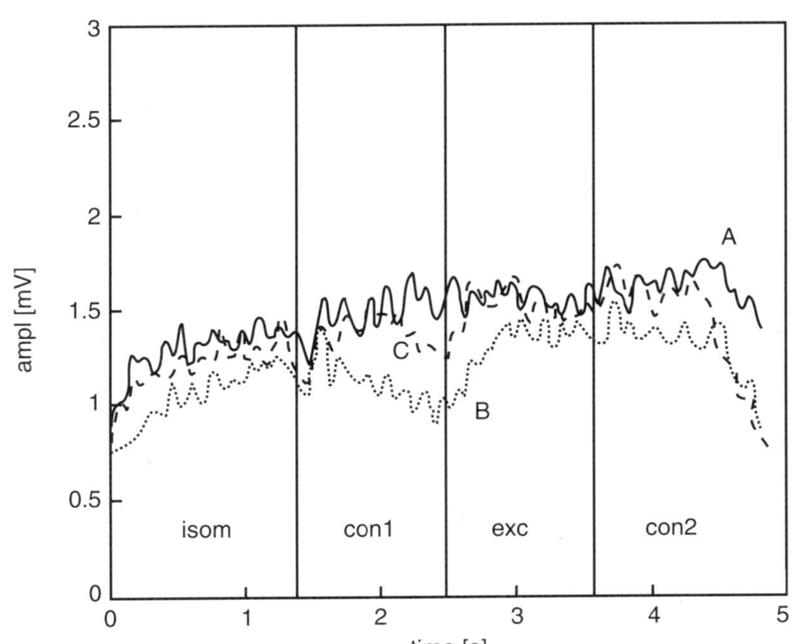

Figure 14.5 Amplitude (filtered and smoothed) of EMG signal of the rectus femoris during test A (–), test B (– ·), and test C (- -).

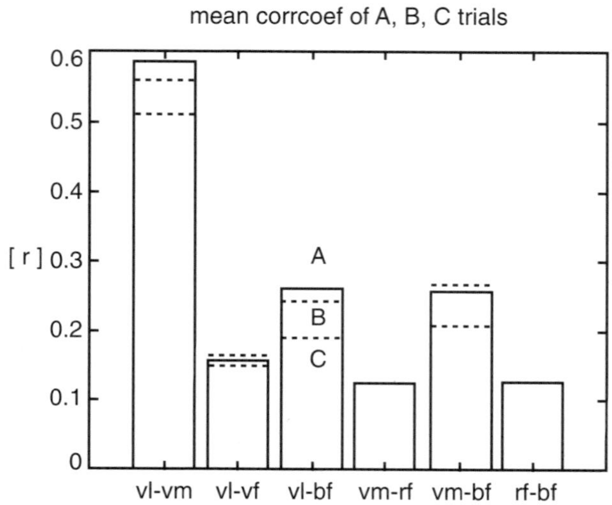

Figure 14.6 Mean coefficient of correlation, *r*, between different muscle groups during tests A, B, and C (vl: vastus lateralis, vm: vastus medialis, rf: rectus femoris, bf: biceps femoris).

written by Bouisset (13), an overview of these early investigations can be found. He concluded that it may be possible to use the value of the surface EMG signal as an indirect and complex indication of the force developed by the muscle. The relation between EMG and force was reported as nonlinear when 0% to 100% of maximal voluntary contraction was considered and as linear for submaximal contraction due to different recruitment of small units first and larger, fast-twitch units in a later phase (90).

Many other investigations (e.g., 77, 78, 97) found a nonlinear relationship for other muscle groups. Philipson and Larsson (69) showed a different relationship according to different quantification algorithms, with the most reliable descriptors of force for the root mean square and average rectified amplitude.

Although Rosentswieg and Hinson (74), in 1972, indicated a difference in EMG activity for different types of contraction, Chaffin and coworkers (17), in 1980, wrote that the estimated maximum EMG allowed the prediction of maximum strength. This has also been reported in earlier papers (25, 45, 61). Attempts have also been made to calculate the number of active motor units from the surface EMG (68).

Another example of the EMG-force relationship is given by Gioux and associates (29). They hoped to establish a direct measure of the mechanical capacities of muscles from the EMG data that would be as reliable as the biopsy technique for selection of sportsmen and training control.

It was seductive to measure the electrical signal and out of that calculate the muscular force during movement. It would have been very simple for modeling purposes. For that reason Lam and others (49) examined the heterogeneity of electromyograms derived from different electrode pairs. Only a limited number of action potentials of motor units surrounding the area of the two electrode tips can be measured. Thus it makes a difference where and how the electrodes are placed in relation to the fiber direction and the motor point. They suggested, therefore, external averaging of multiple pairs of electrodes. Another attempt to calculate the EMG-force relationship was made by Hawkins and Hull (33). They used an activation-recruitment scheme for moderate to large activation levels, taking into account the different muscle fibers. Finally, Herzog and coworkers (34) have presented many basic investigations about the EMG-force relationship in order to analyze quantitatively some physiological properties of the muscle.

Although Bigland and Lippold (6) demonstrated the differences in electrical activity between shortening and lengthening of a muscle as early as 1954, it took almost another twenty years before Komi (44) showed the differences in different types of contractions.

He recorded the tension of the elbow flexor muscles and the integrated EMG of biceps brachii, brachioradialis, and triceps brachii. In all muscles the maximum IEMG activity was about the same at each velocity of contraction and for all types of contraction. This has also been confirmed by the experiments of Seliger and associates (76).

Table 14.2 Median Frequency of EMG During Tests A, B, and C

MF [Hz]	Test A	Test B	Test C
v. lateralis	80	90	85
v. medialis	80	90	85
r. femoris	100	110	100

No differences were found for the different phases of contraction.

Differences in electrical activity of the quadriceps for different angles during maximal concentric and eccentric exercises, as we presented above, have also been shown by Eloranta and Komi (21). Furthermore, a different behavior of EMG signals and muscular force was demonstrated by Hultman and Sjöholm (37). They found that during recovery after a fatiguing electrical stimulation EMG was quickly normalized, whereas force remained at a reduced level. Westing and others (87) found a decrease of EMG activity with decreasing velocities for the knee extensor muscles under concentric loading, while concentric torque increased with decreasing velocities. For all muscles, EMG activity was lower under eccentric loading than velocity matched concentric loading. Each contraction was carried out after an isometric preload.

Again this shows a difference between force and EMG. Differences between concentric and eccentric contractions can be seen, not only at the information sphere, but also on the energy sphere. In an earlier study on a four-extremity ergometer, with constant angular velocities for all great joints (shoulder, elbow, hand and hip, knee, ankle) we have found that the production of lactate is four times higher when the same amount of mechanical output has to be carried out with concentric contraction in contrast to eccentric contraction (12). This is in accordance with earlier experiments mentioned by A.V. Hill (35).

It is doubtful, therefore, whether a biomechanical model for prediction of muscle forces can be proved by measuring the EMG activity (64), especially in the shoulder joints, where muscular activity plays a very important role in fixation as well as movement of the joint system.

Another aspect of a differentiated use of EMG derives from examinations regarding the electromechanical delay at the beginning of contraction and the cessation of torque. Vos and coworkers (85) found the delay between the onset of EMG and the onset of mechanical response to be 81.9 ms and a relaxation delay of 88.8 ms using a bidirectional application of a second order Butterworth filter. Ferris-Hood and others (23) defined the relaxation electromechanical delay as the time between cessation of EMG activity and decrement of torque to 10% of the initial slope of the torque relaxation curve. Average times ranged from 239 ms to 300 ms for the same muscle groups. In another study, however, a much shorter electromechanical delay ranging from 40.4 ms at rest to 63.4 ms at the end of an exercise was reported by Zhou and coworkers (96). This parameter, therefore, is not described consistently enough to be used in standardized situations. In our tests we found that the filtering method used exerted an influence on this parameter that was much greater than any differences found during testing.

In light of all these facts one can suppose that concentric contraction and eccentric load resistance are two situations that are very different from each other. In eccentric contraction an increase of strain can be found, but, simultaneously, one finds a decrease of metabolic cost for a given movement (work). At the same time, electrical activity remains equal, no matter what the mechanical level is doing. Therefore, the EMG signal can be seen just as an indicator for the electrical input and cannot be used as a linear predictor of the mechanical output, although this input determines the mechanical output. On the other hand, the mechanical output determines the electrical input by means of reflectory pathways. Maybe EMG reflects more the metabolic cost of a movement because the metabolic turnover rate is associated more closely with the amount of concentric contraction than with eccentric contraction. EMG activity shows a linear or nonlinear correlation in particular during a concentric contraction.

We can use another picture for understanding muscular function: The electrical activity leads to a linkage of actin and myosin filaments in relation to the central drive. In a maximal voluntary contraction a certain number of linkages exist. To form and to release this linkage is energy consuming and maybe this correlates to the electrical signal. If you put some external strain on this linkage, like in an eccentric load condition, the linkage reacts like a keyed bolt to fix the club in a cylinder. So the musculotendon system behaves according to its elasticity (stiffness). At least for a limited time (500 to 600 ms), we found an exponential increase of strain in our tests during the eccentric phase. During that time, influences of reflexes are assumed. Differences in leveling off were found in the torque signal during the eccentric phase of resistance training among the volunteers, but no differences were found in EMG signals. Influences on the EMG activity were found in the next phase (second concentric phase). No signs of fatigue were noted, because this would have an inhibitory effect on muscular activity (71, 75).

EMG and Muscle Fatigue

The relative proportions of fiber types within a muscle and the characteristics of these muscle fiber types are undoubtedly important determinants of the surface EMG during fatiguing exercise. Normally, type I muscle fibers become recruited at low force levels. When the force level is increased, type II motor fibers become recruited in addition (93), according to Henneman's size principle. Both animal studies (32) and studies in humans (51, 94) have shown that type II fibers are capable of generating more force than type I fibers.

Muscle fatigue may be defined as the reduction in the force generating capacity of the neuromuscular system that occurs during sustained activity (3). Its primary cause has long been the subject of controversy. While it is generally agreed that much of the force loss results from biochemical changes within the muscle fibers, it has also been observed that fatigue of sustained maximum voluntary contractions (MVC) is accompanied by a decline in the surface EMG activity. This suggests that, in voluntary contractions, loss of force may also result from inadequate muscle activation in addition to failure of the contractile mechanism. This reduced activation was found to result from both a reduced motor drive by the central nervous system, a process referred to as "central fatigue," and from failure of the peripheral electrical transmission (8, 9, 38).

When a human subject sustains a submaximal isometric force to the endurance limit, the EMG amplitude of the involved muscle increases (11, 58). Thus, it has been suggested that the central nervous system, in well-motivated subjects, remains capable of fully activating muscle and that the reduction in force results only from failure of the muscle contractile apparatus (11). Therefore, the EMG amplitude is often considered to be a reflection of the descending drive provided by the suprasegmental centers or an impairment of neuromuscular propagation (9, 54).

During submaximal contractions, the increase in amplitude of the surface EMG is thought to result chiefly from additional recruitment of type II fibers and an increasing motor unit firing rate (11, 52, 58, 82). However, the ability of subjects to maintain a sufficient level of neural excitation in the muscle despite a declining force capacity of active motor units probably depends on the interaction of several competing processes: increased excitation of the motor neuron pool by the descending drive, intrinsic adaptation in motor neuron excitability (43), peripheral inhibitory feedback from metabolite sensitive muscle receptors (10), a reduction in muscle spindle (55) and Golgi tendon organ (98) afferent inputs, an increase in recurrent inhibition (56), and impairment of neuromuscular propagation (24). The time course of the voluntary EMG during the fatiguing contraction indicates the net effect of these processes.

A shift to lower frequencies of the power density spectrum is thought to reflect central changes in excitability that originate in response to fatigue-associated metabolite-induced changes in the propagation velocity of the muscle fiber action potentials (10, 16, 52, 79). The shift in the power density frequency spectrum to lower frequencies as a muscle fatigues has been suggested to be caused by two major factors: a decrease in the muscle fiber conduction velocity and a change in the motor unit (MU) firing statistics such as synchronization (59, 60). Relations between the median frequency (MF) shifts and the relative proportions of fiber types within muscles and the characteristics of these muscle fiber types have been discussed as varying in importance. Some have found the MF fatigue pattern to be related to the relative proportions of type I and type II fibers (15), whereas others found this relationship to be of a minor relevance (51). For further information about the role of fatigue on EMG signals we refer to additional articles like those of Bigland-Ritchie (7), Hägg (30), Merletti and Roy (57), and Psek and Cafarelli (72).

EMG and Motor Control

Different roles have been elucidated for monoarticular and biarticular muscles during movement (40, 48, 83). Whereas monoarticular muscles mainly work as force generators, the biarticular muscles, both the agonists and antagonists, are particularly involved in the fine regulation of the net torque over the joints that are crossed. For instance, in a multiarticular movement such as cycling, the SEMG of the monoarticular vastus medialis, vastus lateralis, and glutei muscles appears to be dependent on the position changes and more or less independent of the required moments at the knee and hip joints. In contrast, activity of the biarticular biceps femoris and rectus femoris muscles appears to be a function of the difference between the moments of the agonist and antagonist muscle groups at the hip and knee joints and thus influences both the direction and magnitude of the resultant external force on the bicycle pedal (80, 84).

The different roles of monoarticular and biarticular (agonist and antagonist) muscles were also apparent in the SEMG recorded in simple knee extensions at various loads, even if the biarticular rectus femoris muscle actually functioned as a monoarticular muscle (Ebinbechler and others 1997, submitted). Thus, the EMG of the monoarticular muscles depended upon the load used in the fatigue tasks, whereas in the biarticular muscles, both the agonist rectus femoris and antagonist biceps femoris, it did not. The observed differences between the SEMG of the muscle groups in this very specific monoarticular task imply different neuronal coding mechanisms in the central nervous system. Thus it appears that these different roles of monoarticular and biarticular muscles, as revealed by animal studies (89), may be indicative of two groups of neurons in the cerebral cortex, one coding position (26), the other coding the direction of the resulting net force or net moment (42). Furthermore, the biarticular antagonist will be activated simultaneously with the agonist, according to the "common drive" hypothesis of De Luca and Mambrito (19). According to them, co-contraction may be governed by a central descending "common drive," which suggests that the central nervous system (CNS) controls both the agonist and antagonist muscles as a single motor neuron pool, causing both to be simultaneously active.

Fiber Type

There are only a few articles to our knowledge analyzing the question, can muscle fiber composition be determined by EMG? In several studies of fatigue the decrease of mean power frequency of the EMG signal correlates with the fiber type proportion (31, 63, 81). Therefore, Wretling and associates (91) and Gerdle and others (27) examined whether it is possible to predict the fiber type proportion in the vastus lateralis muscle based on mean power frequency (MPF) during maximum dynamic contractions. They found a significant correlation (r = -.93) between MPF and type I fibers in the vastus lateralis. Similar correlation has been found for different angular velocities of knee extension, although a decrease of this correlation was reported for fast extension (at 180°/s, r = -.644). Correlation between peak torque and proportion of type I was significant only at slow velocity (at 30°/s, r = .80). This is, of course, reasonable because slow movements are predominantly made by slow fibers. The high degree of correlation between MPF and proportion of type I fibers is in part due to the fact that the muscle biopsies were obtained from the same muscle where the EMG was recorded.

In addition to the MPF, Linssen and coworkers (51) examined the action potential conduction velocity (CV) as another parameter and found that muscles composed primarily of fast fibers have a greater CV. To avoid the problems occurring with human tests where limited parts of the muscle can be examined (EMG and biopsy) Kupa and coworkers (47) investigated the whole muscle in an in vitro model. Their findings support the possibility of utilizing surface EMG techniques to obtain an electrophysiological "muscle biopsy" for estimating muscle fiber composition. This could be very helpful in designing different training protocols in rehabilitation as well as in training, especially when using electrotherapy for muscle stimulation. In a recent publication a noninvasive EMG procedure has been demonstrated with high spatial resolution (73). With this technique Rau and associates (73) could demonstrate a deeper insight into the active state of the muscle by detecting the activity of a single motor unit and measuring the conduction velocity in a single muscle fiber, which is affected by the fiber diameter not only of the nerve fiber but also of the muscle fiber.

Stiffness

Inman and Ralston (39) demonstrated the isometric tension-length curve for flexor muscles of the human forearm. The passive tension of the muscles of the lower limb is higher than in the upper limb. Increasing the electrical activity by increasing the amount of voluntary contraction leads to a stiffening of the MTS. The degree of electrical activity therefore determines the elastic behavior of the MTS. Pandy and coworkers (67) described a model for jumping. They related the time rate of change of tendon force (mechanical output) to musculotendon length (l^{MT}), velocity (v^{MT}), muscle activation [$a(t)$], and tendon force (P^T). Thus,

$$\frac{dPT}{dt} = f\left[P^T, l^{MT}, v^{MT}, a(t)\right].$$

Activation was denoted as

$$\frac{da(t)}{dt} = f\left[a, u(t)\right],$$

to describe the time lapse between the incoming neural signal [muscle excitation, $u(t)$] and muscle activation [$a(t)$]. Maybe the EMG signal correlates with $u(t)$. The relation between the neural signal and the muscle activation seems to be nonlinear (see figure 14.7).

Again this illustrates the different behavior of the informational sphere and the structural sphere, as mentioned above. Thus, also in muscle physiology there is a difference between willing to do and acting.

One can expect that an EMG is necessary when examining the stiffness of the musculotendon system. This is of great importance when complex jump

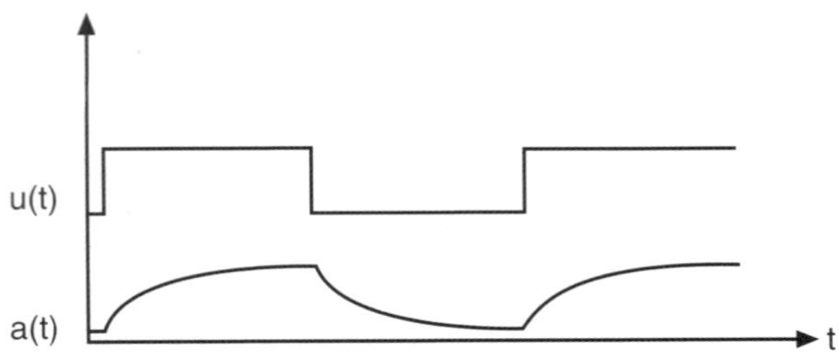

Figure 14.7 Relation between the incoming neural signal *u(t)* and the muscle activation *a(t)*.

exercises are to be investigated, where there is dissipation or consumption of energy that produces oscillations according to resonance phenomenon. A reference comes from the data presented by Nummela and associates (65). They demonstrated that different ground reactions could be measured during sprinting according to different EMG activity prior to the landing phase.

It is speculation to say that the EMG represents the amount of stiffness of the contractile elements, which, together with the stiffness of the elastic elements, determines the overall stiffness of the muscle-tendon system as a part of the stiffness of the body segment (1, 22). The stiffness of the contractile elements, however, is the only parameter that can be regulated voluntarily or reflexively. In addition, this could have an impact on the amount of reflex activity, because different strain production per time causes different reflex activity, and this again causes different stiffness. Furthermore, other influences like vestibular and visual inputs can modify this neuromuscular system, which is well adapted to normal gravity conditions (4).

It seems plausible that EMG can be used as a measurement tool for the excitation and not for the activation of the muscle. It can demonstrate the signal incoming to the neuromuscular system, but it does not seem to be a measurement device in every circumstance to predict the mechanical outcome of the MTS. Maybe it can help to calculate the stiffness of a body segment.

We conclude that in modeling one has to differentiate between the two major functions of the muscle-tendon system: production of "internal" forces and resistance to "external" forces. These two situations can have the same amount of muscular excitation but different amounts of activation. The EMG can be seen as a "magic eye" that is used to look at the exciting excitation of the neuromuscular (sensomotoric) system and in this way to assess neuromuscular control but not as a device to predict muscular force. Maybe it can help to estimate the amount of energy turnover; certainly it can help in the assessment of the interaction of the informational sphere and the structural sphere.

References

1. Alexander R.M., Bennet-Clark H.C.: Storage of elastic strain energy in muscle and other tissues. *Nature* 1977, 265: 114–17.
2. Anderson P.A., Hobart D.J., Danoff J.V. (eds.): *Electrophysiological kinesiology: Excerpta medica*, New York: Oxford University Press, 1991.
3. Asmussen E.: Muscle fatigue. *Med. Sci. Sports Exer.* 1979, 11: 313–21.
4. Avela J., Santos P.M., Kyröläinen H., Komi P.V.: Effects of different simulated gravity conditions on neuromuscular control in drop jump exercises. *Aviat. Space Environ. Med.* 1994, 65: 301–308.
5. Basmajian J.V., DeLuca C.J.: *Muscles alive: Their functions revealed by electromyography.* Baltimore: Williams & Wilkins, 1985.
6. Bigland B., Lippold O.C.J.: The relation between force, velocity, and integrated electrical activity in human muscles. *J. Physiol.* 1954, 123: 214–24.
7. Bigland-Ritchie B.: EMG and fatigue of human voluntary and stimulated contractions. In: *Ciba Foundation Symposium vol. 82. Human muscle fatigue: Physiological mechanisms.* London: Pitman Medical, 1981, 130–56.
8. Bigland-Ritchie B., Johansson R.S., Lippold O.C.J., Woods J.J.: Contractile speed and EMG changes of sustained maximum voluntary contractions. *J. Neurophysiol.* 1983, 50: 313–24.
9. Bigland-Ritchie B., Cafarelli E., Vollestad N.K.: Fatigue of submaximal static contractions. *Acta Physiol. Scan.* 1986, 556(128 suppl.): 137–48.
10. Bigland-Ritchie B., Dawson N.J., Johansson R.S., Lippold O.C.J.: Reflex origin for the slowing of motor neuron firing rates in fatigue of human voluntary contractions. *J. Physiol.* 1986, 379: 451–59.
11. Bigland-Ritchie B., Furbush F., Woods J.J.: Fatigue of intermittent submaximal voluntary contractions: Central and peripheral factors. *J. App. Physiol.* 1986, 61: 421–29.
12. Bochdansky Th., Lechner H., Bachl N.: Veränderungen des Stoffwechsels beim bergang von Kontraktion in Distraktion zur ergometrischen Leistungsbeurteilung. In: *Die trainingsphysiologische und klinische Bedeutung der anaeroben Kapazität,* Wien: Hollinek, 1987, 242–48.

13. Boiusset S.: EMG and muscle force in normal motor activities. In: *New developments in electromyography and clinical neurophysiology,* vol. 1, Desmedt J.E. (ed.). Basel: Karger, 1973, 547–83.
14. Bouissou P., Estrade P.Y., Goubel F., Guezennec C.Y., Serrurier B.: Surface EMG power spectrum and intramuscular pH in human vastus lateralis muscle during dynamic exercise. *J. Appl. Physiol.* 1989, 67(3): 1245–249.
15. Braakhekke J.P., Stegeman D.F., Joosten E.M.G.: Increase in median power frequency of the myoelectric signal in pathological fatigue. *Electroencephal. Clin. Neurophysiol.* 1989, 73: 151–56.
16. Brody L.R., Pollock M.T., Roy S.H., De Luca C.J., Celli B.: The pH-induced effects on median frequency and conduction velocity of the myoelectric signal. *J. App. Physiol.* 1991, 71: 1878–885.
17. Chaffin D.B., Lee M., Freivalds A.: Muscle strength assessment from EMG analysis. *Med. Sci. Sports Exer.* 1980, 12(3): 205–11.
18. Clarys J.P.: Electrology and localized electrization revisited. *J. Electromyogr. Kinesiol.* 1994, 4(1): 5–14.
19. De Luca C.J., Mambrito B.: Voluntary control of motor units in human antagonist muscles: Coactivation and reciprocal activation. *J. Neurophysiol.* 1987, 58: 525–42.
20. DeLuca C.J.: The use of surface electromyography in biomechanics. *J. Appl. Biomechanics* 1997, 13: 135–63.
21. Eloranta V., Komi P.V.: Function of the quadriceps femoris muscle under maximal concentric and eccentric contractions. *Electromyogr. Clin. Neurophysiol.* 1980, 20: 159–74.
22. Ferris D.P., Farley C.T.: Interaction of leg stiffness and surface stiffness during human hopping. *J. Appl. Physiol.* 1997, 82(1): 15–22.
23. Ferris-Hood K., Threlkeld A.J., Horn T.S., Shapiro R.: Relaxation electromechanical delay of the quadriceps during selected movement velocities. *Electromyogr. Clin. Neurophysiol.* 1996, 36: 157–70.
24. Fuglevand A.J., Zackowski K.M., Huey K.A., Enoka R.M.: Impairment of neuromuscular propagation during human fatiguing contractions at submaximal forces. *J. Physiol.* 1993, 460: 549–72.
25. Gans B.M., Noordergraaf A.: Voluntary skeletal muscles: A unifying theory on the relationship of their electrical and mechanical activities. *Arch. Phys. Med. Rehabil.* 1975, 56: 194–99.
26. Georgopoulos A.P., Schwartz A.B., Kettner R.E.: Neuronal population coding of movement direction. *Science* 1986, 233: 1416–419.
27. Gerdle B., Wretling M.L., Henriksson-Larsen K.: Do the fiber type proportion and the angular velocity influence the mean power frequency of the electromyogram? *Acta Physiol. Scan.* 1988, 134: 341–46.
28. Ghori G.M.U., Donne B., Luckwill R.G.: Relationship between torque and EMG activity of a knee extensor muscle during isokinetic concentric and eccentric actions. *J. Electromyogr. Kinesiol.* 1995, 5(2): 109–15.
29. Gioux M., Arne P., Dogui M., Bensch Cl.: Biomechanical and electromyographical characteristics of the human quadriceps in relation with sport performance. In: *Current topics in sports medicine,* Bachl N., Prokop L., Suckert R. (eds.). Baltimore: Urban & Schwarzenberg, 1982, 699–705.
30. Hägg G.M.: Interpretation of EMG spectral alterations and alterations indexes at sustained contraction. *J. Appl. Physiol.* 1992, 73: 1211–217.
31. Häkkinen K., Komi P.V.: Effects of fatigue and recovery on electromyographic and isometric force and relaxation time characteristics of human muscle. *Eur. J. Appl. Physiol.* 1986, 55: 588–96.
32. Hatcher D.D., Luff A.R.: Force-velocity properties of fast-twitch and slow-twitch muscles of the kitten. *J. Physiol.* 1985, 367: 377–85.
33. Hawkins D.A., Hull M.L.: An activation recruitment scheme for use in muscle modeling. *J. Biomechanics* 1992, 25(12): 1467–476.
34. Herzog W., Guimaraes A.C.S., Zhang Y.T.: EMG. In: *Biomechanics of the musculoskeletal system,* Nigg B., Herzog W. (eds.). New York: Wiley, 1994, 308–36.
35. Hill A.V.: The mechanics of voluntary muscle. *Lancet* 1951, 24: 947–51.
36. Holewijn M., Heus R.: Effects of temperature on electromyogram and muscle function. *Eur. J. Appl. Physiol.* 1992, 65: 541–45.
37. Hultman E., Sjöholm H.: Electromyogram, force, and relaxation time during and after continuous electrical stimulation of human skeletal muscle in situ. *J. Physiol.* 1983, 339: 33–40.
38. Housh T.J., DeVries H.A., Johnson G.O., Evans S.A., Housh D.J., Stout J.R., Bradway R.M., Evetovich T.K.: Neuromuscular fatigue thresholds of the vastus lateralis, vastus medialis, and rectus femoris muscles. *Electromyogr. Clin. Neurophysiol.* 1996, 36: 247–56.
39. Inman V.T., Ralston H.J.: The mechanics of voluntary muscle. In: *Human limbs and their substitutes,* Klopsteg, Wilson, (eds.). New York: McGraw-Hill, 1954, 296–317.
40. Jacobs R., Van Ingen Schenau G.J.: Control of an external force in leg extensions in humans. *J. Physiol.* 1992, 457: 611–26.

41. Kabat H., Knott M.: Proprioceptive facilitation techniques for treatment of paralysis. *Phys. Ther. Rev.* 1953, 33: 53.
42. Kalaska J.F., Cohen D.A.D., Hyde M.L., Prud'homme M.: A comparison of movement direction-related versus load direction-related activity in primate motor cortex, using a two-dimensional reaching task. *J. Neurosci.* 1989, 9: 2080–102.
43. Kernell D., Monster A.W.: Motor neuron properties and motor fatigue: An intracellular study of gastrocnemius motor neurons of the cat. *Exp. Brain Res.* 1982, 46: 197–204.
44. Komi P.V.: Relationship between muscle tension, EMG, and velocity of contraction under concentric and eccentric work. In: *New developments in electromyography and clinical neurophysiology,* vol. 1, Desmedt J.E. (ed.). Basel Karger: 1973, 596–606.
45. Komi P.V., Viitasalo J.H.T.: Signal characteristics of EMG at different levels of muscle tension. *Acta Physiol. Scan.* 1976, 96: 267–76.
46. Kostka Ch.E., Cafarelli E.: Effect of pH on sensation and vastus lateralis electromyogram during cycling exercise. *J. Appl. Physiol.* 1982, 52(5): 1181–185.
47. Kupa E.J., Roy S.H., Kandarian S.C., DeLuca C.J.: Effects of muscle fiber type and size on EMG median frequency and conduction velocity. *J. Appl. Physiol.* 1995, 79(1): 23–32.
48. Lagasse P.P.: Prediction of maximum speed of human movement by two selected muscular coordination mechanisms and by maximum static strength. *Percep. Motor Skills* 1979, 49: 151–61.
49. Lam H.S., Morgan D.L., Lampard D.G.: Derivation of reliable electromyograms and their relation to tension in mammalian skeletal muscles during synchronous stimulation. *Electroencephal. Clin. Neurophysiol.* 1979, 46: 72–80.
50. Lechner H., Bochdansky Th., Platner O.: Einrichtung zur Erfassung der Muskelkraft. Patentschrift. Nr. AT 397 033 B, 1994.
51. Linssen W.H.J.P., Stegeman D.F., Joosten E.M.G., Binkhorst R.A., Merks M.J.H., Ter Laak H.J., Notermans S.L.H.: Fatigue in type I fiber predominance: A muscle force and surface EMG study on the relative role of type I and type II muscle fibers. *Muscle & Nerve* 1991, 14: 829–37.
52. Linssen W.H.J.P., Stegeman D.F., Joosten E.M.G., Vant't Hof M.A., Binkhorst R.A., Notermans S.L.H.: Variability and interrelationships of surface EMG parameters during local muscle fatigue. *Muscle & Nerve* 1993, 16: 849–56.
53. Lippold O.C.J.: The relationship between integrated action potentials in human muscles and its isometric tension. *J. Physiol.* 1952, 177: 492–99.
54. Lippold O.C.J., Redffearn J.W.T., Vuco J.: The electromyography of fatigue. *Ergonomics* 1960, 3: 121–31.
55. Macefield G., Hagbarth K.E., Gorman R., Gandevia S.C., Burke D.: Decline in spindle support to alpha motoneurons during sustained voluntary contractions. *J. Physiol.* 1991, 123: 553–64.
56. Mc Nabb N., Frank J.S., Green H.J.: Recurrent inhibition during sustained contractions in humans. *Soc. Neurosci. Abst.* 1988, 14: 948.
57. Merletti R., Roy S.: Myoelectric and mechanical manifestations of muscle fatigue in voluntary contractions. *J. Orthop. Sports Phys. Ther.* 1996, 24(6): 342–53.
58. Merton P.A.: Voluntary strength and fatigue. *J. Physiol.* 1954, 123: 553–64.
59. Miller R.G., Giannini D., Milner-Brown H.S., Layzer R., Koretsky A.P., Hooper D., et al.: Effects of fatiguing exercise on high-energy phosphates, force, and EMG: Evidence of three phases of recovery. *Muscle & Nerve* 1987, 10: 810–21.
60. Mills K.R., Edwards R.H.T.: Muscle fatigue in myophosphorylase deficiency: Power spectral analysis of the electromyogram. *Electroencephal. Clin. Neurophysiol.* 1984, 57: 330–35.
61. Milner-Brown H.S., Stein R.B.: The relation between the surface electromyogram and muscular force. *J. Physiol.* 1975, 246: 549–69.
62. Mizrahi J., Levin O., Aviram A., Isakov E., Susak Z.: Muscle fatigue in interrupted stimulation: Effect of partial recovery on force and EMG dynamics. *J. Electromyogr. Kinesiol.* 1997, 7(1): 51–65.
63. Moritani T., Gaffney F.D., Carmichael T., Hargis J.: Interrelationships among muscle fiber types, electromyogram, and blood pressure during fatiguing isometric contractions. In: *Biomechanics,* vol. IXA, Winter D.A., Norman R.W., Wells R.P., Hayes K.C., Patla A.E. (eds.). Champaign, IL: Human Kinetics, 1985, 287–92.
64. Nieminen H., Niemi J., Takala E.P., Viikari-Juntura E.: Load-sharing patterns in the shoulder during isometric flexion tasks. *J. Biomechanics* 1995, 28(5): 555–66.
65. Nummela A., Rusko H., Mero A.: EMG activities and ground reaction forces during fatigued and nonfatigued sprinting. *Med. Sci. Sports Exer.* 1994, 26(5): 605–609.

66. Oksa J., Rintamaki H., Makinen T., Martikkala V., Rusko H.: EMG activity and muscular performance of lower leg during stretch-shortening cycle after cooling. *Acta Physiol. Scan.* 1996, 157(1): 1–8.
67. Pandy M.G., Zajac F.E., Sim E., Levine W.S.: An optimal control model for maximum-height human jumping. *J. Biomechanics* 1990, 23(12): 1185–198.
68. Parry D.J., Mainwood G.W., Chan T.: The relationship between surface potentials and the number of active motor units. *J. Neurol. Sci.* 1977, 33: 283–96.
69. Philipson L., Larsson P.G.: The electromyographic signal as a measure of muscular force: A comparison of detection and quantification techniques. *Electromyogr. Clin. Neurophysiol.* 1988, 28: 141–50.
70. Piper H.: *Elektrophysiologie menschlicher Muskeln.* Berlin, Germany: Springer, 1912.
71. Potvin J.R.: Effects of muscle kinematics on surface EMG amplitude and frequency during fatiguing dynamic contractions. *J. Appl. Physiol.* 1997, 82(1): 144–51.
72. Psek J.A., Cafarelli E.: Behavior of coactive muscles during fatigue. *J. App. Physiol.* 1993, 74: 170–75.
73. Rau G., Disselhorst-Klug C., Silny J.: Noninvasive approach to motor unit characterization: Muscle structure, membrane dynamics, and neuronal control. *J. Biomechanics* 1997, 30(5): 441–46.
74. Rosentswieg J., Hinson M.M.: Comparison of isometric, isotonic, and isokinetic exercises by electromyography. *Arch. Phys. Med. Rehab.* 1972, 6: 249–52.
75. Sacco P., Newberry R., McFadden L., Brown T., McComas A.J.: Depression of human electromyographic activity by fatigue of a synergistic muscle. *Muscle & Nerve* 1997, 20: 710–17.
76. Seliger V., Dolejs L., Karas V.: A dynamometric comparison of maximum eccentric, concentric, and isometric contractions using EMG and energy expenditure measurements. *Eur. J. Appl. Physiol.* 1980, 45: 235–44.
77. Solomonow M., Guzzi A., Baratta R., Shoji H., D'Ambrosia R.: EMG-force model of the elbow antagonistic muscle pair: The effect of joint position, gravity, and recruitment. *Am. J. Phys. Med.* 1986, 65: 223–43.
78. Solomonow M., Baratta R., Zhou B.H., Shoji H., D'Ambrosia R.: Historical update and new developments on the EMG-force relationships of skeletal muscles. *Orthopedics* 1986, 9(11): 1541–543.
79. Solomonow M., Baten C., Smit J., Baratta R., Hermens H., D'Ambrosia R., Shoji H.: Electromyogram power spectra frequencies associated with motor unit recruitment strategies. *J. App. Physiol.* 1990, 68: 1177–85.
80. Suzuki S., Watanabe S., Homma S.: EMG activity and kinematics of human cycling movements at different constant velocities. *Brain Res.* 1982, 240: 245–58.
81. Tesch P.A., Komi P.V., Jacobs I., Karlsson J., Viitasalo J.T.: Influence of lactate accumulation of EMG frequency spectrum during repeated concentric contractions. *Acta Physiol. Scan.* 1983, 119: 61–67.
82. Thomas C.K., Woods J.J., Bigland-Ritchie B.: Impulse propagation and muscle activation in long maximal voluntary contractions. *J. App. Physiol.* 1989, 67: 1835–842.
83. Van Ingen Schenau G.J., Dorsses W.M.M., Welter T.G., Beelen A., De Groot G., Jacobs R.: The control of monoarticular muscles in multijoint leg extensions in man. *J. Physiol.* 1992, 484: 247–54.
84. Van Ingen Schenau G.J., Boots P.J.M., De Groot G., Snackers R.J., Van Woensel W.W.L.M.: The constrained control of force and position in multijoint movements. *Neuroscience* 1992, 46: 197–207.
85. Vos E.J., Mullender M.G., Van Ingen Schenau G.J.: Electromechanical delay in the vastus lateralis muscle during dynamic isometric contractions. *Eur. J. Appl. Physiol.* 1990, 60: 467–71.
86. Wallinga W., Boom H.B.K., DeVries J. (eds.): *Electrophysiological kinesiology. Excerpta medica,* New York: Oxford University Press, 1988.
87. Westing S.H., Cresswell A.G., Thorstensson A.: Muscle activation during maximal voluntary eccentric and concentric knee extension. *Eur. J. Appl. Physiol.* 1991, 62: 104–108.
88. Winter D.: *Biomechanics and motor control of human movement.* New York: Wiley, 1990.
89. Wise S.P.: Monkey motor cortex: Movement muscles, motor neurons, and metrics. *Trends in Neurosciences* 1993, 16: 46–49.
90. Woods J., Bigland-Ritchie B.: Linear and nonlinear surface EMG-force relationships in human muscles. *Am. J. Phys. Med.* 1983, 62: 287–99.
91. Wretling M.L., Gerdle B., Henriksson-Larsen K.: EMG: A noninvasive method for determination of fiber type proportion. *Acta Physiol. Scan.* 1987, 131: 627–28.
92. Yang J.F., Winter D.A.: Electromyography reliability in maximal and submaximal isometric contractions. *Arch. Phys. Med. Rehabil.* 1983, 64: 417–20.

93. Yoneda T., Oishi K., Fujikura S., Ishida A.: Recruitment threshold force and its changing type of motor units during voluntary contraction at various speeds in man. *Brain Res.* 1986, 372: 89–94.
94. Young A.: The relative isometric strength of type I and type II muscle fibers in the human quadriceps. *Clin. Physiol.* 1984, 4: 23–32.
95. Zakaria D., Kramer J.F., Harburn K.L.: Reliability of nonnormalized and normalized integrated EMG during maximal isometric contractions in females. *J. Electromyogr. Kinesiol.* 1996, 6(2): 129–35.
96. Zhou S., McKenna M.J., Lawson D.L., Morrison W.E., Fairweather I.: Effects of fatigue and sprinting training on electromechanical delay of knee extensor muscles. *Eur. J. Appl. Physiol.* 1996, 72: 410–16.
97. Zuniga E.N., Simons D.G.: Nonlinear relationship between averaged electromyogram potential and muscle tension in normal subjects. *Arch Phys. Med. Rehabil.* 1969, 50: 613–20.
98. Zytnicki D., Lafleur J., Horcholle-Bosavit G., Lami F., Jami L.: Reduction of Ib autogenetic inhibition in motor neurons during contractions of an ankle extensor muscle in the cat. *J. Neurophysiol.* 1990, 64: 1380–389.

CHAPTER 15

A Method for Analyzing Standing and Reactive Balance and Neuromuscular Responses of the Spine and Lower Extremities

Jennifer Ocif
Christine Gardner
John Albright, MD
Malcolm Pope, Dr Med Sci

Introduction

A higher incidence of anterior cruciate ligament (ACL) injuries has been reported in female athletes as compared to their male counterparts (1, 2, 4, 11). Possible causes include deficiencies in muscular strength and coordination, conditioning, and neuromuscular ability, in addition to the inherent physical characteristics of female athletes (3). Although significant research efforts have investigated the causes of ACL injury, only recently has the role of neuromuscular control been addressed. Huston and Wojtys (12) measured the reactive neuromuscular performance of elite female and male athletes by inducing direct anterior tibial translation at the knee joint. They measured the protective responses of the leg muscles to this perturbation in female athletes and found that the quadriceps muscle responded first, before the hamstring or gastrocnemius muscles. This result differed significantly from the results in male athletes.

Among the two sports for which women at the University of Iowa run the highest risk of ACL injury are basketball and gymnastics. Almost all of the ACL injuries have occurred in the absence of any direct blow to the knee. It has been a common observation that the injuries also involved an unplanned move on a planted extremity, an alleged loss of balance, and the sensation of subluxation or hyperextension of the knee. We have also observed that our university women's basketball team members, while gifted players who are capable of very fluid moves, have obvious difficulty simply balancing on one leg, let alone attempting a one-legged squat. On the other hand, our gymnasts have excellent one-legged balance and squat strength that seems appropriate to their ability to accomplish very complex patterned movements with great precision. Other than the pattern of ACL injury, these two groups of athletes appear to have little in common. Neither the gymnasts nor the basketball players, however, appear to be adept at reacting to either an unexpected perturbation or a missed landing, and, consequently, they find themselves at risk when thrown off balance. It is our hypothesis that these elite athletes who are at risk for ACL injury have poor reactive balance that is not adequate for the demands of their sport.

On a more basic level, we have also documented that in an ACL-deficient knee, contraction of the quadriceps unopposed by the hamstrings can cause a rather dramatic pivot shift that the patient describes as a hyperextension episode. This documentation confirms Losee's description of the "slingshot" phenomenon, where the contraction of the quadriceps in a slightly flexed knee allows the patella to push the femoral condyle posteriorly and pull the tibia anteriorly. It is our second hypothesis that this quadriceps-dominant slingshot phenomenon is the cause of many noncontact ACL injuries. Therefore, we have investigated the recruitment order of these muscles to determine the typical firing sequences and the variances that may occur in elite athletes who have a high potential for these injuries. It has been found that typically a hamstring-quadriceps recruitment order, or co-contraction, is common in response to a perturbation (7, 12). However, it is the alteration to the quadriceps-hamstring firing order that puts these athletes at risk.

Since certain body movements such as one-legged cutting maneuvers and sudden stops translate into positions that may predispose the knee joint to injury, we questioned the combined role of balance and motor control in an athlete's ability to safely perform high-performance maneuvers. Years of postural research, by Lewis Nashner (14) and others (10), have established an extensive knowledge base with respect to the human body's automatic response to balance perturbations. By applying these principles to the mechanism of ACL injuries, this study was designed to investigate the automatic postural responses of female athletes during a balance perturbation to upright stance.

The purpose of this study was to demonstrate a new dynamic setup for investigating the ability to maintain balance while standing in a one-legged stance. This setup has the subject standing in a one-limb stance and perturbs the subject by applying a sudden load to the chest. The neuromuscular response of the legs and spinal muscles and the ground reaction forces are recorded through EMG and force plate technology, respectively (see figure 15.1). The recruitment order of the muscles, the timing sequence of the body movements, the magnitude of the muscle responses, and the balance of the subjects can then be analyzed.

Materials and Methods

The protocol for this study was adapted from previous research conducted at the University of Iowa Spine Research Center, ISRC, which has investigated the influence of a sudden load on the muscular responses of healthy subjects and patients with low-back pain (3, 17). In the current study, balance ability and response to a sudden postural perturbation were assessed during one-legged stance. One-legged (as opposed to two-legged) stance was chosen to simulate a weight-bearing position during the stance phase of an athletic maneuver. The postural perturbation was directed anteriorly on the subject's chest (inducing forward sway) to simulate the forward translation of an athlete's center of mass, such as occurs when the athlete is pushed from behind, stops suddenly from a run, or lands off balance from a vault or floor exercise. Previous studies using this test setup have successfully induced enough forward sway to elicit significant muscle responses in the back and lower legs (17).

After removing their shoes, subjects stood on one leg on a stationary force platform with the knee of the stance leg flexed at approximately 15° and the other knee flexed and held at 90°. This position was chosen because it puts significant strain on the ACL in the stance leg, as has been documented in recent literature (6). A sudden load was applied by a "guillotine" mechanism in which a weight of 2 kg was attached to a string and loosely guided to ensure a straight vertical drop. The other string end was threaded through a pulley system and attached to a harness around the subject's shoulders. The weight was dropped from a height of 45 cm above the floor, to apply a sudden forward bending moment at T4 (the 4th thoracic vertebra).

Two conditions were tested: expected and unexpected. For the expected condition, the investigator gave a verbal countdown to the time of weight release. For the unexpected condition, the subject wore music earphones (to mask aural cues to weight release) and closed her eyes (to mask visual cues). Sensory cues to the time of weight release were minimized by two special construction features of the sudden load apparatus. The platform supporting the force plate and the subject were separate from the "guillotine" mechanism and sufficient slack in the string of the pulley system prevented the subject from anticipating weight release. For the unexpected condition, the time to weight release was randomized (between 1–5 s) in order to minimize anticipatory learning effects. Dominance was defined by the subject's preferred hand and leg for daily living and sport activities (handwriting, shooting hand, take-off or landing foot, etc.). The order of side (left or right leg) to be tested was randomized. The following testing sequence was utilized:

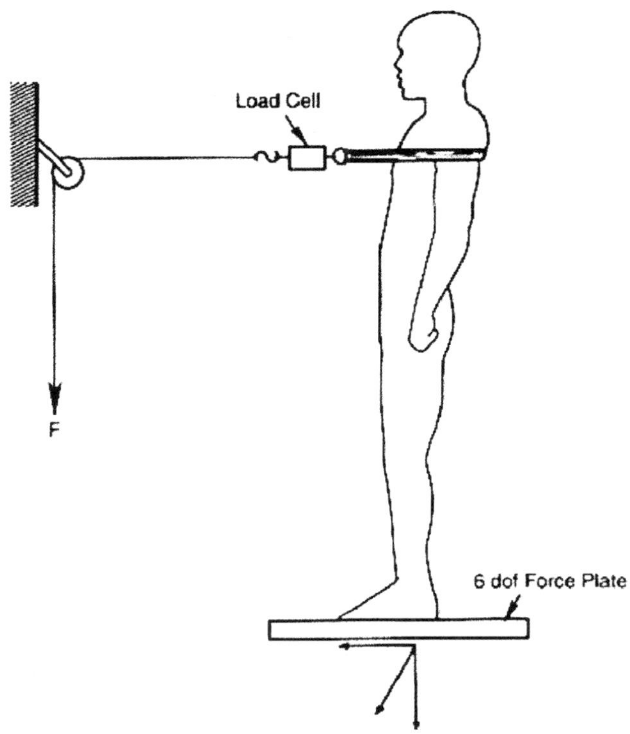

Figure 15.1 Schematic of the sudden load setup.

1. Expected (eyes open), first leg
2. Unexpected (eyes closed), first leg
3. Expected (eyes open), second leg
4. Unexpected (eyes closed), second leg

A piezoresistive (IC sensor) uniaxial accelerometer (weight: 0.5 g) with built-in preamplification was fixed rigidly to the harness to record the time of sudden load application. Ground reaction forces were measured by a Bertec force plate (model #4060) with six degrees of freedom in three planes: sagittal, frontal, and transverse. Force plate data was collected at a sampling rate of 50 Hz for a total of 4 s, beginning at least 500 ms before sudden load application. Surface electromyography (EMG) was used to record muscle activity in three muscle groups of the tested leg—erector spinae, rectus femoris (quadriceps), and biceps femoris (hamstrings). Bipolar electrodes (Therapeutics, Inc., Iowa City, Iowa) with built-in preamplifiers were fixed to the skin at L3 (3d lumbar vertebra), 3 cm lateral to the midline for the right and left erector spinae muscle and at the midpoints of the rectus femoris and biceps femoris muscles on the stance leg. The amplifier equipment was set up for low noise and a gain of 5000. Raw EMG data was collected (via ASYST v4.0, Keithley Instruments, Inc., Taunton, MA) at a sampling rate of 1000 Hz for a total of 4 s, beginning at least 500 ms before sudden load application. All force plate and EMG data were collected simultaneously; sampling was triggered by a computer keystroke, and the data was stored on a personal computer for off-line processing (17).

During off-line processing, accelerometer data was inspected using continuous wavelet transform (CWT) software to determine the onset of sudden load application or the time of stimulus relative to the beginning of data collection (0 ms). The point at which the acceleration curve first significantly deviated from the steady baseline value was defined as the onset of the stimulus.

Force plate data (see figure 15.2) was processed off-line in the time domain only, using Microcal Origin software (Version 4. 1, Microcal Software Inc., Northampton, MA). Ground reaction forces and moments measured during the 4 s duration of the sudden load test were plotted separately in each plane (sagittal, transverse, and frontal). Using the time of sudden load application determined by the accelerometer, manual inspection identified three components of the ground reaction forces that were produced by each subject during balance recovery: onset of force change, peak force, and end of the force response, all relative to the beginning of data collection (0 ms). In addition, the baseline activity 500 ms before the sudden load was applied was recorded to be used for a comparison measure of each subject's balance. These baseline values were defined as the root mean square (*RMS*) average of the region of data being analyzed. This analysis was

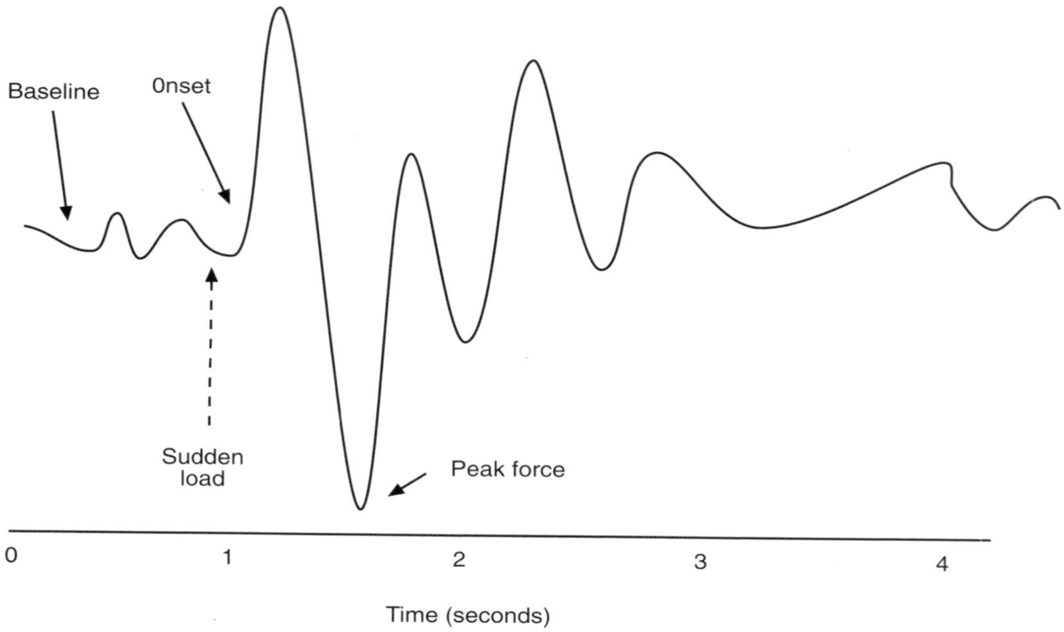

Figure 15.2 Example of force plate signal.

done using Microsoft Excel (Version 6.0, Microsoft Corporation, Seattle, WA) spreadsheet software. All force plate data was normalized by subject body weight (N).

A typical EMG signal (see figure 15.3) recorded during a sudden load test exhibits pronounced muscle activation throughout the entire data collection process. Typically, however, a spike is identified when the sudden load has occurred. The ability to detect the beginning of muscle burst activity with surface electromyography is difficult because of this background muscle activity. There are numerous methods used to analyze EMG data, including rectification/integration (12), *RMS*/filtering (16), and wavelet (18) to name a few. The raw EMG data from this testing was processed in both the time and frequency domains using a custom-designed discrete wavelet transformation (DWT) software program in MATLAB (The Math Works) (11). This custom DWT program has been used in a recent ISRC study that investigated the effects of back belts on trunk muscle activity in normal subjects (18). The raw EMG data was used to find muscle reaction times, or latencies, for each muscle relative to the trigger time determined from the accelerometer data. These latencies were recorded in milliseconds. The latencies could then be used to find the recruitment orders for each subject.

The general linear model (GLM) of analysis of variance (ANOVA) for repeated measures (SAS System, version 6.1.2. OS/2 Warp 4.0) was used to evaluate both the EMG and force plate data. Additional post hoc analyses, including Tukey's Studentized range test, were used to test significance between variables with multiple measures.

A total of 30 college-age females from the University of Iowa were recruited to test the previously described protocol and apparatus. All subjects signed informed written consent before participating, in accordance with university guidelines. Subjects were divided into three groups with 10 subjects per group: elite basketball players (age 21.5 ±2.7 years; weight = 73.7 ±10.9 kg; height = 180.1 ±8.2 cm), elite gymnasts (age = 19.4 ±1.8 years; weight = 56.9 ±8.2 kg; height = 160.5 ±6.9 cm) and age-matched controls (age = 23.4 ±2.4 years; weight 57.0 ±11.0 kg, height = 161.5 ±6.1 cm). Six of the 10 basketball players had no previous knee or ankle injuries, 2 players had ACL reconstruction, 1 had an ACL sprain, and 1 had a meniscus tear. Six of the gymnasts had no previous knee or ankle injuries, 1 had ACL reconstruction, 1 had surgery for patellar tendonitis, 1 had ankle arthroscopy, and 1 had a moderate medial collateral ligament (MCL) sprain. All 10 of the control subjects had no previous knee or ankle injuries.

Results

The force plate data demonstrated that for quiet standing *RMS* values, gymnasts exhibited signifi-

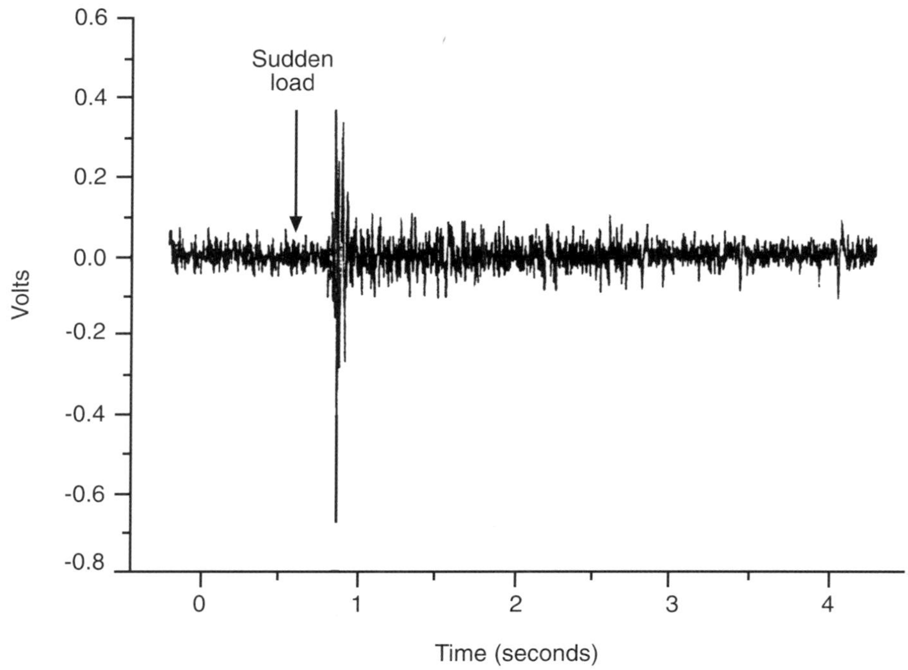

Figure 15.3 Example of EMG signal.

cantly better balance stability in the sagittal plane than basketball players did. In the frontal plane, basketball players exhibited significantly worse balance stability than both the gymnastics and control groups. (See figure 15.4.)

The average onset times of ground reaction times from the force plate showed that the control group always had the fastest onset times compared to both the basketball players and the gymnasts in all three coordinate planes. There was a statistically significant difference between the average onset times of the three groups in the sagittal plane and the transverse plane, but only a moderate trend in the frontal plane. More specifically, in the sagittal plane the onset time for the control group was significantly less than for the gymnasts, and in the transverse plane the onset time for the control group was significantly less than for the basketball players. (See figure 15.5.)

The EMG data showed the following results for recruitment order. The trend demonstrated that a quadriceps-hamstring-erector spinae order was common; however, most subjects exhibited slightly varied muscle recruitment order patterns. There were also no significant differences between subject groups for any of the test conditions for recruitment order. (See figure 15.6.)

Discussion

This study was done to investigate a dynamic setup for testing the postural balance and order of firing of the lower extremities and spinal muscles. Although the test condition has the subject in a stationary position initially, as opposed to a dynamic (running) position, it better mimics the complex reactive movements that occur in basketball and gymnastics than a completely static test setup where the lower limb is immobilized and a force is directly applied to the tibia as done by Huston and Wojtys (12) and Beynnon and coworkers (6).

The data collected showed patterns that were consistent with the literature. The gymnasts demonstrated significantly better forward and backward balance stability than the basketball players while in a one legged stance, and the basketball players demonstrated the lowest balance side-to-side stability even compared to the controls. The gymnast results make intuitive sense considering that gymnasts receive extensive balance training for many years and typically have smaller statures with lower centers of gravity. The poorer reactive balance results from the basketball players confirmed the observations that led to this study.

The onset times of ground reaction forces from the force plate data showed that the control group

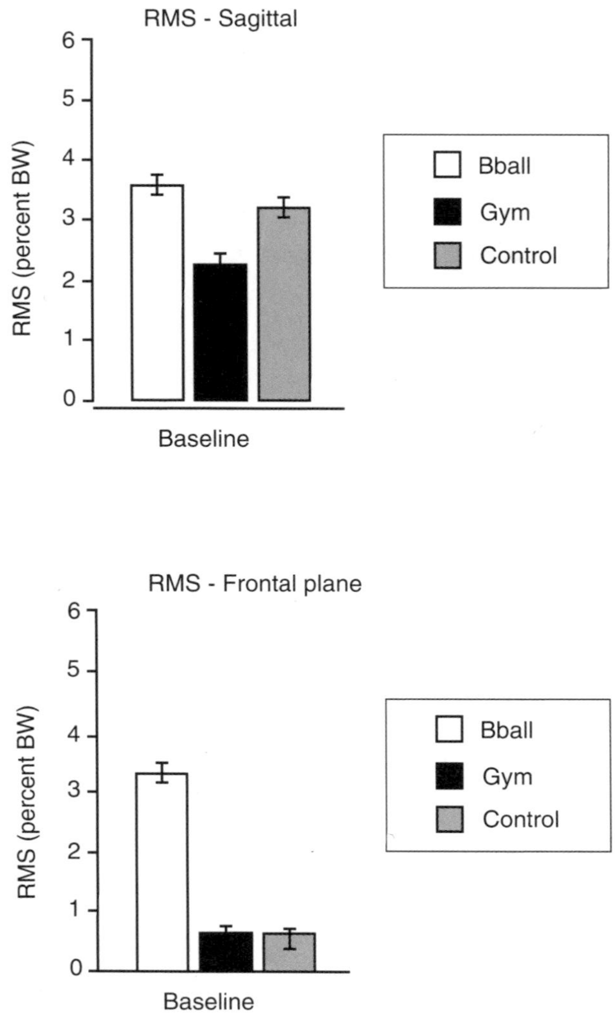

Figure 15.4 Force plate RMS baseline results.

had the fastest onset times compared to both the basketball players and the gymnasts in all three coordinate planes. This result shows that the athletes demonstrate higher resistance to a perturbation than most individuals, which cannot be attributed to their body weight, since the gymnasts and controls weighed approximately the same.

The recruitment order found from the EMG data followed trends of a quadriceps-hamstring firing sequence in our female subjects. These gender-related results are similar to those found by Huston and Wojtys (12).

The outcome of this experiment was positive, although areas in which the protocol could be improved were found. The test setup was found to be an excellent tool for simulating a dynamic perturbation to the spine and lower extremities. It could be used to investigate the neuromuscular response in the lower limbs of persons subject to this sudden load. In order to be more consistent in the testing, however, a few modifications could be made. A varying weight that is a percentage of the subject's body weight needs to be incorporated to perturb subjects of all sizes in a consistent manner. A quick release mechanism should be added to make the height and smoothness of the weight being dropped more repeatable. The strap that goes around the chest should always be perpendicular to the subject; therefore, it needs to be vertically adjustable to compensate for the varying

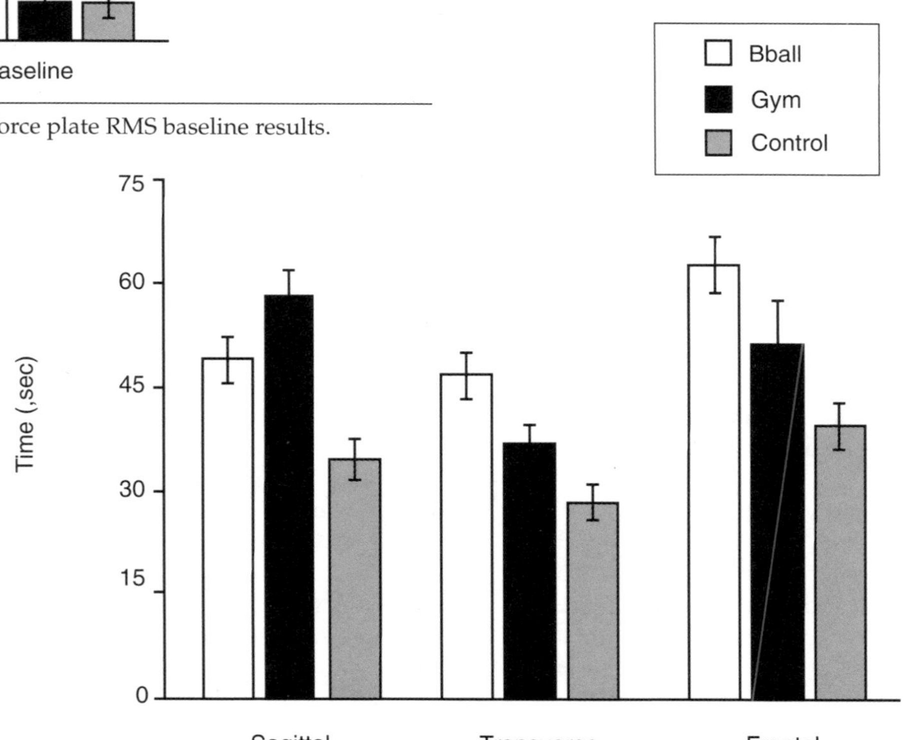

Figure 15.5 Force plate onset times of ground reaction forces.

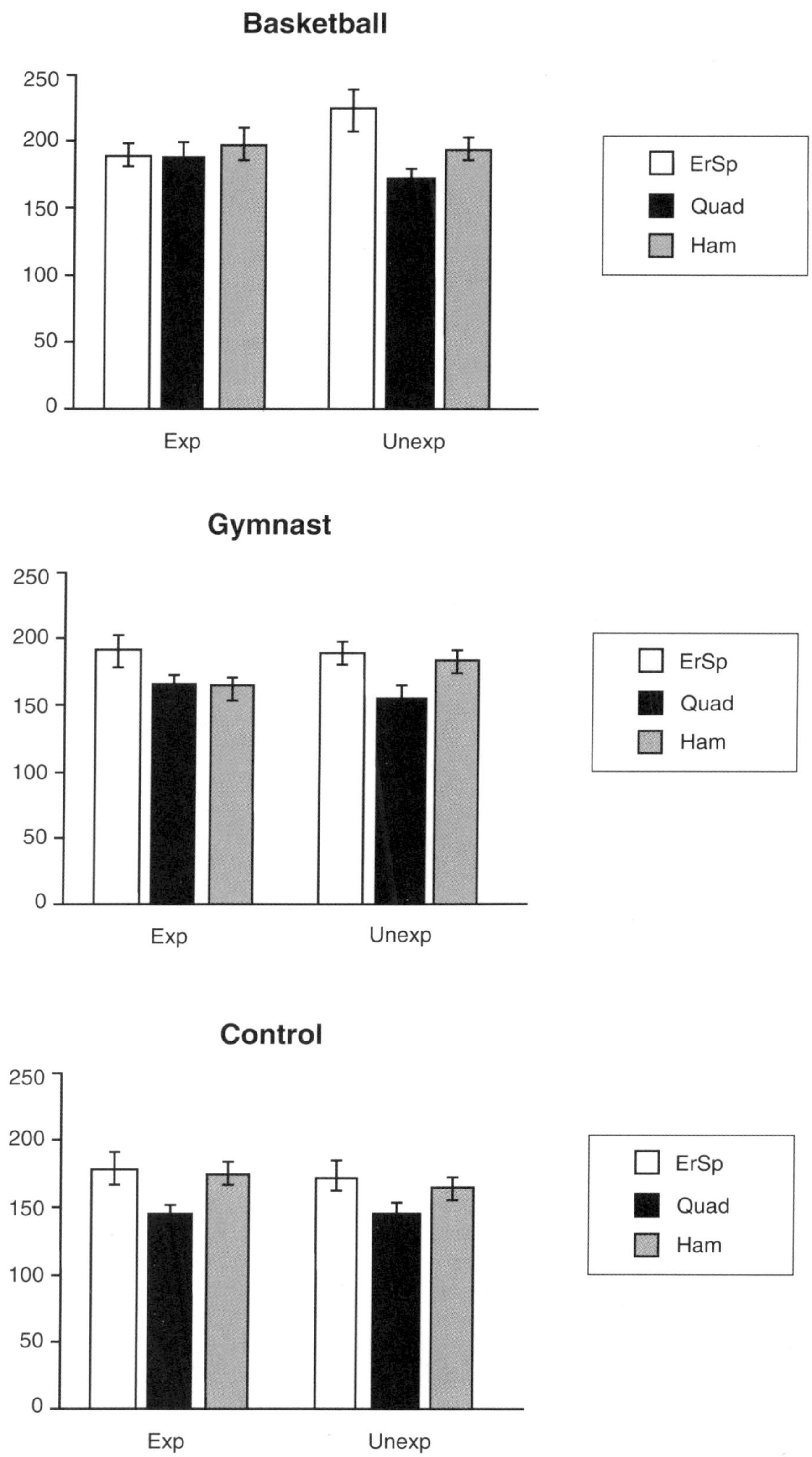

Figure 15.6 EMG recruitment orders.

heights of the subjects. The protocol could also be expanded by applying the sudden load to the subjects in a backward direction as well as in a forward direction. This would test the reactions of the lower limb in each direction and possibly correlate with the likely direction in which an ACL injury may occur. Since we observed that ACL injuries occur when a person is unsuspecting, the unexpected sudden load appears to be a more realistic measure of a possible ACL injury-type blow, and the expected condition does not need to be included in this protocol. Finally, the precision of the EMG placement needs to be solidified in order to obtain consistent, reliable data.

The data analysis that was done provides some interesting results, but an automated collection process would produce more reliability and would be more efficient. The manual data inspection inherent in the wavelet protocol can be subjective and introduces human error.

Balance is a critical part of this study and showed interesting trends in the data collected. For future work, the center of pressure may be an interesting means to analyze force plate activity, both during quiet standing and also while the subject reacts to the perturbation.

This preliminary study demonstrated that this test setup has the potential to be an excellent tool in the analysis of balance and neuromuscular activity in the spine and lower limbs of subjects. The next necessary step is the validation of this test setup through repeatability testing. The protocol and apparatus must be refined and tested to verify that they can produce repeatable data from a sample population twice in one day and over multiple days.

Conclusions

The gymnasts tended to have the best balance stability, whereas the basketball players tended to have the poorest balance stability when compared to both the gymnasts and controls. The trend for recruitment order was found to be quadriceps-hamstrings-erector spinae. The recruitment orders, however, were variable between subjects and between groups.

The results of this study demonstrate that this dynamic setup can be used to obtain neuromuscular and ground reaction force data for the spine and lower limbs of subjects. Future testing will modify the test setup to make it more consistent and investigate applying these methods to ACL-deficient knees.

References

1. Women's soccer injury rates increase in fall 1996 survey. *The NCAA's News* (Overland Park, KS) p. 8, 1997.
2. National Collegiate Athletic Association. *NCAA Injury Surveillance System.* Overland Park, KS: National Collegiate Athletic Association, 1993.
3. Aleksiev A, Pope NM, Hooper DM, Wilder D, Magnusson M, et al: Pelvic unlevelness in chronic low-back pain patients: Biomechanics and EMG time-frequency analyses. *Eur J Phys Med Rehab* 6(l): 3–16, 1996.
4. Arendt E, Dick R: Knee injury patterns among men and women in collegiate basketball and soccer: NCAA data and review of literature. *Am J Sports Med* 23(6): 694–701, 1995.
5. Bartnik EA, Blinowska KJ, and Durka PJ: Single evoked potential reconstruction by means of wavelet transform. *Biological Cybernetics* 67(2): 175–81, 1992.
6. Beynnon BD, Fleming BC, Johnson RJ, Nichols CE, Renström PA, et al: Anterior cruciate ligament strain behavior during rehabilitation exercises in vivo. *Am J Sports Med* 21(l): 24–34, 1995.
7. Ciccotti MG, Kerlan RK, Perry J, Pink M: An electromyographic analysis of the knee during functional activities. *Am J Sports Med* 22(5): 645–58, 1994.
8. Constable R, Thornhill RJ: Using the discrete wavelet transformation for time-frequency analysis of the surface EMG signal. *Biomed Sci Instrumentation* 29: 121–27, 1993.
9. Constable R, Thornhill RJ, Carpenter DR: Time-frequency analysis of the surface EMG during maximum height jumps under altered conditions. *Biomech Sci Instrumentation* 30: 69–74, 1994.
10. Dietz V, Berger W: Spinal coordination of bilateral leg muscle activity during balancing. *Exp Brain Res* 47: 172–76, 1982.
11. Gray J, Taunton JE, McKenzie DC, Clement DB, McConkey JP, et al: A survey of injuries to the anterior cruciate ligament of the knee in female basketball players. *Int J Sports Med* 6: 314–16, 1985.
12. Huston LJ, Wojtys EM: Neuromuscular performance characteristics in elite female athletes. *Am J Sports Med* 24(4): 427–36, 1996.
13. Lee JS: Discrete wavelet transformation: EMG analysis toolkit. (Computer software). Iowa City, Iowa: 1997.
14. Nashner LM: Fixed patterns of rapid postural responses among leg muscles during stance. *Exp Brain Res* 30: 13–24, 1997.

15. Schmidt R: *Motor learning and performance: From principles to practice.* Champaign, IL: Human Kinetics, 1991.
16. Soderberg G: Selected topics in electromyography for use in the occupational setting: Expert perspective. DHHS (NIOSH) Publication Washington, DC: U.S. Government Printing Office, 1992.
17. Wilder DG, Aleksiev AR, Magnusson ML, Pope NM, Spratt KF, et al: Muscular response to sudden load: A tool to evaluate fatigue and rehabilitation. *Spine* 21(22): 2628–639, 1996.
18. Wilder DB, Lee JS, Pope MH, Magnusson ML, Goel VK: Back supports and unexpected load. Paper presented at the meeting of the European Spine Society, Kos, Greece. September 10–13, 1997.

CHAPTER 16

Neuromuscular Performance in the ACL-Deficient Knee

Laura Huston, MS
Edward Wojtys, MD

Background

It is often difficult to predict from a physical examination of the knee which patients will be functionally impaired by the loss of the ACL and which patients will have minimal symptoms (3, 6, 11, 44, 45, 66). In 1983, Noyes and coworkers (45) popularized his "rule of thirds" theory on the prognosis following ACL injury: one-third of patients with ACL tears can continue to participate in their desired sports at preinjury levels, one-third will be satisfied continuing at a less vigorous level after physical therapy and functional bracing, and one-third will experience instability with conservative treatment and opt for surgical intervention. What allows some patients to maintain satisfactory function despite increased laxity is still unknown, but possibilities include uninjured secondary static stabilizers as well as dynamic compensatory mechanisms (61).

Dynamic stability of the knee relies on a complex sensory-motor synergy between passive (ligaments) and active (muscle) restraints designed to control tibiofemoral motion. In addition to its passive mechanical function, the ACL provides important sensory feedback that directly mediates joint position sense and muscular reflex stabilization of the knee joint (24, 33, 53, 57, 58). Varied levels of dynamic stability may help explain the paradox that physicians often see in the clinic: patients with minimal knee laxity presenting with symptoms of instability and, at the same time, ligamentously lax athletes who function at very high levels without any evidence of instability (41, 44, 60, 63). Interestingly, multiple investigators have failed to identify a correlation between the degree of anterior tibial translation and functional outcome in ACL-deficient knees (19, 60, 65). Consequently, neuromuscular control mechanisms may be more effective in predicting functional outcome than passive joint laxity in patients with ACL injuries (12, 63). This functional instability may be due, in part, to deficits in the dynamic system, which are currently less well understood.

The CNS-Dynamic Stabilizer Link

The presence of neuroreceptors in the human knee joint was first described by Raubner in 1874 (55). Abbott and coworkers (2) and Gardner (20–22) reported that the ligaments of the knee had a rich sensory innervation that allowed them to act as the first link in the "kinetic chain." Abbott and his group stated that "impulses arising in the ligaments are transmitted through the central nervous system back to the effector muscles, allowing for maintenance of normal, smooth, coordinated movement of the joint, and abnormally strong impulses, such as those initiated when a ligament is over-stretched, would result in contraction of allied muscle groups, theoretically preventing further subluxation and injury of the knee" (2). In 1956, Cohen and Cohen popularized the idea of an "arthrokinetic reflex" (12). Based on their work with decerebrate cats, they suggested that the origin of important protective afferent input was the knee joint capsule. Cohen and Cohen believed that a quadriceps-hamstrings balance was necessary for knee joint stability. Ivan Palmer theorized that ligaments supplied the central nervous system with the input necessary for dynamic control of the knee (51, 52). He demonstrated reflex contractions of the medial hamstring and vastus medialis in response to stimulation of the deep capsular portion of the medial collateral ligament, and he further showed that this reflex was diminished in the traumatized joint, which loses its selectivity (51, 52).

Solomonow and coworkers reported a direct ligament-muscle reflex arc from their work with ACLs in cats and humans (59). They suggested that ACL injury in humans interrupts the primary ligament reflex arc, triggering a second slower pathway needed to modulate the quadriceps and hamstring muscles from muscle and capsular receptors. Kennedy and coworkers hypothesized that the loss of mechanoreceptor feedback in individuals with torn knee ligaments contributed to progressive instability and recurrent episodes of knee trauma (33, 34). An analysis of these studies suggested that in high-force injury situations, ligaments might be more important for their afferent input to the central nervous system than for their passive mechanical function (24, 33, 53, 57, 58). Unfortunately, a torn ACL disrupts this complex interactive balance between sensory input to the nervous system and the dynamic stabilizers, leading to a diminished capacity for knee joint protection (59). Since tibial-femoral control is desirable regardless of the level of activity with or without an ACL, we should understand the mechanism involved.

Effectiveness of Dynamic Stabilization

The contribution of the dynamic stabilizers should not be underestimated in knee joint stabilization. From their work on subjects with normal and ACL-deficient knees, Aura and Komi concluded that the central nervous system plays an essential role in regulating muscle stiffness (5). In their work on the leg extensor muscles of young men, McNair and Marshall reported that the central nervous system also plays an essential role in regulating muscle stiffness and muscle elasticity during ballistic exercises (43). Louie and Mote investigated the contribution of the knee musculature to rotational stability and torsional stiffness and found that knee joint stiffness could increase up to 400% through quadriceps and hamstring muscle contraction (38). The work of Markolf and associates demonstrated that athletes were able to increase the stiffness of the knee joint 10-fold with muscle contraction (39). Goldfuss and others showed that the stiffness of the medial side of the knee could be increased up to 48% with contraction of the quadriceps and hamstring muscles (23). Wang and Walker demonstrated an 80% reduction in rotatory laxity with 938 N of compressive force (64). Similar findings have been demonstrated by the work of Durselen and coworkers (15), Hagood and others (26), Hsieh and Walker (29), Olmstead and associates (49), and Renstrom and coworkers (56).

Measurement of Tibial-Femoral Control

As discussed in a previous chapter (see Beynnon and associates, chapter 12) elements of neuromuscular function can be measured by a variety of methods. Muscle reaction time (MRT) is one element that has been investigated, utilizing a mechanical stimulus to displace the tibia, which produces anterior tibial translation (ATT), and electromyography to measure the dynamic protective response (see figure 16.1) (8, 32, 65). With this type of testing latency times differ depending on the type and location of the stimulus used, which makes direct comparison of studies difficult (i.e., mechanical stimulus at the proximal calf versus electrical stimulus at the proximal hamstring) (54). Muscle reaction times are typically broken down into spinal and cortical components but can also be subdivided into three phases—spinal, intermediate, and voluntary (see figure 16.2) (35). A spinal cord reflex is monosynaptic, bypasses muscle spindle receptors, and resembles a tendon tap reflex on manual physical examination (35). The intermediate response appears to be a spinal reflex with interneuronal input from centers higher than the spinal cord (16). Voluntary muscle activity is always biphasic, of the largest amplitude, and of longest duration (35).

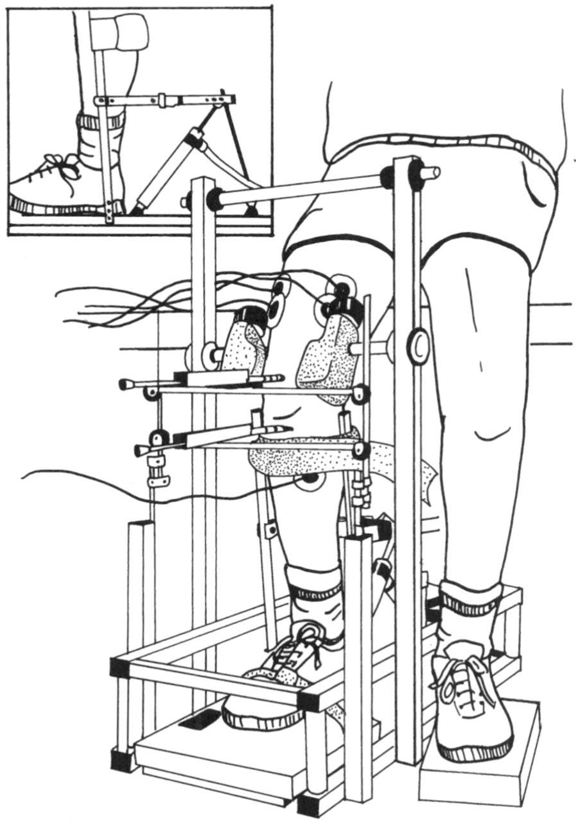

Figure 16.1 Stress testing device for anterior tibial translation testing, with EMG monitoring of the gastrocnemius, quadriceps, and hamstring muscles.

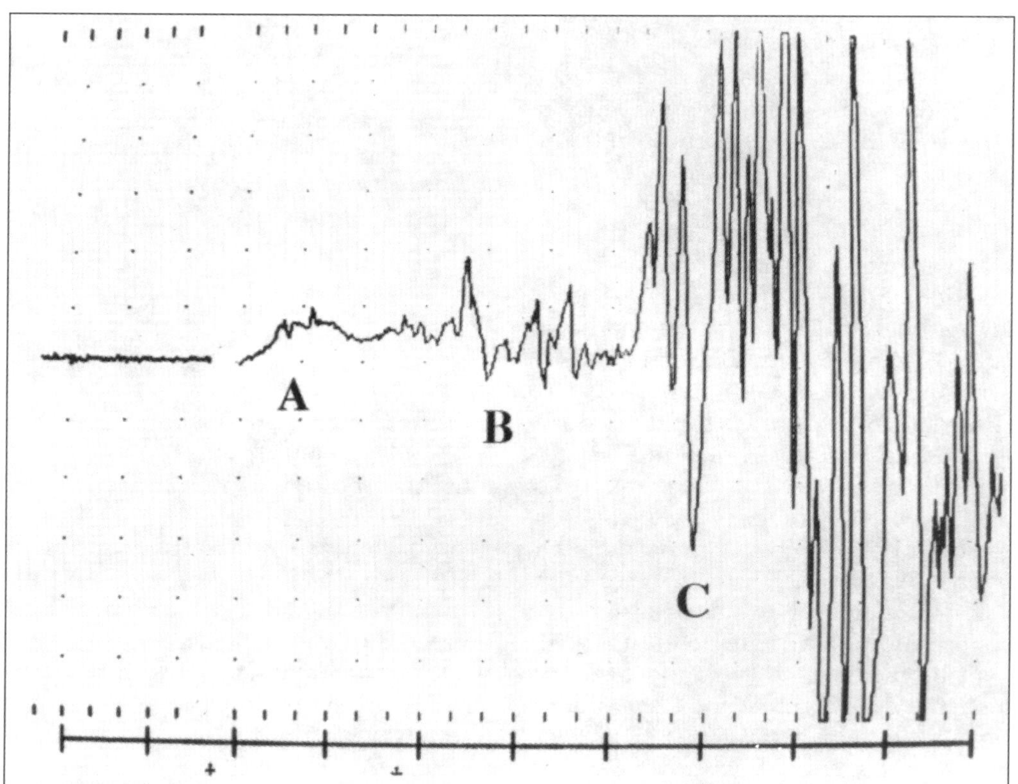

Figure 16.2 Graph depicting the spinal (A), intermediate (B), and voluntary phases (C) of a raw EMG reading.

Table 16.1 MRT of Uninjured Control Group: Dominant vs. Nondominant Average Response Times (ms)

	Dominant	Nondominant	Difference
Spinal reflex			
Gastrocnemius	49.9	54.2	–4.3
Lateral hamstring	73.5	74.0	–0.5
Medial hamstring	73.8	72.4	1.4
Lateral quadriceps	73.8	74.5	–0.7
Medial quadriceps	69.7	70.2	–0.5
Predominant rec. order	G, H, Q	G, H, Q	
Intermediate			
Gastrocnemius	142.8	146.1	–3.3
Lateral hamstring	141.4	139.4	2.0
Medial hamstring	141.1	139.3	1.8
Lateral quadriceps	143.9	146.1	–2.2
Medial quadriceps	142.3	148.8	–6.5
Predominant rec. order	H, Q, G	H, Q, G	
Voluntary			
Gastrocnemius	254.2	255.3	–1.1
Lateral hamstring	234.6	237.3	–2.7
Medial hamstring	226.1	235.7	–9.6*
Lateral quadriceps	233.1	235.7	–2.6
Medial quadriceps	250.9	252.4	–1.5
Predominant rec. order	H, Q, G	H, Q, G	

*Significant difference ($p < .05$).

Muscle Reaction Times of Uninjured Knees

Studying the spinal cord level, Wojtys and Huston found that the initial muscle response to anterior tibial translation (ATT) induced by a mechanical stimulus (applied to the proximal aspect of the posterior calf) was usually first seen in the gastrocnemius muscle an average of 50 ms (range: 41–66 ms) after the initiation of the force (see table 16.1) (65). Initial response times of the quadriceps and hamstrings occurred approximately 20 ms later (70–74 ms after initiation of the mechanical stimulus). During the intermediate phase, the MRT of the quadriceps, hamstrings, and gastrocnemius muscles responded in the time range of 110–188 ms after the mechanical stimulus. Voluntary muscle response times ranged from 172 to 367 ms after the initiation of the 30 lb force. Wojtys and Huston also reported that the dominant extremity exhibited faster voluntary response times in all muscle groups (65). However, only the medial hamstrings muscle of the dominant extremity was significantly faster (dominant = 226 ms; nondominant = 236 ms) (65). These response times correlated well with the work of Beard and others, who also utilized a mechanical stimulus at the same location (8).

Gender Differences

Uninjured males and females exhibited similar muscle reaction times to anterior tibial translation from the quadriceps, hamstrings, and gastrocnemius muscles (see table 16.2) (65). One exception was that females produced statistically faster average voluntary response times in the medial hamstring (females = 211 ms, males = 233 ms) when compared to their uninjured male counterparts. Both the males and females exhibit identical muscle recruitment order patterns for spinal (G, H, Q), intermediate (H, Q, G), and voluntary muscle response times (H, Q, G) (65).

Muscle Reaction Time of ACL-Deficient Extremity

Wojtys and coworkers subdivided 100 ACL-deficient individuals into three groups based on the time from ACL injury to evaluation (65). The acute injury group was defined as those people tested from 0 to 6 mo from the time of injury. In the semiacute injury group, the duration of time from injury to testing was 6 to 18 mo, and in a chronic injury group, it was greater than 18 mo.

Muscle response times were reported to be significantly slower in the ACL-deficient leg compared

Table 16.2 MRT of Control Group: Gender Comparisons

	Males	Females	Difference
Spinal Reflex			
Gastrocnemius	54.4	53.9	0.5
Lateral hamstring	77.2	70.4	6.8
Medial hamstring	73.4	71.4	2.0
Lateral quadriceps	77.0	71.0	6.0
Medial quadriceps	73.8	66.3	7.5
Predominant rec. order	G, H, Q	G, H, Q	
Intermediate			
Gastrocnemius	145.9	138.3	7.6
Lateral hamstring	143.7	137.4	6.3
Medial hamstring	142.2	138.9	3.3
Lateral quadriceps	147.4	137.2	10.2
Medial quadriceps	142.3	142.3	0.0
Predominant rec. order	H, Q, G	H, Q, G	
Voluntary			
Gastrocnemius	252.2	246.9	5.3
Lateral Hamstring	233.0	228.8	4.2
Medial Hamstring	233.1	211.0	22.1*
Lateral quadriceps	229.5	223.9	5.6
Medial quadriceps	253.8	253.7	0.1
Predominant rec. order	H, Q, G	H, Q, G	

*Significant difference ($p < .05$).

to both the uninvolved contralateral limb and to an uninjured control group (65). The spinal response to ATT of the medial and lateral hamstrings in the acute group was slower by an average of 18 ms (range: 13–25 ms) when compared to the uninvolved extremity, while the voluntary response times were slower by an average of 40 ms (range: 24–66 ms; see table 16.3) (65). The muscle response times of the semiacute and chronic ACL-deficient individuals (> 6 mo after ACL injury) were significantly slower compared to the uninvolved extremity in all 5 muscle groups (range: 22–39 ms) (65). This finding is supported by Beard and coworkers (8), who tested 50 patients with unilateral ACL-deficient limbs and 20 normal volunteers using a similar mechanical stimulus. The Beard group found that ACL-deficient patients were significantly slower to contract the hamstrings in the injured limb compared to the unaffected limb and to the uninjured control group (mean 34 ms) (8).

Muscle Reaction Time of Uninvolved Extremity of an ACL-Deficient Individual

The spinal response to ATT of an uninvolved extremity in an ACL-deficient patient was consistent with that seen for an uninjured individual (see table 16.3) (65). The MRT of the gastrocnemius averaged 52 ms (range: 40–74 ms), while the MRT of the hamstrings and quadriceps averaged 70 and 72 ms, respectively (range: 48–110 ms). However, the voluntary responses of the uninvolved extremity in an ACL-deficient person were significantly slower compared to a healthy individual (65). The MRT of the quadriceps and hamstrings were an average of 16 to 24 ms slower (range: 12–30 ms) when compared to an uninjured group (see table 16.3). This poses a significant problem for many investigations that use the uninjured side as a control.

Muscle Recruitment Order: Uninjured Knees

In the spinal response to ATT, the predominant recruitment order in normal, uninjured knees was found to be (1) gastrocnemius, (2) hamstrings, and (3) quadriceps (65). Wojtys and coworkers reported that no significant differences were found in the muscle recruitment between the dominant and nondominant lower extremity (65).

In the voluntary response phase, the hamstrings were the initial muscle group recruited to prevent ATT, while the quadriceps and gastrocnemius muscles usually followed (predominant recruitment order: H, Q, G) (65).

Table 16.3 MRT of Uninvolved Extremity vs. ACL Subgroups

	Uninvolved ext.	Acute	Semiacute	Chronic
Spinal reflex				
Gastrocnemius	52.2	51.7	63.4	55.5
Lateral hamstring	70.4	87.6*	76.1	79.7
Medial hamstring	69.2	88.0*	82.7	86.8*
Lateral quadriceps	72.6	81.7	94.3*	84.3*
Medial quadriceps	70.6	77.8	84.2*	87.1*
Predominant rec. order	G, H, Q	G, H, Q	G, H, Q	G, H, Q
Intermediate				
Gastrocnemius	157.8	161.3*	164.9*	167.3*
Lateral hamstring	146.0	153.4*	148.9	153.9*
Medial hamstring	146.3	153.0*	145.0	153.8*
Lateral quadriceps	145.5	151.2	148.8	155.2*
Medial quadriceps	144.1	147.3	151.9*	159.2*
Predominant rec. order	Q, H, G	Q, H, G	H, Q, G	H, Q, G
Voluntary				
Gastrocnemius	261.8	295.3*	284.4*	284.7*
Lateral hamstring	258.1	297.6*	294.5*	293.8*
Medial hamstring	255.9	296.5*	295.3*	284.1*
Lateral quadriceps	260.0	284.4*	284.8*	288.6*
Medial quadriceps	268.0	268.2*	296.0	301.0*
Predomiannt rec. order	H, G, Q	Q, H, G	G, Q, H	H, Q, G

*Significant difference ($p < .05$) when compared to the control group (leg dominance not considered).

Muscle Recruitment Order: ACL-Deficient Knees

During the spinal response to ATT, an acute ACL-deficient extremity usually exhibited an altered muscle recruitment order compared to the uninjured knee (ACL-deficient leg: G, Q, H; contralateral leg: G, H, Q) (65). However, the muscle recruitment order in an ACL-deficient individual who has had the injury more than 6 mo exhibited an identical recruitment order to both an uninvolved extremity and an uninjured individual (H, Q, G) (65).

During the intermediate response to ATT, an acute ACL-deficient individual was found to rely on the quadriceps for initial knee stabilization (65). For the uninvolved extremity and uninjured limbs individuals usually relied on their hamstrings for initial knee stabilization. It is interesting to note that although muscle reaction time in the leg musculature slowed with ACL injury, the muscle recruitment order 6 mo after injury was usually no different than for uninjured knees.

During the voluntary muscle response to ATT, an ACL-deficient individual within this acute phase (< 6 mo from injury) exhibited altered muscle recruitment patterns, in which the quadriceps muscles fire first for initial knee stabilization (acute: Q, H, G; uninjured control: H, Q, G) (65). After 18 mo (i.e., chronic subgroup) muscle recruitment order in response to ATT returned to an "H, Q, G" muscle recruitment order pattern (65).

Muscle Recruitment Order: Uninvolved Extremity of an ACL-Deficient Knee

The intermediate and voluntary responses to ATT of the contralateral knee in the acute and semiacute phases exhibited altered muscle recruitment orders compared to an uninjured individual (65). The initial muscle response in the intermediate phase was predominantly seen in the quadriceps, followed by the hamstrings and the gastrocnemius (uninjured control: H, Q, G). Initial muscle activity during the voluntary phase was predominantly seen first in the hamstrings, followed by the gastrocnemius and the quadriceps (uninjured control: H, Q, G).

Adaptations in Muscle Recruitment: Initial Compensatory Muscle Mechanisms After ACL Injury

At the spinal level, an acute ACL-deficient individual demonstrates a hamstring response delay when compared to both the uninvolved leg and to an uninjured control group (65). This phenomenon is supported by the work of Solomonow and coworkers, who reported on a direct reflex arc between the ACL and the hamstring muscles (59). Ruptures of the ACL may sever this reflex arc, as evidenced by the longer response times required for the joint capsule-hamstring reflex arc to become active; these responses happen to be slower than the responses generated by the uninjured ACL (average difference: 18 ms) (65).

Muscle Adaptations Over Time

The longest delays in muscle response to ATT are seen in the acute ACL-deficient patient population (65). The hamstring muscles were significantly delayed at the spinal level (by an average of 18 ms) and cortical level (by an average of 40 ms), while the quadriceps usually became the primary muscle used for initial knee stabilization at the voluntary level. Coincidentally, chronic ACL-deficient individuals exhibited identical muscle recruitment orders compared to both the contralateral leg and an uninjured control group (see table 16.3). Several investigators have confirmed that an adjustment in muscle coordination occurs in ACL-deficient individuals and that the central nervous system attempts to compensate for instability of the knee by altering neuromuscular parameters (32, 46, 62).

Diminished Quadriceps Activity

An adjustment in muscle coordination is expected in ACL-deficient patients to maintain knee stability (9, 17, 32, 47). In 1990, Berchuck and coworkers examined the kinematics of walking, jogging, and ascending and descending stairs in two groups of subjects: patients with unilateral ACL deficiency and an uninjured control group (9). Substantial differences from normal function were observed from both limbs of the ACL-deficient patients during level walking and during jogging. A reduction in magnitude of the flexion moment about the knee in ACL-deficient limbs was interpreted as the patient's effort to reduce or avoid contraction of the quadriceps (9). The authors defined this phenomenon as "quadriceps avoidance" gait. Lephart and coworkers recently investigated EMG profiles during gait on "functionally stable" chronic ACL-deficient individuals (36). They reported significantly lower EMG activity of the lateral quadriceps during the swing phase in walking compared to the contralateral leg (36). Similarly, Limbird and coworkers reported that during the swing-to-strike transition phase of gait, the ACL-deficient knee showed significantly less EMG activity in the quadriceps (37). Unfortunately, it may require 12 to 18 mo to develop the protection pattern needed for knee stabilization (65). Therefore, initial muscle response to ATT in an acute group of ACL-deficient individuals may be problematic because unopposed quadriceps activity appears to increase the likelihood of anterior tibial translation and possibly pivot shifting.

Elevated Hamstring Activity

The hamstrings appear to be essential agonists in ACL-deficient patients (1, 14, 26, 43, 48, 50, 59, 63). The balance between the vectors of the quadriceps, hamstrings, and gastrocnemius muscles, which depends upon the activity and angle of flexion, appears to be important, especially in ACL-deficient knees (25, 27, 28). Work by Draganich and coworkers found that the hamstrings coactivate with the quadriceps during the terminal phase of extension in normal knees (14). The Draganich group hypothesized that the hamstrings function synergistically with the ACL to prevent the anterior tibial displacement that is produced by active contraction of the quadriceps (14). O'Connor found that simultaneous contractions of the hamstring and gastrocnemius muscles can unload the cruciate ligaments entirely at flexion angles above 22° (48).

Andriacchi has reported that as knee flexion increases, the ability of the hamstrings to compensate for ACL deficiency increases (4). When the knee is flexed greater than 40°, the hamstrings provide both rotatory stability and resistance to anterior translation (4).

Lephart and coworkers, reporting on "functionally stable" chronic ACL-deficient patients, found that the ACL-deficient limb demonstrated a significant increase in EMG activity of the lateral hamstring compared to the contralateral limb (36). This finding of increased lateral hamstring EMG activity during the stance phase in walking is similar to that reported by Branch and coworkers in ACL-deficient patients during cutting maneuvers (10). Kålund and associates investigated the EMG profiles of ACL-deficient subjects and uninjured controls while walking on a treadmill (32). They found that, while walking uphill, the hamstring muscles in ACL-deficient patients were activated significantly earlier than among controls.

The function of the hamstrings is quite important, as this muscle group has substantial influence in protecting the knee from anterolateral subluxation of the tibia, which occurs during a giving-way episode (40). Increased hamstring activity prevents the knee from excessive tibial translation and rotation, thus providing additional protection to an ACL-deficient knee.

Summary

Recent studies indicate that the function of the knee joint may be the result of a complex synergy between the femur and tibia, ligaments and muscles, and the neuroreceptors contained in these structures (59). When the ACL is torn, it affects not only ligamentous stability, it also appears to affect neuromuscular performance (7, 8, 13, 18, 19, 30, 31, 65). An ACL-deficient individual demonstrates significantly slower muscle reaction times in the quadriceps, hamstrings, and gastrocnemius muscles when compared with both the uninjured knee and uninjured controls. Muscle recruitment patterns are also altered by decreasing quadriceps use. However, in most successful chronic ACL-deficient individuals, the neuromuscular system attempts to adapt to the muscle recruitment patterns seen in uninjured knees (elevated hamstring activity coupled with diminished quadriceps activity). This "auto-conditioning" of protective musculature may be one of the reasons why some patients achieve better function than others do—they may have developed a compensatory mechanism that enhances their dynamic stability. Although beyond the scope of this investigation, it is interesting to speculate if these individuals were predisposed to ACL injury due to these variables. Further studies need to address this intriguing issue.

Conclusions

1. Muscle reaction time is significantly slower in ACL-deficient knees compared to either the uninvolved knee or to uninjured control group knees.
2. Muscle reaction time for the uninjured limb of an ACL-deficient patient is significantly slower than for an uninjured control group, thus making the contralateral limb an unreliable control.
3. The muscle recruitment order of an uninjured control group relies primarily on the hamstrings for initial knee stabilization.
4. Muscle recruitment order is altered with ACL rupture; acute patients generally rely on their quadriceps for initial knee stabilization, while successful chronic patients rely predominantly on their hamstrings for initial knee stabilization.

References

1. Aagaard P, Simonsen EB, Trolle M, Bangsbo J, Klausen K: Isokinetic hamstring/quadriceps strength ratio: Influence from joint angular velocity, gravity correction, and contraction mode. *Acta Physiologica Scandinavica* 154(4): 421–27, 1995.
2. Abbott LC, Saunders JB, Bost FC, Anderson CE: Injuries to the ligaments of the knee joint. *Journal of Bone and Joint Surgery* 26: 503–21, 1944.
3. Andersson C, Odensten M, Good L, Gillquist J: Surgical or nonsurgical treatment of acute rupture of the ACL: A randomized study with long-term follow-up. *Journal of Bone and Joint Surgery* 71A: 965–74, 1989.
4. Andriacchi TP: Dynamics of pathological motion applied to the anterior cruciate deficient knee. *Journal of Biomechanics* 23(suppl): 99–105, 1990.
5. Aura O, Komi PV: Effects of prestretch intensity on mechanical efficiency of positive work and on elastic behavior of skeletal muscle in stretch-shortening cycle exercise. *International Journal of Sports Medicine* 7(3): 137–43, 1986.
6. Barrack RL, Skinner HB: The sensory function of knee ligaments. In: *Knee Ligaments: Structure, Function, Injury, and Repair,* D Daniel, et al. (Eds). New York: Raven Press, 1990, 95–114.
7. Barrack RL, Skinner HB, Buckley SL: Proprioception in the anterior cruciate deficient knee. *American Journal of Sports Medicine* 17: 1–6, 1989.
8. Beard DJ, Kyberd PJ, O'Connor JJ, Fergusson CM, Dodd CA: Reflex hamstring contraction latency in anterior cruciate ligament deficiency. *Journal of Orthopaedic Research* 12: 219–28, 1994.
9. Berchuck M, Andriacchi TP, Bach BR, Reider B: Gait adaptations by patients who have a deficient anterior cruciate ligament. *Journal of Bone and Joint Surgery* 72A: 871–77, 1990.
10. Branch TP, Hunter R, Donath M: Dynamic EMG analysis of anterior cruciate deficient legs with and without bracing during cutting. *American Journal of Sports Medicine* 17: 35–41, 1989.

11. Clancy WG Jr, Ray JM, Zoltan DJ: Acute tears of the ACL: Surgical versus conservative treatment. *Journal of Bone and Joint Surgery* 70A: 1483–488, 1988.
12. Cohen LA, Cohen ML: Arthrokinetic reflex of the knee. *American Journal of Physiology* 184: 433–37, 1956.
13. Corrigan JP, Cashman WF, Brady MP: Proprioception in the cruciate-deficient knee. *Journal of Bone and Joint Surgery* 74B: 247–50, 1992.
14. Draganich LF, Jaeger RJ, Kralj AR: Coactivation of the hamstrings and quadriceps during extension of the knee. *Journal of Bone and Joint Surgery* 71A: 1075–1081, 1989.
15. Durselen L, Claes L, Kiefer H: The influence of muscle forces and external loads on cruciate ligament strain. *American Journal of Sports Medicine* 23: 129–36, 1995.
16. Eccles JC: *Evolution of the Brain.* New York: Routledge & Kegan Paul, 1989, 61–67.
17. Fink C, Hoser C, Benedetto KP, Judmaier W: Neuromuscular changes in the knee-stabilizing muscles after rupture of the anterior cruciate ligament. *Sportverletz Sportschaden* 8: 25–30, 1994.
18. Fridén T, Roberts D, Zätterström R, Lindstrand A, Moritz U: Proprioception in the nearly extended knee: Measurements of position and movement in healthy individuals and in symptomatic anterior cruciate ligament injured patients. *Knee Surgery, Sports Traumatology, Arthroscopy* 4: 217–24, 1996.
19. Friden T, Egund N, Lindstrand A: Comparison of symptomatic versus nonsymptomatic patients with chronic anterior cruciate ligament insufficiency. *American Journal of Sports Medicine* 21: 389–93, 1993.
20. Gardner ED: Reflex muscular responses to stimulation of articular nerves in the cat. *American Journal of Physiology* 161: 133–41, 1950.
21. Gardner ED: The innervation of the knee joint. *Anatomical Record* 101: 109–30, 1948.
22. Gardner ED: The distribution and termination of nerves in the knee joint of the cat. *Journal of Comparative Neurology* 80: 11–32, 1944.
23. Goldfuss AJ, Morehouse CA, LeVeau BF: Effect of muscular tension on knee stability. *Medicine and Science in Sports and Exercise* 5: 267–71, 1973.
24. Gomez-Barrena E, Martinez-Moreno E, Munuera L: Segmental sensory innervation of the anterior cruciate ligament and the patellar tendon of the cat's knee. *Acta Orthopaedica Scandinavica* 67: 545–52, 1996.
25. Gross MT, Tyson AD, Burns CB: Effect of knee angle and ligament insufficiency on anterior tibial translation during quadriceps muscle contraction: A preliminary report. *Journal of Orthopaedic and Sports Physical Therapy* 17: 133–43, 1993.
26. Hagood S, Solomonow M, Baratta R, Zhou BH, D'Ambrosia R: The effect of joint velocity on the contribution of the antagonist musculature to knee stiffness and laxity. *American Journal of Sports Medicine* 18: 182–87, 1990.
27. Hirokawa S, Solomonow M, Lu Y, Lou ZP, D'Ambrosia R: Anterior-posterior and rotational displacement of the tibia elicited by quadriceps contraction. *American Journal of Sports Medicine* 20: 299–306, 1992.
28. Hirokawa S, Solomonow M, Luo Y, et al: Muscular co-contraction and control of the knee stability. *Journal of Electromyography and Kinesiology* 1(3): 199–208, 1991.
29. Hsieh HH, Walker PS: Stabilizing mechanisms of the loaded and unloaded knee joint. *Journal of Bone and Joint Surgery* 58A: 87–93, 1976.
30. Jerosch J, Prymka M: Proprioceptive capacity of the knee joint area in patients after rupture of the anterior cruciate ligament. *Unfallchirurg* 99: 861–68, 1996.
31. Jerosch J, Prymka M: Proprioception and joint stability. *Knee Surgery, Sports Traumatology, Arthroscopy* 4: 171–79, 1996.
32. Kålund S, Sinkjær T, Arendt-Nielsen L, Simonsen O: Altered timing of hamstring muscle action in anterior cruciate ligament deficient patients. *American Journal of Sports Medicine* 18: 245–48, 1990.
33. Kennedy JC, Alexander IJ, Hayes KC: Nerve supply of the human knee and its functional importance. *American Journal of Sports Medicine* 10: 329–35, 1982.
34. Kennedy JC, Weinberg HW, Wilson AS: The anatomy and function of the anterior cruciate ligament, as determined by clinical and morphological studies. *Journal of Bone and Joint Surgery* 56A: 223-35, 1974.
35. Kimura J: *Electrodiagnosis in Diseases of Nerve and Muscle: Principles and Practice.* 2d ed. Philadelphia: Davis, 1989.
36. Lephart SM, Pincivero DM, Giraldo JL, Fu FH: The role of proprioception in the management and rehabilitation of athletic injuries. *American Journal of Sports Medicine* 25: 130–40, 1997.
37. Limbird TJ, Shiavi R, Frazer M, Borra H: EMG profiles of knee joint musculature during walking: Changes induced by anterior cruciate ligament deficiency. *Journal of Orthopaedic Research* 6: 630–38, 1988.
38. Louie JK, Mote CD Jr: Contribution of the musculature to rotatory laxity and torsional stiffness at

the knee. *Journal of Biomechanics* 20: 281–300, 1987.
39. Markolf KL, Mensch JS, Amstutz HC: Stiffness and laxity of the knee—the contributions of the supporting structures: A quantitative in vitro study. *Journal of Bone and Joint Surgery* 58A: 583–94, 1976.
40. Marshall JL, Girgis FG, Zelko RR: The biceps femoris tendon and its functional significance. *Journal of Bone and Joint Surgery* 54A: 1444–450, 1972.
41. McDaniel WJ, Dameron TB: Untreated ruptures of the anterior cruciate ligament. *Journal of Bone and Joint Surgery* 62A: 696–705, 1980.
42. McDonald PB, Hedden D, Pacin O, Sutherland K: Proprioception in anterior cruciate ligament-deficient and reconstructed knees *American Journal of Sports Medicine* 24: 774–78, 1996.
43. McNair PJ, Marshall RN: Landing characteristics in subjects with normal and anterior cruciate ligament deficient knee joints. *Arch Phys Med Rehabil* 75: 584–89, 1994.
44. Noyes FR, Mooar PA, Matthews DS, et al: The symptomatic anterior cruciate-deficient knee: Part I. *Journal of Bone and Joint Surgery* 65A: 154–62, 1983.
45. Noyes FR, Matthews DS, Mooar PA, Grood ES: The symptomatic anterior cruciate-deficient knee: Part II. *Journal of Bone and Joint Surgery* 65A: 163–74, 1983.
46. O'Connor BL, Visco BL, Brandt KD, Albrecht M, O'Connor AB: Sensory nerves only temporarily protect the unstable canine knee joint from osteoarthritis: Evidence that sensory nerves reprogram the central nervous system after cruciate ligament transection. *Arthritis and Rheumatism* 36: 1154–63, 1993.
47. O'Connor BL, Visco DM, Heck DA, Myers SL, Brandt KD: Gait alterations in dogs after transection of the anterior cruciate ligament. *Arthritis and Rheumatism* 32: 1142–147, 1989.
48. O'Connor JJ: Can muscle co-contraction protect knee ligaments after injury or repair? *Journal of Bone and Joint Surgery* 75: 41–48, 1993.
49. Olmstead TG, Wevers HW, Bryant JT, et al: Effect of muscular activity on valgus/varus laxity and stiffness of the knee. *Journal of Biomechanics* 19: 565–77, 1986.
50. Osternig LR, Hamill J, Lander JE, Robertson R: Coactivation of sprinter and distance runner muscles in isokinetic exercise. *Medicine and Science in Sports and Exercise* 18: 431–35, 1986.
51. Palmer I: Pathophysiology of the medial ligament of the knee joint. *Acta Chir Scandinavica* 115: 312–18, 1958.
52. Palmer I: Plastic surgery of the ligaments of the knee. *Acta Chir Scandinavica* 91: 37–48, 1944.
53. Pitman MI, Nainzadeh N, Menche D, et al: The intraoperative evaluation of the neurosensory function of the anterior cruciate ligament in humans using somatosensory evoked potentials. *Arthroscopy* 8: 442–47, 1992.
54. Pratt H, Starr A, Amlie RN, et al: Mechanically and electrically evoked somatosensory potential in normal humans. *Neurology* 29: 1236–244, 1979.
55. Raubner A: Uber die Vater'shen Korper der Gelenkkapseln. *Centr die Med Wissen* 12: 305–306, 1874.
56. Renström P, Arms SW, Stanwyck TS, Johnson RJ, Pope MH: Strain within the anterior cruciate ligament during hamstring and quadriceps activity. *American Journal of Sports Medicine* 14: 83–87, 1986.
57. Schultz RA, Miller DC, Kerr CS, et al: Mechanoreceptors in human cruciate ligaments: A histological study. *Journal of Bone and Joint Surgery* 66A: 1072–1076, 1984.
58. Schutte MJ, Dabezies EJ, Zimny ML, et al: Neural anatomy of the human anterior cruciate ligament. *Journal of Bone and Joint Surgery* 69A: 243–47, 1987.
59. Solomonow M, Baratta R, Zhou BH, et al: The synergistic action of the anterior cruciate ligament and thigh muscles in maintaining joint stability. *American Journal of Sports Medicine* 15: 207–13, 1987.
60. Snyder-Mackler L, Fitzgerald GK, Bartolozzi AR, Ciccotti MG: The relationship between passive joint laxity and functional outcome after anterior cruciate ligament injury. *American Journal of Sports Medicine* 25: 191–95, 1997.
61. Tibone JE, Antich TJ: Electromyographic analysis of the anterior cruciate ligament-deficient knee. *Clinical Orthopaedics and Related Research* 288: 35–39, 1993.
62. Vilensky JA, O'Connor BL, Brandt KD, Dunn EA, Rogers PI, DeLong CA: Serial kinematic analysis of the unstable knee after transection of the anterior cruciate ligament: Temporal and angular changes in a canine model of osteoarthritis. *Journal of Orthopaedic Research* 12: 229–37, 1994.
63. Walla DJ, Albright JP, McAuley E, et al: Hamstring control and the unstable anterior cruciate ligament-deficient knee. *American Journal of Sports Medicine* 13: 34–39, 1985.
64. Wang CH, Walker PS: Rotatory laxity of the human knee joint. *Journal of Bone and Joint Surgery* 56A: 161–70, 1974.
65. Wojtys EM, Huston LJ: Neuromuscular performance in normal and anterior cruciate ligament-deficient lower extremities. *American Journal of Sports Medicine* 22: 89–104, 1994.
66. Wroble RR, Brand RA: Paradoxes in the history of the ACL. *Clinical Orthopaedics* 259: 183, 1990.

CHAPTER 17

Functional Adaptations in Patients With ACL-Deficient Knees

Thomas P. Andriacchi, PhD
Debra E. Hurwitz, PhD
Charles A. Bush-Joseph, MD
Bernard R. Bach, MD

Abstract

The biomechanics of gait adaptations observed in patients with anterior cruciate ligament (ACL)-deficient knees was analyzed. These gait adaptations appear to reduce strains in the secondary restraints to anterior drawer at the knee. Analysis of patients with ACL deficiency suggests that there is a dynamic reprogramming of the locomotor system in some subjects with ACL-deficient knees but not in others. In addition, the development of the gait adaptation appears to take more than one year following the index injury.

From a clinical viewpoint, these results help to explain why some subjects can accommodate an ACL-deficient knee while others have difficulties following loss of the ACL. An understanding of the biomechanics and functional implication of these adaptations can be applied to methods for rehabilitation as well as treatment planning for patients with ACL-deficient knees.

Introduction

Injury to the anterior cruciate ligament (ACL) is among the most frequent of sport-related injuries (20). It has been estimated that skiing alone accounts for over 100,000 ACL injuries in the United States per year (16). In addition, there has been a rapid increase in ACL injuries in women's sports such as basketball, soccer, and volleyball. Not only are there initial functional losses, which occur primarily during more stressful athletic activities, long-term degenerative changes to the knee have been demonstrated in subjects following loss of the ACL. The degenerative changes occur in spite of the fact that active athletic participation has been reduced or abandoned (10, 15, 19, 21). Surgical and nonsurgical (rehabilitation) treatment modalities have demonstrated clinical improvement (1, 7, 14, 30). However, the results are short term, and the long-term efficacy of various procedures to treat ACL deficiency is still unclear. Current methods of clinical examination do not always provide an adequate objective assessment of functional improvement. The ability to assess the probability of future degenerative changes associated with the loss of the ACL would be extremely valuable for treatment planning and the evaluation of various treatment modalities for the ACL-deficient knee. Thus, a better understanding of the functional changes associated with ACL injuries could be extremely important for future improvements in rehabilitation methods and surgical treatment methods.

It is often difficult to predict from passive physical examination of the knee which patients will be functionally impaired by the loss of this ligament and which patients will have minimal symptoms (1, 7, 14, 24, 25, 30). Clinical studies report that approximately one-third of the patients who had an ACL-deficient knee were able to pursue recreational activities, another one-third compensated but had to reduce many activities, and one-third had poor function even after discontinuing sport activities (24, 25). Several studies have reported both degenerative changes and moderate or severe symptoms during stressful activities of daily living in some patients but not in others (15, 17, 21). Perhaps some individuals are better suited to functionally adapt to the loss of the ACL.

Loss of the ACL has been shown to influence the passive mechanics of the knee joint by decreasing overall stiffness of the knee or increasing instability of the knee (13, 18, 22). It is possible, however, to adapt dynamically for the stability lost at the knee through muscular substitution during ambulatory activities (2, 11). The number of surgical reconstructions of the ACL is increasing, yet the management of an ACL-deficient knee still remains controversial. The variable natural history in the progression of degenerative joint disease in some patients and not in others suggests that some patients make appropriate functional adaptations for the loss of the ACL.

The mechanism of gait adaptations observed in some patients with ACL-deficient knees will be discussed in this paper. In addition, the clinical implication of these dynamic adaptations and their relation to muscular substitution for ACL loss will be discussed.

Methods of Gait Analysis

Gait analysis provides unique information not attainable through standard clinical examination, by testing the subject under conditions that replicate activities of daily living and more stressful sports activities. Information from functional testing has the potential to improve treatment planning (23, 26).

The technology and instrumentation to conduct gait analysis with sufficient resolution to provide meaningful measurements are available from a number of sources. The methodological approach in this analysis has been previously described (3–5, 8, 9). Briefly, the lower extremity was idealized as a collection of rigid links with fixed axes of rotation at the joints (12). The ground reaction forces, limb segment masses, and inertia were used to calculate joint moments and forces. The basic components of the measurement system included a force platform, optoelectronic system for motion measurement, and a computer. The external moments were calculated along the axes of flexion-extension, abduction-adduction, and internal-external rotation. In addition, knee motion and temporal measurements were quantified. All moments were normalized to body weight (Bw) and height (Ht) to allow comparison among subjects of different sizes.

There are many measures that can be quantified during functional tests. Thus, it is important to select variables that focus on the measures that directly relate to the physical aspects of the problem. The functional analysis presented here will focus on the moments acting at the knee joint, especially those affecting the function of the ACL. Previous studies have demonstrated that the external moments measured can be interpreted in terms of the loads on muscles, passive soft tissue, and joint surfaces (2–4, 8). In addition, the joint moments have been shown to be sensitive indicators of differences between normal and abnormal function (4, 26, 29).

It is useful to examine the assumptions used as the basis for the interpretation of the joint moments during function. The reader should note that the measurements used to calculate the joint moments are external to the limb and include the ground reaction force, limb segment weight, and limb segment inertia (12). Mechanical equilibrium dictates that external forces and moments must balance internal forces and moments. Internal forces generated by muscle, passive soft tissue, and joint contact force create these internal moments. If muscles act only synergistically when balancing the external moments, then one could directly infer the internal muscle force in synergistic muscle groups. For example, the total force in the quadriceps needed to balance an external moment tending to flex the knee joint could be determined (4). However, if antagonistic muscle activity is present, the external moment reflects the net balance between agonist and antagonist muscles. The force in the synergistic muscle group would be greater under these conditions. The external moment can, however, be used to get a conservative estimate or lower boundary on the synergist muscle force (27). Throughout this presentation, external moments will be described from the measurements taken in the laboratory and inferences will be made in terms of the net muscular moment.

To evaluate the nature of the functional adaptations associated with an ACL-deficient knee, patients with a complete rupture of the ACL were selected. Patients with PCL injury, posterolateral instability, extensive meniscal damage, functionally limiting pain, or the inability to perform simple activities, such as running and cutting or running and stopping maneuvers, were excluded from the study.

The average age of the ACL-deficient patients was 29 yrs and their average height and weight were 1.78 m and 777 N, respectively. The average interval between the injury date and the date of the functional analysis was 4.4 yrs with a range from 2 mo to 18 yrs.

Strength testing and ligament laxity testing were performed on a subset of the ACL-deficient subjects. The deficient side showed a 19% loss in extension strength and a 10% loss in flexion strength when tested at 240°/s. The mean maximum manual difference (using KT-1000) between the deficient and contralateral side was 6 mm.

The ACL-deficient patients and control individuals were studied during level walking, jogging, and stair climbing. The walking and jogging tests were done on a 10 m walkway. Data were collected during the middle stride of several strides, with the measurement starting just before the foot reached the force plate. After the measurement stride, each subject then took several strides of deceleration after the foot or the limb had lifted off the force plate. The measurements during stair climbing were made as the subject stepped onto the bottom step of a three-step staircase. The patients and control subjects were tested with identical protocols. Data were collected on both sides of all subjects.

Results and Discussion: Activities of Daily Living

The greatest variation from normal among the ACL-deficient subjects occurred during level walking. The ACL-deficient subjects walked in a manner that avoided or reduced the moment tending to flex the knee during the middle portion of stance phase. This type of gait has been interpreted as a tendency to avoid or reduce the demand on the quadriceps muscle and has been called a "quadriceps avoidance" gait (4, 8). The pattern of the flexion-extension moment during stance phase was interpreted in terms of the net quadriceps muscle force or net knee flexor muscle force (hamstrings and gastrocnemius) during stance phase. Typically, among the control subjects, at heel strike there was an external moment tending to extend the knee joint (demanding net knee flexor force), as the knee moved into midstance the external moment reversed its direction (demanding net quadriceps force), as the knee passed midstance the moment again reversed its direction (demanding net knee flexor muscle force), and, finally, in the preswing phase the moment tended to flex the knee (demanding net quadriceps muscle force) (see figure 17.1).

Despite the relatively low loads on the knee that occurred during level walking, 75% of the patients studied had the "quadriceps avoidance" gait while 25% had a normal biphasic flexion-extension moment. It is important to note that the magnitude of the difference between the control group and the ACL-deficient patients during walking was large (more than 100%). Thus, the moment was a sensitive indicator of functional changes. The development of the "quadriceps avoidance" gait was found to be dependent on the time-passed index (9).

While the net quadriceps demand was substantially greater during jogging when compared to level walking, the percentage change in the net quadriceps moment between ACL-deficient patients and normal subjects was substantially less. Patients had only a 24% reduction in the flexion moment during jogging as compared to over a 100% reduction during walking. The magnitude of the knee flexion moment (net quadriceps muscle force) increased by more than a factor of 5 during jogging as compared to level walking (see figure 17.2). The flexion-extension moment during jogging was dominated by a moment tending to flex the knee during most of the stance phase of the jogging ac-

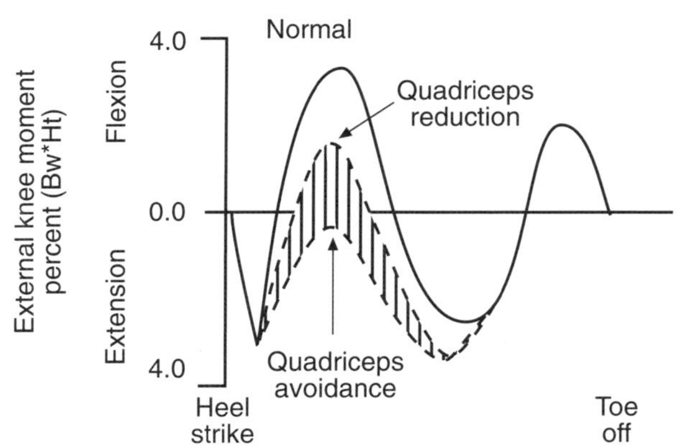

Figure 17.1 The normal flexion-extension moment during the stance phase of gait tended to oscillate between flexion and extension. In patients with ACL-deficient knees, the magnitude of the quadriceps demand was reduced or avoided during stance phase.

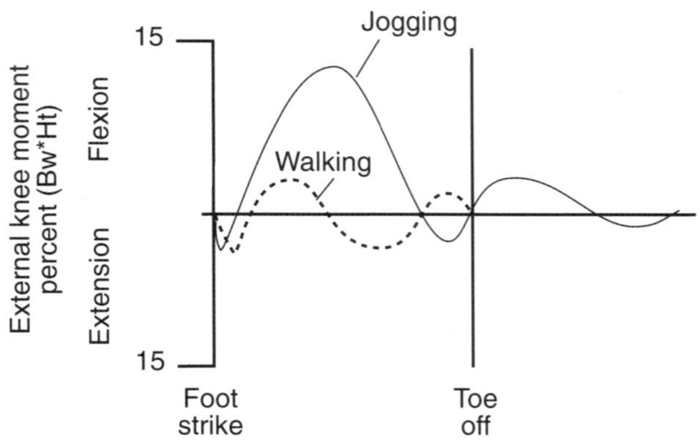

Figure 17.2 A comparison of the pattern of flexion-extension moments during walking and jogging. The illustration shows the limb configuration during jogging.

tivity. It should also be noted that the maximum knee flexion during jogging occurred when the knee was at approximately 40° of flexion as compared to 20° during level walking.

While ascending stairs, the maximum knee flexion occurred at approximately 60° of flexion. Even though the flexion moment during stair climbing was substantially larger than that of level walking, patients with ACL-deficient knees had a greater than normal knee flexion moment while climbing the stairs. The adaptations during the activities of daily living appear to be dependent upon the angle of knee flexion when the greatest knee flexion moment occurred. The adaptations did not appear to be related to the magnitude of the knee flexion moment.

These observations suggest an interaction between the direction of pull of the patellar ligament and the functional role of the ACL. When the knee is near full extension, the patellar ligament places an anterior pull on the tibia. In the absence of the ACL, the tibia would move forward until the forces could be balanced by secondary restraints to anterior displacement. Thus, during level walking when the maximum knee flexion occurred between 0° and approximately 20°, there would have been a greater tendency for the quadriceps contraction to produce an anterior pull on the tibia. The adaptation to avoid quadriceps contraction would have eliminated this anterior force component when the knee was near full extension (see figure 17.3). This

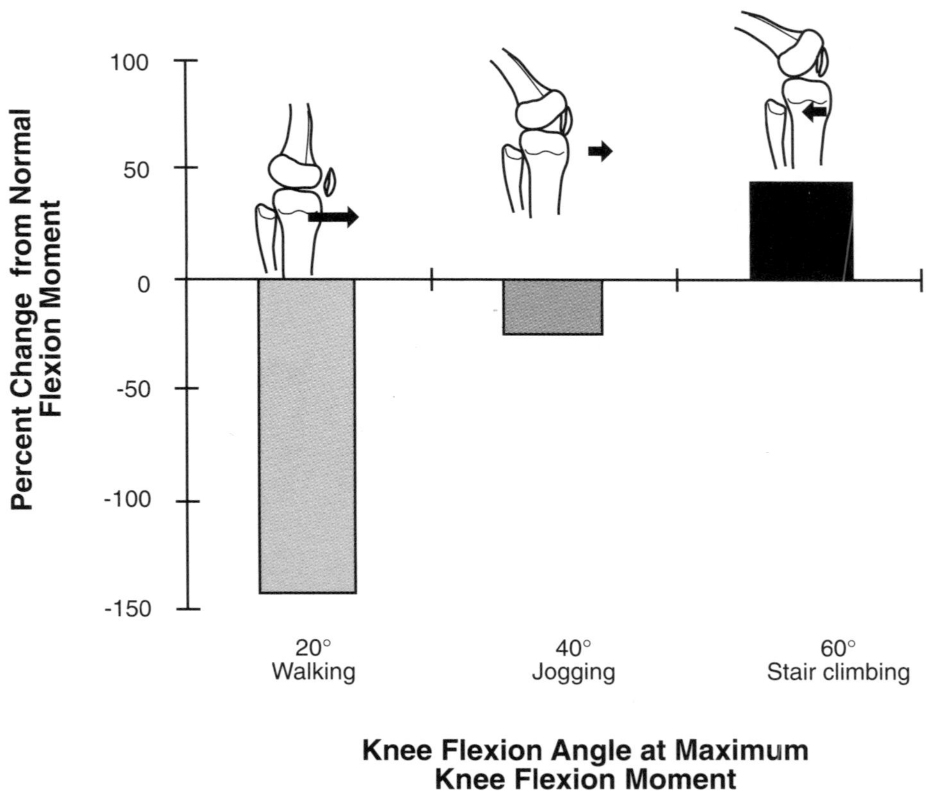

Figure 17.3 A summary of the relationship between the adaptive mechanisms seen in ACL-deficient subjects. The adaptive mechanism appeared to be related to the orientation of the pull of the patellar ligament. The adaptive mechanisms were closely related to the angle of the knee flexion at which the peak knee flexion moment occurred and its associated effect on the direction of the pull of the patellar ligament.

mechanism may explain the large reduction in the knee flexion moment seen among subjects with ACL-deficient knees. More than 2/3 of the subjects with ACL-deficient knees reduced or avoided the knee flexion during the stance phase of walking. During jogging, the maximum quadriceps contraction occurred at approximately 40° of flexion, where the anterior pull of the patellar ligament is substantially less than during level walking, because the orientation of the ligament changes with knee flexion.

As the knee flexes beyond approximately 45 , the orientation of the patellar ligament reverses direction during the quadriceps contraction and now places a posterior pull on the tibia. Thus, at deeper flexion angles, the contraction of the quadriceps would act to compensate for an absent anterior cruciate ligament. Thus, the increased knee flexion moment seen in ACL-deficient subjects during stair climbing suggests that there was an increased use of the quadriceps as a possible means of dynamic muscular substitution for the absent ACL when the knee is at greater flexion angles.

Interestingly, during both the walking and jogging activities, the adaptation in the ACL-deficient limb was also evident in the contralateral limb of the patients who developed the functional adaptations. As a result, the magnitude of the moments about the knee in the affected and unaffected limb did not significantly differ during walking or jogging (8).

These results demonstrated that some patients with ACL-deficient knees adapt their ambulatory function and some do not. The physical characteristics of the adaptations appeared consistent with the hypothesis that patients avoided or reduced quadriceps contraction during angles of knee flexion where the quadriceps produces an anteriorly directed force on the tibia (4, 6, 8). The symmetric nature of this adaptation suggested a reprogramming of the locomotor process. It is not likely that patients instantaneously adapt to instability and the subsequent movement of the tibia during each step (4). It is more likely that the adaptation occurs prior to the instability generated from the muscle contraction so that the abnormal anterior drawer or strain on the secondary restraints does not develop. Perhaps in patients who do not develop this adaptation, there is a continual strain on the secondary restraints to anterior drawer (menisci and collaterals) causing continued stretching of these structures and the eventual degenerative problems that are reported in some ACL-deficient knees.

Results and Discussion: Stressful Activities

Patients with ACL-deficient knees often have sensation of the knee "giving way" or buckling during more stressful activities. Patients with an ACL-deficient knee who tolerate stressful activities are likely to develop some type of functional adaptation to compensate for the structural loss of the ACL. Functionally, when the knee is flexed greater than 40°, the hamstrings are in a position to provide both rotatory stability and resistance to anterior drawer. Thus, it is reasonable that hamstring substitution occurs among ACL-deficient subjects during more stressful activities. Typically, these activities include twisting, pivoting, and stopping from a run.

The patients and control subjects were tested with identical protocols. The protocol for the cutting maneuver had each subject run to a specified location (on the force plate) at approximately 2.5 m/s and then cut laterally away from the supporting leg at 90° to the direction of progression. This maneuver was described as a lateral side step cut. The protocol for the run-to-stop maneuver had each subject running to a specified location (on the force plate) at approximately 2.5 m/s and stopping on one limb as if preparing to jump vertically.

The normal pattern of the flexion-extension moment for both the run-to-stop and run-to-lateral side step cut activities shows a predominant moment tending to flex the knee (demanding net quadriceps forces) during the major portion of stance phase (see figure 17.4). However, during the earlier portion of stance there is an external extension moment (demanding net knee flexor forces). During the early portion of support phase in both the running-and-cutting and running-to-a-stop activities the ACL-deficient patients developed a higher than normal external extension moment. It is possible that the patients activated the hamstring muscles to a greater extent in the early portion of this activity to dynamically stabilize the knee against the higher rotational and abduction-adduction loads that occur during the middle portion of that activity (2). The magnitude of the twisting and adduction moment components during cutting and stopping are substantially higher than those that occur during activities such as level walking. These higher twisting moments may cause the buckling of the knee as often reported by ACL-deficient subject during these activities (2).

The higher extension moment may be a desirable compensation for patients with an ACL-deficient knee. This is likely a method of adaptation that has

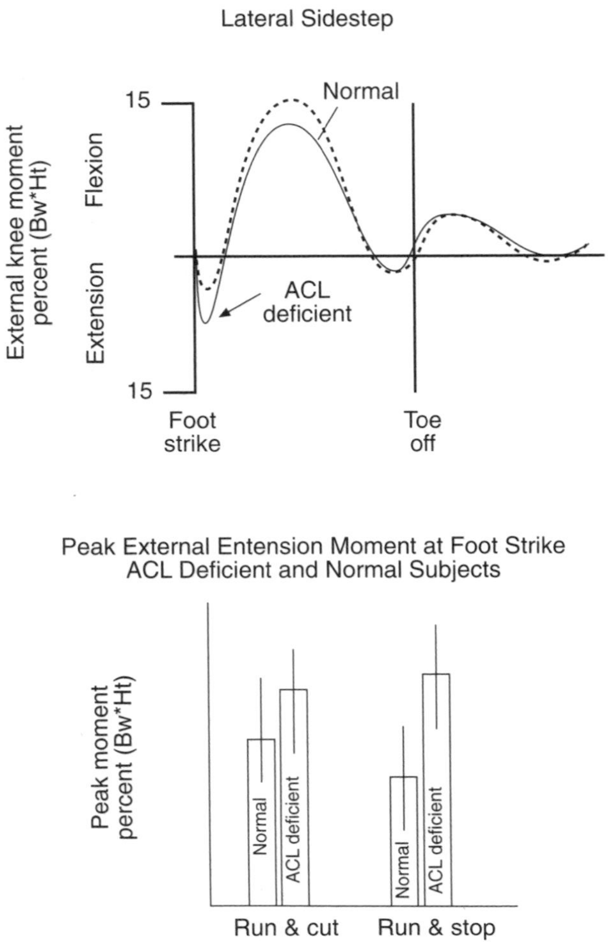

Figure 17.4 Typically, patients with ACL-deficient knees had a higher moment tending to extend the knee (demanding net hamstring forces) during early stance.

been developed prior to the particular activity since it requires anticipation of high loads that occur later in the activity. In most situations muscles cannot contract quickly enough to protect the knee from a sudden destabilizing force. However, if the muscle contracted prior to the initiation of the higher loads, the patients probably would not experience the symptoms associated with the instability since the muscles have provided additional stability.

Reprogramming Theory

The modifications in function identified in this paper and by other studies are presumably adaptations produced by a subconscious protective mechanism to avoid the excessive anterior displacement of the tibia that can occur in the absence of the ACL (11, 28). However, it is not likely that these adaptations are the result of a single stimulus that occurs during each cycle of the activity. It is more likely that these adaptations are the result of repetitive experiences following the loss of the ACL. It is possible that reprogramming of the locomotor process occurs such that the adaptations occur before instability and excessive anterior displacement results. This can be accomplished by altering the pattern of muscle contracture as part of an adaptive locomotor program. The adaptations anticipate the instability and thus avoid the abnormal displacement (see figure 17.5). This general locomotor reprogramming could be part of a learning process that takes place during the early stages following an ACL injury. It would be necessary that the locomotor system be reprogrammed in a manner that would anticipate instability prior to the occurrence of the episode that would produce instability, since the latency time for muscle contraction would be too slow to instantaneously respond to a rapid stimulus.

This reprogramming hypothesis has a number of implications toward the clinical management of patients with ACL-deficient knees. It provides the basis for an explanation as to why some patients adapt while others do not develop an adaptive gait. Perhaps some patients do not have sufficient kinesiological sense of the instability occurring at the knee to provide the appropriate control for modifications in the patterns of muscle firing. Some subjects may have an enhanced ability to fine tune the balance between the quadriceps and hamstring contractions using a higher level of movement coordination. These adaptive mechanisms can be seen both during simple activities such as walking as well as more stressful activities such as the lateral side step cutting maneuvers.

These results suggest that the patients that are capable of adapting their function to the absence of an ACL can protect the secondary restraints such as the medial meniscus during level walking. Thus, even for the individual who reduces sport-related activities, an adaptive gait may be important for protecting against long-term damage to the medial meniscus. A patient who does not develop the adaptive gait will cyclically apply an anterior force to the tibia during each step of walking. These cyclic loads can eventually stretch and damage the medial meniscus. Thus, over time, the degenerative joint changes that are found in patients with ACL-deficient knees are likely to be more prevalent among patients who do not develop an adaptive gait. Similarly, subjects who perform sport activities under more stressful conditions can protect against the rotational and translational stresses at the knee joint by increasing hamstring contraction

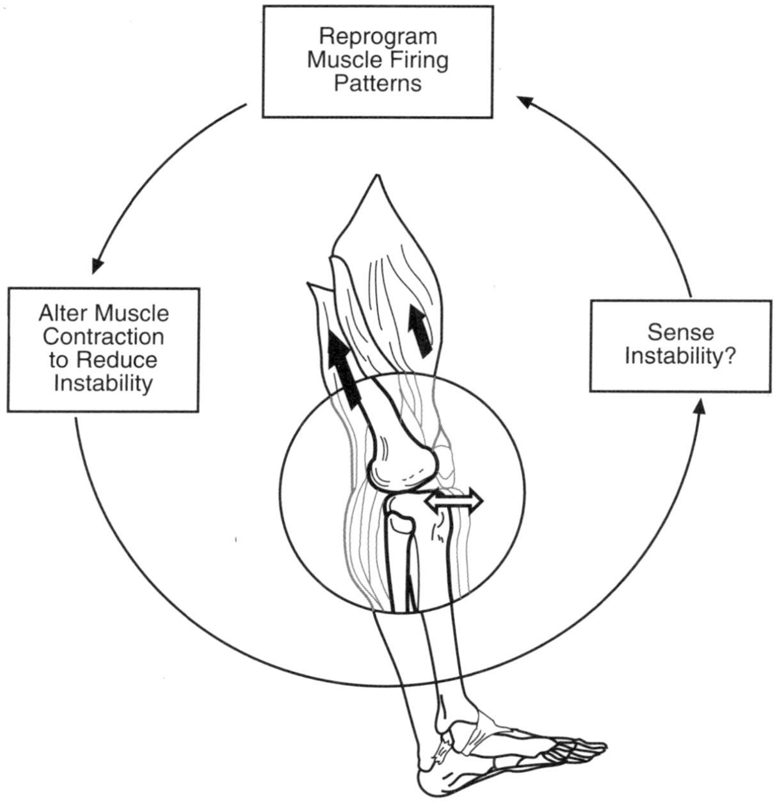

Figure 17.5 The functional adaptations associated with the ACL-deficient subjects can be explained in terms of a reprogramming of the locomotor system. The symmetric and rhythmic nature of the adaptations in patients with ACL-deficient knees suggests there is a reprogramming that takes place in the early period following tear to the ACL. The adaptation observed during locomotion is consistent with one in which the patients have reprogrammed their patterns of muscle contraction in such a manner that the normal patterns of locomotion do not produce an abnormal anterior displacement at the proximal end of the tibia.

as the limb is striking the ground. Again, this muscle contraction must occur before the destabilizing loads occur. As knee flexion increases, the ability of the hamstrings to compensate for ACL deficiency increases. It should be noted that to maintain the knee in this flexed position, one needs strong quadriceps to hold the knee flexed while maintaining co-contraction of the hamstrings. Again, the more coordinated athlete may adopt this process subconsciously, but perhaps rehabilitation and training could enhance these protective mechanisms.

Testing of ambulatory function or gait analysis is particularly relevant to the ACL-deficient population. The appropriate selection of treatment modalities, rehabilitation, and evaluation of patients following treatment can be greatly enhanced through appropriate use of functional testing. These results suggest that all patients do not adapt in the same manner to the loss of the ACL. It has been shown in other studies that the nature of functional adaptations quantified during gait analysis can be extremely useful in the treatment planning and selection of patients for particular procedures (26, 29). It is likely that clinical testing of ambulatory function during both activities of daily living and more stressful athletic activities will improve the treatment outcome and rehabilitation of the ACL-deficient population.

References

1. Andersson, C., Odensten, L.R., Grood, L., Gullquist, J.: Surgical or nonsurgical treatment of fracture rupture of the ACL: A randomized study with long-term follow-up. *J Bone Joint Surg* 71: 965, 1989.
2. Andriacchi, T.P., Kramer, G.M., Landon, G.C.: The biomechanics of running and knee injuries. In the American Academy of Orthopaedic Sur-

geons Symposium on Sport Medicine: *The Knee.* Finerman, G. (Ed.). St. Louis: Mosby, 23–32, 1985.
3. Andriacchi, T.P., Andersson, G.B.J., Fermier, R., Stern, D., Galante, J.O.: A study of lower limb mechanics during stair climbing. *J Bone Joint Surg* 62A: 749, 1980.
4. Andriacchi, T.P.: Dynamics of pathological motion applied to the anterior cruciate deficient knee. *J Biomechanics* 23(Suppl): 99–105, 1990.
5. Andriacchi, T.P.: Biomechanics and orthopedic problems: A quantitative approach. In: *Future Directions in Exercise and Sport Science Research.* Skinner, J.S., Corbin, C.B., Landers, D.M., Martin, P.E., Wells, C.L. (Eds.). Champaign, IL: Human Kinetics, 45–56, 1986.
6. Arms, S.W., Pope, M.H., Johnson, R.J., Fischer, R.A., Arvidsson, I., Eriksson, E.: The biomechanics of anterior cruciate ligament rehabilitation and reconstruction. *Am J Sports Med* 12: 8, 1984.
7. Barrack, R.L., Bruckner, J.D., Kneisl, J., Inman, W.S., Alexander, A.H.: The outcome of nonoperatively treated complete tears of the ACL in active young patients. *Clin Orthop* 258: 192, 1990.
8. Berchuck, M., Andriacchi, T.P., Bach, B.R., Reider, B.R.: Gait adaptations by patients who have a deficient ACL. *J Bone Joint Surg* 72A: 871, 1990.
9. Birac, D., Andriacchi, T.P., Bach, B.R. Jr.: Time-related changes following ACL rupture. *Trans 37th Ann Meet Orthop Res Soc* Sec 1: 231, 1991.
10. Bray, R.C., Dandy, D.J.: Mensical lesions and chronic ACL deficiency: Mensical tears occurring before and after reconstruction. *J Bone Joint Surg* 71B: 128, 1989.
11. Branch, T.P., Hunter, R., Donath, M.: Dynamic EMG analysis of anterior cruciate deficient legs with and without bracing during cutting. *Am J Sports Med* 17: 35, 1989.
12. Bresler, B., Frankel, J.P.: The forces and moments in the leg during level walking. *Trans Am Soc Mech Engng* 48A: 62, 1953.
13. Butler, D.L., Noyes, F.R., Grood, E.S.: Ligamentous restraints to anterior-posterior drawer in the human knee. *J Bone Joint Surg* 62A: 259, 1980.
14. Clancy, W.G., Ray, J.M., Zolton, D.J.: Acute tears of the ACL: Surgical versus conservative treatment. *J Bone Joint Surg* 70A: 1483, 1988.
15. Daniel, D.M., Stone, M.L., Dobson, B.E., Fithian, D.C., Rossman, D.J., Kauman, K.R.: Fate of the ACL-injured patient: A prospective outcome study. *Am J Sports Med* 22(5), 1994.
16. Feagin, J.A., Lambert, K.L., Cunningham, R.R., et al.: Consideration of the anterior cruciate ligament injury in skiing. *Clin Orthop* 216: 13–18, 1987.
17. Finsterbush, A., Frankl, U., Matan, Y., Mann, G.: Secondary damage to the knee after isolated injury of the ACL. *Am J Sports Med* 18: 475, 1990.
18. Grood, E.S., Suntay, W.J., Noyes, F.R., Butler, D.L.: Biomechanics of the knee-extension exercise: Effect of cutting the anterior cruciate ligament. *J Bone Joint Surg* 66A: 725, 1984
19. Jacobsen, K: Osteoarthritis following insufficiency of the cruciate ligament in man: A clinical study. *Acta Orthop Scand* 48: 520, 1977.
20. Johnson, R.J.: The anterior cruciate ligament: A dilemma in sports medicine. *Int J Sports Med* 3: 71, 1982.
21. Kannus, P., Jarvinen, M.: Posttraumatic ACL insufficiency as a cause of osteoarthritis in a knee joint. *Clin Rheumatol* 8(2): 251, 1989.
22. Markolf, K.L., Kochan, A., Amstutz, H.D.: Measurement of knee stiffness and laxity in patients with documented absence of the anterior cruciate ligament. *J Bone Joint Surg* 66A: 242, 1984.
23. Noyes, F.R., Schipplein, O.D., Andriacchi, T.P., Saddemi, S.R., Weise, M.: The anterior cruciate ligament-deficient knee with varus alignment: An analysis of gait adaptations and dynamic joint loadings. *Am J Sports Med* 20(6): 1992.
24. Noyes, F.R., Matthews, D.S., Mooar, P.A., Grood, E.S.: The symptomatic anterior cruciate-deficient knee. Part II: The results of rehabilitation, activity modification, and counseling on functional disability. *J Bone Joint Surg* 65A: 163, 1983.
25. Noyes, F.R., Mooar, P.A., Matthews, D.S., Butler, D.L.: The symptomatic anterior cruciate-deficient knee. Part I: The long-term functional disability in athletically active patients. *J Bone Joint Surg* 65A: 154, 1983.
26. Prodromos, C.C., Andriacchi, T.P., Galante J.O.: A relationship between knee joint loads and clinical changes following high tibial osteotomy. *J Bone Joint Surg* 67A(8): 1188–194, 1985.
27. Schipplein, O.D., Andriacchi, T.P.: Interaction between active and passive knee stabilizers during level walking. *J Orthop Res* 9: 113, 1991.
28. Tibone, J.E., Antich, T.J., Fanton, G.S., Moynes, D.R., Perry, J.: Functional analysis of anterior cruciate ligament instability. *Am J Sports Med* 14: 276, 1986.
29. Wang, J.-W., Kuo, K.N., Andriacchi, T.P., Galante, J.O.: The influence of walking mechanics and time on the results of proximal tibial osteotomy. *J Bone Joint Surg* 72A(6): 905–13, 1990.
30. Wroble, R.R., Brand, R.A.: Paradoxes in the history of the ACL. *Clin Orthop* 259: 183, 1990.

CHAPTER 18

Neuromuscular Profile of the Functionally Stable ACL-Deficient Knee

Christian Fink, MD
Ivan Vassilev, MD
Arthur Kleipool, MD
Freddie H. Fu, MD
Scott M. Lephart, PhD, ATC

Introduction

Treatment of an injury to the anterior cruciate ligament remains controversial despite years of intensive basic and clinical research. Even though it is generally agreed that loss of the ACL results in abnormal biomechanical knee function and kinematics, clinical studies reveal conflicting results. ACL deficiency was found to cause unacceptable performance in sports as well as progressive degenerative changes in a high number of patients (6, 11,15); however, the knees of certain patients, demonstrating the same amount of laxity, function well (4, 7, 13, 15). These factors, and the observation that anterior cruciate ligament reconstruction, which may even restore normal laxity, still is unable to prevent the development of arthritic changes (6, 13), reveal the limitations of a primarily structural view of the problem (9). Neuromuscular control strategies to compensate for joint laxity may be more effective in predicting functional outcome than passive joint laxity, in patients with ACL injuries (14, 38).

Neuromuscular Considerations in the Normal Knee

Recent biomechanical and neuromuscular research has indicated that stabilization of the knee results not only from the mechanical function of ligaments but also from the complex synergism that exists between ligaments, articular structures, muscles, and the nervous system (see figure 18.1). Those structures acting in a coordinate fashion provide both mechanical and dynamic stability to the joints.

The concept of "dynamic stability" with reference to the normal knee has gained increased support as it has been demonstrated that a synergistic relationship exists between the ACL and the muscles of the leg. In histological studies mechanoreceptors have been detected within the ACL as well as at its insertion sides (23, 30, 31). It has been suggested that excitation of these receptors results in a reflex response of the hamstrings (34).

Grüber and coworkers (16) found that the biceps femoris and the semimembranosus act in a synergistic manner to the ACL in preventing anterior

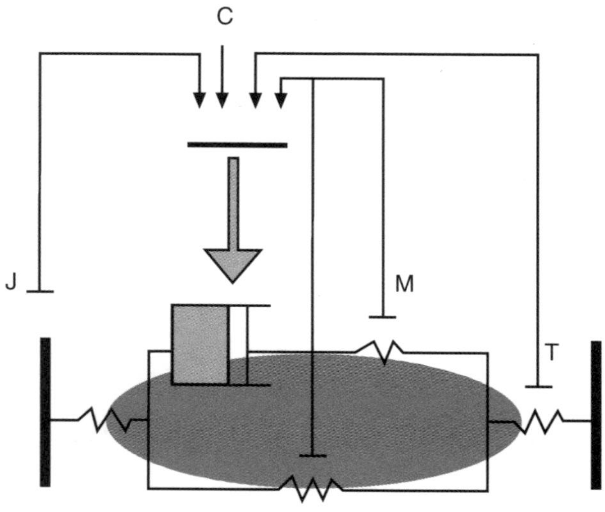

Figure 18.1 Model of neuromuscular control: C = central nervous system, M = muscle receptors, J = joint receptor, T = tendon receptors. From reference 12.

tibial translation. Other investigators have also confirmed this (8, 28, 34). Using an isokinetic electromyographic (EMG) model, Hagood and coworkers (17) concluded that, as the angular velocity of the limb increases, a reflexive increase in the contribution of the antagonist musculature to joint stiffness and laxity occurs. Hirokawa and coworkers (18), in a cadaver model, reported that co-contraction of the hamstring is synergistic to the ACL in avoiding excessive anterior tibial translation. Recent publications have demonstrated that the hamstring-ACL synergism is related to the neurosensory role of the ligament, providing dynamic stability to the knee (19–21). By using EMG in an animal model, Raunest and coworkers (29) demonstrated a reflex arc between hamstrings and ACL, confirming the synergistic relationship between the passive and active restraint to tibial translation. In addition to the quadriceps and hamstrings, the medial gastrocnemius also provides dynamic stability to the knee (24, 32).

Neuromuscular Consideration in the ACL-Deficient Knee

All this data indicate that a complex synergy exists around the anatomical structures of the knee. Therefore, ACL rupture not only results in the loss of a mechanical stabilizer, but it is also accompanied by secondary alterations of the neuromuscular control system (see figure 18.1) (10, 12).

Various studies have profiled muscle activation patterns by the use of electromyography in ACL-deficient subjects across an array of functional tasks; these have resulted in inconsistent findings relative to both levels and duration of muscle activity (3, 5, 22, 26, 36, 39).

There is a large body of data that suggests that ACL rupture acutely diminishes the muscular contribution to knee stability. Beard and coworkers (1) suggested that the reflex capability of the hamstrings becomes insufficient to provide dynamic joint stabilization, because of the deafferentation that may be associated with the ACL rupture. They reported a significantly increased reflex hamstrings contraction latency in ACL-deficient knees. Van Lent and coworkers (37) also reported diminished hamstrings activity in the ACL-deficient limb as a result of mild fatigue.

On the other hand, numerous studies provide evidence that adaptations in this altered neuromuscular mechanism may provide the capability for dynamic stabilization. One reason for the conflicting results of these studies, besides different testing methodology, is patient selection.

Increased Hamstring Activity

In a study performed at the neuromuscular laboratory at the University of Pittsburgh, 17 healthy subjects with a unilateral "functionally stable" ACL-deficient knee were investigated (25). The criteria for subject participation included a minimum age of 18 years, documented chronic unilateral "isolated" ACL deficiency, full range of motion, no concomitant musculoskeletal injuries, no previous neurological disease, and no episodes of giving way with running, cutting, or jumping.

EMG activity from the thigh musculature as well as the medial gastrocnemius was recorded via bipolar Ag/AgCl surface electrodes (see figure 18.2) during walking (see figure 18.3) and hopping (see figure 18.4). Each set of electrodes was connected to a transmitter (Noraxon USA, Inc., Scottsdale, Arizona), which transferred the signals to a computer for further processing.

During the stance phase of walking the ACL-deficient limb demonstrated a significant increase (49%) in EMG activity of the lateral hamstring, and a significant decrease (48%) in vastus lateralis activity was revealed during the swing phase of walking.

The finding of increased lateral hamstring EMG activity during the stance phase of walking is similar to that reported by Branch and associates (3) in

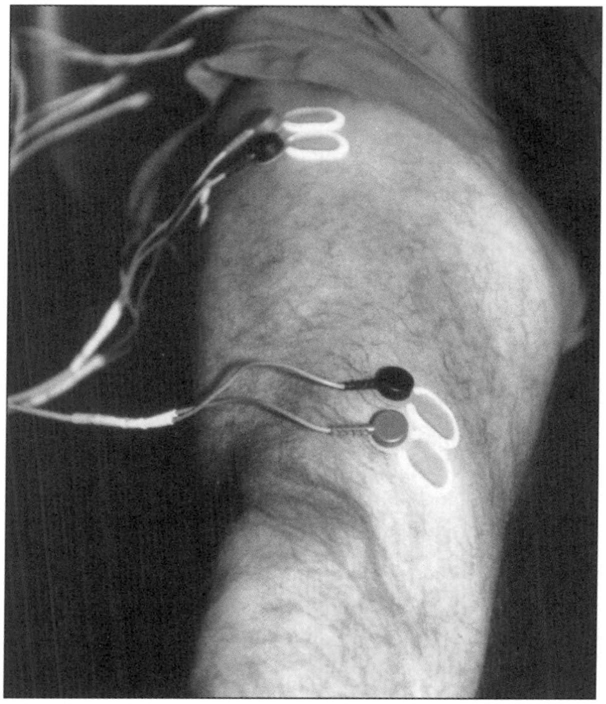

a

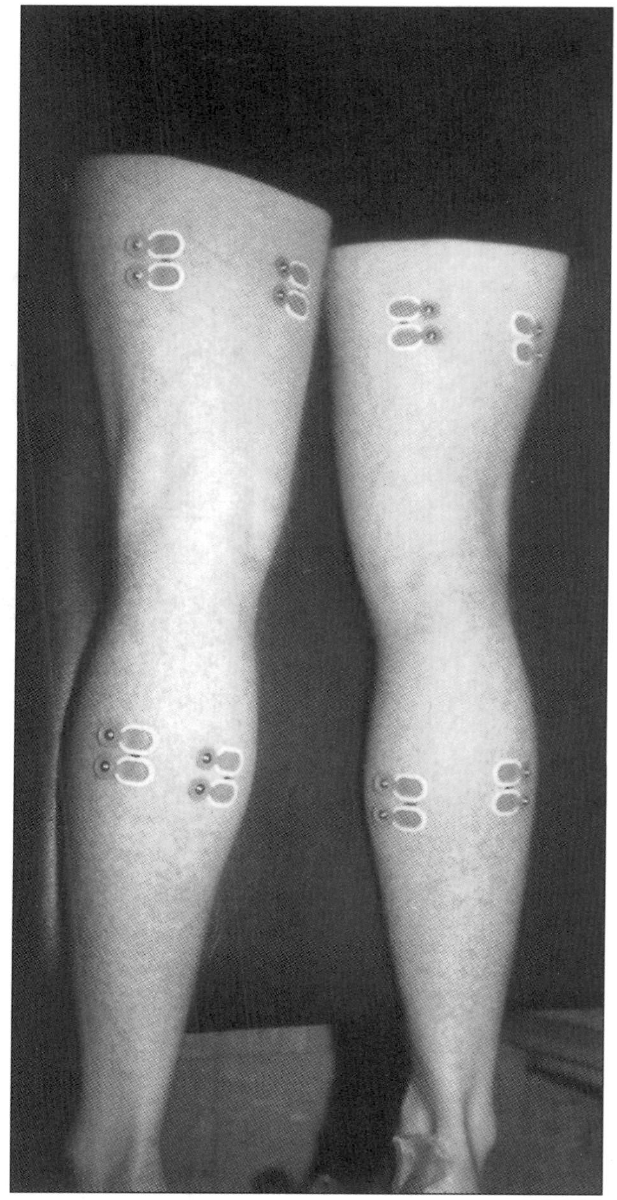

b

Figure 18.2 Electrode placement: *(a)* vastus medialis, vastus lateralis, and rectus femoris; *(b)* medial and lateral hamstrings, medial and lateral gastrocnemius.

ACL-deficient patients during cutting maneuvers and with the findings reported by Ciccotti and coworkers (5) and Kålund and coworkers (22). The function of the lateral hamstring as dynamic stabilizer of the knee is quite important, because this muscle may have substantial influence on protecting the knee from anterolateral subluxation of the tibia, which occurs during a giving-way episode (27). Increased lateral hamstring activity prevents the knee from pivoting and reflects what Ciccotti and coworkers (5) state is a "protective mechanism." Terry and coworkers (35) supported this concept by reporting that the biceps femoris muscle complex is an important static as well as dynamic stabilizer to the lateral side of the knee.

These results imply, therefore, that in the functionally stable ACL-deficient knee, secondary reflex arcs may provide sufficient lateral hamstring activation to oppose tibial subluxation. The findings of enhanced lateral hamstring activity during the stance phase of the normal gait suggest that rehabilitation activities focusing on hamstring activation in a closed kinematic chain position need to be emphasized in order to restore dynamic joint stabilization.

Decreased Quadriceps Activity

Berchuck and coworkers (2), in a gait analyses study, noted a "quadriceps avoidance" pattern in patients with ACL deficiency compared to a group of normal subjects. A reduction in the flexion moment was observed during walking, jogging, and stair climbing, especially when the knee was near full extension. The authors interpreted this as an attempt to avoid excessive quadriceps forces when the knee was in a position susceptible to anterior tibial translation.

In our study, during the swing phase of walking the vastus lateralis demonstrated significantly

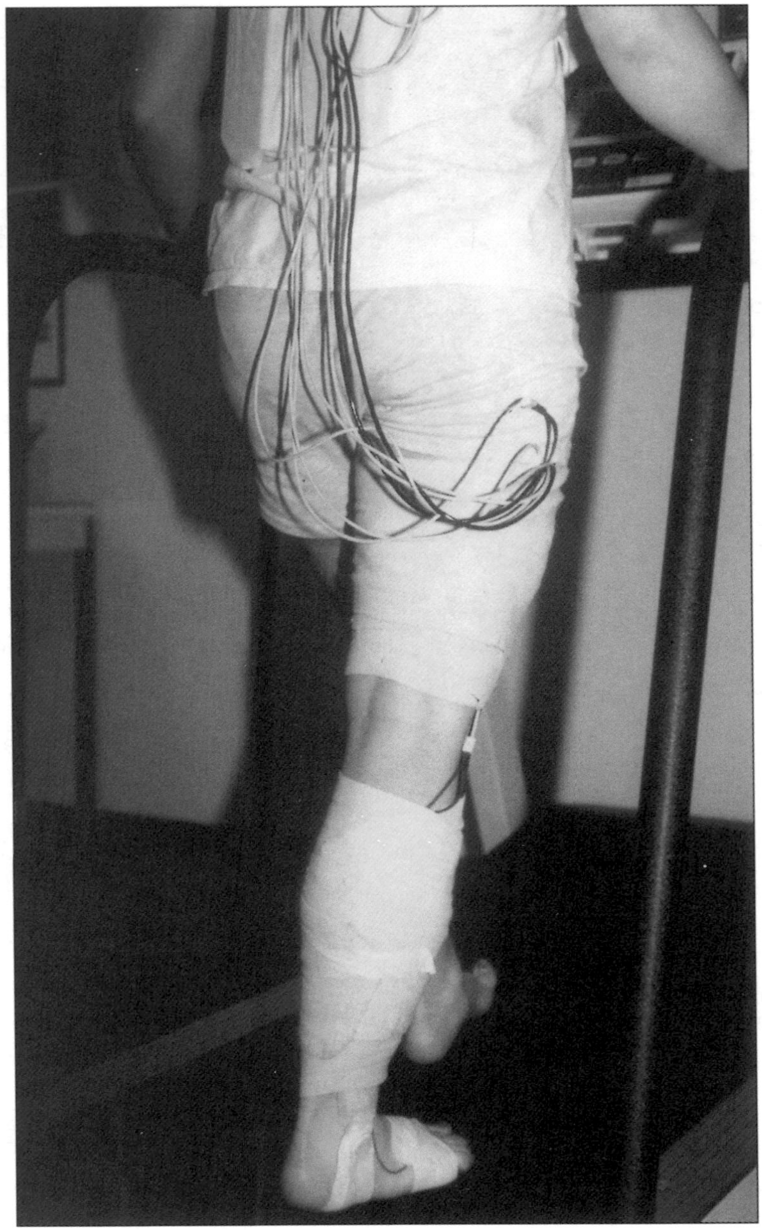

Figure 18.3 Level walking on the treadmill.

lower EMG activity in the ACL-deficient knee when compared to that of the contralateral normal knee (25). Similarly, Limbird and associates (26) reported that, during the swing to strike transition phase of the gait, the ACL-deficient knee showed significantly less activity of the quadriceps.

These findings can be considered as part of the adaptive process of the ACL-deficient knee, in which anterior tibial translation is avoided during the swing phase in preparation for heel strike and the subsequent stance phase of the gait. In the presence of ACL rupture this preparatory inhibition of the vastus lateralis is an attempt to restore more normal kinematics when the knee is loaded as opposed to loading a partially pivoted knee.

Summary

The results of these investigations suggest that adaptations in the neuromuscular activation of the

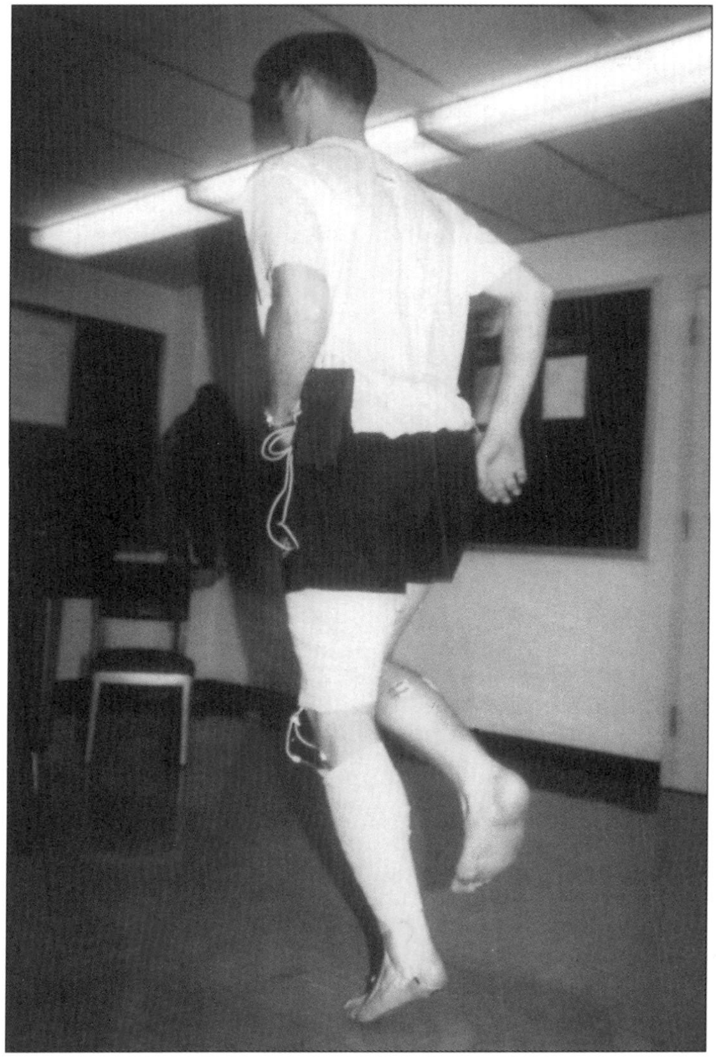

Figure 18.4 Single-leg hopping test.

ACL-deficient knee may enhance the individual's chances for regaining functional stability. In the functionally stable ACL-deficient knee the muscular contribution of the hamstring may contribute to preventing the knee from pivoting during the most vulnerable phases for anterior tibial translation. Furthermore, these results suggest that the quadriceps group, which is an antagonist to the ACL, is selectively inhibited. Consequently, anterior tibial translation is diminished, resulting in a more functionally stable knee.

The ability to change these neuromuscular control patterns, however, seems to vary among individuals. Improvement of current testing methods is required in order to discriminate early after injury between the patient who can cope with ACL deficiency and the one who cannot. This would give us an important objective guidance in selecting the appropriate treatment.

Furthermore, the effects of neuromuscular rehabilitation programs supporting compensatory strategies of the nervous system to the structural changes have to be studied. Up to now EMG and neuromuscular studies still reveal conflicting results. Due to improving technology and better study designs, however, our knowledge will increase rapidly.

References

1. Beard D, Kyberd P, Fergusson C, et al: Proprioception after rupture of the anterior cruciate ligament: An objective indication of the need

for surgery? *J Bone Joint Surg* 75B(2): 311–15, 1993.

2. Berchuck M, Andriacchi TP, Bach BR, Reider B: Gait adaptations by patients who have a deficient ACL. *J Bone Joint Surg* 72A: 871–77, 1990.
3. Branch T, Hunter R, Donath M: Dynamic EMG analysis of the anterior cruciate ligament deficient legs with and without bracing during cutting. *Am J Sports Med* 17(1): 35–41, 1989.
4. Buss DD, Min R, Skyhar M, et al: Nonoperative treatment of acute anterior cruciate ligament injuries in a selected group of patients. *Am J Sports Med* 23: 160–65, 1995.
5. Ciccotti M, Kerlain R, Perry J, et al: An electromyographic analysis of the knee during functional activities. II: The anterior cruciate ligament-deficient knee and reconstructed profiles. *Am J Sports Med* 22(5): 651–58, 1994.
6. Clancy WG, Ray JM, Zoltan DJ: Acute tears of the anterior cruciate ligament. *J Bone Joint Surg* 70A: 1482–488, 1988.
7. Daniel DM, Stone ML, Dobson BE, Fithian DC, Rossman DJ, Kaufmann KR: Fate of the ACL-injured patient: A prospective outcome study. *Am J Sports Med* 22: 632–44, 1994.
8. Draganich LF, Jaeger RJ, Kralj AR: Coactivation of the hamstrings and quadriceps during extension of the knee. *J Bone Joint Surg* 71(7): 1075–1081, 1989.
9. Dye SF: The knee as a biologic transmission with an envelope of function: A theory. *Clin Orthop Rel Res* 323: 10–18, 1996.
10. Elmqvist LG, Lorentzon R, Johansson C, Fugl-Meyer AR: Does a torn anterior cruciate ligament lead to change in the central nervous drive of the knee extensors? *Eur J Appl Physiol* 58: 203–207, 1988.
11. Fetto JF, Marshall JL: The natural history and diagnosis of the anterior cruciate ligament insufficiency. *Clin Orthop* 147: 29–38, 1980.
12. Fink C, Hoser C, Benedetto KP, Judmaier W: (Neuro)muscular changes of the knee stabilizing musculature after ACL injury. *Sportverl Sportschad* 8: 25–30, 1994.
13. Fink C, Hoser C, Benedetto KP, Navarro RA, Pincivero DM: Ten- to 13-year follow-up of nonoperative versus operative treatment of anterior cruciate ligament rupture. Paper presented (No 547) at the American Academy of Orthopaedic Surgeons, 64th Annual Meeting, San Francisco, February 1997.
14. Fridén T, Egund N, Lindstrand A: Comparison of symptomatic versus nonsymptomatic patients with chronic anterior cruciate ligament insufficiency: Radiographic sagittal displacement during weight bearing. *Am J Sports Med* 21: 389–93, 1993.
15. Giove FP, Miller SJ, Kent BE, Sanford TI, Garrick JG: Nonoperative treatment of the torn anterior cruciate ligament. *J Bone Joint Surg* 65: 184–92, 1993.
16. Gruber J, Wolter D, Lierse W: Der vordere Kreuzbandreflex (LCA reflex). *Unfallchirurg* 89: 551–54, 1986.
17. Hagood S, Solomonow M, Baratta R, et al: The effect of joint velocity on the contribution of the antagonist musculature to knee stiffness and laxity. *Am J Sports Med* 18(2): 182–87, 1990.
18. Hirokawa S, Solomonow M, Luo Y, et al: Muscular co-contraction and control of the knee stability. *J Electromyogr Kinesiol* 1(3): 199–208, 1991.
19. Johansson H, Sjölander P, Sojka P, et al: A sensory role for the cruciate ligaments. *Clin Orthop* 268: 161–78, 1991.
20. Johansson H, Sjölander P, Sojka P: Receptors in the knee joint ligaments and their role in the biomechanics of the joint. *Biomed Engineering* 18(5): 341–68, 1991.
21. Johansson H: Role of knee ligaments in proprioception and regulation of muscle stiffness. *J Electromyogr Kinesiol* 1(3): 158–79, 1991.
22. Kålund S, Sinkjær T, Arendt-Nielsen A, et al: Altered timing of hamstring muscle action in anterior cruciate ligament deficient patients. *Am J Sports Med* 18(3): 245–48, 1990.
23. Kennedy JC, Alexander IJ, Hayes KC: Nerve supply of the human knee and its functional importance. *Am J Sports Med* 10: 329–35, 1982.
24. Lass P, Kaalund S, LeFevre S, et al: Muscle coordination following rupture of the anterior cruciate ligament. *Acta Orthop Scand* 62(1): 9–14, 1991.
25. Lephart SM, Kleipool A, Vassilev I, Lee HM, et al: EMG profile of the functional ACL-deficient patient during dynamic activities. Paper presented at the AOSSM Specialty Day, American Academy of Orthopaedic Surgeons, 64th Annual Meeting, San Francisco, February 1997.
26. Limbird T, Shiavi R, Frazer M, et al: EMG profiles of the knee musculature during walking: Changes induced by anterior cruciate ligament deficiency. *J Orthop Res* 6(5): 630–38, 1988.
27. Marshall JL, Girgis FG, Zelko RR: The biceps femoris tendon and its functional significance. *J Bone Joint Surg* 54A(7): 1444–450, 1972.
28. Osternig LR, Caster BL, James CR: Contralateral hamstring (biceps femoris) coactivation patterns and anterior cruciate ligament dysfunction. *Med Sci Sports Exerc* 27(6): 805–808, 1995.
29. Raunest J, Sager M, Burgener E: Proprioceptive mechanisms in the cruciate ligaments: An elec-

tromyographic study on reflex. *J Trauma* 41(3): 488–93, 1996.

30. Schultz RA, Miller DC, Kerr CS, et al: Mechanoreceptors in human cruciate ligaments. *J Bone Joint Surg* 66A: 1072–1076, 1984.
31. Schutte MJ, Dabezies EJ, Zimny ML, et al: Neural anatomy of the human anterior cruciate ligament. *J Bone Joint Surg* 69(A): 243–47, 1987.
32. Sinkjær T, Arendt-Nielsen L: Knee stability and muscle coordination in patients with anterior cruciate ligament injuries: An electromyographic approach. *J Electromyogr Kinesiol* 1(3): 209–17, 1991.
33. Snyder-Mackler L, Fitzgerald GK, Bartolozzi AR, Ciccotti MG: The relationship between passive joint laxity and functional outcome after anterior cruciate ligament injury. *Am J Sports Med* 25: 191–95, 1997.
34. Solomonov M, Baratta R, Zhou BH, et al: The synergistic action of the anterior cruciate ligament and the thigh muscles in maintaining joint stability. *Am J Sports Med* 15(3): 207–13, 1987.
35. Terry G, LaPrade R: The biceps femoris muscle complex at the knee: Its anatomy and injury patterns associated with acute anterolateral-anteromedial rotatory instability. *Am J Sports Med* 24(1): 2–8, 1996.
36. Tibone J, Antich TJ, Fanton G, et al: Functional analysis of anterior ligament instability. *Am J Sports Med* 14(4): 276–84, 1986.
37. Van Lent MET, Drost MR, Wildenberg FAJM v.d: EMG profiles of ACL-deficient patients during walking: The influence of mild fatigue. *Int J Sports Med* 15(8): 508–14, 1994.
38. Walla D, Albright JP, McAuley E, et al: Hamstring control and the unstable anterior cruciate ligament-deficient knee. *Am J Sports Med* 13(1): 34–39, 1985.
39. Yang J, Winter D: Surface EMG profiles during different walking cadences in humans. *Electroencephalomyogr Clin Neurophys* 60(6): 485–91, 1985.

CHAPTER 19

Effects of Knee Ligament Injury and Reconstruction on Proprioception

Robert L. Barrack, MD
Barry G. Munn, MD

Introduction

Recent literature has continued to suggest the importance of proprioception in maintaining normal joint kinematics in the knee, as well as in other joints. A more complete understanding of both the anatomy and the neurophysiology of proprioception has been possible using new techniques. In addition, a greater appreciation of the process in both the normal and abnormal joint has been facilitated. The concepts of proprioception and the importance of intraarticular neuroreceptors are not new. The presence of neuroreceptors in the human knee joint was described by Rauber in 1874, (91) and the term proprioception was first coined in 1906 by Sherrington. (95) Duchenne was among the first to recognize the clinical importance of articular sensations in the latter part of the nineteenth century. (88) Abbott and coworkers (1) and Gardner (39–41) reported that the ligaments of the knee had a rich sensory innervation that allowed them to act as the first link in the "kinetic chain." The Abbott group went on to state that "impulses arising in the ligaments are transmitted through the central nervous system back to the effector muscles, allowing for maintenance of normal, smooth, coordinated movement of the joint, and that abnormally strong impulses, such as those initiated when a ligament is over-stretched, would result in contraction of allied muscle groups, thereby protecting further injury and subluxation of the knee" (1).

In the 1950s, Palmer demonstrated reflex contraction of the medial hamstring and vastus medialis in response to stimulation of the deep capsular portion of the medial collateral ligament (MCL) and further showed that this reflex was diminished in the traumatized joint and loses its selectivity. (86) (See figure 19.1.) Kennedy and coworkers hypothesized that the loss of mechanoreceptor feedback in individuals with torn knee ligaments contributed to a progressive instability and recurrent episodes of major and minor trauma. (68, 69) Freeman and Wyke (35–37) and

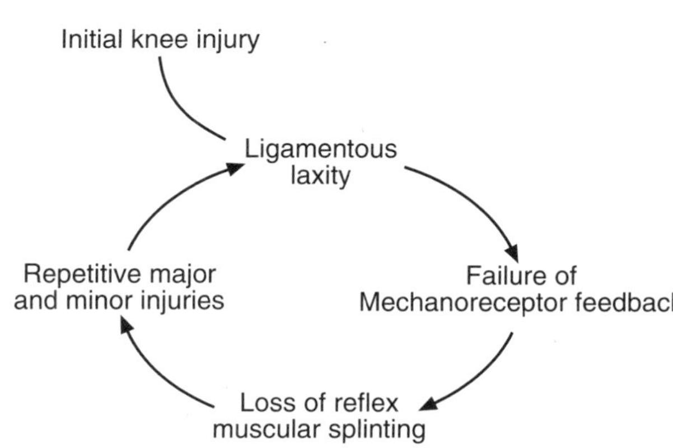

Figure 19.1 Knee injury cycle.

later Johansson and coworkers (62–64) proposed that symptoms such as functional instability or a feeling of giving way, which often persisted after reconstruction of damaged cruciate ligaments, might be the result of a partial deafferentation of the injured joint. If it is assumed that different motor programs are adapted to receive specific sensory input for the execution of various motor tasks, then ligament injury probably causes an alteration in the normal sensory feedback, which does not fit existing motor programs. This, in turn, may induce errors in the normal coordination pattern of the muscles and result in disturbances in functional joint stability. (62–64) Noyes and associates demonstrated that active persons with ACL-deficient knees have symptoms of instability and degeneration with significant long-term implications. (82) O'Connor and coworkers demonstrated that the effect of sectioning the afferent nerves to a ligamentously unstable knee joint in dogs was to accelerate the development of osteoarthrosis. (84) Noyes and coworkers, (81) Insall and coworkers, (58) and DuToit (31) all advocated certain reconstructive techniques, in part, to increase afferent preservation. More recent anatomic studies have demonstrated a variety of mechanoreceptors in intraarticular structures including the cruciate ligaments, the menisci, and the patellar tendon. (29, 30, 51, 67, 70, 83, 93, 94, 108–111) The purpose of this chapter is to review the previous knowledge of joint sensation, including the basic anatomy and physiology, and to review current research in the area, especially as it relates to injuries, rehabilitation, and reconstruction.

Terminology and Basic Principles

Awareness of the body and its relationship with the surrounding environment is mediated through the phenomenon of sensation. The senses are broadly divided into special (sight, hearing, taste, smell) and somatic, or somesthetic, (pain, temperature, touch). Each specific type of sensation is called a modality. Every sensory modality has a specific end organ that responds to a stimulus in a characteristic way. The stimulus is converted to an electrical potential and is conducted along nerve fibers specific to each sensory modality. The impulses are carried along established neural pathways to either elicit an appropriate reflex or reach the cortical level (and thus conscious awareness) of a stimulus. (8)

Proprioception can be considered a specialized variation of the sense of touch and encompasses the sensation of joint movement (kinesthesia) and joint position in space (joint position sense). (71) These modalities originate by stimulation of specialized nerve endings referred to as mechanoreceptors. These specialized end organs function as transducers, converting mechanical energy of physical deformation into the electrical energy of a nerve action potential. Grigg and Hoffman correlated mechanoreceptor afferent discharge with strain energy density and have calibrated mechanoreceptors as in vivo load cells in the posterior capsule of the feline knee. (44–47, 53) Mechanoreceptors can be classified as either rapidly adapting or slowly adapting. All receptors are maximally stimulated (i.e., they generate the maximal number of electrical impulses) immediately after a new stimulus is detected. If a stimulus is continually applied, receptors differ as to how they continue to respond. Rapidly adapting receptors such as Pacinian corpuscles and hair receptors respond to small changes in pressure with a sudden burst of high frequency impulses followed by a rapid deterioration even though the stimulus is maintained. They are, therefore, very sensitive to the onset of changes in movement but not to slow or constant pressures. Slowly adapting receptors such as joint receptors, Ruffini endings, and muscle spindles are always generating impulses depending on the relative position of muscles and joints, delivering steady state information on joint position as well as sensing motion and angle of rotation. (8)

Impulses from mechanoreceptors are conducted to the central nervous system through different nerve fiber types specific to each modality. Proprioceptive impulses are carried along large diameter myelinated nerve fibers that have higher conduction velocities, whereas fibers that transmit pain are smaller diameter and unmyelinated with associated lower conduction velocities. The majority of sensory impulses reaches the central nervous system via the articular nerves and ascends to the cerebral cortex via the dorsal column-lemniscal (posterior column) system. The postcentral gyrus of the cerebral cortex has a high degree of spatial organization, which accounts for the conscious awareness of position sense of the extremities. (See figure 19.2.) Muller has noted that there is a disproportionately high cortical representation of the lower limb, which he interprets as evidence for the importance of proprioceptive input from the lower extremity. (79)

Mechanoreceptor Function

Specialized end organs in the joint capsules and ligaments are thought to serve at least two func-

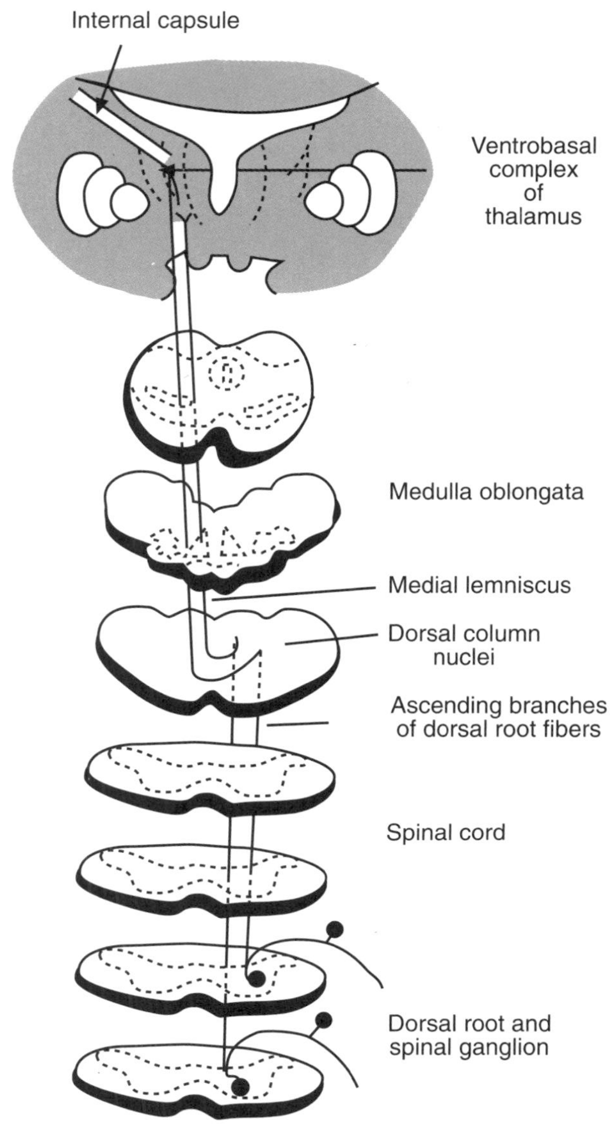

Figure 19.2 The postcentral gyrus of the cerebral cortex has a high degree of spatial organization, which accounts for the conscious awareness of position sense of the extremities.

tions. They provide position sense or conscious awareness of the joint in space, and they initiate protective reflexes that help to stabilize the joint and avoid injury. Ruffini and Golgi tendon organs are slow adapting and have been previously described as the dominant receptor type in joint capsules. (2, 83, 100) They respond to active or passive motion and generate impulses throughout the range of motion. (48) Maximal responses, however, have consistently been demonstrated at the extremes of motion. (44, 45, 47, 99) Friden and coworkers reported that proprioceptive sensitivity improved with greater degrees of knee extension, (38) and Borsa and coworkers found that proprioceptive ability improved near full extension and was more sensitive moving into further degrees of extension. (18) External rotation also has been shown to accentuate discharge from these receptors. (21, 24, 44, 100) Since these are positions in which the cruciate ligaments are vulnerable to injury, it is reasonable to conclude that these receptors may play a role in signaling impending injury. (8)

Clinically, the threshold to detection of passive motion (TTDPM) has been used to measure the response from these ligamentous and capsular receptors. (6–11, 54, 66, 97–99) Although these slowly adapting receptors have been thought to play a dominant role in conscious awareness of joint position, stimulation of these same receptors has elicited reflex muscular contractions important in stabilizing the affected joint. (32, 35) Rapidly responding receptors such as Pacinian corpuscles have been described in high densities near the insertions of ligaments, especially the ACL. (See figure 19.3.) Since they respond to changes in acceleration, they too would be in a position to initiate protective reflexes. (8)

Ruffini end organs, Golgi tendon organs, and Pacinian corpuscles have repeatedly been found in knee joint capsules, ligaments, menisci, and patellar tendons in a number of animal dissections. (19, 21, 36, 41, 83) Receptors in these organs have also been shown to have the capacity to initiate reflex muscle contraction. (5) The reflex pattern most often elicited is one of inhibition of knee extension and facilitation of knee flexion. (100) The exact mechanism by which muscular reflexes are initiated is still a subject of debate. It is uncertain whether some impulses generated from the mechanoreceptors result directly in stimulation of alpha motor neurons or whether the effect is mediated primarily by the gamma efferent muscle spindle system. An extensive investigation by Johansson and coworkers concluded that knee ligament mechanoreceptors increased the response in the gamma efferent muscle receptors, which was primarily responsible for the firing of appropriate muscles necessary to help stabilize the joint and protect it from injury under moderate loads. (62–64) Grigg has suggested that muscles that cross a joint can activate afferent joint receptors when they contract. (44) Anatomically, the close association of muscle and tendinous insertions with the joint capsule has been well demonstrated. Hughston and coworkers described the capsular arms of the semimembranosus and the effect of muscle contraction in tightening the capsule. (55, 56)

It has been questioned whether reflex muscular contraction initiated by stress on the knee joint could

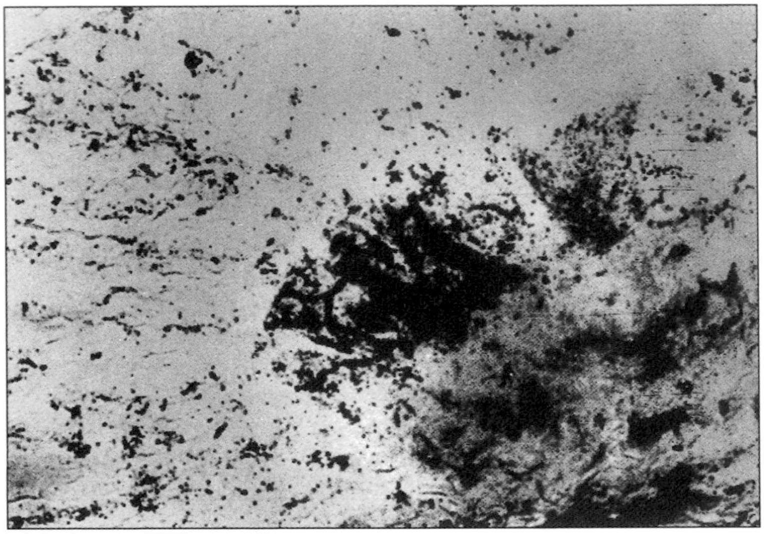
a

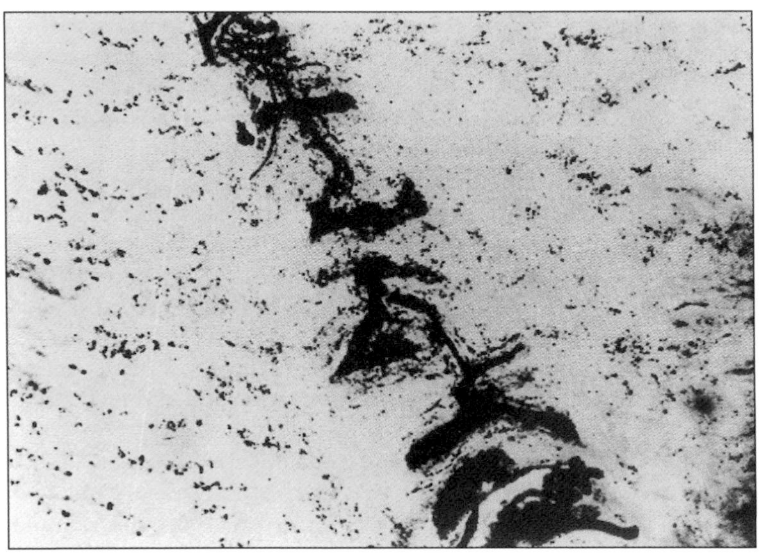
b

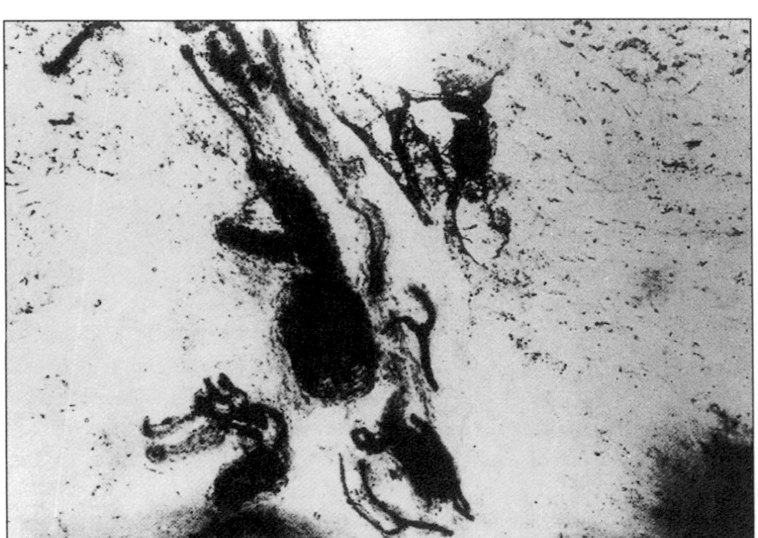
c

Figure 19.3 Pacinian corpuscles near the insertions of ligaments.

occur in time to prevent knee injury. This question was examined by Pope and coworkers, who showed that contraction of the medial hamstring muscles and the quadriceps significantly increased the valgus stiffness of the medial knee ligaments by 104% and 164%, respectively, providing substantial protection from injury. (89) In response to visual or tactile stimulation, protective muscle activity occurred in insufficient time to be of value in protecting the knee from injury. (See figure 19.4.) This study assumed, however, that the origin of a protective reflex was from pain fibers or through voluntary contraction. Free nerve endings responsible for pain mediation, however, have been found to be sparse or absent in knee ligaments, especially the cruciates, compared with the population of mechanoreceptors, and pain is not elicited when the mechanoreceptors are maximally stimulated. (94) Reflex muscle contraction is more likely the result of impulses resulting from the physical deformation of Golgi, Ruffini, or Pacinian mechanoreceptors. These impulses are carried by the larger diameter myelinated fibers with conduction velocities one or two magnitudes faster than those of the unmyelinated fibers associated with free nerve endings. Guyton emphasized the great speed of these large-fiber proprioceptive nerves and their probable importance in modulating muscle tension in high-demand activities such as running. (48) The high energy imparted in many contact sports, however, exceeds the maximal stiffness of the ligament even with maximal muscle contraction. In addition, the high speed of many contact injuries exceeds the conduction velocities of even the large myelinated fibers. It is likely, therefore, that proprioceptive input is adequate to protect or stabilize the knee during normal daily functions such as walking or running, but the high energy of many catastrophic injuries exceeds the ability of any level of muscle contraction to prevent ligament injury. (7, 8)

Innervation of the Knee Joint

Hilton stated that joints are innervated by articular branches of the nerves that supply the muscles that cross the joint. (52) Proprioceptive responses have been recorded from the knee joint through monitoring the posterior articular nerve (19, 21, 24, 39) as well as the medial and lateral articular nerves. (23, 100) The innervation of the knee joint has been described by Jeletsky (59) and Gardner. (41) Our current state of

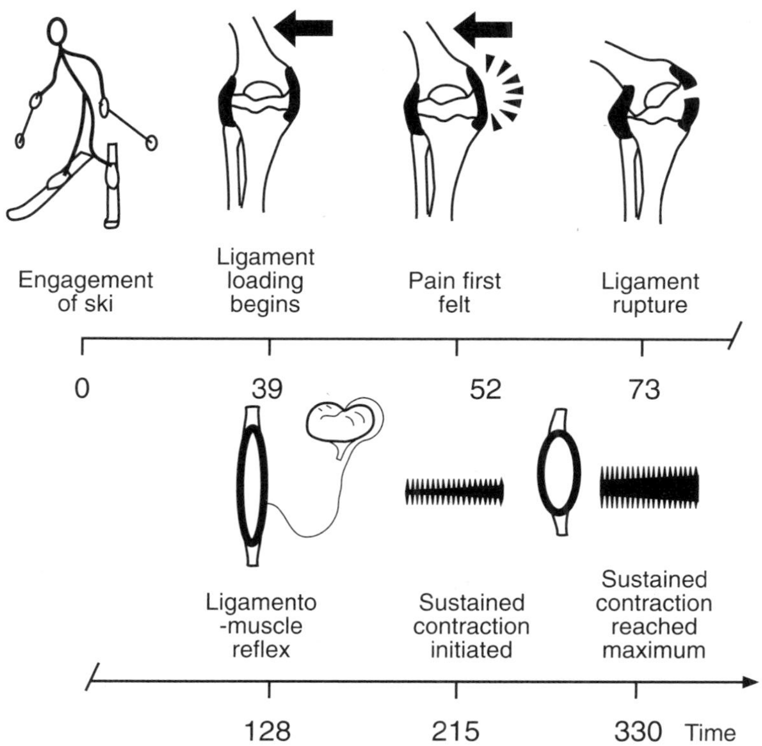

Figure 19.4 Timeline of knee ligament injury in milliseconds.

understanding of the innervation of the human knee joint was summarized by Kennedy and coworkers, who described two groups of articular nerves. (68) The first, a posterior group, consisted of a prominent posterior articular nerve that is a branch of the tibial nerve and a second, smaller nerve that was a terminal branch of the obturator nerve. The anterior group consisted of articular branches of the femoral, peroneal, and saphenous nerves. Consistent with the findings of many previous examiners, the most prominent nerve was the posterior articular nerve. This is commonly felt to be the primary nerve supply to the posterior capsule and the cruciate ligaments. This nerve arises in the popliteal fossa and penetrates the posterior capsule. (68)

On a microscopic level, articular mechanoreceptors have been demonstrated in both animal and human studies. Neuroanatomical studies by Kennedy and coworkers revealed variability in the innervation of the human knee and found mechanoreceptors within multiple clefts in the tibial origin of the ACL and within its vascular synovial covering. None, however, was found within the substance of the ligament. (68) In 1984, Schultz and coworkers reported on the presence of mechanoreceptors in human cruciate ligaments, in ligaments obtained at the time of total knee replacement. (93) Histology of ligaments from younger patients without evidence of degenerative arthritis showed higher density populations, which is consistent with the findings of Skinner and coworkers (97) and Kaplan and coworkers, (66) who found that proprioception declines as a part of the normal aging process.

Subsequently, Schutte and coworkers performed a more detailed histological analysis of the human ACL.[94] These researchers performed semi-quantitative analysis of the population densities of various receptor populations and found receptors that were morphologically similar to Ruffini endings, Golgi tendon organs, and Pacinian corpuscles, with relatively few free nerve endings being demonstrated. The highest densities of receptors were clustered at the tibial and femoral attachments, which is consistent with the previous work done by Kennedy and associates. (69) Neural elements constituted 1% of the total area of the anterior cruciate ligament. (94)

Similar findings have been reported by Yahia and Newman, (109) and by Zimny and Wink. (110, 111) The highest densities were again reported near the bony attachments. More recent studies have utilized more specific immunohistological techniques to confirm the earlier authors' findings. Haus and coworkers (51) examined 21 ACLs with both light and electron microscopy and found populations of Ruffini corpuscles, Pacinian corpuscles, and free nerve endings similar to those described by Zimny and Wink and Yahia and Newman. Rivard and coworkers used antineurofilament protein as well as antisera to substance P to examine the ACL. (92) Substance P is thought to be fairly specific for free nerve endings or pain fibers, while neurofilament protein would be more likely to be found in specialized nerve endings such as mechanoreceptors. The technique detected significant numbers of mechanoreceptors and indicated virtually no uptake of the substance P marker. This is consistent with a previous study by Biedert and coworkers, which showed that the ACL had a lower number of free nerve endings than any of the knee structures they examined. (17)

Other authors have examined specimens obtained after ACL injury and reconstruction. Denti and coworkers took biopsies of the ACL remnants after a rupture had occurred, and for several weeks after injury mechanoreceptors persisted in the ACL remnant. At 6 mo, however, without reconstruction there was marked atrophy or complete absence of receptors. (30) Conversely, Tsujimoto and coworkers examined patellar tendon grafts following ACL reconstruction in an animal model utilizing goats. Few, if any receptors were present prior to 6 mo postreconstruction. (106) Goertzen and coworkers reported similar results in a dog model utilizing ACL allograft with receptors being absent until at least 6 mo after reconstruction. (43)

More recent studies have advanced the understanding of the neural pathway between the ACL and the central nervous system. Madey and coworkers utilized a dynamic histological technique to establish definitively a connection between the dorsal root ganglion and the anterior cruciate ligament. By injecting a peroxidase stain transported by axonal flow into the dorsal root ganglion, they were later able to demonstrate the presence of the dye in Ruffini and Pacinian receptors in the posterior capsule and Golgi tendon organs in the ACL. (77) Kraupse and others also recently demonstrated a direct link between the ACL and the posterior articular nerve and sciatic nerve. (70) Pitman and coworkers utilized somatosensory-evoked potentials to establish a link from the ACL to the cerebral cortex. (87) By electrically stimulating the ACL during routine arthroscopy they consistently were able to detect cortical response. Stimulation of the medial meniscus has also been shown to elicit a cortical-evoked response. (33) A variety of histological and neurophysiological techniques have consistently demonstrated a direct link between knee ligaments and the spinal cord and brain.

Clinical Measurement of Proprioception

Proprioception has been measured clinically by at least two techniques: the threshold to detection of passive motion(TTDPM) or the ability to reproduce passive joint positioning. Several devices with similar designs have been developed to measure these parameters in a variety of populations, including normal subjects, athletic individuals, elderly patients with degenerative joint disease, and patients with ACL-deficient knees and postreconstructed knees. Subjects undergoing proprioceptive testing are seated comfortably in the apparatus and all external cues to motion are removed. To test reproduction of passive positioning, the device passively positions the leg at various positions from the starting position, and the subjects are asked to reproduce this angle after returning to the starting position. In tests to detect threshold to detection of passive motion, the subjects are asked to determine when the position of the extremity is changed as the apparatus moves the extremity at a slow rate. Despite the hypothesized role of sensory input from the intraarticular and extraarticular structures of the knee, until recently, few studies had been done measuring knee joint proprioception and position sense. Horch and coworkers measured position sense in the knee and found that the threshold to the detection of slow passive motion was reported as 2–4° in normal subjects at angular velocities of 0.5°/s. (54) Under these conditions, the slowly adapting Ruffini or Golgi mechanoreceptors are thought to be selectively stimulated.

Age and arthrosis were found to adversely affect a subject's proprioceptive ability. Skinner and associates and Kaplan and associates discovered that propriceptive ability as measured by these tests declined in older patients. (66, 97, 98) It has been suggested that a loss of proprioceptive input may play a role in geriatric orthopedic problems, such as hip fractures that result from an increased incidence of falls, along with a lack of reflex muscular splinting. (8, 66) Other groups have studied subjects with degenerative arthritis of the knee and those having undergone total knee arthroplasty. The decline in proprioception, found to occur secondary to the arthritic process, was not found to be significantly different following joint replacement. (8, 11) This decline can be explained histologically in a study by Schultz and coworkers, who noted a relative absence of mechanoreceptors in ligament specimens retrieved during total knee arthroplasty. (93) This decrease in proprioceptive feedback may explain the abnormal gait patterns noted by Andriacchi, in patients following total knee arthroplasty. (4)

Conversely, athletic training has been shown to improve proprioceptive function. Barrack and coworkers studied ballet dancers and Lephart and coworkers studied collegiate gymnasts and both groups reported significantly improved proprioceptive ability in the highly trained athletes. (9, 71, 72) Caraffa and coworkers prospectively followed a group of soccer players for three seasons and found that players who had undergone specific proprioceptive training sustained fewer knee injuries than those players who had not received the proprioceptive training. (22) Giove and coworkers reported a high clinical success rate in returning athletes to competitive sports after ACL injury simply by achieving hamstring control. (42) Walla and coworkers found that active hamstring control was successful in reducing the pivot shift in 95% of patients who had successfully avoided surgery following ACL injury. (107) They concluded that the results were related to "reflex level" control and not to improved strength. Finally, Ihara and Nakayama described the beneficial effects of "dynamic joint control." (57) Patients received specific proprioceptive training on a tilt board and achieved a significant improvement in hamstring reactive time and strength of contraction.

EMG and Reflex Studies

In addition to measuring proprioception using the means described above, several authors have used both neural response times, reflected in EMG and reflex muscle contraction, and gait analysis as ways to evaluate the functional changes in proprioception in injured and diseased joints. Solomonow and coworkers found that a direct stress on the anterior cruciate ligament inhibits the quadriceps and stimulates the hamstrings, establishing the presence of a direct ACL reflex. (101) D'Ambrosia and coworkers performed EMGs during normal daily activities and found that the hamstrings were active during such functional activities as walking, stair climbing, and arising from a seated position, implying that the hamstrings were potential stabilizers of the knee during daily activities. (28) Kalund, Sinkjaer, Simonsen, and Arendt-Nielson demonstrated early recruitment and prolonged activity in the lateral hamstrings and medial gastrocnemius during ambulation, especially on an incline, which supports the findings of earlier researchers that the hamstrings act as potential stabilizers. (65, 96)

An alteration in the normal muscle firing pattern can lead to abnormalities in gait, which can be studied biomechanically. In an early study, Stauffer and coworkers described a number of gait abnormalities in patients with rheumatoid arthritis and osteoarthritis of the knees. (102) Compared to age-matched controls, patients with diseased knee joints walked with an exaggerated medial to lateral displacement of the body center resulting in a "waddling" type of gait. The authors suggested that the wider-based gait might offer better balance and improve proprioceptive feedback from the diseased knee joint.

Prodromos and coworkers utilized gait analysis to study patients undergoing high tibial osteotomy for medial gonarthrosis. (90) Patients who walked with a high adduction moment preoperatively tended to maintain this gait pattern postoperatively, and they had a poorer clinical result. A proprioceptive neural mechanism was again suggested as a means by which some patients utilized a compensatory gait pattern.

Andriacchi and coworkers examined patients following total knee arthroplasty with implants of various prosthetic designs. (4) Patients with implants who retained the cruciate ligaments performed better than those with cruciate-sacrificing prostheses. It was not clear whether this was due to better maintenance of mechanical restraint, better joint kinematics, or afferent sensory input from the cruciates. The authors did suggest, however, that loss of proprioceptive input might be a factor in the results. (4)

Effect of Ligament Injury and Reconstruction on Proprioception

A number of recent studies have evaluated the effect of ACL injury and ACL reconstruction on clinical proprioceptive measurement. Barrack and coworkers showed an increase in the TTDPM in the majority of patients with ACL rupture and functional instability. (10) This finding was subsequently confirmed by Corrigan and coworkers who also found diminished proprioception after ACL injury. (27) Barrett reported a defect in the accuracy of a visual analogue test in 10 ACL-deficient and 45 ACL-reconstructed patients compared with a control group. (12) Co and coworkers reported no significant differences in reproduction error between a normal population and the injured limb and contralateral normal limb in 10 patients with ACL reconstruction. (26) In threshold measurements both limbs of the patients were more accurate than controls, and the ACL-reconstructed limb was less accurate than the patient's uninjured extremity. Harter and coworkers found no difference between the injured and uninjured knee in a group of 51 patients after reconstruction. (49) Newberg, also with the uninjured limb serving as an internal control, observed deficits after ACL reconstruction in 35 patients in reproduction tests. (80) MacDonald and coworkers showed a significant difference between the injured and uninjured knees in patients with ACL insufficiency, as well as between the reconstructed knees and normal knees in two different groups of patients who had had different techniques of reconstruction. (76) Oeffenger and coworkers also stressed the positive influence of ACL reconstruction on joint coordination sense. (85) Jerosch and Prymka reported on 25 patients with ACL-deficient knees, 14 preoperatively and 11 after ACL reconstruction. (61) They found that the patients in the reconstructed group had significantly better proprioception than the preoperative group. The addition of an elastic bandage improved proprioception in both ACL-deficient patients and in normal volunteers. In a related study the authors showed a decrease in the proprioceptive function in patients with a history of recurrent dislocation of the patella. (60) Clark and coworkers reported a significant difference between knees in TTDPM in 8 patients with unilateral injuries to their posterior cruciate ligament. (25)

Several groups have examined the effects of joint effusions on proprioceptive capabilities, with varying results. Excessive joint fluid can be related to variety of degenerative and inflammatory conditions as well as acute trauma. Decreased joint proprioception has been noted in patients with osteoarthrosis, rheumatoid arthritis, and Charcot arthropathy. McNair and coworkers created effusions by injecting saline intraarticularly. They did not find a significant difference in ability to actively track a passively positioned contralateral limb after intraarticular injection of saline and suggested that the long time interval or inflammatory nature of the fluid were contributory in the decline in proprioception seen in patients with chronic effusions, secondary to injury, or degenerative or inflammatory arthritis. (78)

A number of studies have examined proprioception after ACL reconstruction. Barrett and coworkers measured proprioception after autogenous graft procedures, and they found that the proprioception was better than the average ACL-deficient patient but significantly worse than in the normal knee. (13) They found that patients' satisfaction more closely correlated with their proprioceptive ability than with their clinical knee scores. Harter and coworkers, conversely, could not demonstrate a difference between the operative and nonoperative knee at an average of 3 yrs after ACL reconstruction. (49) They utilized the reproduction of passive positioning rather than the threshold to detection of passive motion, which has generally been found to be a less sensitive test of proprioceptive ability. Lephart and coworkers examined 12 patients postoperatively utilizing the threshold measurement technique and found that significant asymmetry persisted after ACL allograft or autograft. (73, 74) Co and coworkers examined patients after ACL reconstruction and found that the reconstructed knee continued to have a proprioceptive deficit postoperatively. (26) The consensus among most investigators performing proprioceptive clinical testing is that a proprioceptive deficit occurs in most patients after an ACL rupture who have functional instability and that this deficit persists to some degree after ACL reconstruction.

Functional Testing in ACL-Deficient Knees

Several authors have studied patients after ACL rupture using both EMG and gait analysis methodology. An initial block to effective rehabilitation is the presence of a knee effusion, which causes reflex inhibition of the quadriceps muscle. (34, 68) Tibone and coworkers demonstrated changes in muscle firing patterns, particularly during cutting activities, following ACL injury. They found that quadriceps and hamstring strengthening alone was not sufficient to avoid ACL reconstruction. (103, 104) Limbird and coworkers monitored EMG during walking and showed numerous differences in muscle energy patterns in ACL-deficient patients. (75) They also noted increased activity in the hamstrings and decreased activity in the quadriceps during joint loading. Beard and coworkers measured the latency of the ACL-hamstring reflex after ACL rupture; they found that the reflex was significantly prolonged compared to controls, and there was a direct correlation between the prolongation of this reflex and the functional instability the patients experienced. (15) Branch and coworkers performed dynamic EMG analysis in ACL-deficient knees and showed similar results. (20) They also noted that the addition of a derotation brace did not affect muscle firing patterns. Andriacchi and Birac found that ACL-deficient patients had a higher than normal net hamstring activity during normal functional activities such as walking, stair climbing, and jogging. (3) This is consistent with a study by Barrack and coworkers, which showed that many ACL-deficient patients experienced functional disability with normal daily activities. (10) Hasan and coworkers found that the ground reaction force of ACL-deficient patients was significantly different from controls in walking and pivoting activities and that these differences were most significant during the stance phase of gait. (50) Berchuck and coworkers also showed that 75% of patients had a dramatically decreased net flexion moment during normal walking as well as during jogging. (16) The magnitude of this was 140% less than normal during walking and 30% less than normal during jogging. This pattern of decreased quadriceps activity resulting in a lower flexion moment was termed the quadriceps avoidance gait. This was not present in 25% of patients, which may to some degree explain Noyes' rule that one-third of patients seem to function well in the absence of an ACL. (82) This corresponds to the 30% good and excellent results in young active patients with ACL deficiency that were reported by Barrack and coworkers. (10)

While there is general agreement that changes in gait pattern occur after ACL injury, the effect of successful ACL reconstruction on these abnormalities had not investigated until recently. Timoney and coworkers, utilizing the methods of Andriacchi and Birac, found that there was quadriceps activity during stance phase and that these patients had a net flexion moment. (105) The quadriceps avoidance gait had been reversed to some extent, but there was still a significant decrease in flexion moments when compared to normal patients. In a follow-up study to their previous work, Beard and coworkers demonstrated an improvement in proprioception after ACL reconstruction. Most of the improvement in contraction latency and function was found to occur in the first 3 mo after surgery. (14) The results of proprioceptive and gait studies following ACL reconstruction seem to indicate that sensory function is improved but not uniformly returned to normal following surgical intervention.

Neurophysiological Testing

Proprioception testing, including detection of the threshold to detection of passive motion (TTDPM) and reproduction of knee joint angles, has been pivotal in initiating interest in research into the sensory function of knee ligaments. These types of proprioceptive testing, however, do have some inherent difficulties. Results of these tests represent a composite of input from the entire extremity, including knee ligament mechanoreceptors as well as muscles, tendon, skin, and other tissue that may contribute a variable degree of sensory input. These proprioceptive tests do not necessarily isolate input from the structures in question. In addition, there is significant variability in results that is difficult to overcome, because such testing requires a high degree of patient understanding and cooperation in order to illicit consistent responses. These difficulties may, in part, explain some of the variability in results reported from this type of proprioceptive testing. In an attempt to overcome these difficulties some recent studies have focused on neurophysiological testing that does not require any input or interpretation on the part of the test subject. One recent study examined graft reinnervation following ACL reconstruction utilizing the patellar tendon in a canine model. Reinnervation was defined as a return of histological evidence of mechanoreceptors and a return of a somosensory-evoked potential (SSEP) following patellar tendon reconstruction. (6, 7)

Barrack and coworkers define the relative type and quantity of mechanoreceptors in the canine patellar tendon versus the ACL. It was discovered that the patellar tendon contained approximately 90% free nerve endings and only 10% mechanoreceptors while, conversely, the ACL contained approximately 90% mechanoreceptors and 10% free nerve endings. If reinnervation of the patellar tendon graft were to take place in a way that would allow the graft tissue to function similar to an ACL, the distribution of receptor types would have to change. In addition, SSEPs were performed on the native ACL, and a consistent response was obtained. The ACL was then excised and patellar tendon reconstruction performed. Immediately following the reconstruction no SSEP could be elicited, as was expected since it was a free graft and all nerve endings would have been severed. Six months later an SSEP was elicited in 3 of 6 cases. Histological examination of the graft at this point revealed a population of mechanoreceptors that was intermediate between that of the patellar tendon and ACL. There were approximately 50% mechanoreceptors and 50% free nerve endings. The results of this study indicate that in at least some cases, reinnervation of free patellar tendon grafts does occur. It was uncertain why this response was variable. Patellar tendon graft is a much more demanding procedure in the canine. In addition, six months may have been an inadequate time for reinnervation to occur. The results of these neurophysiological tests are consistent with previous proprioceptive, EMG, and gait studies, in the sense that there was evidence of reinnervation; however, this did not occur in every case. (See figure 19.5.)

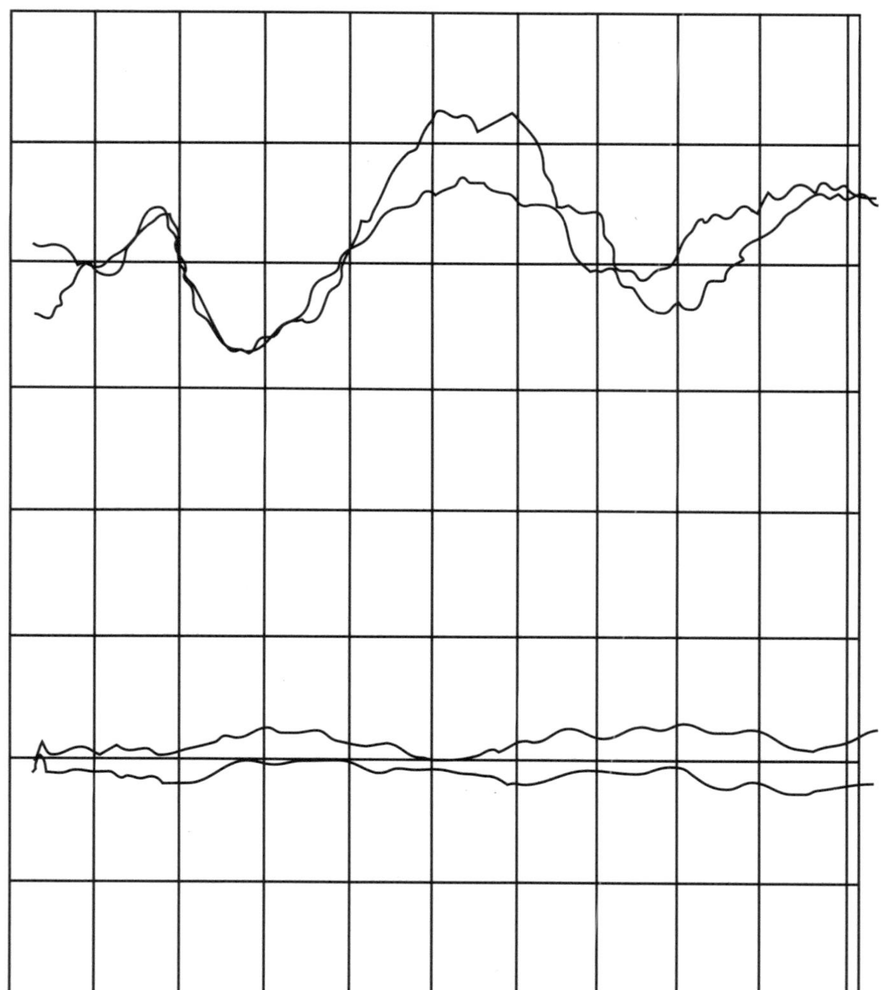

Figure 19.5a EMG of reinnervation of patellar tendon graft.

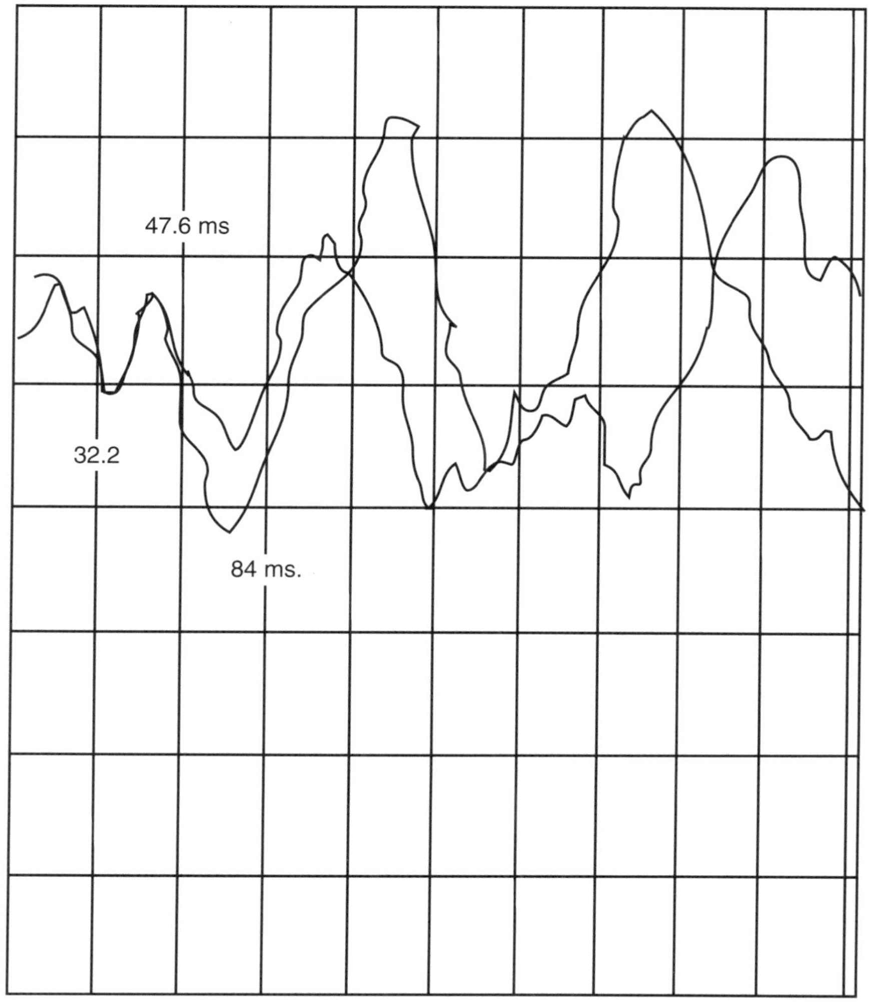

Figure 19.5b EMG of reinnervation of patellar tendon graft.

References

1. Abbott LC, Saunders JB, Dec M, et al.: Injuries to the ligaments of the knee joint. *J Bone Joint Surg* 26: 503–21, 1944.
2. Adams JA: Feedback theory of how joint receptors regulate the timing and positioning of a limb. *Psychol Rev* 84: 504–23, 1977.
3. Andriacchi TP, Birac D: Functional testing in the anterior cruciate ligament-deficient knee. *Clin Orthop* 288: 40–47, 1993.
4. Andriacchi TP, Galante JO, Fermier RW: The influence of total knee-replacement design on walking and stair climbing. *J Bone Joint Surg* 64A: 1328–335, 1982.
5. Arnoczky SP: Anatomy of the anterior cruciate ligament. *Clin Orthop* 172: 19–25, 1983.
6. Barrack RL, Lund PJ, Munn BG, et al.: Evidence of reinnervation of free patellar tendon autograft used for anterior cruciate ligament reconstruction. *Am J Sports Med* 25: 196–202, 1997.
7. Barrack RL, Lund PJ, Skinner HB: Knee joint proprioception revisited. *J Sport Rehab* 3: 18–42, 1994.
8. Barrack RL, Skinner HB: The sensory function of knee ligaments. In: *Knee Ligaments: Structure, Function, Injury, and Repair*, D Daniel, et al. (Eds.). New York: Raven Press, 1990, pp. 95–114.
9. Barrack RL, Skinner HB, Brunet ME, Cook SD: Joint kinesthesia in the highly trained knee. *J Sport Med Phys Fitness* 24: 18–20, 1983.
10. Barrack RL, Skinner HB, Buckley SL: Proprioception in anterior cruciate deficient knee. *Am J Sports Med* 17: 1–6, 1989.

11. Barrack RL, Skinner HB, Cook SD, Haddad RJ: Effect of articular disease and total knee arthroplasty on knee joint position sense. *J Neurophysiol* 50: 684–87, 1983.
12. Barrett, DS: Proprioception and function after anterior cruciate ligament reconstruction. *J Bone Joint Surg* [Br] 73B: 833–37, 1991.
13. Barrett DS, Cobb AG, Bentley G: Joint proprioception in normal, osteoarthritic, and replaced knees. *J Bone Joint Surg* [Br] 73B: 53–56, 1991.
14. Beard DJ, Dodd CAF, Simpson AH: The effect of reconstruction on proprioception in the anterior cruciate ligament-deficient knee. Paper presented at the 42d annual meeting of the Orthopaedic Research Society, Atlanta, GA, 1992.
15. Beard DJ, Kyberd PJ, Fergusson CM, et al.: Proprioception after rupture of the anterior cruciate ligament. *J Bone Joint Surg* [BR] 75B: 311–15, 1993.
16. Berchuck M, Andriacchi TP, Bach BR, et al.: Gait adaptations by patients who have a deficient anterior cruciate ligament. *J Bone Joint Surg* 72A: 871–77, 1990.
17. Biedert RM, Stauffer E, Friedrich NF: Occurrence of free nerve endings in the soft tissue of the knee joint: A histological evaluation. *Am J Sports Med* 20: 430–33, 1992.
18. Borsa PA, Lephart SM, Irrgang JJ, et al.: The effects of joint position and direction of joint motion on proprioceptive sensibility in anterior cruciate deficient athletes. *Am J Sports Med* 25: 336–40, 1997.
19. Boyd IA: The histological structure of the receptors in the knee joint of the cat correlated with their physiological response. *J Physiol* 124: 476–88, 1954.
20. Branch TP, Hunter R, Donath M: Dynamic EMG analysis of anterior cruciate deficient legs with and without bracing during cutting. *Am J Sports Med* 17: 35–41, 1989.
21. Burgess PR, Clark FJ: Characteristics of knee joint receptors in the cat. *J Physiol* 203: 317–35, 1969.
22. Caraffa A, Cerulli G, Projetti M, et al.: Prevention of anterior cruciate ligament injuries in soccer: A prospective randomized controlled study on proprioceptive training. *Knee Surg Sports Traumatol Arthroscopy* 4: 19–21, 1996.
23. Clark FJ: Information signaled by sensory fibers in medial articular nerve. *J Neurophyiol* 38: 1464–472, 1975.
24. Clark FJ, Burgess PR: Slowly adapting receptors in the cat knee joint: Can they signal joint angle? *J Neurophysiol* 38: 1448–463, 1975.
25. Clark P, MacDonald PB, Sutherland K: Analysis of proprioception in the posterior cruciate ligament-deficient knee. *Knee Surg Sports Traumatol Arthroscopy* 4: 225–27, 1996.
26. Co FJ, Skinner HB, Cannon WD: Effect of ACL reconstruction on proprioception of the knee and the heel strike transit. *Trans Orthop Res Soc* 16: 603, 1991.
27. Corrigan JP, Cashman WF, Brady MP. Proprioception in the cruciate deficient knee. *J Bone Joint Surg*[Br] 74B: 247–50, 1992.
28. D'Ambrosia RD, Solomonow M, Baratta R. Do the hamstrings provide for knee stability while performing daily functions? Paper presented at the 106th annual meeting of the American Orthopaedic Association, Coronado, CA, 1993.
29. DeAvila GA, O'Conner BL, Visco DM, Sisk TD. The mechanoreceptor innervation of the human fibular collateral ligament. *J Anat* 162: 1–7, 1989.
30. Denti M, Montleone M, Beradi A, et al.: Anterior cruciate ligament mechanoreceptors. *Clin Orthop* 308: 29–32, 1994.
31. DuToit GT: Knee joint cruciate ligament substitution: The Lindemann (Heidelberg) operation. *S Afr J Surg* 5: 25–30, 1967.
32. Ekholm J, Eklund G, Skoglund S: On the reflex effects from the knee joint of the cat. *Acta Physiol Scand* 50: 167–74, 1960.
33. Facini R, Traina GC, Graziani S, et al.: Electrophysiological study of meniscal innervation in arthroscopy. *J Sports Trauma* 12: 33–39, 1990.
34. Fahrer H, Rentsch HU, Gerber NJ, et al.: Knee effusion and reflex inhibition of the quadriceps: A bar to effective retraining. *J Bone Joint Surg* [Br] 70B: 635–38, 1988.
35. Freeman MAR, Wyke BD: Articular contributions to limb muscle reflexes: An electromyographic study of the influence of ankle joint mechanoreceptors upon reflex activity in the gastrocnemius muscle of the cat. *J Physiol* 171: 20P–21P, 1964.
36. Freeman MAR, Wyke BD: The innervation of the knee joint: An anatomical and histological study in the cat. *J Anat* 101: 505–32, 1964.
37. Freeman MAR, Wyke BD: Articular reflexes of the ankle joint: An electromyographic study of normal and abnormal influences of ankle-joint mechanoreceptors upon reflex activity in leg muscles. *Br J Surg* 54: 990–1001, 1967.
38. Friden T, Roberts D, Zatterstrom R, et al.: Proprioception in the nearly extended knee: Measurements of position and movement in healthy individuals and in symptomatic anterior cruciate ligament injured patients. *Knee Surg Sports Traumatol Arthroscopy* 4: 217–24, 1996.

39. Gardner ED: Reflex muscular responses to stimulation of articular nerves in the cat. *Am J Physiol* 161: 133–41, 1950.
40. Gardner ED: The distribution and termination of nerves in the knee-joint of the cat. *J Comp Neurol* 80: 11–32, 1944.
41. Gardner ED: The innervation of the knee joint. *Anat Rec* 101: 109–30, 1948.
42. Giove TP, Miller SJ, Kent BE, et al.: Nonoperative treatment of the torn anterior cruciate ligament. *J Bone Joint Surg* 65A: 1984–992, 1983.
43. Goertzen M, Gruber J, Dellman A, et al.: Neurohistological findings after experimental anterior cruciate ligament allograft transplantation. *Arch Orthop Trauma Surg* 111: 126–29, 1992.
44. Grigg P: Mechanical factors influencing response from joint afferent neurons from cat knee. *J Neurophysiol* 38: 1473–484, 1975.
45. Grigg P, Hoffman AH: Properties of Ruffini afferents revealed after stress analysis of isolated sections of cat knee capsule. *J Neurophysiol* 47: 41–54, 1982.
46. Grigg P., Hoffman AH: Calibrating joint capsule mechanoreceptors as in vivo soft tissue load cells. *J Biomechanics* 22: 781–85, 1989.
47. Grigg P, Hoffman AH, Fogarty KE: Properties of Golgi-Mazzoni afferents in cat knee joint capsule as revealed by mechanical studies of isolated joint capsule. *J Neurophysiol* 47: 31–40, 1982.
48. Guyton AC: *Textbook of Medical Physiology*, 7th ed. Philadelphia: Saunders, 1986.
49. Harter RA, Osternig LR, Singer KM, et al.: Long-term evaluation of knee stability and function following surgical reconstruction for anterior cruciate ligament insufficiency. *Am J Sports Med* 16: 434–42, 1988.
50. Hasan SS, Edmondstone MA, Limbird TJ, et al.: Reaction forces of injured and uninjured knees during walking and pivoting. *J Electromyogr Kinesiol* 1: 218–28, 1991.
51. Haus J, Halata Z, Refior HJ: Proprioception in the human anterior cruciate ligament: Basic morphology. *Z. Orthop* 130: 484–94, 1992.
52. Hilton J: On the influence of mechanical and physiological rest in the treatment of accidents and surgical diseases and the diagnostic value of pain. *A Course of Lectures.* London: Bell and Daldy, 1863.
53. Hoffman AH, Grigg P: Measurement of joint capsule tissue loading in the cat knee using calibrated mechanoreceptors. *J Biomechanics* 22: 787–91, 1989.
54. Horch KW, Clark FJ, Burgess PR: Awareness of knee joint angle under static conditions. *J Neurophyiol* 388: 1436–447, 1975.
55. Hughston JC, Barrett GR: Acute anteromedial rotatory instability: Long-term results of surgical repair. *J Bone Joint Surg* 65A: 145–53, 1983.
56. Hughston JC, Eilers AF: The role of the posterior oblique ligament in repairs of acute medial (collateral) ligament tears of the knee. *J Bone Joint Surg* 55A: 923–40, 1973.
57. Ihara H, Nakayama A: Dynamic joint control training for knee ligament injuries. *Am J Sports Med* 14: 309–15, 1986.
58. Insall J, Joseph DM, Aglietti P, Campbell RD: Bone-block iliotibial-band transfer for anterior cruciate insufficiency. *J Bone Joint Surg* 63A: 560–69, 1981.
59. Jeletsky AG. On the innervation of the capsule and epiphysis of the knee. *Vestn Khir* 22: 74–112, 1931.
60. Jerosch J, Prymka M: Knee joint proprioception in patients with posttraumatic recurrent patella dislocation. *Knee Surg Sports Traumatol Arthroscopy* 4: 14–18, 1996.
61. Jerosch J, Prymka M: Proprioception and joint stability. *Knee Surg Sports Traumatol Arthroscopy* 4: 171–79, 1996.
62. Johansson H: Role of knee ligaments in proprioception and regulation of muscle stiffness. *J Electromyog Kinesiol* 1: 158–79, 1991.
63. Johansson H, Sjolander P, Sojka P: A sensory role for the cruciate ligaments. *Clin Orthop* 268: 161–78, 1991.
64. Johansson H, Sjolander P, Sojka P: Receptors in the knee joint ligaments and their role in the biomechanics of the joint. *Crit Rev Biomed Eng* 18: 341–67, 1991.
65. Kalund S, Sinkjaer T, Arendt-Nelson L, Simonsen O: Altered timing of hamstring muscle action in anterior cruciate ligament deficient patients. *Am J Sports Med* 18: 245–48, 1990.
66. Kaplan FS, Nixon JE, Reitz M, et al.: Age-related changes in joint proprioception and sensation of joint position. *Acta Orthop Scand* 56: 72–74, 1985.
67. Katonis PG, Assimakopoulos, et al.: Mechanoreceptors in the posterior cruciate ligament. *Acta Orthop Scand* 62: 276–78, 1991.
68. Kennedy JC, Alexander IJ, Hayes KC: Nerve supply of the knee and its functional importance. *Am J Sports Med* 10: 329–35, 1982.
69. Kennedy JC, Weinberg HW, Wilson AS: The anatomy and function of the anterior cruciate ligament as determined by clinical and morphological studies. *J Bone Joint Surg* 56A: 223–35, 1974.
70. Kraupse R, Schmidt M, Schaible H: Sensory innervation of the anterior cruciate ligament. *J Bone Joint Surg* 74A: 390–97, 1992.
71. Lephart SM, Fu FH, Borsa PA, et al.: Proprioception of the knee and shoulder joint in normal, athletic, capsuloligamentous pathological,

and postreconstruction individuals. *Orthop Trans* 18: 1157, 1995.
72. Lephart SM, Giraldo JL, Borsa PA, Fu FH: Knee joint proprioception: A comparison between female intercollegiate gymnasts and controls. *Knee Surg Sports Traumatol Arthroscopy* 4: 121–24, 1996.
73. Lephart SM, Kocher MS, Fu FH, et al.: Proprioception following ACL reconstruction. *J Sport Rehab* 1: 188–96, 1992.
74. Lephart SM, Pincivero DM, Giraldo JL, Fu FH: The role of proprioception in the management and rehabilitation of athletic injuries. *Am J Sports Med* 25: 130–40, 1997.
75. Limbird TJ, Shiavi R, Frazer M, Borra H: EMG profiles of knee joint musculature during walking: Changes induced by anterior cruciate ligament deficiency. *J Orthop Res* 6: 630–38, 1988.
76. MacDonald PB, Hedden D, Pacin O, Sutherland K: Proprioception in anterior cruciate ligament-deficient and reconstructed knees. *Am J Sports Med*, 24: 774–78, 1996.
77. Madey SM, Wolff AJ, Rand RA, et al.: Characterization of ACL neural endings with wheat-germ agglutination horseradish immunoperoxidase. *Trans Orthop Res Soc* 18: 322, 1993.
78. McNair PJ, Marshall RN, Maguire K, Brown C: Knee joint effusion and proprioception. *Arch Phys Med Rehabil* 76: 566–68, 1995.
79. Muller W: *The Knee: Form, Function, and Ligament Reconstruction*. New York: Springer-Verlag, 1983.
80. Newberg TA: Examining joint position sense in knees having undergone anterior cruciate ligament reconstruction. Unpublished master's thesis, University of Oregon, Eugene, 1986.
81. Noyes FR, Butler DL, Paulos LE, Grood ES: Intraarticular cruciate reconstruction. I: Perspectives on graft strength, vascularization, and immediate motion after replacement. *Clin Orthop* 172: 71–77, 1983.
82. Noyes FR, Matthews DS, Mooar PA, Grood ES: The symptomatic anterior cruciate-deficient knee. II: The effects of rehabilitation, activity modification, and counseling on functional disability. *J Bone Joint Surg* 65A: 163–74, 1983.
83. O'Connor BL: The mechanoreceptor innervation of the posterior attachments of the lateral meniscus of the dog knee joint. *J Anat* 138: 15–26, 1984.
84. O'Connor BL, Viscoe DM, Brandt KD, et al.: Neurogenic acceleration of osteoarthrosis: The effects of previous neurectomy of the articular nerves on the development of osteoarthrosis after transection of the anterior cruciate ligament in dogs. *J Bone Joint Surg* 74A: 367–76, 1992.
85. Oeffenger D, Shapiro R, Nyland J, et al.: Proprioception in ACL-reconstructed knees varies among allografts, autografts, and normals. Paper presented at the 42d annual meeting of the Orthopaedic Research Society, Atlanta, GA, 1996.
86. Palmer I: Pathophysiology of the medial ligament of the knee joint. *Acta Chir Scand* 115: 312–18, 1958.
87. Pitman MI, Nainzadeh N, Menche D, et al.: The intraoperative evaluation of neurosensory function of the anterior cruciate ligament in humans using somatosensory evoked potentials. *Arthroscopy* 8: 442–47, 1992.
88. Poore GV: Paralysis of the muscular and articular sensibility. In : *Selections from the Clinical Works of Dr. Duchenne*. London: New Sydenham Society, 1883, pp. 378–98.
89. Pope MH, Johnson RJ, Brown DW, Tighe C: The role of the musculature in injuries to the medial collateral ligament. *J Bone Joint Surg* 61A: 398–402, 1979.
90. Prodromos CC, Andriacchi TP, Galante JO: A relationship between gait and clinical changes following high tibial osteotomy. *J Bone Joint Surg* 67A: 1188–194, 1985.
91. Rauber A: Uber die Vater'schen Korper der Gelenkkapseln. *Centr Med Wiss* 12: 305–306, 1874.
92. Rivard CH, Yahia LH, Rhalmi S, Newman N: Immunohistochemical demonstration of sensory nerve fibers and endings in human anterior cruciate ligaments. *Trans Orthop Res Soc* 18: 61, 1993.
93. Schultz RA, Miller DC, Kerr CS, Micheli L: Mechanoreceptors in human cruciate ligaments: A histological study. *J Bone Joint Surg* 66A: 1072–1076, 1984.
94. Schutte MJ, Dabezies EJ, Zimny ML, Happel LT: Neural anatomy of the human anterior cruciate ligament. *J Bone Joint Surg* 69A: 243–47, 1987.
95. Sherrington CS: On the proprioceptive system, especially in its reflex aspect. *Brain* 29: 467–82, 1906.
96. Sinkjaer T, Arendt-Nelson L: Knee stability and muscle coordination in patients with anterior cruciate ligament injuries: An electromyographic approach. *J Electromyog Kinesiol* 1: 209–17, 1991.
97. Skinner HB, Barrack RL Cook SD: Age-related decline in proprioception. *Clin Orthop* 184: 208–11,1984.
98. Skinner HB, Barrack RL Cook SD, Haddad RJ: Joint position sense in total knee arthroplasty. *J Orthop Res* 1: 276–83, 1984.
99. Skinner HB, Wyatt MP, Stone ML, Hodgdon JA, Barrack RL: Exercise-related knee joint laxity. *Am J Sports Med* 14: 30–34, 1986.

100. Skoglund ST: Joint receptors and kinesthesis. In: *Handbook of Sensory Physiology*, A Iggo (Ed.). New York: Springer-Verlag, 1973, pp. 111–36.
101. Solomonow M, Baratta BH, Zhou BH, et al.: The synergistic action of the anterior cruciate ligament and thigh muscles in maintaining joint stability. *Am J Sports Med* 15: 207–13, 1987.
102. Stauffer RN, Chao EY, Gyory AN: Biomechanical gait analysis of the diseased knee joint. *Clin Orthop* 126: 246–55.
103. Tibone JE, Antich TJ: Electromyographic analysis of the anterior cruciate deficient knee. *Clin Orthop* 288: 35–39, 1993.
104. Tibone JE, Antich TJ, Funton GS, et al.: Functional analysis of anterior cruciate ligament instability. *Am J Sports* Med 14: 276–84, 1986.
105. Timoney JM, Inman WS, Quesad, PM, Sharkey PF, et al.: Return of normal gait patterns after anterior cruciate ligament reconstruction. *Am J Sports Med* 21: 887–89, 1993.
106. Tsujimoto K, Andrish JT, Kambic HE, et al.: An investigation of the neurohistology and biomechanics of ACL reconstruction in goats: A comparison of primary repair and augmentation versus primary reconstruction alone. *Trans Orthop Res Soc* 18: 26, 1993.
107. Walla DJ, Albright JP, McAuley E, et al.: Hamstring control and the unstable anterior cruciate ligament-deficient knee. *Am J Sports Med* 13: 34–39, 1985.
108. Wojtys EM, Beaman DN, Glover RA, Janda D: Innervation of the human knee joint by substance P fibers. *Arthroscopy* 6: 254–63, 1990.
109. Yahia LH, Newman N: Mechanoreceptors in the canine anterior cruciate ligament. *Anat Anz* 173: 233–38, 1991.
110. Zimny ML: Mechanoreceptors in articular tissues. *Am J Anat* 182: 16–32, 1988.
111. Zimny ML, Wink CS: Neuroreceptors in the tissues of the knee joint. *J Electromyog Kinesiol* 1: 148–57, 1991.

CHAPTER 20

Effects of ACL Reconstruction on Proprioception and Neuromuscular Performance

David Beard, PhD, PT
Kathryn Refshauge, PT

Introduction

Surgical reconstruction of the ligament is increasingly preferred over conservative management for the patient with an injured anterior cruciate ligament (ACL), and the results of surgery are encouraging; several studies have shown that the operation is successful in restoring function in patients with unstable knees (1, 2, 44, 49). The exact mechanism of functional restoration remains elusive, however, as does an explanation as to why some patients continue with abnormal functions, despite a seemingly satisfactory operation. Therefore, exploration into the mechanism of joint stability, particularly restoration of stability following ACL reconstruction, continues.

Although most research has focused on the properties of passive structures involved in ligament reconstruction, that is, graft tensile strength and graft placement (3, 15, 16, 60), it is acknowledged that stabilization is unlikely to be achieved by fortification of passive joint restraints alone; studies have shown a lack of association between measures of passive joint laxity (anterior translation) and function (9, 48, 57). It may be that elements of the sensorimotor system, including physiological control mechanisms, are as important, if not more so, than the mechanical alterations to the passive structures of the joint. It is safe to assume that joint stability following ACL reconstruction is achieved by an intricate and complex interplay between the active and passive control systems of the musculoskeletal system.

One aspect of the sensorimotor system that is closely associated with stability and neuromuscular performance is proprioception, and a number of questions arise concerning proprioception and ACL reconstruction:

- Is proprioception affected by ACL injury?
- Can proprioception be changed by ACL reconstruction?
- If so, by what mechanism is it changed?
- What is the clinical significance of any change in proprioception following reconstruction?

The objective of this paper is to address each of these questions and achieve some tentative conclusion using the evidence that is available to date.

Is Proprioception Affected by ACL Injury?

The remit of this paper is to examine only the effects of reconstruction. The issues surrounding change in proprioception after initial ACL injury and the possible mechanisms involved are addressed elsewhere in this book. However, it should be stated that the evidence for sensorimotor deficits following ACL injury is far from conclusive and some controversy remains as to whether proprioception is indeed affected. Such prior evidence is obviously essential for any further exploration of the effects of intervention, such as reconstruction, on proprioception. Therefore, the following arguments presented in this paper should be interpreted in the context of such limitations.

Is Proprioception Changed by ACL Reconstruction?

The lack of a universal definition of proprioception is problematic and has possibly hampered progress in this area of research. There are many proposed definitions. Proprioception and kinesthesia are now often used interchangeably, despite the differences of meaning intended by their originators, Sherrington (50) and Bastian (8). Originally, kinesthesia was used to describe perceived sensations of joint position and movement (both active and passive), including velocity of movement, the impressions not necessarily being perceived (8, 40). Proprioception had a wider meaning and included vestibular sensation (50). Today, proprioception does not usually include vestibular sensations but may include sensory input utilized in orientating reflexes for the control of both voluntary and involuntary movement and is not necessarily consciously perceived (56). Researchers have developed various measurement techniques to indicate different aspects of proprioceptive ability. In itself, this is not unexpected, as the identification of the relative contribution of individual afferent structures to physiological events, such as proprioception, has occupied the minds of a number of eminent researchers over many years (17, 21, 36–40, 51, 55). Unfortunately, the variability in the methods of proprioceptive assessment precludes any direct comparison between studies and makes it difficult to obtain overall conclusions; the different experimental constructs likely test entirely different variables. Broadly speaking, the studies assessing proprioception can be separated into three categories: those that measure (i) joint position sense; (ii) kinesthesia, and (iii) muscle activation. Each type of study will be examined with specific reference to changes in proprioception following ACL reconstruction.

(I) Joint Position Sense

Measurement of joint position sense involves identification of a static joint angle by methods of analogy or replication. It is generally considered a reliable test and has been used in several experiments investigating proprioception of the knee (7, 17, 35, 53, 58). Most experiments have been based upon the methods of Goodwin (23), although it was Ferrell and coworkers (19, 20) who examined position sense of the human finger in great detail. In agreement with other researchers (31, 40), it was considered that the afferent input for "proprioception" is obtained from varied sources, namely, skin, joint, and muscle receptors.

The team of Barrack and Skinner and associates pioneered assessment of joint position sense as a measure of proprioception of the knee (4, 5, 53, 54). In their early papers (5, 54) they describe a simple, but innovative method in which the subject reproduces a previous knee angle set passively by an examiner. Later work showed that aging, ACL disruption, arthritis, and total knee replacement were all associated with deficits in joint position sense (53). More relevant to this discussion was the finding that there was no difference in joint position sense between limbs, in patients who had undergone ACL reconstruction (including rehabilitation). They concluded that the surgical procedure was successful in restoring joint position sense. Since no preintervention data is presented, however, this conclusion should be interpreted cautiously even though some later work, which will be outlined in subsequent sections, gives some support to this proposal.

Such a limitation is not unique, as most studies assessing proprioception after ACL reconstruction assume a proprioceptive deficit prior to intervention. Single-point measures designs show association, not cause; namely, whilst they are adequate to demonstrate differences in proprioception at one point in time, they are incapable of demonstrating effects over time due to intervention such as reconstruction.

A similar technique has been used by Barrett to examine changes in joint position sense in a group of patients 3 yrs after ACL reconstruction (6). He devised an experiment in which a blindfolded subject had a leg held in a splint and was then asked to represent the perceived angle of flexion using a visual analogue model incorporating a goniometer. The angles were set between 0° and 30°. Three groups of subjects were examined: subjects with an intact ACL (normal control subjects), patients with ACL deficiency, and patients who had undergone ACL reconstruction. A significant difference in joint position sense was found among all 3 groups. The subject with the normal intact knee was more accurate than the patient with the reconstructed knee, who was better than the patient with the ACL-deficient knee. Barrett concluded that reconstruction of the ACL improved joint position sense but not to the level of a normal uninjured limb. The lack of preintervention data limits interpretation, although this study does provide data from both control and ACL-deficient groups that can be used to demonstrate proprioceptive improvement over time in the ACL-reconstructed group.

Similar measurements of joint position sense were performed by Harter and coworkers (27). They examined joint position sense between 15° and 35° flexion in 48 ACL-reconstructed patients at 2 yrs follow-up. In contrast to the findings of Barrett (6), they found no significant difference between reconstructed and control contralateral knees and concluded that any preexisting proprioceptive deficit had been corrected at follow up. It may be of interest that subject accuracy of joint position sense for both injured and uninjured knees fell between that for subjects with ACL-intact and reconstructed knees in Barrett's work. This suggests that there may be differences in either methodology or sample characteristics between the two studies and close comparison may not be appropriate.

More recently, Co, Skinner, and Cannon (18) used reproduction of both active and passive motion methods to test for differences in joint position sense between normal uninjured, uninjured contralateral control, and ACL-reconstructed knee joints. Whilst their findings were similar to those of Harter and coworkers (27) (no difference between groups), the power of the study to detect such small differences, as the authors correctly state, is low, and therefore it provides limited evidence for a change in proprioception due to reconstruction.

There are four major papers investigating joint position sense after anterior cruciate ligament reconstruction. Three of these report no difference in proprioception between limbs (18, 27, 53); the other (6) suggests that the reconstructed limb may be improved over an ACL-deficient limb but does not achieve the accuracy of a control uninjured limb. Most of the studies can be considered comparable in terms of the joint ranges assessed (0–30°) and measurement techniques. Together, these papers provide some evidence that minimal difference exists in proprioception after reconstruction, but a lack of preintervention data limits the conclusions that can be drawn about changes over time. There is little to show that any reduced joint position sense (resulting from ACL deficit) is corrected or at least compensated by this operative procedure, which aims to restore the correct mechanical environment.

(II) Kinesthesias

Assessment of kinesthesia by measuring the threshold to detection of passive movement is a widely recognized method of assessing proprioception. The technique has been used extensively in studies of ankle proprioception (22, 25, 26, 32, 47) but has since been employed successfully to examine the ACL-deficient knee (33). The protocol involves the lower limb shank being passively moved through an angular displacement, usually at a constant velocity and with the knee joint as center of rotation. Extraneous cues and sensory information from the skin are minimized by various means. Two types of design have been used: those which assess (a) the time taken or distance moved before a subject is able to reliably perceive the direction of movement or (b) the number of times the subject can correctly identify the direction of imposed movement, from several repeated trials.

The results of studies assessing kinesthesia after reconstruction are more consistent than those examining joint position sense. In contrast to the latter studies, the evidence appears to support the premise that surgical reconstruction does not restore kinesthetic sense.

Lephart and colleagues (33) examined twelve subjects who had undergone patellar tendon-ACL reconstruction using either autograft or allograft prostheses. Two different starting positions were examined, 15° and 45° flexion. Up to 2 yrs after surgery significant kinesthetic deficits were found in the reconstructed knee compared to the uninvolved knee when starting at 15° flexion (from full extension). Interestingly, these differences were not evident when a starting position of 45° was employed, and no difference was found between autograft and allograft groups for any of the test conditions.

This difference in kinesthetic sense between normal and ACL-reconstructed knees was also found by Skinner and Barrack (53), MacDonald and coworkers (34), and Co and coworkers (18). The first two studies have shown that a deficit in kinesthetic awareness persists after surgery. However, results from the study of MacDonald and associates are difficult to interpret. Four groups of patients were tested for their ability to detect movement: subjects who were ACL deficient (*n* = 10), subjects who had undergone ACL reconstruction using a bone-patellar tendon bone graft (*n* = 8), subjects who had undergone ACL reconstruction using a hamstrings-tendon ligament graft with augmentation (*n* = 8), and a group of control uninjured subjects (*n* = 6). All 3 experimental groups showed a significantly increased threshold to detection of movement when compared to their uninvolved limb but between group analysis (which included the control group) revealed no significant differences. This unusual finding may have been due to an inability to detect differences between groups owing to low statistical power.

Regardless of the above evidence, it is still cannot be stated with certainty that reconstruction has no effect on kinesthesia. The debate is fueled by studies such as that performed by Co and coworkers (18). In addition to the aforementioned joint position sense experiments, they also examined kinesthesia after reconstruction and found a difference between limbs in ACL-reconstructed subjects (with a deficit existing in the involved limb at 31 mo). Interestingly, the threshold to detection was lower in both knees of the experimental subjects compared to that for control uninjured subjects. This leads to the unlikely suggestion that reconstruction promotes kinesthetic ability in the nonaffected limb also. A more sensible suggestion, as provided by the authors, is that the rehabilitation following surgical reconstruction cannot be ignored as a factor when attempting to establish changes in proprioception.

It appears, therefore, that a kinesthetic deficit persists after reconstruction of the ACL. However, the effect of ACL reconstruction on kinesthesia is unclear because again there is no preintervention data. It is possible that reconstruction, and rehabilitation, improves proprioception but this remains speculative until demonstrated by longitudinal studies.

(III) Hamstring Activation Studies

A further variable that has been included under the umbrella of proprioception is muscle activation pattern. By rights, such studies should be described under the sensorimotor heading rather than proprioception, as they address both sensory and motor components as opposed to purely afferent events. There are two studies that have examined hamstrings activation using EMG to give an indication of proprioceptive ability after reconstruction (10, 24).

Recent work by Beard (10) examined hamstring contraction latency before and after ACL reconstruction. Twenty-five unilateral, chronic ACL-deficient (ACLD) patients had measures of contraction latency obtained prior to, and 3 and 6 mo after reconstruction. Contraction latency was measured as the time taken for hamstrings to respond to an anteriorly directed translating force applied to the tibia whilst in standing position. The response of the hamstring muscles was recorded using surface EMGs and movement of the tibia indicated by an accelerometer attached to the tibia (14). A significant (> 9 ms) prolongation in hamstring contraction latency was found in 11 subjects (mean 34 ms) prior to intervention. All other patients had slight or no significant differences between limbs. Change in contraction latency difference over time was examined in subjects who exhibited a deficit (n = 11) and was found to significantly decrease (indicating improvement) following surgery (see figure 20.1). It was concluded that the prolonged hamstring contraction latency of cruciate-injured subjects, a measure of sensorimotor performance, could change after surgical reconstruction. However, because the first postoperative measurements

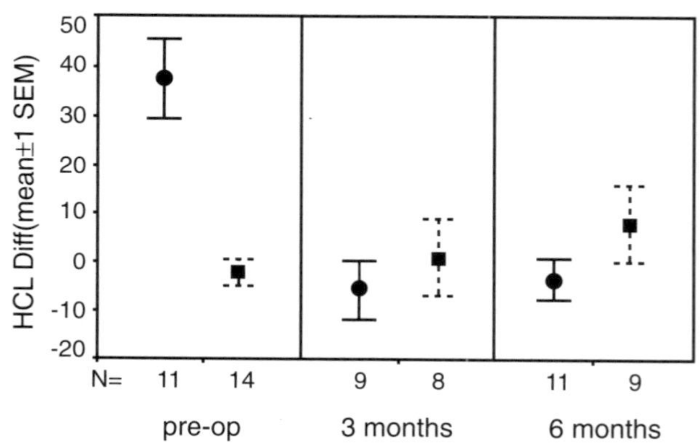

Figure 20.1 Mean ±1SEM of the difference in hamstring contraction latency (HCL) between limbs for a group of ACL-injured patients who underwent reconstruction. In addition to preop measurement, the difference at two other time intervals postreconstruction (3 and 6 mo) is shown. Subjects are classified into two groups: those with prolonged HCL prior to surgery (> 9 ms difference) λ and those who had no difference between limbs prior to surgery [ν]. The preop difference observed in some subjects (n = 11) is not evident at 3 or 6 mo. (From Beard et al. 1996.) (12).

were taken 3 mo after surgery, it could be stated that the changes were directly due to reconstruction. They may have been due to other maturation or rehabilitation.

A separate study by Grabiner and Weiker (24) recorded the recruitment pattern of the thigh muscles in a group of ACL-deficient and reconstructed patients (time since operation 6 mo to 9 yrs) during isometric knee extension exercises. Rather than studying temporal features, as in the previous study, the researchers explored the activation levels of muscle recruitment. It was found that the recruitment pattern for ACL-deficient subjects was similar to that of ACL-reconstructed patients but different from that of control uninjured subjects. Although it appeared that the reconstruction had no effect on proprioception, the lack of baseline measures suggests caution in interpreting the results.

Section Summary

Overall, it appears that selected aspects of the sensorimotor system are normal postreconstruction (i.e., joint position sense and hamstring contraction latency), whereas other aspects are impaired (kinesthesia). Further, reconstruction and rehabilitation have been shown to improve hamstring contraction latency. However, the evidence for an alteration in the sensorimotor system and proprioception due to ACL reconstruction is insubstantial. Normative and preintervention data are required before the effect of reconstruction can be established.

By What Mechanism?

Selected aspects of the sensorimotor system appear to be normal following reconstruction. The inference is that existing sensorimotor and proprioceptive deficits are restored by surgery. Unfortunately, the lack of agreement on the existence of preoperative deficit somewhat constrains any discussion on the proposed mechanism for changes following reconstruction. Nevertheless, if the evidence from the above studies is combined with information derived from associated research, including basic science, it is possible to propose some explanation.

Before taking this line of argument it is necessary to discuss the work that has shown a continued deficit in the sensorimotor system following reconstruction (i.e., work showing that reconstruction has not improved proprioception or muscle activation) (6, 24, 33, 34, 53). The most common theory explaining the sensorimotor deficit after reconstruction is based on the premise that the ACL contains receptors whose afferent output is used by the central nervous system to signal movement. Hence, rupture of the ligament interrupts this output, producing a proprioceptive deficit. Reconstruction with deinnervated tissue should do nothing to restore the interrupted sensory pathways, and the proprioceptive deficit should persist after surgery. However, such a model is controversial for two reasons. Firstly, there is now evidence for reinnnervation of ACL autograft, and secondly, the model assumes that sensory information is primarily obtained from articular structures. Whilst it is acknowledged that the origin of sensory information is from three sources (muscles, ligaments, and skin), evidence suggests that muscle receptors, rather than articular receptors, provide the most proprioceptive information at the knee (29, 32, 39).

The study of Barrett (6) is unique in that it indicates that proprioception is restored after surgery, yet not to the level of control uninjured subjects. He suggests that sensory information after ACL rupture is maintained by undamaged capsular and collateral ligaments, but the information is disorganized due to the knee moving in a nonphysiological axis. Mechanical restoration of the joint by reconstruction then enhances cortical interpretation and can result in improved joint position sense and stability. The proposal is compelling but again relies on the premise that the ACL is the primary receptor in joint position sense. A strong feature of this work is that it makes an explicit connection between the mechanics of the knee and neuromuscular control, including proprioception.

The kinesthetic studies of Harter and coworkers (27) and Co and associates (18) are more consistent with current thinking that the majority of proprioceptive feedback is muscular in origin. Again accepting the possibility that there may have been no proprioceptive deficit originally, their proposed mechanism implies that, as muscle receptors are the primary afferents, they will be unaffected by both the original injury and surgical intervention. This would then account for the similarity between limbs in proprioception following reconstruction.

However, the finding by Co and colleagues (18) that patients, after reconstruction, had better proprioception compared to uninjured controls, is more problematic. They suggest that such an effect is due to rehabilitation and the "training" of muscle receptors. The proposal would seem to suggest that after surgery muscle receptors increase their proprioceptive output to a level above that of normal limbs. As most training is bilateral, it is difficult to provide theoretical support for these findings, and even though other work (13) has shown similar findings (enhanced proprioception in ACLD limbs above that of normal limbs), the results should be interpreted with caution.

The work on hamstring contraction latency, although an indicator of the entire sensorimotor system rather than true proprioception, is especially useful in the discussion of mechanisms for change after reconstruction because the studies have preintervention data. In view of this, the work is discussed in more detail.

Hamstring Contraction Latency: Controlled Experiments

Since a change in the sensorimotor system following reconstruction was widely proposed, a series of controlled experiments was performed by Beard (10) to further investigate such changes. These experiments demonstrated that (i) the muscle response was likely to be a spinal reflex, (ii) the afferent information originated from hamstrings muscles, and (iii) hamstring contraction latency was related to the magnitude of tibial excursion occurring during the experiment, thereby suggesting a mechanical mechanism for sensorimotor loss and restoration.

(I) A Spinal Reflex?

The stretch reflex of the hamstrings (a reflex known to be monosynaptic) was recorded for normal uninjured subjects with the knee in 30° flexion using an instrumented tendon hammer. The mean latency for this stretch reflex obtained using the tendon hammer was found to be 36 ms, the order expected for a monosynaptic spinal reflex of the hamstrings. This value was comparable to the average hamstring contraction latency for normal limbs (30–40 ms), hence the event under investigation in hamstring contraction latency experiments is most likely to be a monosynaptic spinal reflex.

(II) Which Receptors?

The afferent source for the spinal reflex noted above (as found in contraction latency experiments) could have originated from skin, muscle, or articular receptors. Selected experiments were performed to exclude both the skin and articular receptors as a source of afferent information for the observed response.

Skin was excluded as the source of information by performing an experiment in which stimulation of hamstring muscle or articular receptors was deliberately avoided. In this experiment, rather than being unconstrained anteriorly as in the standard setup, the tibia was blocked and the force applied distal to the attachment of the hamstrings muscles. No muscle response was observed. This suggests that the skin was not a significant contributor of sensory information for observed response.

Other controlled experiments were required to verify that the response was hamstring muscle stretch reflex as opposed to an ACL or articular response. Although there is substantial evidence that proprioceptive information is likely to be derived from muscle receptors rather than articular receptors (29, 32, 39), further experiments were considered necessary to verify that the response was a hamstring muscle stretch reflex for this particular set of experiments. In addition, these controlled experiments showed that the latency of contraction was dependent upon the length and tension of the hamstring muscles.

Hamstring contraction latency was measured in 6 normal, uninjured knees in 3 different flexion angles: (1) the standard measurement angle, 30° flexion, (2) 0° flexion, and (3) 70° flexion. A fourth recording was then made with the knee at 30° but with the hip flexed as much as possible (approximately 90°). A similar set of experiments was then repeated on five ACLD patients.

The results for both the normal knees and ACLD knees showed a trend for prolongation of hamstring contraction latency with increasing knee flexion angle (as the hamstrings become more slack). The hip flexion angle was kept constant. This trend was more pronounced in the ACLD subjects, who had increased latency. As the contraction latency was found to decrease when the hip was flexed (hamstrings tightened) and the knee maintained in 30 , it can be concluded that the latency was independent of changes at the knee (i.e., articular structures) but was related to length and tension changes in the hamstrings. This provides evidence that the response examined in these experiments was a muscle- rather than articular receptor-generated response. (See figure 20.2.)

(III) Proposed Mechanisms

It should be noted that any proposed mechanism for change in proprioception following ACL recon-

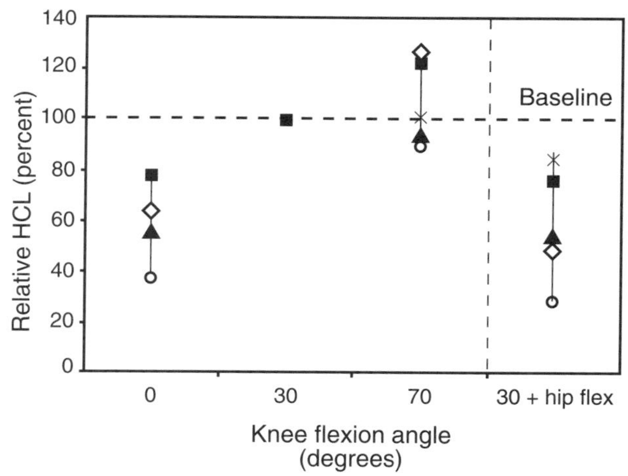

Figure 20.2 Hamstring contraction latency (HCL) at different knee flexion angles in 5 ACLD knees. Each symbol represents an individual subject (HCL normalized; HCL at 30° = 100%). (From Beard 1996).

struction is probably related to the mechanism for change in proprioception following ACL rupture. Therefore, mechanisms for change in proprioception following ACL rupture are addressed first:

Change in proprioception following ACL rupture. From the above, it is argued that the increased hamstring contraction latency is an effect of ACL injury on a spinal reflex of hamstring muscle origin. The observed delay could have been the result of (a) a prolonged neurological reflex (i.e., the time taken from stimulation of afferent receptors to motor response) or (b) a delay in stimulating the afferent receptors. Further work demonstrated that the increased latency was due to the latter.

Comparisons were made between HCL values (obtained with the apparatus) and the latency of simple stretch reflexes of the hamstrings (obtained with an instrumented tendon hammer) in five different ACLD patients. Whilst increased latency was confirmed in the ACLD limb using the HCL setup, no significant difference existed between limbs in the stretch reflexes. The delayed muscle activation in ACLD subjects would therefore seem to result from a delay in reaching the muscle receptor discharge threshold, that is, a mechanical delay in stretching the muscle, rather than deficiencies of the intrinsic neuromuscular system, such as muscle wasting, or afferent nerve conduction velocities. The question that then arises is how the condition of the ACL deficiency is responsible for producing a mechanical delay that manifests itself as a prolonged contraction latency. At this point the discussion becomes somewhat speculative.

A physical elongation of the hamstring muscles could be considered as one explanation; the hamstrings may undergo a change in muscle fiber resting length or optimal muscle fiber length (L_0), as described by Zajac (61), following ACL loss. It is feasible that such a change in muscle length could occur if the hamstrings, over time, were repeatedly stretched. Hence the delay observed in ACLD patients would result from the added time taken to achieve a critical length change of the muscle (and spindle) in the ACLD limb; in effect "taking up the slack" in the physically elongated muscle.

The arguments in support of this mechanism include the following:

1. Repeated stretching of hamstring muscles is likely in a sagittally lax knee.
2. It has been shown that the passive properties of the muscle adapt to a gradual stretch (42, 52, 59). Sarcomeres (in series) are added to the muscle in response to chronic stretch, and this would produce an increase in the optimal length (L_0) of a muscle.
3. The delays in HCL that were observed are of an appropriate magnitude to be accounted for by a physical increase in muscle length, that is, 22 ms for 1 mm increase in length, 71 ms for 10 mm increase in length (10).
4. The observed changes in HCL following both rehabilitation and reconstruction can be explained in terms of this alteration in the muscle length model.

The argument against such a mechanism is that no evidence exists for a change in the length of the muscle following ACL rupture. Muscle length changes after ACL injury and intervention have yet to be investigated.

Additional support for the change in HCL being dependent upon *mechanical* differences existing between normal and ACLD knees was obtained by examining the relationship between HCL and the anterior tibial translation occurring during the experiment. A plot combining ACLD and normal knees shows that the greater the tibial displacement, the longer the latency (see figure 20.3). As the response is a spinal reflex of the hamstrings, it could be argued that these findings give further credence to a mechanism based on alterations of muscle properties, suggesting that the muscles adjust their length according to the existing mechanical parameters of the joint.

Change in proprioception following ACL reconstruction: The results reported earlier show that the between limb difference in contraction latency

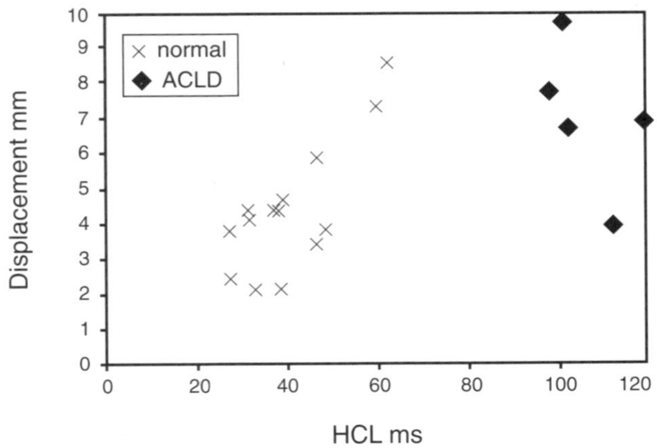

Figure 20.3 Plot of hamstring contraction latency (HCL) against forced tibial displacement (FTD) for 14 normal knees and 5 ACLD knees. (From Beard 1996).

decreased over time, possibly due to reconstruction. In accordance with the muscle receptor model and arguments given previously, reduction in HCL could have occurred by physical change in the muscle length. Following cruciate rupture sarcomeres may have been added to the muscle in response to chronic stretch. It is possible that, after ACL reconstruction, a change in the optimal length (L_0) of the muscle towards its preinjury level occurred by reduction in the number of sarcomeres.

(IV) Which Intervention: Rehabilitation or Reconstruction?

An important issue remains unresolved. Regardless of the mechanism, because all patients underwent rehabilitation following surgery, it still remains uncertain which *intervention* was responsible for the improvement in HCL. The improvement could have resulted from

1. maturation,
2. surgical restoration of joint mechanics, or
3. rehabilitation following surgery.

Maturation: Although unlikely due to the magnitude of the changes in HCL, maturation cannot be fully ruled out as a reason for the improved contraction latency after reconstruction. Further work should include a control group that does not undergo reconstruction.

Surgical restoration of the joint mechanics: Restoration of joint mechanics following reconstructive surgery could produce a readjustment of the hamstrings muscles to the new working parameters of the joint. It may be that surgery, by constraining anterior translation and preventing repeated stretching of the muscle, resulted in a physical shortening (restoration of normal length) of the muscle.

The mean forced tibial displacement for the ACL-reconstructed knee (5.9 mm) was found to be less than in the ACL-deficient knee (7.0 mm), and although the sample size was small, there was a weak relationship between tibial displacement and HCL. (See figure 20.4) This provides some support for the reduction in HCL being due to a restoration of joint mechanics.

Although a mechanism based on changes in muscle spindle threshold due to increased or decreased gamma fiber activity (30) had been effectively ruled out for this experiment (because of the disparity between HCL and simple stretch reflex obtained with the tendon hammer), it should not be dismissed for all proprioceptive changes. As Barrett (6) has stated, if mechanical integrity is a prerequisite for meaningful sensory information, then restoration of mechanics may have allowed previously uninterpretable sensory signals to be of value once again, thus producing a faster response.

It was concluded that restoration of joint kinematics may well contribute to the changes in HCL following ACL reconstruction, but the mechanism remains somewhat speculative in the absence of strong evidence.

Rehabilitation following surgery: The rehabilitation (as distinct from reconstruction) should also be considered as a possible source for the changes in the sensorimotor system: specific exercise programs have already been shown to improve contraction latency and proprioception (13, 28). However, because the intensity and difficulty of exercises were gradually increased with increasing time since surgery, any effects of rehabilitation on HCL would perhaps be more likely seen later in the study, that is, between 3 and 6 mo. Most changes were found to occur between reconstruction and 3 mo, hence the argument for the sensorimotor changes being due to rehabilitation rather than reconstruction is weak. Further investigation is warranted into the time at which changes occur following surgery.

What Is the Clinical Significance of Any Changes?

There are several clinical implications of changes in the sensorimotor system following injury. One issue is the relationship between function and proprioception. Although studies have used different experimental constructs, there is some evidence of

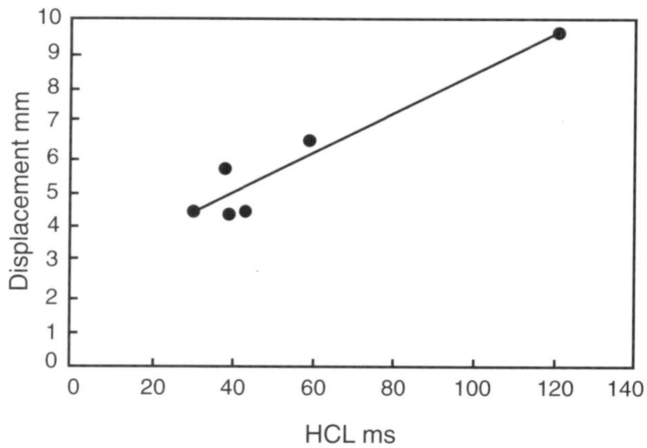

Figure 20.4 Forced anterior tibial displacement (FTD) versus hamstring contraction latency in 6 ACL-reconstructed knees. (From Beard et al. 1996).

a positive relationship between functional outcome and selected aspects of proprioception in both the ACL-injured and reconstructed knee (6, 11, 41). This suggests that proprioception should always be considered in the overall management of ACL-injured patients. However, the magnitude of deficit that constitutes a clinical significance remains unknown.

If successful outcome following surgical reconstruction (i.e., functional stability) is dependent on the sensorimotor system and proprioceptive ability around the knee joint, then efforts should be made to enhance and facilitate proprioception during and following the operation. If articular receptors are considered to contribute, then consideration should be given to the procedure itself, including limitation of tissue damage and the provision of an optimum environment for nerve regeneration. Interestingly, recent research has shown that the preservation of the ACL stump at reconstruction is not necessarily beneficial in terms of normalizing proprioception or outcome (34).

It may be suggested that, in addition to merely obtaining a mechanical block of excessive translation, aims of surgery should be to provide the optimal mechanical environment for afferent feedback. Such a proposition is upheld by the documented lack of association between passive joint laxity (as measured by an arthrometer) and functional outcome following ACL injury (9, 48, 57). Whilst a similar association is less obvious for ACL reconstruction, there is some anecdotal evidence that a joint with decreased laxity compared to the uninvolved knee (too tight a graft) can lead to decreased function.

In terms of rehabilitation, exercises to enhance the sensorimotor system (particularly contraction latency) should be prescribed early in the management after reconstruction. Such exercises have already been explored to some extent in the ACL knee and these may be generalized to the reconstructed knee (13, 28). Furthermore, the limited evidence that knee orthoses can improve proprioceptive ability (7, 45, 46) may indicate that postsurgical bracing should focus upon a sensory, rather than mechanical role.

As reported by Lephart and coworkers (33), it remains unclear whether proprioceptive deficits in ACL-injured patients contribute to degenerative joint conditions. However, the animal work of O'Connor and coworkers (43) provides substantial evidence that proprioceptive ability is a factor in joint degeneration, and results of longer-term follow-up studies that employ measures of proprioception will show whether such findings can be extrapolated to ACL-reconstructed subjects.

One final clinical implication is the use of proprioception as a milestone in rehabilitation and return to athletic activity. Harter and colleagues (27) have recommended that patients should not be released from the postoperative rehabilitation program (with return to sport) until any proprioceptive deficits have been restored. The suggestion is that patients will be better able to protect their graft and may avoid re-injury.

Whilst investigations into proprioception are valuable, care must be taken not to overemphasize the importance of sensorimotor performance, and especially proprioception, for this condition. In one study (11), the functional gains achieved following ACL reconstruction occurred without an improvement in muscle contraction latency. In addition, some patients who underwent reconstruction had minimal sensorimotor deficit prior to surgery but still required operative intervention. The function of these patients, which was *poor* prior to reconstruction, improved after operation. This does suggest that sensorimotor performance (in this case hamstring contraction latency) is perhaps not as significant for functional outcome following ACL reconstruction as for ACL-deficient patients. It may be that overall improvement in function following ACL reconstruction is likely to be a combined effect of rehabilitation and kinematic restoration, and although these may *affect* the sensorimotor performance and proprioception, improvement is not necessarily *dependent* on changes in the sensorimotor system and proprioception.

Summary

1. Studies examining sensorimotor performance and proprioception after ACL reconstruction

are often incomparable and their results conflict.
2. Most studies are limited in that they have no preintervention data. Observed differences could be attributed to the effects of maturation or other interventions such as exercise.
3. The research that provides stronger evidence of change following reconstruction does not address truly afferent "proprioception" but examines sensorimotor performance, which includes both afferent and efferent components.
4. Providing there is a preexisting sensorimotor deficit following ACL rupture, only weak evidence exists to support a change in sensorimotor performance following ACL reconstruction.
5. The aforementioned uncertainty about sensorimotor changes following rupture or reconstruction limits any discussion of a proposed mechanism.
6. Studies proposing mechanisms fit into two main categories: those that consider the ACL receptors as the primary afferent receptor and those that take muscle receptors as the primary receptor.
7. Most evidence to date supports a mechanism in which the muscle receptor is the primary afferent receptor. Thus if change in sensorimotor performance occurs following reconstruction, it is likely to be due to the effect of surgery (or time) on these muscle receptors.
8. The following observations relate specifically to hamstring contraction latency experiments:
   - A simple mechanical delay in stretching the hamstring muscle appears to be the most likely mechanism for increased hamstring contraction latency found in the ACLD limb.
   - Increased contraction latency of ACLD limbs may be accounted for by alterations in the optimum length (L_0) of the muscle (i.e., a true change in length).
   - Changes in contraction latency following re construction may have resulted from further alteration in the resting or optimum length (L_0) of the muscle.
9. Because reconstruction is never performed without comprehensive rehabilitation, it is not possible to delineate their relative contributions to sensorimotor change (if present).
10. In view of the limited evidence for sensorimotor changes, clinical implications are restricted. However, sensorimotor performance and proprioception should be considered in the surgical technique and rehabilitation for ACL-injured patients.

References

1. Anderson AF, Snyder RB, Lipscomb AB: Anterior cruciate ligament reconstruction using the semitendinosus and gracilis tendons augmented by the Losee iliotibial band tenodesis. *Am J Sports Med* 22(5): 620–31, 1994.
2. Andersson C, Odensten M, Gillquist J: Knee function after surgical or nonsurgical treatment of acute rupture of the anterior cruciate ligament: A randomized study with long-term follow-up period. *Clin Orthop* 264: 255–63, 1991.
3. Arms SW, Pope MH, Johnson RJ, Fischer RA, Arvidsson I, Eriksson E: The biomechanics of anterior cruciate ligament rehabilitation and reconstruction. *Am J Sports Med* 12(1): 8–18, 1984.
4. Barrack RL, Skinner HB, Buckley SL: Proprioception in the anterior cruciate-deficient knee. *Am J Sports Med* 17(1): 1–6, 1989.
5. Barrack RL, Skinner HB, Cook SD: Perception of the knee joint. *Am J Phys Med* 63: 175–81, 1984.
6. Barrett DS: Proprioception and function after anterior cruciate ligament reconstruction. *J Bone Joint Surg* [Br] 73B(5): 833–37, 1991.
7. Barrett DS, Cobb AG, Bentley G: Joint proprioception in normal, osteoarthritic, and replaced knees. *J Bone Joint Surg* [Br] 73B(1): 53–56, 1991.
8. Bastian HC: The functions of the kinesthetic area of the brain. *Brain* 32: 327–41, 1909.
9. Beard DJ: An investigation into the relationship between knee joint laxity and knee function in anterior cruciate ligament-deficient subjects. MSc thesis, Kings College, London. 1992.
10. Beard DJ: Hamstring contraction latency following anterior cruciate ligament rupture, rehabilitation, and reconstruction. Doctoral dissertation, Oxford, London. 1996.
11. Beard DJ: Hamstring contraction latency following anterior cruciate ligament rupture, rehabilitation, and reconstruction (abstract). *Physiotherapy* 82(9): 540, 1996.
12. Beard DJ, Dodd CAF, Simpson AHRW: The effect of reconstruction on proprioception in the anterior cruciate ligament-deficient knee. Paper presented at the 2d World Congress on Sports Trauma/American Orthopaedic Society for Sports Medicine (AOSSM), Lake Buena Vista, Florida, USA, 1996. 13. Beard DJ, Dodd CAF, Trundle H, Simpson AHRW: Proprioceptive enhancement for anterior cruciate ligament deficiency: A prospective randomized trial of two physiotherapy regimes. *J Bone Joint Surg* [Br] 76B(4): 654–59, 1994.

14. Beard DJ, Kyberd PJ, O'Connor JJ, Fergusson CM, Dodd CAF: Reflex hamstring contraction latency in anterior cruciate ligament deficiency. *J Orthop Res* 12(2): 219–28, 1994.
15. Beynnon B, Braden C, Fleming B, Johnson R, Nichols C, Renström P, Pope M: Anterior cruciate ligament strain behavior during rehabilitation exercises in vivo. *Am J Sports Med* 23: 24–33, 1995.
16. Beynnon B, Howe J, Pope M, Johnson R, Fleming B: The measurement of anterior cruciate ligament strain in vivo. *Orthopedics* 16: 1–12, 1992.
17. Clark FJ, Horch KW, Bach SM, Larson GF: Contributions of cutaneous and joint receptors to static knee-position sense in man. *J Neurophysiol* 42: 877–88, 1979.
18. Co HF, Skinner HB, Cannon WD: Effect of reconstruction of the anterior cruciate ligament on proprioception of the knee and the heel strike transient. *J Orthop Res* 11: 696–704, 1993.
19. Ferrell W, Gandevia S, McCloskey D: The role of joint receptors in human kinesthesia when intramuscular receptors cannot contribute. *J Physiol* 386: 63–71, 1987.
20. Ferrell WR, Smith A: Position sense at the proximal interphalangeal joint of the human index finger. *J Physiol* 399: 49–61, 1988.
21. Gandevia SC: Kinesthesia: Roles for afferent signals and motor commands. In *Integration of Motor, Circulatory, Respiratory, and Metabolic Control During Exercise.* American Physiological Society, 1996, 128–72.
22. Garn SN, Newton RA: Kinesthetic awareness in subjects with multiple ankle sprains. *Phys Ther* 68(11): 1667–671, 1988.
23. Goodwin GM: The sense of limb position and movement. *Exer and Sport Sci Rev* 4: 87–124, 1976.
24. Grabiner MD, Weiker GG: Anterior cruciate ligament injury and hamstrings coactivation. *Clin Biomech* 8: 215–19, 1993.
25. Gross MT: Effects of recurrent lateral ankle sprains on active and passive judgments of joint position. *Phys Ther* 67(10): 1505–509, 1987.
26. Gurfinkel VS, Lipshits MI, Popov KE: Kinesthetic thresholds in the orthograde posture. *Agressologie* 20B: 133–34, 1979.
27. Harter RA, Osternig LR, Singer KM: Knee joint proprioception following anterior cruciate ligament reconstruction. *J Sport Rehab* 1: 103–10, 1992.
28. Ihara H, Nakayama A: Dynamic control joint training for knee ligament injuries. *Am J Sports Med* 14(4): 309–15, 1986.
29. Johansson H: Role of knee ligaments in proprioception and regulation of muscle stiffness. *J Electromyogr Kinesiol* 1(3): 158–79, 1991.
30. Johansson H, Sjölander P, Sojka P: Receptors in the knee joint ligaments and their role in the biomechanics of the joint. *CRC Crit Rev in Biomed Eng* 18(5): 341–68, 1991.
31. Johansson H, Sjolander P, Sojka P: A sensory role for the cruciate ligaments. *Clin Orthop* 268: 161–78, 1991.
32. Konradsen L, Ravn J, Sørensen A: Proprioception at the ankle: The effect of anaesthetic blockade of ligament receptors. *J Bone Joint Surg* [Br] 75B(4): 433–36, 1993.
33. Lephart SM, Kocher MS, Fu FH, Borsa BA, Harner CD: Proprioception following anterior cruciate ligament reconstruction. *J Sport Rehab* 1: 188–96, 1992.
34. MacDonald PB, Hedden D, Pacin O, Sutherland K: Proprioception in anterior cruciate ligament-deficient and reconstructed knees. *Am J Sports Med* 24(6): 774–78, 1996.
35. Marks R: Repeatability of position sense measurements in persons with osteoarthritis of the knee: A pilot study. *Clin Rehab* 9: 314–19, 1995.
36. Marsden C, Merton P, Morton H: Stretch reflex and servo action in a variety of human muscles. *J Physiol* 259: 531–68, 1976.
37. Marsden C, Merton P, Morton H: New observations on the human stretch reflex. *J Physiol* 360: 51P, 1985.
38. Matthews PBC: Where does Sherrington's muscular sense originate? *Ann Rev Neurosci* 5: 189–218, 1982.
39. Matthews PBC: Proprioceptors and their contribution to somatosensory mapping: Complex messages require complex processing. *Can J Physiol Pharmacol* 66: 430–37, 1988.
40. McCloskey DI: Kinesthetic sensibility. *Physiol Rev* 58: 763–820, 1978.
41. McNair PJ, Wood GA, Marshall RN: Stiffness of the hamstrings muscles and its relationship to function in anterior cruciate ligament-deficient individuals. *Clin Biomech* 7: 131–37, 1992.
42. Moseley AM: The effect of casting combined with stretching on passive ankle dorsiflexion in adults with traumatic head injuries. *Phys Ther* 77(3): 240–59, 1997.
43. O'Connor BL, Visco DM, Brandt KD, Albrecht M, O'Connor AB: Sensory nerves only temporarily protect the unstable canine knee joint from osteoarthritis. *Arthritis and Rheumatism* 36(8): 1154–163, 1993.
44. Odensten M, Hamburg P, Nordin M, Lysholm J, Gillquist J: Surgical or conservative treatment of the acutely torn anterior cruciate ligament—

a randomized study: Term follow-up observations. *Clin Orthop* 198: 88–93, 1995.

45. Osternig LR, Robertson RN: Effects of prophylactic knee bracing on lower extremity joint position and muscle activation during running. *Am J Sports Med* 21(5): 733–37, 1993.
46. Perlau R, Frank C, Fick G: The effect of elastic bandages on human knee proprioception in the uninjured population. *Am J Sports Med* 23(2): 251–55, 1995.
47. Refshauge KM, Fitzpatrick RC: Perception of movement at the human ankle: Effects of leg position. *J Physiol* 488(1): 243–48, 1995.
48. Seto JL, Orofino AS, Morrissey MC, Medeiros JM, Mason WJ: Assessment of quadriceps and hamstring strength, knee ligament stability, functional and sports activity levels five years from ACL reconstruction. *Am J Sports Med* 16(2): 170–79, 1988.
49. Shelbourne KD, Klootwyk TE, Wilckins JH, De Carlo MS: Ligament stability two to six years after anterior cruciate ligament reconstruction with autogenous patellar tendon graft and participation in accelerated rehabilitation program. *Am J Sports Med* 23(5): 575–79, 1995.
50. Sherrington CS: The muscular sense. In *Textbook of Physiology*, vol 2. Edinburgh: Pentland, 1900, 1002–1025.
51. Sherrington C: On the proprioceptive system, especially in its reflex aspects. *Brain* 29: 467, 1906.
52. Simpson AHRW, Williams PE, Kyberd PJ, Goldspink G, Kenwright J: The response of muscles to stretch. *J Bone Joint Surg* [Br] 77B: 630–36, 1995.
53. Skinner HB, Barrack RL: Joint position sense in the normal and pathologic knee joint. *J Electromyog and Kines* 1(3): 180–90, 1991.
54. Skinner HB, Barrack RL, Cook SD: Age-related decline in proprioception. *Clin Orthop* 184: 208–11, 1984.
55. Skoglund S: Anatomical and physiological studies of knee joint innervation in the cat. *Acta Physiol Scand* 36(suppl 124): 1–101, 1956.
56. Swash M: Position sense in a damaged knee [letter]. *J Neurol Neurosurg Psych* 49: 100, 1986.
57. Walla DJ, Albright JP, McAuley E, Martin RK, Eldridge V, El-Khoury G: Hamstring control and the unstable anterior cruciate deficient knee. *Am J Sports Med* 13(1): 34–40, 1985.
58. Warren PJ, Olanlokun TK, Cobb AG, Bentley G: Proprioception after knee arthroplasty: The influence of prosthetic design. *Clin Orthop* 297: 182–87, 1993.
59. Williams PE, Simpson AHRW, Kyberd P, Kenwright J, Goldspink G: Physiological and structural changes in the rabbit anterior tibialis muscle following surgical limb lengthening. *J Physiol* 344: 571, 1992.
60. Woo S-Y, Young E, Kwan M: Fundamental studies in knee ligament mechanics. In *Knee Ligaments: Structure, Function, Injury, and Repair.* New York: Raven Press, 1990, 115.
61. Zajac F: Muscle and tendon: Properties, models, scaling, and application to biomechanics and motor control. *Crit Rev in Biomed Eng* 17(4): 359–411, 1989.

CHAPTER 21

Effects of Injury and Reconstruction of the Posterior Cruciate Ligament on Proprioception and Neuromuscular Control

Marc R. Safran, MD
Christopher D. Harner, MD
Jorge L. Giraldo, MD
Freddie H. Fu, MD
Scott M. Lephart, PhD, ATC

Introduction

Our current understanding of the posterior cruciate ligament (PCL) lags behind that of the ACL by 10 years. Many reasons for this exist, including greater difficulty in making the correct diagnosis, infrequency of isolated injury to the PCL, and the presumed benign course following PCL injury. As such, previous research has concentrated on more common knee ligamentous injuries such as the medial collateral ligament (the most commonly injured knee ligament) and anterior cruciate ligament (the ligament most commonly injured resulting in residual pathological laxity). PCL injuries are being recognized more frequently, stimulating interest in the biomechanics of this ligament as well as the biomechanical and neurosensory contribution of this ligament to knee function. This is particularly true in light of the known neurosensory and mechanical contributions of the anterior cruciate ligament (ACL) in knee function. Further, the natural history, treatment, and techniques of reconstruction of the PCL are topics of great debate at this time. Critical analysis of the documented clinical results after different treatment protocols (including nonoperative) has been handicapped by heterogeneous patient populations, and the lack of uniform criteria to assess and document the results of treatment has resulted in this debate and controversy.

One of the main reasons for controversy about the treatment of isolated posterior cruciate ligament (PCL) injuries is the unclear fate of the isolated PCL-injured knee. Many authors and surgeons note that often patients function well, even in high level sports, with a torn posterior cruciate ligament. This is in direct contradistinction with the ACL-injured knee. The reason for this difference is not clear, as the PCL is a larger and stronger ligament as compared with the ACL.

For years, knee surgeons have postulated that the sensory loss associated with ACL injury may affect the results of ACL repair and reconstruction (2, 7, 34). DuToit (20), Insall and coworkers (31), and others (36, 42, 48) have all advocated certain reconstructive techniques, in part, to increase afferent preservation. A proprioceptive deficit has been demonstrated following ACL disruption (2, 4, 7, 14); however, little research exists evaluating proprioception in the PCL-deficient or reconstructed knee.

Unlike combined ligament injuries involving the PCL, there is much more debate about the natural history and treatment of the "isolated" PCL-deficient knee (10, 15, 17, 19, 22, 33, 46, 52, 58). It is well known that in the ACL-deficient knee, instability and reinjury can lead to arthritis over time (9, 23, 29, 41, 43, 49, 53, 56). Further, authors suggest that function in the ACL-deficient and reconstructed knee is more reliably predicted by proprioceptive ability than physical examination or knee test scores (4, 7, 14, 30). Several studies have shown that proprioceptive deficits that exist in ACL-deficient knees can be partially restored by surgical reconstruction (2, 4, 13). While the relationship of reduced proprioception in the arthritic knee is not known, some suggest that proprioceptive loss results in arthritis (5, 55).

Many authors note that patients with "isolated" PCL deficiency initially function well, while progression to degenerative arthritis over time is less well defined (10, 19, 46, 52). To our knowledge, the University of Pittsburgh Neuromuscular Research Laboratory is the only lab to study the potential proprioceptive deficits in the PCL-deficient knee and assess the neuromuscular effects of PCL reconstruction. The following summarizes our protocol and the results of proprioceptive testing in subjects with isolated PCL injuries and those who underwent PCL reconstruction.

PCL-Injured Subjects

We prospectively studied 18 subjects with isolated ruptures of the PCL. These subjects ranged in age from 19 to 51 yrs (average: 32 yrs). The time from injury to examination and proprioception testing averaged 29 mo (range: 1–226 mo). No patient could have an inner ear or equilibrium disorder, previous neurological disease, or contralateral knee injury.

All subjects underwent a complete history and thorough knee examination. Examination of the posterior cruciate ligament begins with the knowledge that the medial tibial plateau normally is 10 mm anterior to the medial femoral condyle with the knee in 90° flexion. Posterior drawer testing is then graded as follows. In a grade I injury there is asymmetry side to side, but the medial tibial plateau remains anterior to the medial femoral condyle (less than 10 mm). In a grade II injury the posterior drawer at 90° pushes the tibial plateau to the level of the medial femoral condyle (approximately 10 mm). In a grade III PCL injury, the medial tibial plateau can be pushed posterior to the medial femoral condyle (more than 1 cm). The posterior sag is similarly graded: grade I is when the medial tibial plateau sits further posteriorly than the "normal" contralateral knee but still anterior to the medial femoral condyle with the knee flexed approximately 90°; in a grade II the tibial plateau is at the level of the medial femoral condyle, and a grade III step-off is when the medial tibial plateau rests posterior to the medial femoral condyle. To be an isolated PCL tear, no anterior cruciate or collateral ligament injury is noted. Further, posterior lateral rotatory instability (dial test) at 30° must be symmetric. Many so-called grade III PCL injuries have concomitant capsular and posterolateral corner involvement.

A standard radiographic knee series, including flexion weight-bearing PA view, lateral and sunrise views, and a magnetic resonance imaging scan were obtained on all subjects. KT-1000 (KT-1000, MEDmetric; San Diego, California) instrumented knee testing was also performed to assess the degree of laxity of both knees for comparison.

PCL-Reconstructed Subjects

Ten men with unilateral PCL injury, who underwent PCL reconstruction by the senior author, were evaluated. These subjects ranged in age from 23 to 54 yrs (average: 31 yrs). Five left knees and 5 right knees were involved. Seven patients had an isolated PCL rupture and no other knee disorder. One patient had concomitant medial tibiofemoral chondrosis, 1 had lateral patellar and tibiofemoral chondrosis (this patient underwent an open lateral meniscal transplantation), and another had tricompartmental arthrosis. The time from reconstruction to proprioceptive testing ranged from 6 to 44 mo (average: 27 mo). Patients were examined clinically and with the knee ligament arthrometer (KT-1000, MEDmetric; San Diego, California).

All subjects were tested on the proprioceptive testing device developed at the University of Pittsburgh (modeled after that of Barrack) (see figure 21.1). Subjects with isolated PCL-deficient knees were tested for threshold to detect passive motion (kinesthesia) and the ability to passively reproduce passive positioning (joint position sense). Based on the results of this study, those patients who underwent PCL reconstruction had proprioception kinesthesia testing by studying the threshold to detect passive motion only.

A proprioceptive testing device (PTD) was used to measure kinesthesia as the threshold to detec-

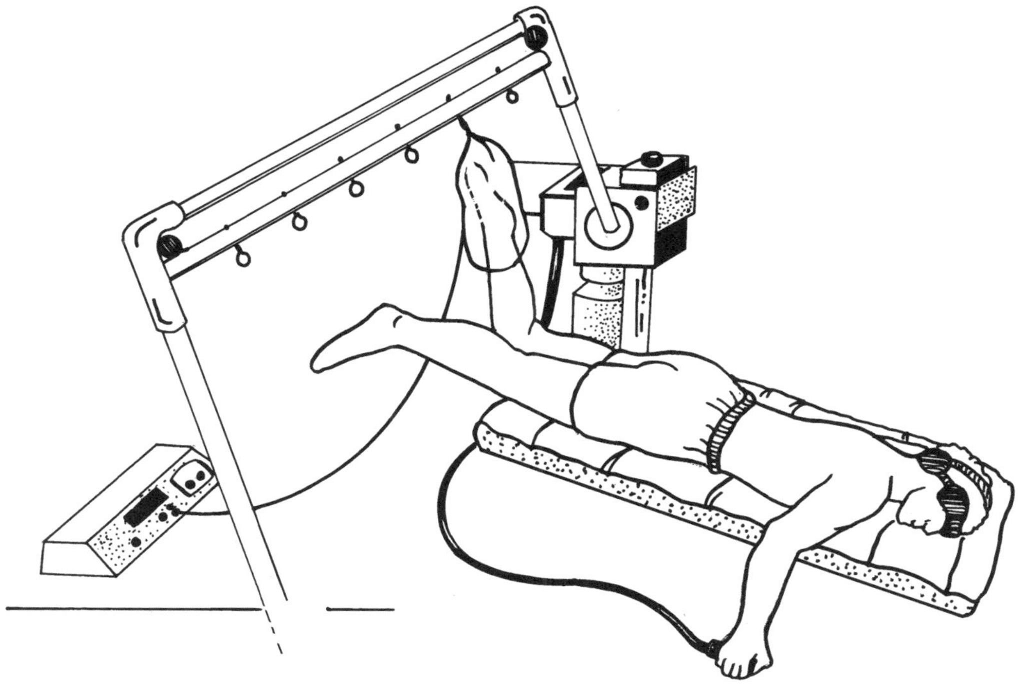

Figure 21.1 Proprioception testing device for PCL proprioception.

tion of passive movement (TTDPM) and joint position sense by the ability to passively reproduce passive joint positioning (RPP). This device has been used previously to assess proprioceptive awareness (38). The PTD rotates the knee into flexion and extension through the axis of the joint. A rotational transducer interfaced with a digital microprocessor counter provided the angular displacement values directly. A pneumatic compression boot was placed on each foot to reduce cutaneous input. One pneumatic boot was attached to the moving bar of the PTD, the other to a stationary bar. Patients were tested in the prone position to reduce the likelihood of cutaneous input of their upper calf hitting the testing bench in higher degrees of flexion, as would occur if they were seated upright.

The knee was tested moving into flexion and extension from two starting positions. These positions were 45° and 110° of knee flexion. The midrange of knee motion (45°) was chosen as a starting position because there, the capsule, ACL, and PCL are relatively relaxed, and, thus, the poorest proprioceptive sensory results should be noted. No difference should exist, therefore, between the injured and uninjured knees. Knee flexion of 110° was chosen, since tension on the PCL should play a role in proprioception, and thus some difference in afferent input might be identified. This is based on the findings of Wascher and coworkers, who showed a low to intermediate resultant force in the substance of the PCL in 45° flexion, and significantly greater resultant force with increasing knee flexion (60).

Two familiarity trial tests were performed prior to the subjects being blindfolded and having a headset placed over the ears to negate visual and auditory cues. Testing was performed in a single session with test order of injured and uninjured knee, starting position, and direction of movement being randomized and counterbalanced. The PTD tester was blinded as to the normal and PCL injured knee. Instrument reliability was established previously as intraclass correlations (ICC) were calculated using a fixed model and ranged from ICC = .87 to ICC = .92.

Threshold to detection of passive motion: TTDPM assessment was started with the motor and shaft of the PTD disengaged. Subjects were blindfolded and had earphones placed over their ears. The subject gave a thumbs-up to indicate readiness to perform the test. At a random point during the subsequent 20 s, knee movement was engaged by the tester. The subject disengaged the PTD by pressing a handheld switch upon perception of sensation of movement at the knee. The PTD rotated the knee at a constant angular velocity of 0.5°/s. This slow speed was chosen to minimize contribution from muscle receptors while maximally stimulating slow adapting joint mechanoreceptors. Three trials from a starting position of 45° and 110° knee flexion moving into both flexion and extension were performed. Both the injured and uninjured knees were tested. Mean TTDPM values were calculated for the 4 test conditions.

Reproduction of passive positioning: The subjects were blindfolded but permitted to communicate with the PTD tester during RPP testing. As with the TTDPM testing, 45° and 110° knee flexion were used as starting positions (reference angle). After confirmation of the subject's readiness, the knee was moved passively 10° into further flexion or extension (presented angle) by the tester. The angles were presented at variable velocities in order to reduce any time-associated cues. The limb was held in the presented angle position for 10 s and the subject was asked to concentrate on this position. The limb was then returned passively to the reference angle by the examiner. The subject was then instructed to manipulate the on/off switch to reproduce the previously presented angle at an angular velocity of 0.5°/s. This was recorded and repeated for each of the 3 starting positions moving into flexion and extension. The difference between the presented angle and the angle that was repositioned by the subject was calculated as the error of reproduction. The mean of 3 trials was calculated for the 4 test conditions.

PCL-injured and uninjured knee mean differences were analyzed using a paired *T* test for both TTDPM and RPP testing. A p value of .05 was considered to indicate a significant difference. Pearson product moment correlation coefficients were established between all dependent variables.

Results for PCL-Injured Subjects

Eighteen subjects met the criteria for inclusion—isolated PCL injury without contralateral knee injury, surgery, or other concomitant knee injury. These 13 males and 5 females averaged 32 yrs of age. The patients averaged 29 mo from time of injury to proprioception testing. There were 10 right knees injured and 8 left knees. All individuals except 3 (including the one who underwent PCL reconstruction 1 mo after the injury) underwent physical therapy stressing quadriceps rehabilitation.

On physical examination, 15 patients (83%) had a grade II posterior drawer test on physical examination, while the remaining 3 patients (17%) had a grade III posterior drawer test. Two subjects had minimal laxity of the medial collateral ligament, while there was no other ligamentous injury (ACL, MCL, LCL, rotatory instability) identified on physical examination of any of the subjects. Nine patients (50%) returned to their previous level of sporting activity, 5 participate in sports at a lower level, and 4 do not participate in sports at all (2 did not participate in sports prior to injury).

KT-1000 instrumented testing revealed an average corrected posterior displacement of 7.5 mm (range: 2.5–12.5 mm), manual maximum side-to-side difference at 90°, and 3.1 mm manual maximum side-to-side difference at 20° of knee flexion. Plain radiographs showed no degenerative changes in any of the 18 subjects. Magnetic resonance imaging of all 18 subjects revealed an isolated PCL tear with no meniscal or chondral injuries.

For TTDPM starting at 45°, the PCL-injured knee averaged 1.5° ±0.2°, while the uninjured knee averaged 1.2° ± 0.1° (p = .051) as the knee was moving into extension. TTDPM at 45° moving into flexion averaged 1.9° ±0.4° for the involved knee and 1.2° ±0.2° for the uninvolved knee (p = .022) (see figure 21.2). At 110°, TTDPM was not statistically significantly different between the PCL-injured and normal knees moving into flexion and into extension (see figure 21.3).

Testing RPP at 110°, the injured knee averaged 2.3° ±0.4° error from the true test angle, and the uninjured knee averaged 3.1° ±0.6° error as the test angle was brought into more extension (p = .050). RPP at 110° testing into flexion showed an average

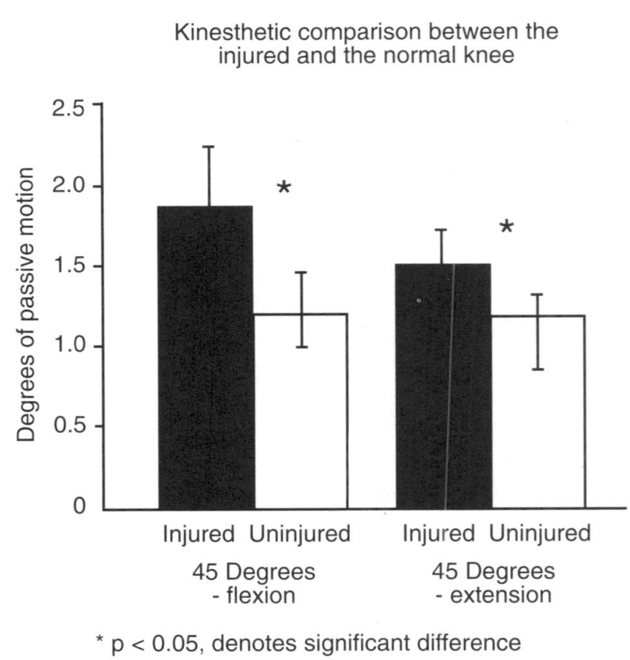

Figure 21.2 Mean total magnitude of degrees before sensation was detected. Kinesthesia (angular displacement) for the PCL-injured versus uninvolved knee from a starting position of 45° of knee flexion, moving into flexion and extension (±SE, p = .02 for flexion, p = .05 for extension).

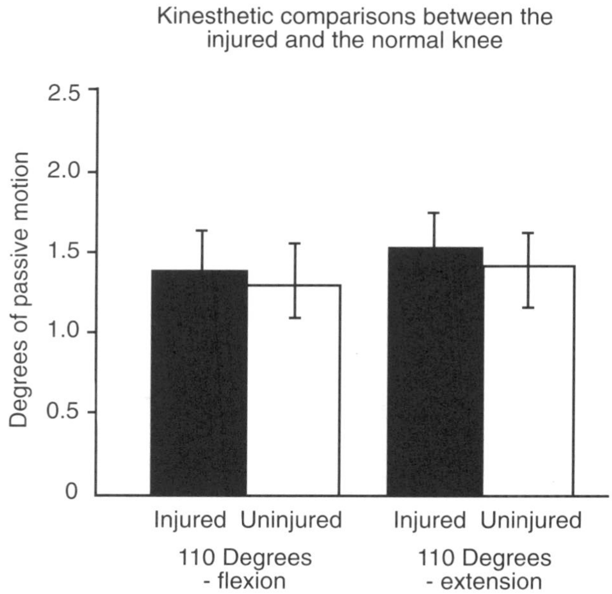

Figure 21.3 Mean total magnitude of degrees before sensation was detected. Kinesthesia (angular displacement) for the PCL-injured versus uninvolved knee from a starting position of 110° of knee flexion, moving into flexion and extension (±SE, $p = .29$ for flexion, $p = .12$ for extension).

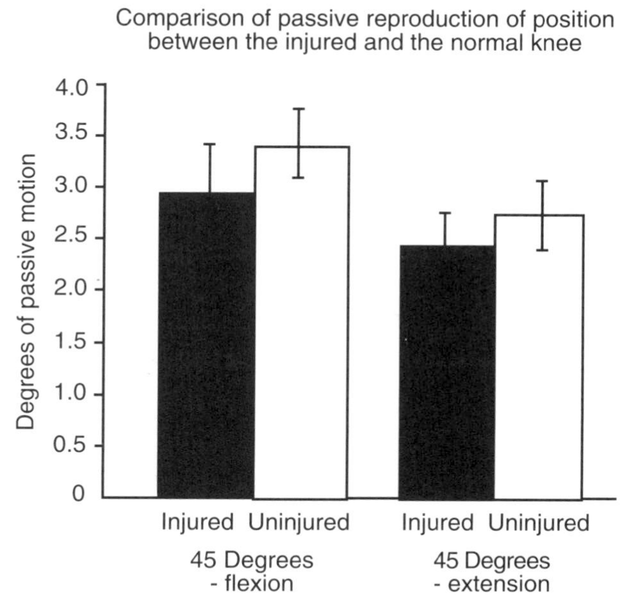

Figure 21.4 Mean difference in degrees of error between the presented angle and patient's positioning. Joint position sense (angular displacement) for the PCL-injured versus uninvolved knee from a starting position (reference angle) of 45° of knee flexion, moving into flexion and extension (±SE, $p = .16$ for flexion, $p = .22$ for extension).

error of 2.2° ±0.3° for the involved knee and 3.0° ±0.4° for the uninvolved knee ($p = .050$) (see figure 21.5). Testing RPP in 45° was not significantly different between the PCL-deficient and normal knee with the test angle in more flexion or extension (see figure 21.4 and table 21.1).

A correlation matrix revealed a significant correlation between the time from injury and the ability to passively reproduce a joint angle at 110° flexion moving into extension ($r = .687$).

Results for PCL-Reconstructed Subjects

Ten men met the criteria for inclusion: unilateral PCL injury and PCL reconstruction by the senior author. These subjects ranged in age from 23 to 54 yrs (average: 31 yrs). Five left knees and 5 right knees were involved. Seven patients had an isolated PCL rupture and no other knee disorder. One patient had concomitant medial tibiofemoral chondrosis, 1 had lateral patellar and tibiofemoral chondrosis (this pa-

Table 21.1 Summary of Results for PCL Proprioception Testing in PCL-Injured Subjects

Test	Injured knee	Uninjured knee	*p* Value
TTDPM 45°: ext	1.51° ± 0.19°	1.19° ± 0.10°	.05*
TTDPM 45°: flex	1.87° ± 0.35°	1.21° ± 0.22°	.02*
RPP 45°: ext	2.43° ± 0.33°	2.75° ± 0.33°	.22
RPP 45°: flex	2.97° ± 0.47°	3.42° ± 0.30°	.16
TTDPM 110°: ext	1.54° ± 0.22°	1.43° ± 0.18°	.12
TTDPM 110°: flex	1.38° ± 0.24°	1.29° ± 0.25°	.29
RPP 110°: ext	2.28° ± 0.37°	3.11° ± 0.56°	.05*
RPP 110°: flex	2.15° ± 0.28°	2.96° ± 0.36°	.05*

Proprioception results are for kinesthesia testing, which is measured as the angular displacement, in degrees, prior to sensing joint motion, and joint position sense, the angular displacement error between the true angle to which the knee was bent and the angle to which the subject moved the knee, measured in degrees. The starting knee flexion angle was 45° or 110°. (TTDPM = threshold to detect passive motion, RPP = ability to reproduce passive positioning, ext = moving into extension, flex = moving into flexion.)

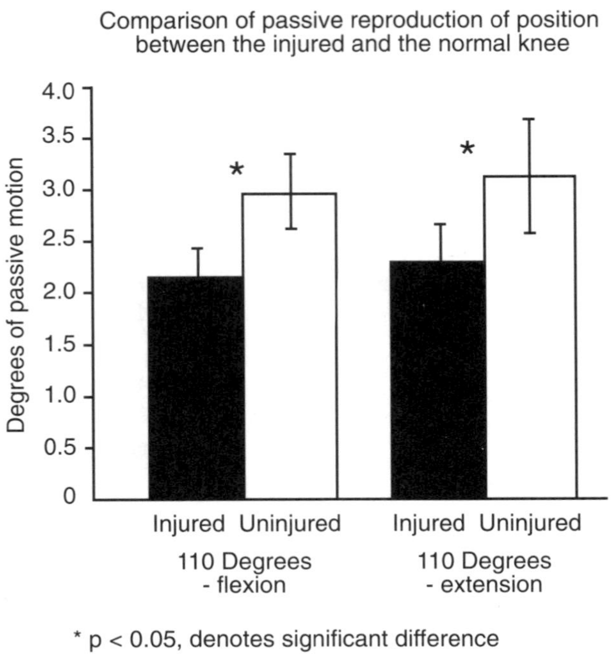

Figure 21.5 Mean difference in degrees of error between the presented angle and patient's positioning. Joint position sense (angular displacement) for the PCL-injured versus uninvolved knee from a starting position (reference angle) of 110° of knee flexion, moving into flexion and extension (±SE, p = .05 for flexion, p = .05 for extension).

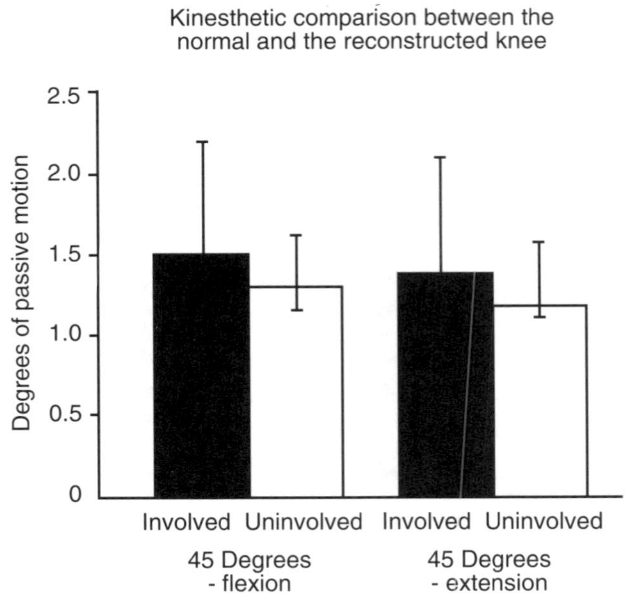

Figure 21.6 Mean total magnitude of degrees before sensation was detected. Kinesthesia (angular displacement) for the PCL-reconstructed versus uninvolved knee from a starting position of 45° of knee flexion, moving into flexion and extension (±SE, p = .6 for flexion, p = .2 for extension).

tient underwent an open lateral meniscal transplantation), and another had tricompartmental arthrosis. The time from reconstruction to proprioceptive testing ranged from 6 to 44 mo (average: 27 mo). KT-1000 results identified a corrected posterior displacement of 1.2 ±0.8 mm of the normal (unaffected) knee and 4.7 ±2.6 mm laxity of the reconstructed knee (p = .0018). All patients remained active in sports, though four had changed to a less demanding sport, and 6 returned to their preinjury level of activity.

The results for kinesthesia from starting positions of 45° and 110° of flexion revealed no statistically significant difference between the uninvolved and reconstructed knees, as they were passively moved into flexion and extension from both starting angles. From 45° moving into flexion, the uninvolved knee averaged 1.35° prior to the subject detecting motion, while the reconstructed knee averaged 1.50° (p = .6). From 45° moving into extension, the uninvolved knee averaged 1.25° and the reconstructed knee averaged 1.45° (p = .2). (See figure 21.6.) Testing from the 110° starting position and moving into flexion, the uninvolved knee averaged 1.50° and the reconstructed knee averaged 1.63° prior to the subject detecting motion (p = .5). Alternatively, starting at 110° and moving into extension, the uninvolved knee averaged 1.60° and the reconstructed knee averaged 1.95° (p = .3) (See figure 21.7 and table 21.2).

Discussion

Proprioception is considered a specialized variation of the sensory modality of touch and encompasses the sensations of joint movement (kinesthesia) and joint position (joint position sense). Conscious proprioception is essential for proper function in activities of daily living, sports, and occupational tasks. Unconscious proprioception modulates muscle function and initiates reflex stabilization. Much effort has been dedicated to elucidating the mechanical function of knee articular structures and the corresponding mechanical deficits that occur secondary to disruption of these structures. Knee articular structures may also have a significant sensory function that plays a role in dynamic joint stability, acute and chronic injury, pathologic wearing, and rehabilitation training.

Extrinsic innervation of joints follows Hilton's law (61), which states that joints are innervated by articular branches of the nerves supplying the muscles that cross that joint. The afferent innerva-

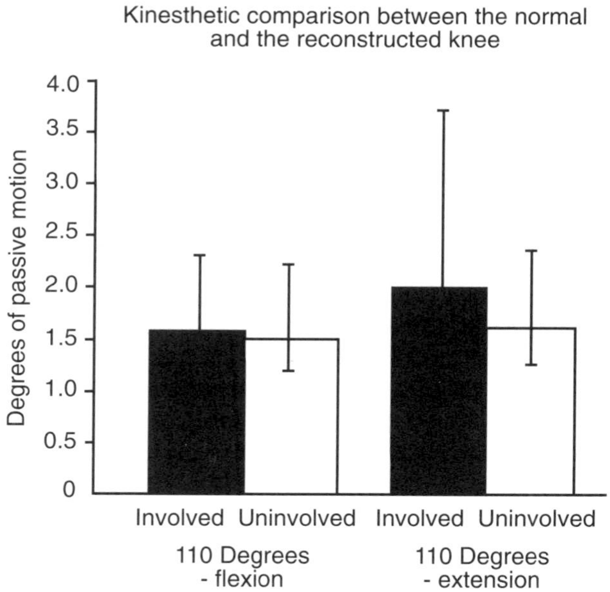

Figure 21.7 Mean total magnitude of degrees before sensation was detected. Kinesthesia (angular displacement) for the PCL-reconstructed versus uninvolved knee from a starting position of 110° of knee flexion, moving into flexion and extension (±SE, p = .5 for flexion, p = .3 for extension).

tion of joints is based on peripheral receptors located in articular, muscular, and cutaneous structures. Articular receptors include nociceptive free nerve endings and proprioceptive mechanoreceptors. Ruffini endings, Pacinian corpuscles, and Golgi tendon organs are mechanoreceptors that have been histomorphologically identified in the ACL (28, 34–36, 47, 50, 51), PCL (32, 51), meniscus (40, 44, 45, 62), lateral collateral ligament (18), and infrapatellar fat pad (37).

There is considerable debate over the relative contribution of muscle receptors versus joint receptors to proprioception, with traditional views emphasizing muscle receptors (11, 16, 24–26). Recent work suggests that muscle receptors and joint receptors are probably complementary components of an intricate afferent system in which each receptor modifies the function of the other (6, 21, 27).

Functionally, kinesthesia is assessed by measuring threshold to detection of passive motion (TTDPM), and joint position sense is assessed by measuring reproduction of passive positioning (RPP). In patients with unilateral joint involvement, the contralateral knee serves as an internal control, and uninjured knees in a normative population serve as external controls. Using these measures in the knee, investigators have found proprioceptive deficits with aging (3, 5, 54), arthrosis (3, 5, 55), and ACL disruption (2, 4, 7, 14). These processes damage articular structures containing mechanoreceptors and are thus hypothesized to result in partial deafferentation with resultant proprioceptive deficits. Proprioceptive enhancement was found to occur in ballet dancers (1) and also with the use of an elastic knee sleeve (4, 38), suggesting that training and bracing may have proprioceptive benefits.

The use of the threshold to detect passive motion as a measure of kinesthesia has been established by previous studies. Slow, passive motion was used in this investigation, as this is thought to maximally stimulate slow adapting joint mechanoreceptors while minimally stimulating muscle receptors (2). Although we were primarily focusing on joint receptors in joint injury, muscle receptors are an integral component of a complex afferent system and may also play a role in kinesthetic awareness of slow, passive motion. In addition to reflex pathways, joint mechanoreceptors have been shown to have cortical pathways that account for conscious appreciation of joint movement and position.

As with other information about the knee ligaments, information about PCL proprioception lags behind that of ACL proprioception. We have studied the proprioceptive function of a selective group of human subjects with isolated injuries to the posterior cruciate ligament and those who have undergone PCL reconstruction. Other than studies iden-

Table 21.2 Summary of Results for PCL Proprioception Testing in PCL-Reconstructed Subjects

Test	Reconstructed knee	Uninjured knee	p Value
TTDPM 45°: ext	1.45° ± 0.7°	1.25° ± 0.4°	.2
TTDPM 45°: flex	1.5° ± 0.7°	1.35° ± 0.3°	.6
TTDPM 110°: ext	1.95° ± 1.7°	1.62° ± 0.7°	.3
TTDPM 110°: flex	1.63° ± 0.4°	1.5° ± 0.4°	.5

Proprioception results are for kinesthesia testing, measured as the angular displacement, in degrees, prior to sensing joint motion. The starting knee flexion angle was 45° or 110°. (TTDPM = threshold to detect passive motion, ext = moving into extension, flex = moving into flexion.)

tifying proprioceptive mechanoreceptors within the substance of the PCL, few studies have attempted to assess the clinical function of these mechanoreceptors within the PCL.

One previous study found better joint position sense in patients undergoing total knee arthroplasty using a PCL-retaining prosthesis as compared with a PCL-sacrificing implant (59). Joint position sense was measured by having the subjects move a handheld knee model to replicate the perceived amount of passively placed knee flexion. Twenty-five subjects tested underwent a total knee replacement with a PCL-retaining prosthesis more than 1 year prior to testing and were compared with 9 age-matched controls and 30 patients with PCL-sacrificing knee arthroplasties (59). However, Tibone and coworkers, in the only other PCL proprioception-related study in the English literature that we have found, reported no electromyographic differences between PCL-deficient (some with posterolateral corner injury) and PCL-reconstructed knees (using medial head of the gastrocnemius) during functional tasks (57). Both groups had abnormal findings during gait (57). It may be that those with PCL reconstruction, who were quite symptomatic preoperatively, may have had greater proprioceptive deficits. Thus, the discrepancy as compared with our data may be due to many possible factors such as nonanatomic reconstruction (medial head of gastrocnemius using muscles that may affect proprioceptive input versus our intraarticular reconstruction of the anterolateral bundle of the PCL), large preoperative proprioceptive deficits that may be only incompletely restored, or their testing protocol, which is functional, requiring input from muscle and other fibers as compared with our slow moving, passive model.

One published study more similar to ours studied the threshold to detect passive positioning in 8 patients with isolated PCL-deficient knees (12). Their 8 patients averaged 34 yrs of age, 7 were men, and the average time from injury to testing was 3 years (range: 8 mo to 6 yrs). These patients were tested for TTDPM in the sitting position with their knee moved at 0.5°/s into flexion or extension from 37°. These authors found statistically significantly reduced ability to detect passive motion in the PCL-injured knee as compared with the normal, contralateral knee (12). We also found statistically significant differences in the TTDPM at a similar range (45° moving into both flexion and extension), though we did not find the reduced TTDPM at 110° of knee flexion. Clark and coworkers did not study this greater degree of extension, nor did they study the ability to passively reproduce passive positioning.

Those with isolated PCL disruption in our study are, for the most part, examples of the best clinical case scenario. These are subjects who have been treated nonoperatively for isolated grade II and III posterior laxity of the knee. Subjects with more significant injury are more likely to undergo early knee ligament reconstruction. Therefore, individuals who undergo early ligament reconstruction may be expected to exhibit more significant proprioceptive differences. These subjects, by nature of not already having undergone a reconstructive procedure, are people who mostly have adapted or compensated to their PCL-deficient state. They function well enough for activities of daily living, and in many cases, sports.

Proprioceptive deficits have been identified in the ACL-deficient knee (2, 38). These proprioceptive losses are reduced more significantly at 15° than at 45° flexion in the ACL-deficient knee. This is expected since the ACL has more force at 15° flexion and thus more input in functioning mechanoreceptors. Further, in a study of ACL-reconstructed patients, Barrett (4) showed that patient satisfaction and function appeared to correlate with proprioceptive function rather than with clinical examination and knee scores.

We have shown that isolated PCL deficiency in the human knee does result in reduced kinesthesia, as tested by the threshold to detect passive positioning and enhanced ability to reproduce passive positioning. Thus, the proprioceptive mechanoreceptors within the PCL do appear to have some function. Proprioceptive deficits in studies of patients with ACL disruption reveal greater proprioceptive deficits, both in magnitude and over a greater range of motion, as compared with the findings presented here for PCL deficiency. The proprioceptive deficits in kinesthesia identified in PCL-deficient knees are eliminated (or reduced to a nonsignificant level) by PCL reconstruction.

It has been argued that proprioception may play a protective role in acute injury through reflex muscular splinting (38). The protective reflex arc initiated by mechanoreceptors and muscle spindle receptors occurs much more quickly than the reflex arc initiated by nociceptors (70–100 m/s vs. 1 m/s). Thus, proprioception may play a more significant role than pain sensation in preventing injury in the acute setting. More importantly, proprioceptive deficits may play a more significant role in the etiology of chronic injuries and reinjury. Initial knee injury results in partial deafferentation and sensory deficits that can predispose to further injury (34). Proprioceptive deficits may also contribute to the etiology of degenerative joint disease through pathological wearing of a joint with poor sensation. It is unclear whether the proprioceptive deficits that accompany degenerative joint disease are a result of the underlying pathological process or contribute to the etiology of the pathological process. It may be surmised then, that the apparent loss of proprioception over a greater range of motion in the ACL-deficient knee helps explain why the so-called isolated PCL-deficient knee has a relatively more "benign course." It has yet to be proven that PCL deficiency leads to degenerative arthritis, and yet to be reported is whether PCL reconstruction can prevent or delay the onset of degenerative change within the operative knee.

We do not attempt to explain why TTDPM is reduced only at 45° and why RPP appears to be better at 110°. There are many possible explanations, including the altered kinematics of the PCL-deficient knee, variable coordinated input between the ACL and PCL at varying degrees of flexion (the ACL may have significant resultant force when flexed) (60), or even that the PCL may still contribute proprioceptive information as it may heal in a lengthened position. Further, the effect of physical therapy following injury may enhance proprioceptive function of the remaining mechanoreceptors, or it may be that kinesthesia and joint position sense are mediated through different pathways.

Looking specifically at the threshold to detect passive motion, PCL reconstruction appears to provide a kinesthetic pattern similar to that of the contralateral, normal knee. The deficit seen in nonoperated knees with PCL tears does not exist in knees following PCL reconstruction. This is in light of the fact that 3 patients who underwent PCL reconstruction and proprioceptive testing had some degree of degenerative joint disease. Knees with degenerative joint disease have previously been shown to have worse proprioception than the contralateral knee and age-matched controls. Thus, it is likely that PCL reconstruction did significantly improve kinesthesia at 45° of knee flexion (at 110°, no significant difference was observed between the involved and noninvolved knee in either study).

The most plausible explanation for the restoration of proprioception following reconstructive surgery appears to be related to the ligamentous and capsular tension of the joint (8, 39). Excessive laxity of those structures that contain proprioceptive mechanoreceptors results in diminished mechanical deformation of joint structures and reduces the afferent signal that mediates proprioception.

Regardless of the many possible explanations, the fact remains that mechanoreceptors within the PCL do have proprioceptive function and may play a role in the clinical function of patients with PCL injuries, and proprioception may be normalized (or deficits reduced) by PCL reconstruction. Future research in this area will help delineate the exact clinical function of proprioceptive mechanoreceptors within the posterior cruciate ligament.

References

1. Barrack RL, Skinner HB, Brunet ME, Cook SD: Joint kinesthesia in the highly trained knee. *J Sports Med Phys Fitness* 24: 18–20, 1983.
2. Barrack RL, Skinner HB, Buckley SL: Joint proprioception in the anterior cruciate ligament-deficient knee. *Am J Sports Med* 17: 1–6, 1989.
3. Barrack RL, Skinner HB, Cook SD, Haddad RJ Jr: Effect of articular disease and total knee arthroplasty on knee joint-position sense. *J Neurophysiol* 50: 684–87, 1983.
4. Barrett DS: Proprioception and function after anterior cruciate reconstruction. *J Bone Joint Surg* 73B: 833–37, 1991.
5. Barrett DS, Cobb AG, Bentley G: Joint proprioception in normal, osteoarthritic, and replaced knee. *J Bone Joint Surg* 73B: 53–56, 1991.
6. Baxendale RA, Ferrell WR, Wood L: Responses of quadriceps motor units to mechanical stimulation of knee joint receptors in the decerebrate cat. *Brain Res* 453: 150–56, 1988.
7. Beard DJ, Kyberd PJ, Fergusson CM, Dodd CAF: Proprioception after rupture of the anterior cruciate ligament: An objective indication of the need for surgery? *J Bone Joint Surg* 75B: 311–15, 1993.
8. Blaiser R, Carpenter J, Huston L: Shoulder proprioception: Effect of joint laxity, joint position, and direction of motion. *Orthop Rev* 23: 45–50, 1994.
9. Chick RR, Jackson RW: Tears of the anterior cruciate ligament in young athletes. *J Bone Joint Surg* 60A: 970–73, 1978.
10. Clancy WG Jr, Shelbourne KD, Zoellner GB, Keene JS, Reider B, Rosenberg TD: Treatment of knee joint instability secondary to rupture of the posterior cruciate ligament. *J Bone Joint Surg* 65A: 310–22, 1983.
11. Clark FJ, Burgess PR: Slowly adapting receptors in cat knee joint: Can they signal joint angle? *J Neurophysiol* 38: 1448–463, 1975.

12. Clark P, MacDonald PB, Sutherland K: Analysis of proprioception in the posterior cruciate ligament-deficient knee. *Knee Surg Sports Traumatol Arthroscopy* 4: 225–27, 1996.
13. Co FH, Skinner HB, Cannon WD: Proprioception of the knee following ACL reconstruction and its relation to heel strike impulse. Transactions of the 37th annual meeting of the Orthopaedic Research Society, Anaheim, CA, 1991, p. 603.
14. Corrigan JP, Cashman WF, Brady MP: Proprioception in the cruciate-deficient knee. *J Bone Joint Surg* 74B: 247–50, 1992.
15. Cross MJ, Powell JF: Long-term follow-up of posterior cruciate ligament rupture: A study of 116 cases. *Am J Sports Med* 12: 292–97, 1984.
16. Cross MM, McCloskey DI: Position sense following surgical removal of joints in man. *Brain* 55: 443–45, 1973.
17. Dandy DJ, Pusey RJ: The long-term results of unrepaired tears of the posterior cruciate ligament. *J Bone Joint Surg* 64B: 92–94.
18. DeAvila GA, O'Connor BL, Visco DM, Sisk TD: The mechanoreceptor innervation of the human fibular collateral ligament. *J Anat* 162: 1–7, 1989.
19. Dejour H, Walch G, Peyrot J, Eberhard P: The natural history of rupture of the posterior cruciate ligament. *Fr J Ortho Surg* 2: 112–20, 1988.
20. DuToit GT: Knee joint cruciate ligament substitution: The Lindemann (Heidelberg) operation. *S Af J Surg* 5: 25–30, 1967.
21. Ferrell WR: The response of slowly adapting mechanoreceptors in the cat knee joint to tetanic contraction of hind limb muscles. *Quar J Exp Physiol* 70: 337–45, 1985.
22. Fowler PJ, Messieh SS: Isolated posterior cruciate ligament injuries in athletes. *Am J Sports Med* 15: 553–57, 1987.
23. Giove TP, Miller SJ III, Kent BE, Sanford TL, Garrick JG: Nonoperative treatment of the torn anterior cruciate ligament. *J Bone Joint Surg* 65A: 184–92, 1983.
24. Goodwin GM, McCloskey DI, Matthews PB: The persistence of appreciable kinesthesia after paralyzing joint afferents but preserving muscle afferents. *Brain Res* 37: 326–29, 1972.
25. Goodwin GM, McCloskey DI, Matthews PB: The contribution of muscle afferents to kinesthesia shown by vibration induced illusions of movement and by the effects of paralyzing joint afferents. *Brain* 95: 705–48, 1972.
26. Grigg P: Mechanical factors influencing response of joint afferent neurons from cat knee. *J Neurophysiol* 38: 1473–484, 1975.
27. Grigg P: Response of joint afferent neurons in cat medial articular nerve to active and passive movements of the knee. *Brain Res* 118: 482–85, 1976.
28. Halata Z, Haus J: The ultrastructure of sensory nerve endings in human anterior cruciate ligament. *Anat Embryol* 179: 415–21, 1989.
29. Hawkins RJ, Misamore GW, Merritt TR: Follow-up of the acute nonoperated isolated anterior cruciate ligament tear. *Am J Sports Med* 14: 205–10, 1986.
30. Ihara H, Nakayama A: Dynamic joint control training for knee ligament injuries. *Am J Sports Med* 14: 309–15, 1986.
31. Insall J, Joseph DM, Aglietti P, Campbell RD: Bone-block iliotibial-band transfer for anterior cruciate insufficiency. *J Bone Joint Surg* 63A: 560–69, 1981.
32. Katonis PG, Assimakopoulos AP, Agapitos MV, Exarchou EI: Mechanoreceptors in the posterior cruciate ligament: Histological study on cadaver knees. *Acta Orthop Scand* 62: 276–78, 1991.
33. Keller PM, Shelbourne D, McCarroll JR, Rettig AC: Nonoperatively treated isolated posterior cruciate ligament injuries. *Am J Sports Med* 21: 132–36.
34. Kennedy JC, Alexander IJ, Hayes KC: Nerve supply of the human knee and its functional importance. *Am J Sports Med* 10: 329–35, 1982.
35. Kennedy JC, Weinberg HW, Wilson AS: The anatomy and function of the anterior cruciate ligament as determined by clinical and morphological studies. *J Bone Joint Surg* 56A: 223–35, 1974.
36. Krauspe R, Schmidt M, Schaible HG: Sensory innervation of the anterior cruciate ligament: An electrophysiological study of the response of single identified mechanoreceptors in the cat. *J Bone Joint Surg* 74A: 390–97, 1992.
37. Krenn V, Hofmann S, Engel A: First description of mechanoreceptors in the corpus adiposum infrapatellare of man. *Acta Anatomica* 137: 187–88, 1990.
38. Lephart SM, Kocher MS, Fu FH, Borsa PA, Harner CD: Proprioception following ACL reconstruction. *J Sports Rehabil* 1: 188–96, 1992.
39. Lephart SM, Warner JJP, Borsa P, Fu FH: Proprioception of the shoulder joint in healthy, unstable, and surgically repaired shoulders. *J Shoulder Elbow Surg* 3: 371–80, 1994.
40. MacKenzie WG, Shim SS, Day B, Leung G: The blood and nerve supply of the knee meniscus in man. *Anat Rec* 211: 115–16A, 1985.
41. McDaniel WJ, Dameron TB Jr: The untreated

anterior cruciate ligament rupture. *Clin Orthop* 172: 158–63, 1980.

42. Noyes FR, Butler DL, Paulos LE, Grood ES: Intraarticular cruciate reconstruction. Part I: Perspectives on graft strength, vascularization, and immediate motion after replacement. *Clin Orthop* 172: 71–77, 1983.
43. Noyes FR, Mooar PA, Matthews DA, Butler DL: The symptomatic anterior cruciate ligament deficient knee. Part I: The long-term functional disability in athletically active individuals. *J Bone Joint Surg* 65A: 154–62, 1983.
44. O'Connor BL: The histological structure of dog knee menisci with comment on its possible significance. *Am J Anat* 147: 407–17, 1976.
45. O'Connor BL, McConnaughey JS: The structure and innervation of cat knee menisci and their relation to a "sensory hypothesis" of meniscal function. *Am J Anat* 153: 431–42, 1978.
46. Parolie JM, Bergfeld JA: Long-term results of nonoperative treatment of isolated posterior cruciate ligament injuries in the athlete. *Am J Sports Med* 14: 35–38, 1986.
47. Rivard CH, Yahia LH, Rhalmi S, Newman N: Immunohistochemical demonstration of sensory nerve fibers and endings in human anterior cruciate ligaments. Transactions of the 39th annual meeting of the Orthopaedic Research Society, San Francisco, CA, 1993, p. 61.
48. Safran MR, Caldwell GL Jr, Fu FH: Proprioception considerations in surgery. *J Sports Rehab* 1: 105–15, 1994.
49. Satku K, Kumar VP, Ngoi SS: Anterior cruciate ligament injuries: To counsel or to operate? *J Bone Joint Surg* 68B: 458–61, 1986.
50. Schultz RA, Miller DC, Kerr CS, Micheli L: Mechanoreceptors in human cruciate ligaments: A histological study. *J Bone Joint Surg* 66A: 1072–1076, 1984.
51. Schutte MJ, Dabezies EJ, Zimny ML, Happel LT: Neural anatomy of the human anterior cruciate ligament. *J Bone Joint Surg* 69A: 243–47, 1987.
52. Shelbourne, KD, Patel DV: The natural history of acute isolated nonoperatively treated posterior cruciate ligament injuries of the knee: A prospective study. Transactions of the 64th annual meeting of the American Academy of Orthopaedic Surgeons, 1997, pp. 77–78.
53. Sherman MF, Warren RF, Marshall JL, Savatsky GJ: A clinical and radiographical analysis of 127 anterior cruciate insufficient knees. *Clin Orthop* 227: 229–37, 1988.
54. Skinner HB, Barrack RL, Cook SD: Age-related decline in proprioception. *Clin Orthop* 184: 208–11, 1984.
55. Skinner HB, Barrack RL, Cook SD, Haddad RJ Jr: Joint position sense in total knee arthroplasty. *J Orthop Res* 1: 276–83, 1984.
56. Sommerlath K, Lysholm J, Gillquist J: The long-term course after treatment of acute anterior cruciate ligament ruptures. *Am J Sports Med* 19: 156–62, 1991.
57. Tibone JE, Antich TJ, Perry J, Moynes D: Functional analysis of untreated and reconstructed posterior cruciate ligament injuries. *Am J Sports Med* 16: 217–23, 1988.
58. Torg JS, Barton TM, Pavlov H, Stine R: Natural history of the posterior cruciate ligament-deficient knee. *Clin Orthop* 246: 208–16, 1989.
59. Warren PJ, Olanlokun TK, Cobb AG, Bentley G: Proprioception after knee arthroplasty: The influence of prosthetic design. *Clin Orthop* 297: 182–87, 1993.
60. Wascher DC, Markolf KL, Shapiro MS, Finerman GAM: Direct in vitro measurement of forces in the cruciate ligaments. Part I: The effects of multiplane loading in the intact knee. *J Bone Joint Surg* 75A: 377–86, 1993.
61. Wyke BD: The neurology of joints. *Ann Royal Coll Surg* 41: 25–49, 1967.
62. Zimny ML, Albright DJ, Dabezies E: Mechanoreceptors in the human medial meniscus. *Acta Anatomica* 133: 35–40, 1988.

CHAPTER 22

Proprioception and Sensorimotor Control in the Functionally Unstable Ankle

Lars Konradsen, MD
Bruce D. Beynnon, PhD
Per A. Renström, MD, PhD

Proprioceptive Function of the Ankle

Research into ankle proprioception has been of interest to investigators in neurophysiology, where the concern is primarily the human reaction to changes in body equilibrium, and to investigators in sport traumatology, who are concerned with chronic functional ankle instability.

In the former line of research, the reaction of lower limb muscles to sudden but small perturbations around a dorsal/plantar flexion axis has been studied under various conditions. This has led to an understanding of the different elements of the reflex EMG response (short, medium, and long latency loop responses), to an understanding of the role of peripheral and higher center strategies on different response patterns, and to an understanding of the effect of repetition and learning on the modulation of perturbation responses.

In the latter line of research, the proprioceptive function and sensorimotor control of the ankle-foot complex in the inversion-eversion plane has been studied with special reference to the maintenance and loss of functional ankle stability.

This chapter reviews findings from research in sport traumatology. We review inversion injury mechanisms, the central and peripheral elements that secure functional ankle stability, and the source of peripheral afferent information relevant for maintaining functional stability. We then turn to functional ankle instability and consider (1) the evidence suggesting a proprioceptive predisposition to functional instability, (2) the evidence showing an effect of acute injury on sensorimotor control factors, and (3) the evidence connecting deficiencies in sensorimotor function and functional ankle instability. Finally, we present models connecting sensorimotor deficits with the increased frequency of inversion injuries.

Inversion Injury Mechanisms

Inversion injuries are by far the most common ankle distortion injury (2), and we will therefore concentrate on the pathodynamics of this entity.

The axially loaded ankle-foot complex is very stable, especially in the neutral flexion-extension position. As shown by Stormont and coworkers (39), the axially loaded talocrural joint is stable against inversion due to the bony restrictions of the joint. The subtalar joint has an axis that passes lateral in relation to the axially compressive forces that are generated during activities like walking, running, and jumping. This will cause the joint to evert when loaded and thus protect it from inversion (44).

Inversion sprains are thus the result of two connected events. First, an inversion rotation (or a combination of inversion and plantar flexion) (36) of the unloaded joint that (1) will place the talotibial joint in a position where bony stability is lost (39), and (2) invert the subtalar joint so that the point of contact between the foot and the ground surface will be moved medial to the subtalar axis (40, 41). With the ankle-foot complex in this vulnerable position the subsequent application of a compressive force (like a heel strike) will produce an inversion torque that will strain the lateral constraints and, depending on the magnitude of the compressive force and the contact of the articular surfaces of the situation, cause lateral ligament and capsule injury.

Maintaining Functional Ankle Stability

Maintaining functional ankle stability can theoretically be divided into two major entities based on the considerations of inversion injury mechanisms discussed above:

1. the ability to avoid situations where the foot-ankle complex is forced into inversion past the limit that secures stability prior to loading with a compressive force, and
2. the ability to prevent unstable situations, where the ankle is subject to an inversion torque, from progressing to injury of the lateral ligaments and capsule of the ankle-foot complex.

In other words: (1) a person who does not get the ankle complex into situations of excessive plantar flexion and inversion is not at risk, and (2) if the ankle has become subject to an inversion torque, injury can still be prevented if the reaction to counteract the inversion torque is sufficiently fast and strong.

First, we consider the reaction patterns applied by individuals in case of sudden inversion. After that we discuss the ability to avoid inversion-prone situations. Finally, we review studies considering the source of peripheral afferent information for securing ankle stability.

Reaction to Sudden Inversion

The basic strategy that results from a sudden forced inversion of the ankle seems to be consistent between individuals (25). The reaction is a combination of a peripheral response and of higher center strategies.

Peripheral Response

The first reaction measured after sudden inversion of the ankle is a short-to-medium latency EMG response in the peroneal muscles (25, 35). Different studies have reported this response to occur from 49 to 90 ms after the sudden inversion (3, 17, 20, 21, 23, 31, 34, 40). In the study performed by Löfvenberg and coworkers (31) (49 ms reaction time) this may suggest a short loop reaction. In most other studies the response has been considered a medium latency reflex (40). This signal is followed by a cortical signal of substantial magnitude and length that can voluntarily be suppressed (25) (Konradsen 1997, unpublished). Ten to 20 ms after the beginning of the medium latency reflex, an EMG response can be measured in the thigh muscles (23), while EMG signals in the unilateral tibialis anterior muscle are seen at the same time (31) or later (3) than the peroneal signal. As can be seen, the range of the reflex reaction times between different studies is very large. This can be explained to some extent by differences in equipment, different techniques to filter the raw signal, and by differences in the technique used to detect the first EMG signal. Some have used a threshold level of $2 \times SD$ (standard deviation) (24) of the activity level prior to perturbation, others go up to $10 \times SD$ of the preperturbation activity level (32). This may cause some investigators to see the middle loop latency signal as the first EMG signal, while others register the cortical signal as the first response. The time until the first EMG response is detected, however, may not be an important indicator as to the productive mechanism against inversion trauma. Far more important is the time from perturbation and until a substantial eversion force can be produced in the appropriate muscles. This will dictate how efficiently the muscles can counteract the inversion. Using a 6 degrees-of-freedom force platform combined with a tilt platform, we have found that eversion torque begins approximately 150 ms after the start of a sudden ankle inversion, and 75% of the maximal torque output was reached after 250–300 ms (Konradsen et al. 1997, unpublished). When subjects were asked not to react to the sudden inversion stimulus, they could eliminate the major part of the eversion torque response, which suggests that the production of a maximal eversion torque is centrally controlled and is not dependent on short or median loop latencies.

Higher Center Responses

Parallel to the response of the peroneal, the involved limb, as well as the body as a whole, shows a reaction pattern designed to reduce the inversion torque on the inverting ankle. Flexion of the hip averaging 25°, of the knee averaging 30°, and of the ankle averaging 20° (25) decreases the compressive forces on the ankle-foot complex in a standing sudden inversion simulation (23). In a walking simulation the contralateral limb is accelerated to the area of the center of gravity of the body to provide support for the body weight (25). All of these reactions, however, are delayed more than 0.2–0.3 s after the start of the inverting stimulus.

The Time Frame of the Response to Sudden Inversion

As mentioned, a substantial active eversion torque is first seen 150 ms after sudden inversion, and reactions that can be seen as central mediated strategies are seen even later. This has to be compared to the 80 ms it takes the ankle-foot complex to evert 40° from a standing position on a tilt platform. Mathematical simulations with the compressive forces of real-life situations suggest that the limit of normal range of motion may be reached after only 40 ms (40). Thus, it does not seem possible to establish an active response to a sudden inversion in time to protect the lateral capsule and ligaments. This interpretation, however, is based on the assumption that (1) the inversion proceeds without any external restriction (changes in ground surface configuration can slow down the rotation), and (2) the event that forces the ankle into inversion is followed immediately by the compressive force that causes the substantial inversion torque. This would be the case if, for example, a basketball player in landing from a jump stepped on the foot of a fellow player, sustaining the inversion rotation of the foot immediately before landing with his weight on the affected limb. If, however, the inversion rotation of the foot was caused by stumbling during walking, the time of ankle loading that coincides with the time of heel strike might be separated in time from the inversion episode, thus allowing the active protective response to be established.

Avoiding Inversion-Prone Situations: Strategies for Securing Stability During Locomotion

Securing functional stability is also characterized by the ability to avoid situations where the ankle loses its intrinsic passive stability. As for the previous situation of reacting to sudden ankle inversions, both central strategies and peripheral information combine to secure this goal.

During the stance phase of walking the ankle-foot complex is loaded and inversion stable. During the swing phase the foot-ankle complex is brought forward in a great percentage of strides without measurable activity in the peroneal muscles until just before heel strike (11, 24, 43). In the normal stride on a level surface and with intact lateral soft tissue structures, the foot is brought forward in approximately 10° degrees of inversion, and this balance of passive inversion-eversion restraints provides a stable situation even though the lateral border of the foot passes just 5 mm above the ground surface in the latter part of the swing phase (44). In a cadaver study, where the swing phase of the lower limb was simulated, we have found that if an impact occurs between the lateral border of a 10° inverted foot and the ground surface, it results in rotation of the foot into 40° of inversion, 40° of plantar flexion, and 30° of internal tibial rotation, which was the limit of our setup (Konradsen et al. 1997, unpublished). The foot-ankle complex would thus be susceptible to injury if the body weight loaded the foot at that moment.

The risk of creating an unstable situation can be avoided by applying several central strategies:

- The choice of motion pattern can be changed. This includes lifting the foot higher during the swing phase. This is seen as an extreme situation in patients with peroneal nerve palsy. To avoid catching the foot during swing phase they lift their feet high after toe-off and set them down nearly vertically at heel strike.
- Another centrally mediated strategy could be to preactivate the peroneal muscles before situations that are perceived or known from experience to be dangerous. This has not been investigated, but, anecdotally, experienced cross-country runners can report that they pretense their lateral muscle groups when anticipating areas of rough terrain.
- Peripheral afferent information relaying the position of the joint can also change the execution of a single stride. If the degree of inversion is perceived to be too great for safety in midswing phase, lateral muscle contractions can be instituted to produce a correction. This has not been shown directly, but indirect evidence points to such a regulatory mechanism (24). The frequency of midswing phase peroneal muscle activity was measured during 100 gait cycles of vigorous walking. Application of an ankle support that held the ankle in a neutral position of

inversion-eversion reduced the frequency of peroneal activity significantly. It was proposed that the reduced need for eversion corrections was responsible for this reduction in the frequency of peroneal muscle activation (24).

The Source of Peripheral Afferent Information: Relevant for Maintaining Functional Ankle Stability

Mechanoreceptors are present in many structures about the lateral aspect of the ankle (ligaments, capsule, and tendon tissue). With the abundance of afferent information available from the area, it would not seem reasonable that the body would rely on input solely from one anatomical structure, for example, the lateral ligaments. In agreement with this conclusion, studies of proprioceptive ankle function in healthy subjects following injection of local anesthetics in the area of the anterior talofibular and calcaneofibular ligaments have not been able to show any deterioration in single-limb stability or joint position sense under anesthesia (4, 5).

In a study where a Bier block was applied at the level of the malleoli to obtain a total block of afferent information from the ankle and foot, changes in various aspects of proprioception occurred to varying degrees (24). The reproduction of passive positioning of the joint was greatly affected by the block suggesting that afferent information for this proprioceptive ability is supplied by receptors close to the ankle joint area. This is in agreement with results from studies of other joints (33). If, however, positioning of the joint with muscles proximal to the block was allowed, a near-normal sense of ankle positioning was accomplished. The reaction of the muscles to sudden inversion was unchanged by the block. These findings suggest that the afferent information for the latter proprioceptive abilities could be mediated by receptors in the muscle-tendon system. This is in accord with previous research on other joints (12).

Proprioception and Functional Ankle Instability

The interest in ankle sensorimotor control in connection with functional ankle instability evolved from the observations that subjects with complaints of repeated ankle inversion injuries also showed an increased degree of sway during single-limb stance (6, 38). The primary thrust of research in this field since then has concentrated on proving or disproving coexistence between functional ankle instability and deficits in different measurements of ankle sensorimotor control.

To establish a causal relationship between a sensorimotor deficit and the development of functional instability, several requirements need to be met. These are (1) a cause-effect relationship between the first acute inversion ankle injury and a deficit in the sensorimotor control parameter that is measured, (2) a coexistence between functional ankle instability and the sensorimotor deficit, and (3) a model that can explain how a measured deficit in the given sensorimotor control factor can cause the increased frequency of ankle inversion injuries and "giving-way" situations. The requirement of a first-time effect of an ankle inversion injury on the sensorimotor parameter in question can be modified based on different theories on the etiology of functional instability. If it is assumed that certain subjects are predisposed to functional instability due to an inherent defect in sensorimotor control ability, such a subgroup must be identified in the population, and an increased frequency of inversion injuries must be shown as the group is followed. If it is believed that it is the effect of the repeated injuries that gradually creates the sensorimotor control deficit, such a cumulative effect must be substantiated.

Definition of Functional Instability

There is no universally agreed-upon definition for functional ankle instability. The term is used to describe the repeated ankle inversion injuries and "giving-way" feelings that certain subjects experience. There are no requirements as to how often distortions need to be sustained, how long the disability has had to be present, at what level of activity injuries are sustained, or at what degree of external provocation. As shown by Leanderson and coworkers (28), over 90% of the players on a division-level basketball team have sustained at least one major ankle inversion injury. They would not all be considered, however, to have a functionally unstable ankle. Rather, it would be considered that the sport in itself was the primary risk factor, and the inversion injuries would be seen as a normal consequence of this risk. In defining functional instability, it is therefore of great importance that the inversion injuries and the giving-way episodes are experienced in situations where ankle-stable subjects would not normally sustain injuries.

Nonmechanical Predisposition to Repeated Ankle Inversion Injuries

As most factors concerned with the human body are more or less normally distributed, it is a reasonable thought that a group of individuals in the tail of the distribution could present a less efficient neuromuscular controlling ability of the ankle area.

To support this view, Tropp (41) found that subjects with unilateral functional instability showed increased postural sway when standing on both the unstable and the stable foot. Furthermore, he found that in a population of 127 soccer players, subjects with a postural sway exceeding 2 × *SD* of the values for normal controls had a significantly higher frequency of ankle inversion injuries during the following season compared to players with normal postural sway. This occurred regardless of their history of previous ankle injuries.

Contrary to these findings, Beynnon and coworkers (1) did not find that an increase in the mean displacement of the center of pressure in the AP plane during single-limb stance or an increase in the latency of the EMG reflex of the triceps surae to sudden ankle dorsiflexion was an ankle inversion injury risk factor. They prospectively tested 116 college athletes and followed them during an athletic season. Sixteen sprains were encountered during the season, and the sensorimotor control measurements could not predict that these athletes would sustain injuries.

Acute Ankle Injury

To make definite statements on the effect of acute ankle inversion injuries on ankle sensorimotor control, studies would be required to test a large group of subjects for baseline measurements, follow this group over an athletic season, and perform the sensorimotor measurement on those subjects who were injured as well as those who were uninjured.

Two prospective studies following groups of preinjury-tested subjects have been reported. Leanderson and coworkers (27) studied ballet dancers, and Kleinrensink and coworkers (22) studied army recruits. Six ballet dancers and 7 army recruits provided new cases of acute inversion injury for follow-up in these studies (out of a base population of 53 and 118, respectively). In order to reach greater subject numbers, other investigations have had to settle for designs where results from the involved ankles were compared to the contralateral healthy ankles at the time of injury. Bilateral measurements on healthy subjects with the sensorimotor control tests employed in these studies, however, have not shown any differences between sides (right-left, dominant-nondominant) (5, 7, 14, 19) (Konradsen et al., 1997, unpublished), and therefore it was assumed that the involved ankle would have performed as the contralateral ankle.

The two prospective studies have shown a causal relationship between acute ankle inversion injuries and changes in sensorimotor control factors measured as an increase in peroneal nerve conduction velocity for two segments of the deep peroneal nerve (22) and as an increase by mean 45% in the magnitude of single-limb postural sway over 60 s (26). In studies where preinjury baseline tests were not performed, but where the results for the acutely injured ankles were compared to the normal contralateral side, Friden and coworkers (7) showed increased sway in the frontal plane during single-limb stance on the injured leg in 14 subjects. The time of measurement was 25.6 s. Using a less objective measurement of sway, Freeman and coworkers (6) found increased sway in 34% of 85 patients with an acute ankle sprain; 16% had normal sway, while the test was inconclusive in the rest of the subjects. Sway was judged by an observer as better, worse, or equal to the healthy contralateral side. An effect of acute ankle injury on postural sway was not found by Tropp (41).

We have found the passive ankle position replication error to be increased by approximately 100% one week after an acute ankle injury in 46 previously ankle-stable subjects. After 12 weeks a 33% increase in error was still present (Konradsen et al., submitted for publication 1997).

Chronic Functional Instability

As mentioned earlier, there are a number of concerns when comparing the sensorimotor control values of a functionally unstable group with those of a functionally stable group. These include the lack of a definition of functional instability, the etiologic complexity of functional instability (mechanical vs. functional, intrinsic vs. extrinsic), the variation of techniques employed even within the same method, and the lack of validation of the methods. All of these factors make it difficult to compare studies.

Postural Sway and Functional Instability

Using postural sway during single-limb stance with open eyes over a 60 s period, Tropp (42) found that 29 soccer players with a history of functional ankle instability showed a 27% increase in postural sway when compared to 18 controls. The same results using the same method were seen by Gauffin and coworkers (9). They also found that the functionally unstable subjects showed an impaired postural correction pattern that could be improved towards a normal pattern with training.

Leanderson and coworkers (28) tested the balance of 38 basketball players on a computer-assisted force plate. They found that players with previously injured ankles differed significantly from a control group. These players had a larger mean frontal plane postural sway and used a larger sway area.

Using less objective measurements, Freeman and coworkers (6) found that 7 of 14 subjects who complained of repeated inversion injuries had increased sway, which compared to no subjects with increased sway among 17 who did not complain of functional instability. Single-limb balance with eyes open and closed was compared to the contralateral side and noted by the observer as better, worse, or unchanged. With a similar outcome measure Lentell and coworkers (30) found increased sway on the involved side in 33 subjects with unilateral chronic ankle instability. Chronic ankle instability was defined as a history of one grade 3 ligament sprain with a persistent feeling of weakness, pain, or function deficiency compared to the contralateral side at the time of testing. In 20 subjects with repeated inversion injuries (mean: 6 inversion injuries per subject), Garn and Newton (8) found that 67% presented with increased postural sway when standing on the affected limb compared to the normal side.

One report did not find a relationship between functional instability and increased postural sway. Isakov and Mizrahi (16) tested 8 competitive gymnasts with at least 3 distortion injuries to only one foot. All had an increased anterior drawer sign. They used the mean foot-ground reaction force in medial-lateral and anterior-posterior direction, seen as a percentage of the body weight, as sway measurement.

Allowing subjects to balance on a soft surface, Jerosch and Bischof (18) used the number of touchdowns of the contralateral foot as the instability measurement. They found a significant difference between the stable and unstable limbs in 16 unilaterally unstable subjects.

To assess the effect on sensorimotor control of a combination of functional instability and mechanical instability, Gottlieb and coworkers (13) measured postural sway in 14 subjects with functional instability and 9 subjects with both functional and mechanical instability. Increased sway was found in the latter group when compared to the former for force but not for displacement measurements characterizing sway. Thus the standard deviation of the vertical force and standard deviation of the medial-lateral force were increased by 65%, while sway amplitude and sway magnitude of the center of pressure did not show any differences.

Soderberg and coworkers (37) measured EMG activity of the peroneal muscles during balancing on a tilt board and found no difference in the magnitude of the mean peroneal EMG signal in 14 subjects with chronic ankle instability when compared to 14 normal controls.

Ankle Kinesthesia and Functional Ankle Instability

Measuring kinesthesia or movement threshold has not been studied as intensively as in proprioceptive knee research. Garn and Newton (8) found a significantly increased frequency of error ($p < .01$) when 20 functionally unstable subjects had to answer the question whether or not an ankle had been moved from 0° to 5° of plantar flexion at a rate of 0.3°/s. Lentell and coworkers (29) found that the amount of motion necessary to register movement was increased by 1° ($p = .044$) when comparing inversion threshold for the uninjured and the injured ankles of 42 subjects.

Ankle Position Assessment and Functional Ankle Instability

Glencross and Thornton (10) found an increase in the error with which plantar flexion angles were passively replicated in 24 subjects with one previous sprain. They found that severe sprains seemed to result in greater degrees of replication error than mild sprains and that the replication error was greatest with the ankle plantar flexed.

Jerosch and Bischof (18) also found an increased absolute error when replicating 3 inversion angles (5°, 15° and 20°) in 16 unilaterally functionally unstable subjects when comparing the stable and the unstable side. The difference between sides was approximately 0.9°. In a setup where the inversion angles 10°, 15°, and 20° were replicated 10 times each, a significant difference of 0.9° between the results of 23 functionally and mechanically unstable subjects and 40 stable controls was also found (Konradsen et al. 1997, unpublished), with the unstable subjects showing the greatest error. In contrast, Gross (14) could not find a difference between 14 stable and 14 unstable subjects in an inversion setup of both passive and active angle replications. The angles 10° eversion, 10° inversion, and 20° inversion were replicated twice.

Peroneal Muscle Reaction Time and Functional Ankle Instability

The time from a sudden inversion of the ankle to a measurable EMG reaction in the peroneal muscles is usually measured as the peroneal reaction time. The methods for subjecting people to a sudden ankle inversion are quite uniform. It is most often the body weight that drives the rotating platform and the rotational speed is often around 200 to 400°/s. Most investigators agree that the first EMG signal is a medium latency loop response; however, these reaction times vary greatly from study to study (see table 22.1).

Based on these results it still seems unclear whether or not an increased peroneal reaction time to sudden ankle inversion is present in functional ankle instability.

Functional Tests and Functional Ankle Instability

Jerosch and Bischof (18) tested 16 subjects with unilateral functional instability on a single-limb hopping course. This test is considered to be a measure of the functional ability of the ankle and of the activity of the foot, knee, hip, and upper extremity, as well as the ability of the visual and the vestibular systems. They found a significant increase of 10% in the time used for the hopping course for the injured leg ($p < .01$).

The Influence of a Measured Sensorimotor Deficiency on Functional Instability

Some of the tests described above suggest that the neuromuscular function of the ankle or of the body as a whole is altered in subjects with functional ankle instability. Tests like sway during single-limb stance provide easy tools for testing patients for their overall neuromuscular function and can be very effective in helping patients realize the need for rehabilitation. The tests do not, however, suggest a cause-effect relationship between the measured deficiency and the increased frequency of inversion injuries, which characterizes functional ankle instability. For some of the measured sensorimotor deficiencies a cause-effect relationship can be modeled. We will discuss the consequence of an increased peroneal reaction time to sudden inversion and an increased degree of error in inversion angle replication.

The reaction of the peroneal muscles is the first dynamic response to sudden ankle inversion (25). An increased reaction time, as seen by some in functionally unstable groups, would thus suggest that the dynamic defense against inversion is recruited later, resulting in an increased risk of injury in case of ankle inversion. It should be remembered, however, that it is not an EMG signal but the build up of eversion force in the peroneal muscles that dictates the efficiency of the dynamic defense. As mentioned early in this chapter, we found that an active eversion torque was first seen after approximately 150 ms and 75% of maximum eversion moment was reached, at the earliest, 180 ms after perturbation (Konradsen et al. 1997, unpublished). This has to be compared to the 40–50 ms it would take the ankle to reach the anatomical limit of about 40° of inversion in a walking situation. The response is still the body's dynamic response to a potentially dangerous situation, however, and it seems reasonable to assume that the faster the reaction is, the greater the degree of protection achieved.

The consequence of a deficient sense of ankle positioning can also be modeled. As mentioned earlier in the chapter, ankle inversion injuries are seen if the ankle is inverted past the point where bony

Table 22.1 Peroneal Reaction Time to Sudden Ankle Inversion for Functionally Ankle-Stable and Unstable Groups From Different Studies

Authors	Publ. year	Number of subjects	Unstable Subjects: Injured ankle ms	Unstable Subjects: Uninjured ankle ms	Stable controls	p
Isakov et al.[17]	1986	11	64	—	68	n.s.
Konradsen et al.[23]	1990	15	82	—	65	0.01
Karlsson et al.[21]	1989	20	83	68	—	0.001
Johnson & Johnson[20]	1993	7	65	68	72	n.s.
Löfvenberg et al.[31]	1995	13	65	—	49	0.001
Huber et al.[15]	1996	19	86	90	87	n.s.

stability is lost and then loaded with the weight of the body. Studying the walking cycle, we have identified two situations where the ankle seems to be at risk. One is the time of heel strike, where the transition from an unloaded to a loaded condition happens with every stride. Based on a cadaver study, we found, however, that the subtalar joint had to invert approximately 30°, combined with an internal rotation of the tibia of 20°, before an inversion torque would be generated upon impact (Konradsen et al., 1997, unpublished). With an ankle position sense deficit of about 1° when comparing functionally unstable subjects with stable subjects, reaching position errors of a magnitude as suggested above would be unrealistic. During the late swing phase of the gait cycle there is, however, the period where the lateral edge of the foot passes close to the ground with only a clearance of 5 mm (44) and where an impact between the lateral edge of the foot and the supporting surface would cause the ankle to invert, plantar flex, and internally rotate (Konradsen et al. 1997, unpublished). This could potentially create a stumbling situation. The degree of inversion position error necessary to cause an impact between the lateral edge of the foot and the ground is approximately 8°. The greater position assessment error seen in functionally unstable subjects combined with the increased variance of the results in this group (18) would make the risk of an unsuspected impact statistically much greater in a functionally unstable group when compared to a stable group.

Conclusion

Maintaining functional ankle stability is seen as a combination of two primary capabilities:

1. to prevent situations of ankle-foot inversion that would promote an ankle inversion torque during ankle loading, and
2. to prevent a hyperinversion situation from progressing into lateral ligament and capsule injury.

Each ability is secured by peripheral and central mechanisms.

To secure the first ability, central performance strategies, especially for the swing phase of the gait cycle, combined with an exact sense of position are seen as important. To secure the second ability, afferent information from the lateral ankle, and especially from tendons transversing the ankle, is thought to generate the peripheral response that stimulates a force buildup in the peroneal muscles, resisting further inversion. Furthermore, a central strategy is triggered with the goal of reducing the compressive force on the inverting ankle-foot complex.

There is considerable evidence that acute ankle inversion injuries cause damage to sensorimotor control as registered by the outcome measures: postural sway, joint position sense, and nerve conduction velocity.

In chronic functional ankle instability the evidence of concomitant sensorimotor control deficiencies is not as strong as might have been expected. For the outcome measure postural sway, a great part of the clinical evidence is built on subjective assessment of the magnitude of sway. Of the studies with an objective sway measurement, the number of studies that show a connection between functional instability and increased sway outnumber the studies that do not show a connection. This also seems to be the case for the measurements of ankle kinesthesia and ankle position awareness.

References

1. Beynnon BD, Renström PA, Alosa DM, Vacek PM, Baumhauer JF. A prospective study of ankle injury risk factors. *Proceedings of the Orthopaedic Research Society*, 43d annual meeting, 1997.
2. Broström L. Sprained ankles. I: Anatomic lesions in recent sprains. *Acta Chir Scand* 1964; 128: 483–95.
3. Brunt D, Andersen JC, Huntsman B, Reinhert LB, Thorell AC, Sterling JC. Postural responses to lateral perturbation in healthy subjects and ankle sprain patients. *Med Sci Sports Exerc* 1992; 24(2): 171–76.
4. DeCarlo MS, Talbot RW. Evaluation of ankle proprioception following injection of the anterior talofibular ligament. *JOSPT* 1986; 8(2): 70–76.
5. Feuerbach JW, Grabiner MD, Koh TJ, Weiker GG. Effect of an ankle orthosis and ankle ligament anesthesia on ankle joint proprioception. *Am J Sports Med* 1994; 22(2): 223–29.
6. Freeman MAR, Dean MRE, Hanham IWF. The etiology and prevention of functional instability of the foot. *J Bone Joint Surg* [Br] 1965; 47B: 678–85.
7. Fridén T, Zätterström R, Lindstrand A, Moritz U. A stabilometric technique for evaluation of lower limb instabilities. *Am J Sports Med* 1989; 17(1): 118–22.

8. Garn SN, Newton RA. Kinesthetic awareness in subjects with multiple ankle sprains. *Phys Ther* 1988; 68(11): 1667–671.
9. Gauffin H, Tropp H, Odenrick P. Effect of ankle disk training on postural control in patients with functional instability of the ankle joint. *Int J Sports Med* 1988; 9(2): 141–44.
10. Glencross D, Thornton E. Position sense following joint injury. *J Sports Med Phys Fitness* 1981; 21: 23–27.
11. Glick JM, Gordon RB, Nashimoto D. The prevention and treatment of ankle injuries. *Am J Sports Med* 1976; 4: 136–41.
12. Goodwin GM, McCloskey DI, Matthews PBC. The persistence of appreciable kinesthesia after paralyzing joint afferents but preserving muscle afferents. *Brain Res* 1972; 38: 326–29.
13. Gottlieb DJ, Huber BM, Roos EM, Renström PA, Beynnon BD. Stabilometry in unilateral, chronic ankle instability. *ORS* 1996.
14. Gross MT. Effects of recurrent lateral ankle sprains on active and passive judgement of joint position. *Phys Ther* 1987; 67: 1505–509.
15. Huber BM, Gottlieb DJ, Roos EM, Alosa D, Renström PA, Beynnon BD. Muscle reaction and joint motion changes in chronically unstable ankles. *ORS* 1996.
16. Isakov E, Mizrahi J. Is balance impaired by recurrent sprained ankle? *Br J Sports Med* 1997; 31: 65–67.
17. Isakov E, Mizrahi J, Solzi P, Susak Z, Lotem M. Response of the peroneal muscles to sudden inversion of the ankle during standing. *Int J Sports Biomech* 1986; 2: 100–109.
18. Jerosch J, Bischof M. Proprioceptive capabilities of the ankle in stable and unstable joints. *Sports Exerc Inj* 1996; 2: 167–71.
19. Jerosch J, Hoffstetter I, Bork H, Bischof M. The influence of orthoses on the proprioception of the ankle joint. *Knee Surg Sports Traumatol Arthroscopy* 1995; 3(1): 39–46.
20. Johnson MB, Johnson CL. Electromyographic response of peroneal muscles in surgical and nonsurgical injured ankles during sudden inversion. *JOSPT* 1993; 18: 497–501.
21. Karlsson J, Andreasson GO. The effect of external ankle support in chronic lateral ankle joint instability: An electromyographic study. *Am J Sports Med* 1992; 20(3): 257–61.
22. Kleinrensink G, Dijkstra P, Boerboom A, Stoeckart R. Reduced motor conduction velocity of the peroneal nerve caused by inversion damage: A prospective longitudinal study. *Acta Orthop Scand* 1996; 67(Suppl 272): 83.
23. Konradsen L, Ravn JB. Ankle instability caused by prolonged peroneal reaction time. *Acta Orthop Scand* 1990; 61(5): 388–90.
24. Konradsen L, Ravn JB, Sørensen AI. Proprioception at the ankle: The effect of anesthetic blockade of ligament receptors. *J Bone Joint Surg* [Br] 1993; 75(3): 433–36.
25. Konradsen L, Voigt M, Højsgaard C. Ankle inversion injuries: The role of the dynamic defense mechanism. *Am J Sports Med* 1997; 25(1): 54–58.
26. Leanderson J. *Ankle sprain: Subjective and objective measures of functional impairment and treatment*. Stockholm: University of Stockholm, 1996.
27. Leanderson J, Eriksson E, Nilsson C, Wykman A. Proprioception in classical ballet dancers: A prospective study of the influence of an ankle sprain on proprioception in the ankle joint. *Am J Sports Med* 1996; 24(3): 370–74.
28. Leanderson J, Wykman A, Eriksson E. Ankle sprain and postural sway in basketball players. *Knee Surg Sports Traumatol Arthroscopy* 1993; 1(3–4): 203–205.
29. Lentell G, Baas B, Lopez D, McGuire L, Sarrels M, Snyder P. The contributions of proprioceptive deficits, muscle function, and anatomic laxity to functional instability of the ankle. *JOSPT* 1995; 21(4): 206–15.
30. Lentell GL, Katzman LL, Walters MR. The relationship between muscle function and ankle stability. *JOSPT* 1990; 11(12): 605–11.
31. Löfvenberg R, Kärrholm J, Sundelin G. Prolonged reaction time in patients with chronic lateral instability of the ankle. *Am J Sports Med* 1995; 23: 414–17.
32. Lynch SA, Eklund U, Gottlieb D, Renström PA, Beynnon B. Electromyographic latency changes in the ankle musculature during inversion moments. *Am J Sports Med* 1996; 24(3): 362–69.
33. McCloskey DI, Gandavia SC. Role of inputs from skin, joints, and muscles and of corollary discharges, in human discriminatory tasks. In *Active touch—The mechanism of recognition of objects by manipulation: A multidisciplinary approach.* Gordon G, ed. Oxford: Pergamon Press, 1977: 177–88.
34. Nawoczenski DA, Owen MG, Ecker ML, Altman B, Epler M. Objective evaluation of peroneal response to sudden inversion stress. *JOSPT* 1985; 7(3): 107–109.
35. Nishikawa T, Grabiner MD. Ankle braces influence the reflex amplitude of muscle in response to stretch. *Proceedings of the Orthopaedic Research Society*, 42d annual meeting, 1996.

36. Renström P, Wertz M, Incavo S, et al. Strain in the lateral ligaments of the ankle. *Foot & Ankle* 1988; 9(2): 59–63.
37. Soderberg GL, Cook TM, Rider SC, Stephenitch BL. Electromyographic activity of selected leg musculature in subjects with normal and chronically sprained ankles performing on a BAPS board. *Phys Ther* 1991; 71(7): 514–22.
38. Staples OS. Result study of ruptures of lateral ligaments of the ankle. *Clin Orthop Rel Res* 1972; 85: 50–58.
39. Stormont DM, Morrey BF, An KN, Cass JR. Stability of the loaded ankle: Relation between articular restraint and primary and secondary static restraints. *Am J Sports Med* 1985; 13(5): 295–300.
40. Thonnard JL, Plaghki L, Willems P, Benoit JC, DeNayer J. La Pathogenie de l'entorse de la cheville: Test d'une hypothese. *Medica Physica* 1986; 9: 141–46.
41. Tropp H. Functional instability of the ankle joint. Linköping, Sweden: Linkoping University, 1985.
42. Tropp H. Pronator muscle weakness in functional instability of the ankle joint. *Int J Sports Med* 1986; 7(5): 291–94.
43. Van Linge B. Activity of the peroneal muscles, the maintenance of balance, and prevention of inversion injury of the ankle: An electromyographic and kinematic study. *Acta Orthop Scand* 1988; 59(Suppl 227): 67–68.
44. Winter DA. *The biomechanics and motor control in human gait: Normal, elderly and pathological.* Ontario: University of Waterloo Press, 1991.

CHAPTER 23

Effects of Shoulder Instability on Joint Proprioception

Joerg G. Jerosch, MD

Introduction

The stability of the glenohumeral joint is based on the integrity of the ligamentous structures, the muscular stabilization, and the osseous congruity of the corresponding joint structures. The glenohumeral joint presents a relatively small glenoid fossa facing a large humeral head like a golf ball on the tee. According to Resch and coworkers (72) minimum requirements regarding the diameter, the radius, and the inclination of the glenoid fossa must be met to provide a stable base for the humeral head. The anterior and posterior glenohumeral ligaments and the coracohumeral ligament, as well as the joint capsule, are considered to be of main importance for passive shoulder stabilization (17, 18, 35, 42, 66, 97). This capsular-ligamentous stabilization ensures the congruity of the corresponding joint structures at rest, and it restricts the range of motion in extreme positions. The musculature, however, supports and stabilizes these passive structures and balances the joint (43, 66, 75, 79, 80, 95). The recent literature emphasizes mainly the ligamentous stabilization and presents studies of three different types:

1. Anatomic studies with selective preparation of the glenohumeral ligaments (18, 20, 21, 27, 82, 95, 97)
2. Clinical studies with description of the intraarticular pathology (3, 4, 16, 39, 77, 79)
3. Biomechanical studies based on selective section of ligaments or direct measurements of the strain on the ligaments in different positions (34, 40, 42, 85, 97, 99)

These studies have demonstrated the strain on different capsule-ligament structures in different functional positions. However, the small diameter of different ligaments found in anatomic preparations or arthroscopic interventions is striking to the critical observer. In contrast to other major joints, for example, the knee joint, where the cruciate ligaments make up a strong central column and the collateral ligaments facilitate an efficient lateral stabilization, the glenohumeral joint ligaments are rather weak structures.

On the other hand, it is well known that an injury to the anterior capsule-ligament complex is associated with a high risk of recurrent anterior shoulder instability. Despite their relative weakness, the capsular structures seem to play an important role for joint stability. Therefore, the proprioceptive capability of these structures was investigated recently by different groups. In anatomic, biomechanical, neurophysiological, histological and clinical studies different aspects of proprioception were evaluated:

- Where is the proprioceptive tissue located (36, 44–46, 75)?
- Which kinds of mechanreceptors have the greatest influence on proprioceptive capabilities (5–8, 12, 13, 22–25, 46, 58, 86, 87, 90)?

- What influence does proprioception have on the static and dynamic stability of different joints (7, 15, 22, 23, 46, 58, 86–88)?
- How do degenerative joint disease and joint injury affect proprioceptive capabilities (5, 6, 23, 30, 32, 47, 48, 50, 51, 57, 58, 81, 86–88)?
- What effect does age have on the proprioception (7, 14, 38, 64, 86, 87)?
- By which mechanisms can proprioceptive deficits be compensated (7, 15, 24, 55, 60–62)?

Our own interest in proprioception of the shoulder was in histological investigations and neurophysiological evaluations, as well as clinical studies.

Histological Investigation: Material and Methods

We examined 12 fresh shoulder specimens aged 25 to 59 yrs (5 male, 7 female) with special focus on proprioceptive tissue within the glenohumeral ligaments (46). We harvested the joint capsule and the glenohumeral ligaments 3 to 12 hrs after death. After opening the glenohumeral joint by a dorsal approach the ligaments were completely excised. The tissue was marked according to its origin and direction, allowing the orientation to be maintained throughout processing. The material was fixed in 10% formaldehyde solution for 6 wks. Dehydration and paraffin embedding was carried out according to usual techniques.

Transversally serial sections of 15 μm were performed using a rotation microtome. Then the slices were dewaxed, watered, and one out of three slices was hematoxylin-eosin and van Giesson stained for light microscopic evaluation. When a possible neural structure, such as a possible nerve ending, was detected, the adjacent cuts were dehydrated and preserved with DePeX and cover glass. Then, for specific identification of neural elements, we made use of a special silver impregnation technique described by Novotny and Gommert-Novotny for staining peripheral axons (63). This technique proved to be highly sensitive for neural structures and gives reproducible results. With this technique axons appeared dark brown to black on a clear yellowish-brown background. Large axons were frequently less intensely impregnated but were always unmistakable. Very fine axons (0.2 μm diameter or less) appear as thin gray lines. Muscle and collagen fibers have a reddish-brown color. Second opinion for the control of interpretation of the silver-impregnated stained cuts was performed in 8 out of 12 specimens by Novotny himself.

Histological Investigation: Results

The glenohumeral ligaments were found to have an extensive intraligamentous neural network. We discovered axons of different diameters ranging from 0.2 μm to 70 μm, mainly in the inferior glenohumeral ligament. Close to the humeral site the axons run parallel to small vessels, representing neurovascular bundles. Within the ligaments, however, these axons have no relation to vessels or vessel walls. Most of these axons show a serpentine configuration, oriented in line with collagen fibers (see figure 23.1). This may be due to artifacts during fixation, processing, and preparation of the specimens. However, because of the uniform longitudinal configuration, almost parallel, within the collageneous tissue of the ligaments, it seems to be a regular pattern of these intraligamenteous axons, which gives extra length and may allow stretching of the nerve tissue during motion and elongation of the collagen tissue.

Most of the discovered axons were located in the subsynovial layer of the ligaments. Generally the diameter of these subsynovial axons does not exceed 10 μm. In addition to these axonal structures, we detected nerve endings that could be classified according to Freeman and Wyke as type II mechanoreceptors (Pacinian corpuscles) (25) (see figure 23.2). These mechanoreceptors had a diameter of approximately 150 μm. They were also positioned directly beneath the synovial membrane (see figure 23.3). Both the nerve network and the mechanoreceptors could be clearly correlated to the ligaments and were not part of the rotator cuff tendons. A quantitative analysis to compare the nerve network, nerve density, or the amount of nerve endings in different regions of the capsule or the ligaments could not be performed on the base of the evaluated material.

Neurophysiological Investigation: Material and Methods

Subjects: Intraoperative EMG responses were experimentally measured in 10 patients with subacromial pathology (52). The patients' ages ranged from 25 to 67 yrs; none suffered from any kind of shoulder instability. Diagnostic arthroscopy did not reveal any intraarticular pathologic findings indicating an unstable glenohumeral joint.

Anesthesia: In order to exclude possible influences on the EMG response by narcotics, we used a modified neuroleptanalgesia (tranquanalgesia). This was an analgesic-based anesthesia without narcotic gases,

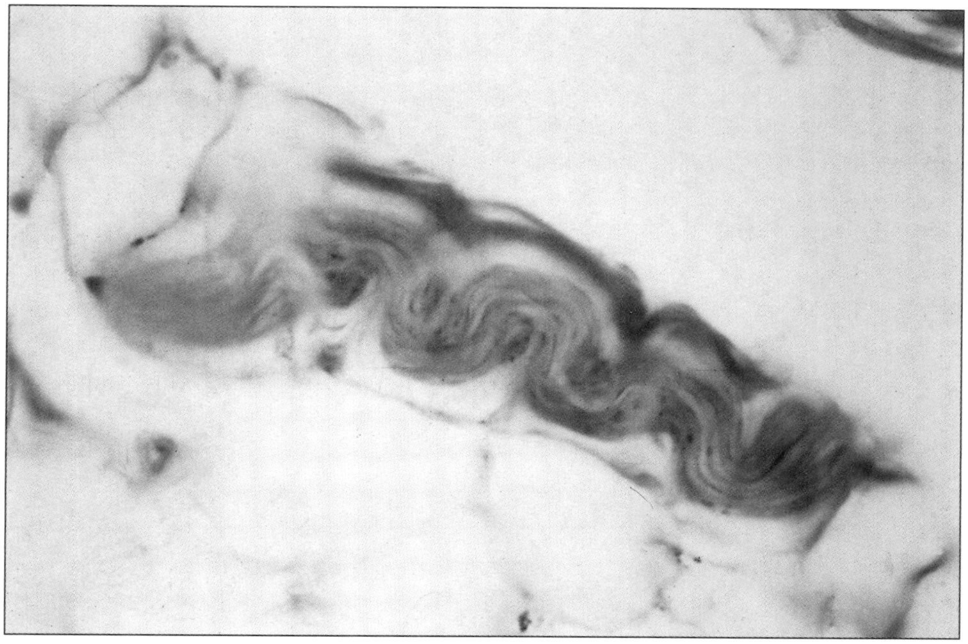

Figure 23.1 Nerve fiber within the glenohumeral ligaments.

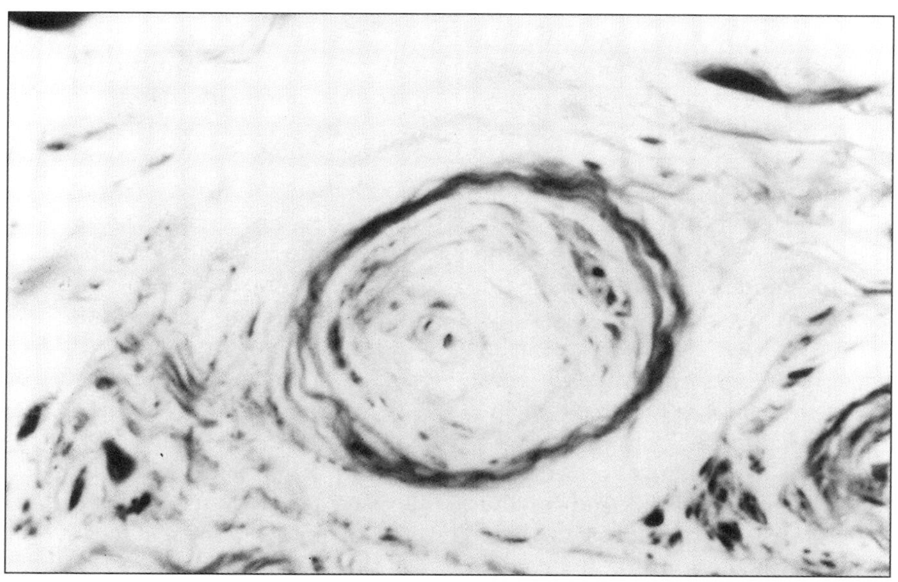

Figure 23.2 Pacinian corpuscle in the glenohumeral ligaments.

based mainly on fentanyl and benzodiazepines. In one subject, serving as an internal control, we blocked the neural pathway by plexus anesthesia.

Arthroscopy: Arthroscopy was performed in the beach-chair position. The glenohumeral joint was entered via a standard dorsal portal. After complete joint inspection an anterosuperior portal was developed in an outside-in technique. The intraarticular stimulation electrode was inserted through this portal. This electrode was a screw electrode that was placed in the anteroinferior capsule. During the whole procedure the joint was filled with a nonconducting fluid in order to avoid unselected stimulation of glenohumeral structures (see figure 23.4).

Intraoperative response: Stimulation was performed with a stimulation frequency of 1–2 Hz (Schwarzer EMG 2002). The value of the electric cur-

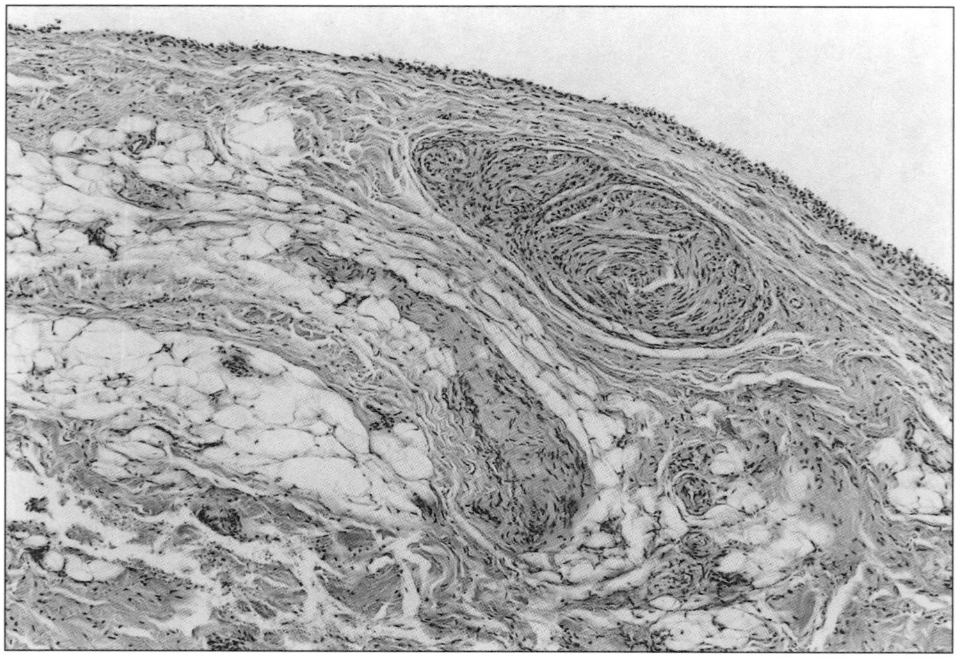

Figure 23.3 Mechanoreceptor located directly beneath the synovial membrane.

rent was automatically set by the EMG device between 100 and 200 V in accordance with the individual needs and reactions of each individual, but was limited to 90 mA. With this stimulation technique adapted to each subject, we attempted to generate the minimum receptor potential leading to a muscle response. With this setup each muscle was tested in every subject. The generated muscle potentials were recorded with needle electrodes for the following muscles: trapezius muscle, pectoralis muscle, deltoid muscle with its three parts, biceps brachii muscle, teres minor muscle, subscapularis muscle, supraspinatus muscle, and infraspinatus muscle (see figure 23.5).

Stimulation electrode: A cardiological pacemaker electrode (Modell Y, Biotronics) was used for the intraarticular stimulation. The electrode was screwed into the joint capsule with its helicoidal apex. The head of the screw electrode had a surface area of 12 mm^2, and the ring electrode had a surface area of 48 mm^2.

Neurophysiological Investigation: Results

The results of EMG recording in the first two subjects tested were too irregular, due to technical difficulties. Except for the one patient with plexus anesthesia, alterations of the membrane potential were detected in all other subjects in the superficial and in the deep muscle groups after intraarticular stimulation (see figure 23.6).

The EMG response in the different muscle groups occurred with a clearly demonstrable latency period between 100 and 516 ms, ruling out an immediate transmission of the impulse. The shortest latency periods could be demonstrated in the anterior part of the deltoid muscle. In increasing order, the EMG-response times of the other muscles were as follows: pectoralis major, posterior part of the deltoid, teres minor, infraspinatus, trapezius, subscapularis, biceps brachii, supraspinatus, and the lateral part of the deltoid (see table 23.1). No significant differences were noted. We did not perform a quantitative or qualitative differentiation of individual muscle groups. In the one patient with plexus anesthesia no EMG response after stimulation of the glenohumeral joint capsule was detected. This excluded the direct overflow in this setup.

Clinical Investigation: Material and Methods

Evaluation technique: For documentation of the joint position sense (JPS) we used an active angle reproduction test (ART) (49). A motion analyzing system with passive reflecting markers was used for measuring the joint position. The low weight of the

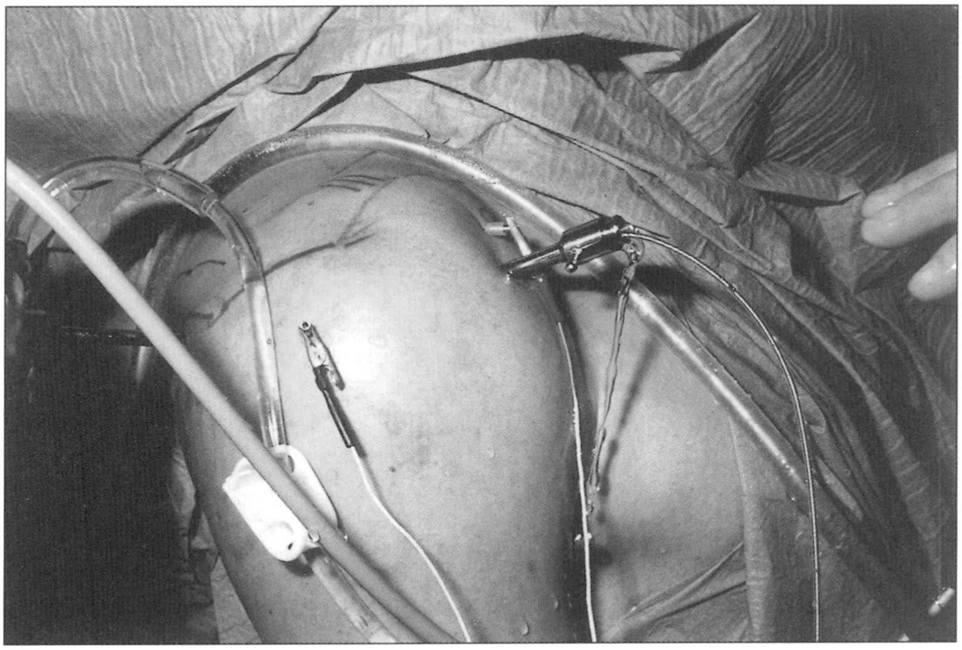

Figure 23.4 Arthroscopic set-up.

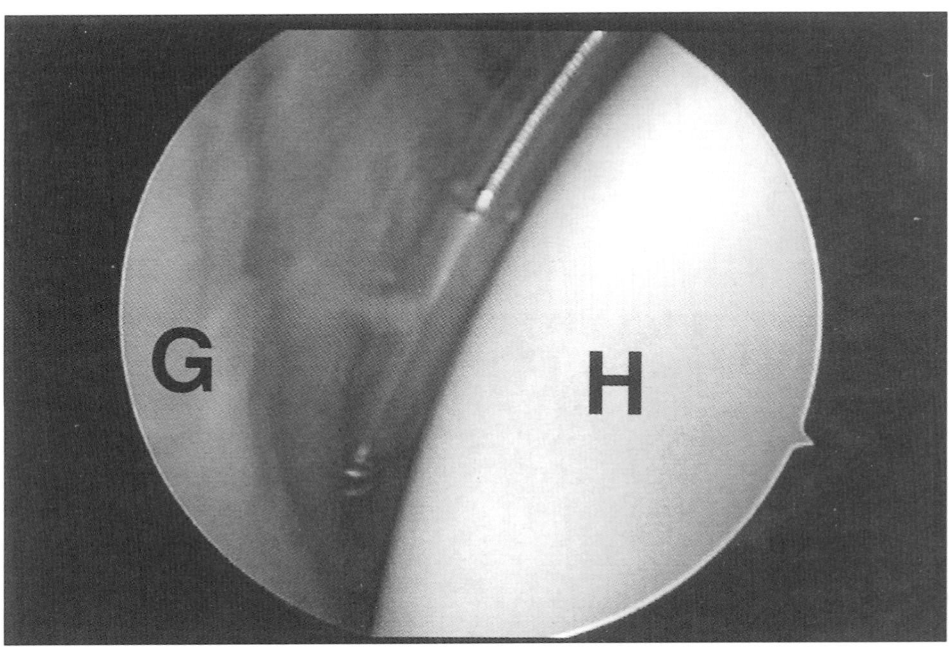

Figure 23.5 Stimulation electrode at the anteroinferior capsule.

markers did not influence the motion pattern of the tested subjects (see figure 23.7). The markers were illuminated by infrared light. The picture was recorded by a CCD camera under normal light conditions and the signal was stored by a PC.

The scanning frequency of the system was 50 Hz. The maximal accuracy of the measuring system depends on the marker size and the distance between the camera and measured object. With reference to our setup (distance to object: 5 m; marker size: 2 cm in

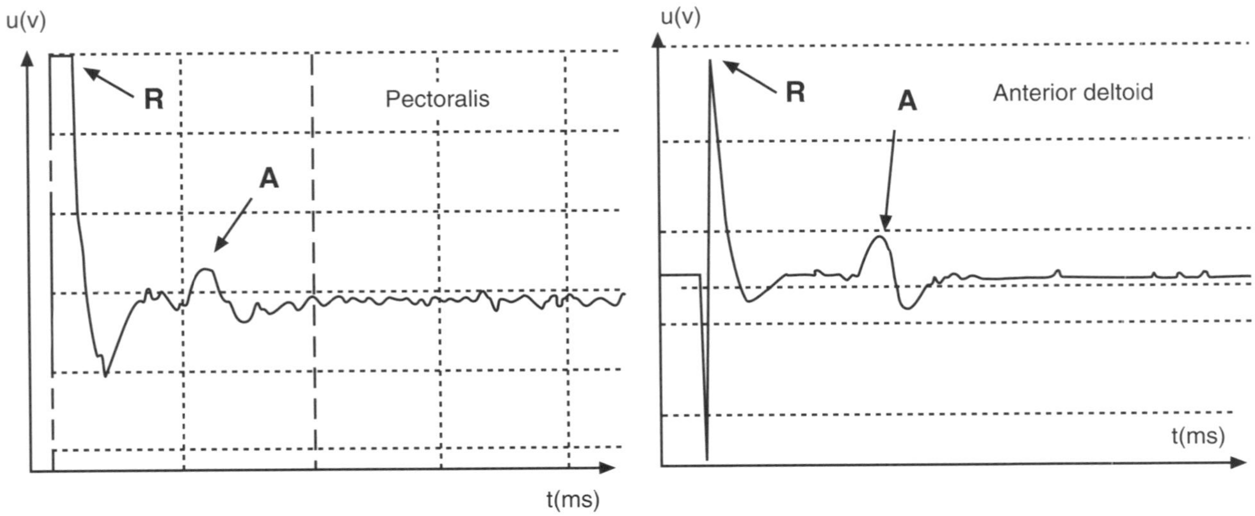

Figure 23.6 EMG signal (A) after intraarticular stimulation (R) of the joint capsule; pectoralis muscle, anterior deltoid muscle.

Table 23.1 Latency Periods of Different Muscle Groups After Intraarticular Stimulation of the Shoulder Joint Capsule (in ms)

	Minimum	Maximum	Mean	Standard deviation
Trapezius	286	324	302.0	18.3
Delt. ant.:	100	372	215.5	90.0
Delt. post:	232	269	251.6	15.2
Delt. lat:	433	510	470.6	31.5
Pect.:	110	353	229.3	88.0
Infras.:	132	425	287.8	104.3
Supra.:	377	516	424.5	54.7
Subscap.:	304	377	349.3	28.3
Biceps:	356	416	386.0	24.5
Tr. min.:	142	352	252.6	86.1

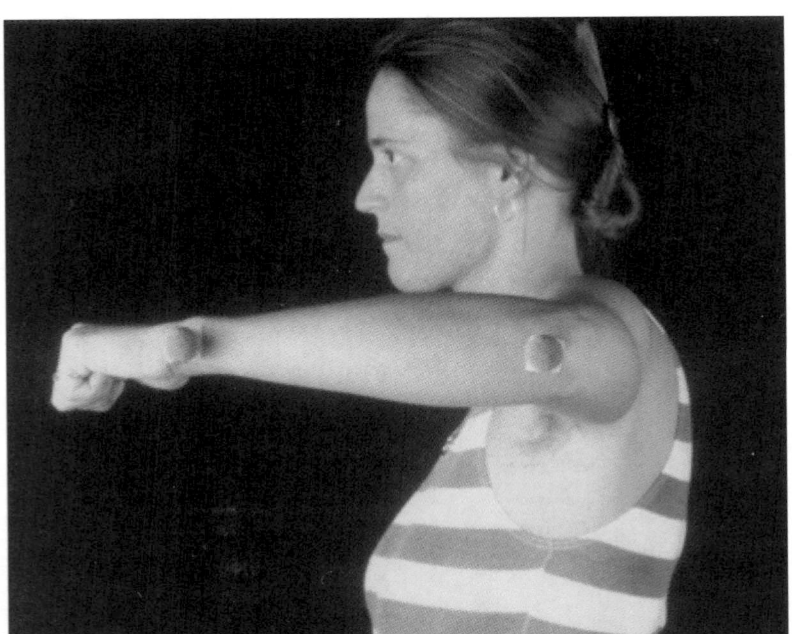

Figure 23.7 The angle reproduction test (ART) for documentation of the joint position sense.

diameter; resolution of the camera chip: 512 × 312 pixel; using a normal camera objective), the accuracy was 3 mm. The two markers necessary for angle calculation in the horizontal or vertical plane have a distance of approximately 30 cm (elbow to end of ulnar bone). For this case, our motion analysis system ("Kinemetrix") has a maximum error regarding angle calculation of less than 0.6%. Adding the error that results by skin movement and joint position adjustment error by the examiner, the total error was ≤ 0.98%.

After a standardized warm-up the volunteers were asked to actively reproduce 9 standardized joint position angles with and without visual control. Prior to each measurement the appropriate joint position was adjusted by the volunteer and controlled by the examiner. In order to avoid influences on the perception by skin receptors, the measurements were performed stripped to the waist among male volunteer and with a bikini top among the female volunteers.

Other environmental influences (draft, noise) were excluded by using a special room and creating reproducible standardized conditions. The measurements were performed for the dominant as well as for the nondominant extremity with and without visual control.

Starting from the neutral position, the following joint positions were measured: 50°, 100°, and 150° abduction in the plane of the scapula, 50°, 100°, 150° flexion, +45°, 0°, –45° rotation in 90° abduction. In total, 36 measurements for each volunteer were performed.

Control group: A group of 30 healthy volunteers (12 females, 18 males) with an age range of 22 to 36 yrs served as control. According to the past history none of the subjects suffered from previous acute shoulder injuries or any chronic complaints. On clinical examination there were no pathological findings.

Patient group: With the same setup, we examined 28 patients (15 female, 13 male) with posttraumatic anterior shoulder instability. The ages ranged from 21 to 35. The number of redislocations ranged from 4 to 32. All patients underwent subsequent surgery and all had Bankart lesions on arthroscopic examination.

Statistical evaluation: The results of each measurement were determined by means of angle-time-diagrams. Multivariate analysis of variance was used to examine statistical differences in the data tables. Student's *t* tests were performed to analyze the differences in normally distributed variables (paired and unpaired). In addition, the comparison of more than two independent random samples were carried out by an univariate analysis of variance (ANOVA). A level of $p < .05$ was accepted for statistical significance.

Clinical Investigation: Results

Control group: As expected, the highest differences could be documented by comparing the measured values between tests carried out with and without visual control. Without visual control the protocol showed worse results below the shoulder level (50°) for flexion as well as for abduction. This means that the differences of the angle reproduction tests with and without visual control were highly significant.

Similar results could be demonstrated for rotation above shoulder level as well. While external rotation in 90° abduction did hardly reveal any difference between the reproducing angles with and without visual control, there were significant differences in neutral rotation as well as in internal rotation.

The analysis of the results regarding the dominant versus the nondominant extremity did not reveal any statistical difference. The analysis concerning the influence of the volunteer's gender did also not show any differences except in 50° abduction at the nondominant extremity, in 150° flexion at the dominant side, as well as in 100° abduction at the nondominant side.

Patient group: In the patient group again there was a significantly better JPS with visual control than without. When comparing the patients to the controls there were differences in most of the ARTs with worse results in the patient group. These differences were significant in 150° flexion with and without visual control, in 150° abduction without visual control, and in 100° abduction with visual control. For rotation there were trends for almost all joint positions; however, the differences were significant only in the –45° position (see tables 23.2–23.4).

When comparing the noninjured contralateral shoulder of the patients with the control group, there still were differences. Again these differences were not significant in all joint positions, but significantly worse JPS could be demonstrated for 150° abduction without visual control, 50° flexion without visual control, –45° rotation without visual control, and 0° rotation with visual control (see tables 23.5–23.10).

Joint Position Sense in Elite Adolescent Tennis Players

Volunteers: A group of 60 adolescent volunteers (27 females, 33 males) aged 8 to 16 yrs were examined (mean age: 12.58 ±2.41 yrs). Of these, 40 volunteers

Table 23.2 Injured Group vs. Healthy Group Shoulder Abduction

	Without visual control			With visual control		
	50°	100°	150°	50°	100°	150°
Injured group	7.5	8.6	9.1	5.1	6.7	7.2
Control group	8.7	7.7	5.9	3.8	4.1	5.0
SD	5.0	7.6	5.2	4.8	5.9	5.6
SD	6.7	7.4	4.9	4.0	3.5	4.2
p	0.395	0.61	0.013	0.199	0.043	0.105

Table 23.3 Injured Group vs. Healthy Group Shoulder Flexion

	Without visual control			With visual control		
	50°	100°	150°	50°	100°	150°
Injured group	10.3	8.7	9.4	5.7	5.6	7.4
Control group	10.4	6.4	5.4	6.5	4.4	3.9
SD	8.1	5.5	6.6	3.8	4.8	7.1
SD	7.7	5.7	4.2	5.7	3.0	4.2
p	0.947	0.081	0.001	0.551	0.158	0.040

Table 23.4 Injured Group vs. Healthy Group Shoulder Rotation

	Without visual control			With visual control		
	45°	–45°	0°	45°	–45°	0°
Injured group	7.8	15.1	8.2	5.0	8.2	5.2
Control group	6.0	6.9	7.7	4.9	4.2	3.8
SD	4.9	10.1	4.8	4.6	7.0	4.3
SD	5.0	5.4	6.3	5.3	3.9	3.2
p	0.143	0.001	0.755	0.899	0.021	0.116

Table 23.5 Healthy Side of Injured Group vs. Control Group Shoulder Abduction

	Without visual control			With visual control		
	50°	100°	150°	50°	100°	150°
Injured group	7.3	7.5	10.3	5.1	6.0	7.4
Control group	8.7	7.7	6.0	3.8	4.1	5.0
SD	6.6	4.7	7.1	4.9	7.0	6.1
SD	6.6	7.4	4.9	0.2	3.5	4.2
p	0.377	0.91	0.006	0.202	0.185	0.076

Table 23.6 Healthy Side of Injured Group vs. Control Group Shoulder Flexion

	Without visual control			With visual control		
	50°	100°	150°	50°	100°	150°
Injured group	7.7	6.4	6.8	6.1	4.4	5.8
Control group	10.4	6.4	5.4	6.5	4.4	3.9
SD	4.5	4.6	5.4	5.6	4.0	5.7
SD	7.7	5.7	4.2	5.7	3.0	4.2
p	0.039	0.995	0.173	0.783	0.996	0.128

Table 23.7 Healthy Side of Injured Group vs. Control Group Shoulder Rotation

	Without visual control			With visual control		
	45°	–45°	0°	45°	–45°	0°
Injured group	7.2	9.9	6.9	4.9	5.7	5.5
Control group	6.0	6.9	7.7	4.9	4.2	3.8
SD	5.5	7.3	4.1	6.7	4.4	3.1
SD	5.0	5.4	6.3	5.3	3.9	3.2
p	0.298	0.036	0.487	0.994	0.115	0.022

Table 23.8 Healthy vs. Injured Side Shoulder Abduction

	Without visual control			With visual control		
	50°	100°	150°	50°	100°	150°
Injured side	7.5	8.6	9.1	5.1	6.7	7.2
Healthy side	7.3	7.4	10.0	5.1	6.3	6.5
SD	5.0	7.6	5.2	4.8	5.9	5.6
SD	6.6	4.6	6.9	4.9	7.2	5.6
p	0.910	0.437	0.57	1.000	0.793	0.486

Table 23.9 Healthy vs. Injured Side Shoulder Flexion

	Without visual control			With visual control		
	50°	100°	150°	50°	100°	150°
Injured side	10.3	8.7	9.4	5.7	5.6	7.4
Healthy side	7.5	6.4	7.2	5.9	4.4	5.5
SD	8.1	5.5	6.6	3.8	4.8	7.1
SD	4.5	4.7	5.6	5.6	4.1	6.1
p	0.050	0.123	0.186	0.831	0.253	0.293

Table 23.10 Healthy vs. Injured Side Shoulder Rotation

	Without visual control			With visual control		
	45°	–45°	0°	45°	–45°	0°
Injured side	7.8	15.1	8.2	5.0	8.2	5.2
Healthy side	6.7	10.4	6.7	5.0	5.3	5.7
SD	4.9	10.1	4.8	4.6	7.0	4.3
SD	4.5	7.7	3.8	7.2	4.3	3.4
p	0.445	0.002	0.278	1.000	0.123	0.661

were national elite tennis players (18 females, 22 males). The remaining 20 subjects (11 males, 9 females) within the age range of 14 to 16 yrs (mean age: 15.05 ±0.76 yrs) served as controls. According to the rules of the German Tennis Federation the players at state or national level were obliged to participate in a yearly routine physical and medical checkup. All volunteers of the control group attended the examination voluntarily; a written informed consent was signed by their parents. None of the subjects suffered from any acute injuries or chronic complaints of the shoulder (50). For documentation of JPS we used the above-described ART.

Results

Angle reproduction of all volunteers was best in the midrange of shoulder motion (100° flexion, 100° abduction, neutral rotation in 90° abduction). Angle reproduction capability was worst below shoulder level (50° flexion, 50° abduction, internal rotation in 90° abduction). A correlation of proprioceptive capabilities to sex or dominant extremity could not be found. Subjects older than 12 yrs have a tendency for better angle reproduction compared to younger subjects. Tennis players older than 12 yrs showed significantly better capabilities for angle reproduction in tennis-specific movements of the shoulder complex.

Discussion

In the 19th century, the neurologist Duchenne stressed the importance of sensory impulses from articular structures (69). Physiologists also considered the sensory information from periarticular structures to be an important source for proprioceptive and kinesthetic information (2, 89, 90). In 1944 Abbott (1) discovered sensory innervations in knee ligaments. He concluded that signals transferred to the central nervous system regulate the joint-stabilizing muscles.

In a study of patients who had undergone cruciate ligament reconstruction, Kennedy and coworkers (56) found that good short-term results always deteriorate in the long run. According to their opinion the loss of the feedback mechanism by the mechanoreceptors would explain this phenomenon, rather than reduction of the mechanical stability of the ACL transplant itself. In the following years many ultrastructural histological studies concentrated on the knee joint.

Schultz and coworkers (83) and Schutte and coworkers (84) detected mechanoreceptors in the anterior cruciate ligament. In a microscopic study using light, electron, scanning electron, and transmission electron microscopy, Haus and coworkers (37) classified 3 types of nerve endings:

1. Pacinian corpuscles, transferring fast alterations of forces, showing a fast adaptation and low stimulation threshold
2. Ruffini corpuscles, signaling slowly changing dimensions of effecting forces and showing a slow adaptation and a low stimulation threshold
3. Free nerve endings, reacting as nociceptors and signaling pain and possibly mechanical and thermal stimuli as well

Does the Shoulder Joint Follow Mechanisms Comparable to Those in the Knee Joint?

Injury to the anteroinferior ligament complex is the main predisposing factor for shoulder instability. According to the literature, the incidence of accompanying Bankart lesions ranges from 27% to 100% (76). Baker and coworkers (3) arthroscopically examined patients after traumatic shoulder dislocation within 10 days after the initial injury. Besides different intraarticular injury patterns, they found the most unstable shoulder joints in patients with a complete avulsion of the anterior labrum complex, which is termed a Bankart lesion (4). Wheeler and coworkers (101) found a redislocation rate of 92% after a traumatic anterior shoulder dislocation in young athletes. After arthroscopic labrum fixation in comparable subjects, the redislocation rate could be reduced to 22%. These clinical observations of the Baker and Wheeler groups emphasize the clinical relevance of the traumatic disruption of the anterior capsule-labrum complex in the pathogenesis of the posttraumatic shoulder instability.

The concept attributing neurological synergy between ligaments and muscles to the common purpose of maintaining joint stability was first described in 1990 by Payr (68). Even nature shows that loss of sensation leads to shoulder instability, for example, in patients with syringomyelia (73). It is thought that involvement of deep pain fibers early in the course of this disease allows for the development of neuropathic joints even before the recognition of other deficits (71). As a general rule, involvement of the anterior horn cells and the lateral horn of the spinal cord gray matter occurs later in the disease process (96). It is also thought that loss of protective joint sensitivity and the secondary relaxation of the glenohumeral ligaments can allow advertent overload of the shoulder joint and may eventually produce joint damage (10, 26).

Rudinger (78) described in the first detailed microscopic dissection of the shoulder capsule extensive innervation from articular branches of the axillary, musculocutaneous, and suprascapular nerves terminating within the capsule. Wrete (102) performed histological serial sections of 5 silver-impregnated fetus shoulders, and he described multiple innervations of the capsule by sensory branches from the axillary, musculocutaneous, suprascapular, and subscapular nerves. Gardner (29) described innervation patterns similar to those given by Wrete (102), with the exception of a possible articular innervation by the radial nerve. Furthermore, Glousman and coworkers (31) found in EMG studies significantly increased activity in the supraspinatus muscle in subjects with unstable glenohumeral joints. These findings showed the importance of active stabilizing mechanisms of the rotator cuff.

The neurological structures in the glenohumeral joint capsule that were detected (44, 46), therefore seem to be of clinical significance. These histological studies demonstrated mechanoreceptors (Pacinian corpuscles) in the glenohumeral ligaments. The receptors are considered to belong to the fast adapting type (9, 25, 103) called "acceleration receptors" (90). Other authors pointed out that these mechanoreceptors are activated by each movement, regardless of the starting position of the joint, and they found that the answer of the receptors was a function of the motion velocity (11, 19). In the following years different groups also reported on the presence of mechanoreceptors in the glenohumeral joint capsule (36, 67, 74 ,91, 98) or in paraarticular structures (41, 65).

Our histological and neurophysiological findings suggest that the joint capsule probably contains PD receptors, which are a combination of proportional (intensity detectors) and differential (velocity detectors) receptors. An electrical stimulation will depolarize all receptor structures of the joint capsule. A receptor potential will be generated since an electrical stimulus adequately addresses each type of receptor. This may be a reason for the response of almost all muscles of the shoulder girdle.

The different response time in different shoulder muscles is also not surprising, taking into account that during shoulder motion different EMG patterns of the surrounding musculature can be obtained. This shows that each muscle has its own function in different shoulder positions.

The long latency reflexes of the EMG response corresponds to similar findings in the knee joint (53, 70). Johansson and coworkers (53) stated that the long latency in response excludes a direct protective reflex at the knee joint. They postulated an indirect influence on the discharge of the alpha motoneurons via the gamma spindle system by alteration of the sensitivity of the muscle spindles. By this mechanism the mechanoreceptors cause a certain pretension of the musculature and, therefore, an increase in joint stability. A direct muscle reflex, therefore, can no longer be supported.

Guanche and coworkers (33) proved the existence of an indirect reflex arc from the glenohumeral capsule to several muscles crossing the shoulder joint in a feline model. They found three branches of the axillary nerve terminating in the glenohumeral capsule.

Tibone and coworkers (94) evaluated the sensorimotor pathway in patients with stable and unstable shoulder joints with somatosensory cortical evoked potentials. They were able to generate consistent waveforms when stimulating different intraarticular structures (inferior glenohumeral ligament, middle glenohumeral ligament, subscapularis tendon, biceps tendon, supraspinatus tendon, glenoid labrum) with a monopolar electrode.

Taking all these findings into account, proprioception is considered to play an important role in the stabilization and coordination of the shoulder joint (8, 15, 60, 61). Blasier and coworkers (8) adopted our histological findings and also regarded the tension of the capsule as the responsible mechanism of the shoulder proprioception. Cohen (12, 13) emphasized that the main contribution to a precise position sense is created by joint receptors; the skin and muscle-tendon receptors, however, have smaller but important and independent responsibilities regarding position sense.

In our clinical studies we measured joint position sense (JPS) by an angle reproduction test (ART). Abduction was performed in the plane of the scapula to reproduce the true physiological abduction plane (55). A motion analyzing system with passive reflective markers was used. The advantage of this technique, compared to mechanic or electronic devices, is that a supporting surface is not needed (8, 15, 46, 60, 61, 92). Therefore, the measurements could be performed free of contact with the subject, and the subjects did not receive any information from tactile receptors. The weight of the markers was so low that the proprioceptive information was not influenced.

Other Test Designs for the Measurements of the Proprioception

Smith and Brunolli (92) used a "shoulder wheel" device. The volunteers were placed in a supine position, with a 90° abduction of the shoulder joint and a flexed elbow joint. In order to avoid skin sensation, the extremity was placed into an air splint, which was fixed at a wheel. Furthermore, the subjects were blindfolded and headphones were put on. By means of surface electrodes the electrical activity of the pectoralis major muscle was checked. Three different tests were performed (threshold to sensation of movement test, angle reproduction test, end range reproduction test). The shoulder wheel was connected to a motor in such a way that the arm could be well balanced and rotated in a passive manner. For the angle reproduction test the volunteers were put into a position that was maintained for a period of 30 s. After that the wheel rotated back to the baseline position and moved after a short time toward the direction of the given position. The volunteers were asked to signal when they thought the arm had reached the previously given angle. The pectoralis major muscle must stay relaxed during the entire test in order to minimize the influence of the muscle receptors.

Lephart and coworkers (60) performed an angle reproduction test and a threshold to sensation of movement test. The test protocol was similar to that of Smith and Brunolli (92). During this test the arm of the subject was passively rotated to a defined position. This given position, however, had to be actively reproduced by the subject. In the threshold to sensation of movement test, the shoulder is passively rotated internally and externally from different baseline position, and the subject gives a signal when a motion, as well as the corresponding direction of motion, is detected.

Blasier and coworkers (8) performed a threshold to sensation of movement test. An electrogoniometer served as a measuring device. The test protocol was similar to that of Lephart and coworkers (60); however, there was a significant difference in the position of the subjects. At given positions (0°, 60°, 90°) the forearm stayed in a vertical position toward the measuring device, and the backrest of the seat was set at 0°, 60° and 90°. The purpose of this setup was to minimize skin sensation, which could be created by the weight of the forearm (8).

Davies and Dickhoff-Hoffmann (15) applied an angle reproduction test in shoulder flexion, abduction, and internal and external rotation in 100 healthy male subjects. For that purpose they used a Cybex system, but they did not describe how the measurements were performed.

A study with a completely different setup was undertaken by Cohen (12, 13) in 1957. In the frontal plane in front of the subjects a target with four concentric circles was placed. On each of these circles 12 points were marked, which corresponded to the positions of the dial of a clock. With closed eyes the subjects, who were acoustically directed by the examiner, placed the index finger of the extended arm exactly on one of these points. After that the subjects moved their arms into the relaxed starting position and then tried to reproduce the previous position. One advantage of this setup was the contact-free evaluation. Secondly, a quite large range of motion can be easily evaluated with this design. However, this can be also considered as a limitation of his study, because, when performing the movements, the subjects always used combinations of abduction, horizontal flexion, and vertical flexion (anteversion). Considering the accuracy, this test design is, of course, inferior to computer assisted measuring devices as used in more recent studies (8, 15, 47, 48, 60).

The validity of the proprioceptive test procedures is certainly a problem, which was recognized by Blasier and coworkers (8). They have already stated that the measured sensitivity for motion has its origin not only in the glenohumeral joint. Lephart and coworkers (60), Blasier and coworkers (8), and

Smith and Brunolli (92) tried to minimize the tactile perceptions of the extremity by air splints, elastic bandages, or the preservation of the vertical position of the forearm. But they did not take into consideration that during rotation of the glenohumeral joint, significant motion of the scapula occurs, which in the supine position possibly leads to proprioceptive sensation.

Comparison With Results of Other Studies

Our JPS studies demonstrated that in abduction and flexion the subjects reproduced substantially above the given angles in the lower range of motion and substantially below the given angles in the higher range of motion, especially for the tests without visual control. Furthermore, it became obvious that the lowest deviations occurred at 100° flexion and the highest at 50° flexion.

Cohen (12, 13) showed that, in general, the average error in the smallest circle was smaller than the average error in any other circle. Because the circles were in a concentric formation and the movements were performed as combinations of abduction and horizontal and vertical flexion, the result of the present study could be confirmed.

Lephart and coworkers (60) compared the angle reproduction of unstable shoulders with the contralateral stable shoulders. Commencing with 0° and 30° external rotation, 10° positions had to be reproduced. In this setup the internal rotation showed higher deviations than the external rotation.

Blasier and coworkers (8) demonstrated that the sensation of movement during external rotation was significantly more sensitive ($p < .001$) than during internal rotation. The sensitivity of the external rotation increased more clearly the further the limit of the rotation ability was approached. Furthermore, these studies demonstrated very significant proprioceptive deficits ($p < .002$) for subjects with general laxity and highly significantly greater sensitivity of external rotation movements, which caused a tightening of the glenohumeral capsule, than internal rotation movements, which led to a loosening of the capsule.

The question that still remains is why the most accurate proprioceptive capability was found in the present study at the neutral rotation and, according to the results of Cohen (12, 13), at the innermost circle. During external rotation from –45° to 0°, tightening of the glenohumeral joint capsule results, but it is certainly not as distinct as during external rotation from 0° to 45°. In the present study the best proprioceptive sensitivity of the abduction and flexion position was registered in the midrange of motion, and the lowest sensitivity of the flexion position was measured in the lower motion sectors. These findings are in accordance with previous studies (48, 49).

Based on the hypothesis that tightening of the capsule is one of the mechanisms responsible for shoulder proprioception, the results of abduction and flexion can be explained. At 110° the maximal abduction position in the scapular plane of the glenohumeral joint is reached. Therefore, at the 100° position the joint capsule is almost maximally tightened and a high stimulation of the mechanoreceptors that are responsible for proprioception can be detected. This capsular tension is far from being achieved at 50° abduction and, therefore, because of the substantially lower stimulation of the mechanoreceptors, the proprioceptive capacity is decreased.

The question that now arises is why the results in the 150° position are worse compared to those at 100°, because the glenohumeral capsule is maximally tightened at an angle of 150°. A possible explanation for this finding may be that the proprioceptive demand is higher in abduction of 150° than at 100°. The reason could be that the 100° abduction position is mainly a glenohumeral movement, while the 150° abduction is performed with the involvement of the acromioclavicular and sternoclavicular joints as well as the rotation of the scapula. Therefore, the 150° abduction is a more complex movement and requires the coordination of proprioceptive information derived from different articular structures. With respect to the findings for the flexion positions, a similar explanation can be applied.

The assumption is that an increased proprioceptive requirement arises with involvement of the clavicular joints and the scapula, but this involvement does not have any influence on the rotation, because in the present study the rotation was carried out only in an area between –45° and +45°. The glenohumeral joint, however, includes an area between –60° and +60°. Although Blasier and coworkers (8) detected that the proprioceptive capability increased by approaching the limit of the external rotation, the findings of the present study revealed that more precise results could be achieved at 60° external rotation compared to 90° external rotation. These results could be possibly explained by the assumption that the clavicular joints and the shoulder blades are involved in the external rotation movement between 60° and 90°.

Angle reproductions of the dominant and nondominant extremities: In the present study the comparison of the dominant and nondominant extremity did not reveal any significant differences. These findings are in accordance with those of Blasier and coworkers (8), Lephart and coworkers (60), Smith and Brunolli (92), as well as Jerosch and coworkers (48, 49).

Sex-Dependent Differences

The results of the present study, as well as those of Blasier and coworkers (8) and Jerosch, Thorwesten and coworkers (48, 49), showed that the proprioceptive capability does not depend on the sex of the subjects. Proprioceptive advantages of one gender over the other could not be demonstrated, either when comparing men and women, or boys and girls.

Age-Dependent Differences

When comparing age groups, the older group (age > 12yrs) attained more accurate results in almost all measurements, but only four joint positions showed statistically significant differences. Nevertheless, it can be concluded that children up to 11 yrs of age have certain proprioceptive disadvantages compared to adolescents older than 11 yrs. Crowe and coworkers (14) and Hearn and coworkers (38) found substantial age-dependent differences in their study of a group of 137 in the age range of 8 to 24 yrs; accuracy increased slowly but significantly with increasing age.

The comparison between tennis players and control group revealed that the proprioception of the shoulder of adolescent tennis players under the age of 11 yrs is not different from that of other adolescents. Older tennis players, however, achieved better results at tennis-specific movements compared to the control group. Therefore, the conclusion can be drawn that the improved proprioceptive abilities can be learned and are not inherited.

Proprioceptive Capability in Subjects With Unstable Glenohumeral Joints

Our results of angle reproduction capability showed decreased proprioception in the unstable as well as in the contralateral glenohumeral joint. These findings are comparable to the results of Lephart and coworkers (60, 61), who measured kinesthesia and joint position sense in healthy, unstable, and surgically repaired shoulders. They found reduction in all tested proprioceptive capabilities in the unstable subjects and restoration after surgical repair.

Many factors point, therefore, to a kind of sensory function (biological strain gauge). Through this mechanism the shoulder stabilizing musculature may be partially regulated. A traumatic disruption of the capsule-labrum structure may lead to a decrease of this feedback mechanism, causing a deterioration of the active muscular stabilization that is of such great importance, especially for the glenohumeral joint. The increased translation strain on the hyaline cartilage and the repetitive micro- and macrotrauma to the joint lead to early joint degeneration and to further decompensation of the passive stabilizers. Although we still do not know everything about the mechanisms of proprioception, we know the proprioceptive capabilities are in-fluenced by many factors. Proprioception is part of the afferent pathways of the sensorimotor system.

Future Influence on Clinical Practice

For prevention of joint injuries, proprioceptive training should be performed. A standardized proprioceptive test should be included in the diagnostic evaluation of patients suffering from acute joint injuries or chronic joint complaints. Not only the injured, but also the contralateral noninjured extremity should exercise proprioceptive capabilities during postoperative rehabilitation or conservative treatment. When looking for new surgical techniques or when evaluating classical operations we should focus not only on anatomic but also on neurophysiological ways for restructure in order to restore the neurophysiological feedback mechanism.

There still are plenty of questions to answer in the future:

1. What is the mechanism of proprioception?
2. Does the incidence of shoulder dislocation, ACL injury, or ankle sprain correlate with decreased proprioception, or does the injury itself lead to a generalized decrease in proprioceptive capabilities?
3. Is proprioception a congenital or acquired factor?
4. Can we restore proprioception with surgical procedures?
5. Is proprioceptive prophylaxis cost effective?

Acknowledgments

I would like to acknowledge the following people who made the studies mentioned in this manuscript possible: H. Clashed, M. Schmitz-Nahrath, A. Grosse-Hackmann, L. Thorwesten, J. Steinbeck, T. Teigelkötter, M. Schröder, and M. Westhues.

References

1. Abbott LC, Saunders JB, Dec M. Injuries to the ligaments of the knee joint. *J Bone Joint Surg* 1944, 26: 503–21.
2. Adams JA. Feedback theory of how joint receptors regulate the timing and positioning of a limb. *Psychol Rev* 1977, 84: 504–23.
3. Baker CL, Uribe JW, Whitman C. Arthroscopic evaluation of acute initial anterior shoulder dislocation. *Am J Sports Med* 1990, 18: 25–28.
4. Bankart ASB. Recurrent or habitual dislocation of the shoulder joint. *Br Med J* 1923, 2: 1132–133.
5. Barrack RL, Skinner HB, Cook SD. Proprioception of the knee joint. *Am J Phys Med* 1984, 63: 175–81.
6. Barrack RL, Skinner HB, Cook SD, Haddad RJ Jr. Effect of articular disease and total knee arthroplasty on the knee joint position sense. *J Neurophysiol* 1983, 50: 684–87.
7. Barrett DS, Cobb AG, Bentley G. Joint proprioception in normal, osteoarthritic, and replaced knees. *J Bone Joint Surg* 1991, 73B: 53–56.
8. Blasier RB, Carpenter JE, Huston LJ. Shoulder proprioception: Effect of joint laxity, joint position, and direction of motion. *Orthop Rev* 1994, 23: 45–50.
9. Boyd IA. The histological structure of the receptors in the knee joint of the cat correlated with their physiological response. *J Physiol* 1954, 124: 476–88.
10. Brower AC, Allman RM. Pathogenesis of the neurotrophic joint: Neurotraumatic vs. neurovascular. *Radiology* 1981, 139: 349–54.
11. Burgess PR, Clarke FJ. Characteristics of the knee joint receptors in the cat. *J Physiol* 1969, 203: 317–35.
12. Cohen LA. Analysis of position sense in human shoulder. *J Neurophysiol* 1958, 21: 550–62.
13. Cohen LA. Contributions of tactile, musculotendinous and joint mechanisms to position sense in human shoulder. *J Neurophysiol* 1958, 21: 563–68.
14. Crowe A, Keessen W, Kuus W, van Vliet R, Zegeling A. Proprioceptive accuracy in two dimensions. *Percept Mot Skills* 1989, 69: 831–46.
15. Davies GJ, Dickoff-Hoffmann S. Neuromuscular testing and rehabilitation of the shoulder complex. *J Orthop Sports Phys Ther* 1993, 18: 449–58.
16. Davis AG. A conservative treatment for habitual dislocations of the shoulder. *JAMA* 1936, 107: 1012.
17. Delorme L. Die Hemmungsbänder des Schultergelenks und ihre Bedeutung für die Schulterluxation. *Arch Klin Chir* 1910, 92: 79–101.
18. Detrisiac DA, Johnson LL. *Arthroscopic shoulder anatomy.* Thorofare, NJ: Slack, 1986, pp. 95–114.
19. Ecklund G, Skoglund S. On the specificity of the Ruffini-like joint receptors. *Acta Physiol Scand* 1970, 49: 184–91.
20. Fick R. *Handbuch der Anatomie und Mechanik der Gelenke unter Berücksichtigung der bewegenden Muskeln.* Jena, Germany: Fischer, 1904, pp. 51–65.
21. Flood V. Discovery of a new ligament of the shoulder joint. *Lancet* 1829, 672–73.
22. Freemann MAR. Treatment of ruptures of the lateral ligament of the ankle. *J Bone Joint Surg* 1965, 47B: 661–68.
23. Freeman MAR. Instability of the foot after injuries to the lateral ligament of the ankle. *J Bone Joint Surg* 1965, 47B: 669–77.
24. Freeman MAR, Dean MRE, Hanham JWF. The etiology and prevention of functional instability of the foot. *J Bone Joint Surg* 1965, 47B: 678–85.
25. Freeman MAR, Wyke BD. The innervation of the knee joint: An anatomical and histological study in the cat. *J Anat* 1967, 101: 505–32.
26. Frewin DB, Downey JA, Feldman F, Myers SJ. Neuropathic arthropathy: A report of two cases. *Aust NZ J Med* 1973, 3: 587–92.
27. Galenus. *On the usefulness of the parts of the body.* Vol. 2. May MT, Trans. and Ed. Ithaca, NY: Cornell University Press, 1968, pp. 263–76.
28. Gandevia SC, McCloskey DI. Joint sense, muscle sense, and their combination as position sense, measured at the distal interphalangeal joint of the middle finger. *J Physiol* 1976, 260: 387–407.
29. Gardner E. The innervation of the shoulder joint. *Anat Rec* 1948, 102: 1–18.
30. Glencross D, Thornton E. Position sense following joint injury. *J Sports Med* 1981, 21: 23–27.
31. Glousman R, Jobe F, Tibone J. Dynamic electromyographic analysis of the throwing shoulder with glenohumeral instability. *J Bone Joint Surg* 1988, 70A: 220–26.

32. Gross MT. Effects of recurrent lateral ankle sprains on active and passive judgement of joint position. *Phys Ther* 1987, 10: 67–69.
33. Guanche C, Knatt Th, Solomonow M, Lu Y, Baratta R. The synergistic action of the capsule and the shoulder muscles. *Am J Sports Med* 1995, 23: 301–306.
34. Hammon DJ, France EP, Terry GC. Stabilizing function of passive shoulder restraints. *Trans Orthop Res Soc* 1987, 12: 77.
35. Harryman DT, Sidles JA, Harris SL, Masten FA. Laxity of the normal glenohumeral joint: A quantitative in vivo assessment. *J Shoulder Elbow Surg* 1992, 1: 66–76.
36. Hashimoto T, Hamada T, Suzuki K. Immunohistochemical approach to investigate the nerve distribution in shoulder joint capsule. Paper presented at the 3rd Scandinavian-Japanese Congress on Shoulder Surgery, Aarhus, Denmark, July 7–9, 1993.
37. Haus J, Halata Z, Refior HJ. Propriozeption im vorderen Kreuzband des menschlichen Kniegelenkes—morphologische Grundlagen. *Z Orthop* 1990, 130: 484–94.
38. Hearn M, Crowe A, Keessen W. Influence of age on proprioceptive accuracy in two dimensions. *Percept Mot Skills* 1989, 69: 811–18.
39. Hovelius L, Eriksson K, Fredin H, Hagberg G, Hussenius A, Lind B, Thorling J, Weckström J. Recurrences after initial dislocation of the shoulder. *J Bone Joint Surg* 1983, 65A, 343–48.
40. Howell SM, Galinat BJ, Renzi AJ, Marone PJ. Normal and abnormal mechanics of the glenohumeral joint in the horizontal plane. *J Bone Joint Surg* 1988, 70A: 227–32.
41. Ide K, Shirai Y, Ito H, Sibasaki T, Takayama A, Hashiguchi H, Ito H, Yoshimoto H. The neurohistological study in the subacromial bursa. Paper presented at the 20th annual meeting of the Japan Shoulder Society, Nagasaki, Japan, Oct 1–2, 1993.
42. Jerosch J, Moersler M, Castro WHM. Über die Funktion der passiven Stabilisatoren des glenohumeralen Gelenkes: Eine biomechanische Untersuchung. *Z Orthop* 1990, 128: 206–12.
43. Jerosch J, Marquardt M. Sonographische Untersuchung zur AP Translation des Humeruskopfes bei der aktiven Bewegung bei traumatischer anteriorer Schulterinstabilität. *Z Orthop* 1990, 128: 637–41.
44. Jerosch J. Über die Funktion der passiven Stabilisatoren des glenohumeralen Gelenkes. In: Kohn D, Wirth CJ, Eds, *Die Schulter: Aktuelle operative Therapie.* Stuttgart: Thieme, 1992, pp. 2–15.
45. Jerosch J, Castro WHM, Halm H, Drescher H. Does the glenohumeral joint capsule have proprioceptive capability? *Knee Surg Sports Traumatol Arthroscopy* 1993, 1: 80–84.
46. Jerosch J, Steinbeck J, Clahsen H, Schmitz-Nahrath M, Grosse-Hackmann A. Function of the glenohumeral ligaments in active stabilization of the shoulder joint. *Knee Surg Sports Traumatol Arthroscopy* 1993, 1: 152–58.
47. Jerosch J, Castro WHM, Hoffstetter I, Bischof M. Propriozeptive Fähigkeiten bei Probanden mit stabilen und instabilen Sprunggelenken. *Dtsch Z Sportmed* 1994, 45: 380–89.
48. Jerosch J, Thorwesten L. Propriozeption des Schultergelenkes bei gesunden Probanden. In: Jerosch J, Steinbeck J, Eds, *Aktuelle Konzepte der Diagnostik und Therapie des instabilen Schultergelenkes.* Aachen, Germany: Shaker, 1994, pp. 31–45.
49. Jerosch J, Thorwesten L, Steinbeck J, Reer R. Proprioceptive function of the shoulder girdle in healthy volunteers. *Knee Surg Sports Traumatol Arthroscopy* 1995, 3: 219–25.
50. Jerosch J, Thorwesten L, Teigelkötter T. Propriozeption des Schultergelenkes bei jugendlichen Tennisspielern. *Sportverl-Sportschad* 1997 11: 1–9.
51. Jerosch J, Schmidt K, Prymka M. Beeinflussung propriozeptiver Fähigkeiten von Kniegelenken mit einer primären Gonarthrose. *Unfallchirurg* 1997, 100: 219–24.
52. Jerosch J, Steinbeck J, Schröder M, Westhues M, Reer R. Intraoperative EMG response of the musculature after stimulation of the glenohumeral joint capsule. *Acta Orthop Belg* 1997, 63: 8–14.
53. Johansson H, Sjölander P, Sojka P. A sensory role for cruciate ligaments. *Clin Orthop* 1991, 268: 161–75.
54. Kapandji IA. *Funktionelle Anatomie der Gelenke.* Bd., Stuttgart: Enke, 1984, pp. 2–71.
55. Karlsson J, Andreasson GO. The effect of external ankle support in chronic lateral ankle joint instability: An electromyographic study. *Am J Sports Med* 1992, 20: 257–61.
56. Kennedy JC., Alexander IJ, Hayes KC. Nerve supply of the human knee and its functional importance. *Am J Sports Med* 1982, 10: 329–35.
57. Konradsen L, Ravn JB. Ankle instability caused by prolonged peroneal reaction time. *Acta Orthop Scand* 1990, 61: 388–90.
58. Konradsen L, Ravn JB, Sørensen AI. Proprioception at the ankle: The effect of anesthetic blockade of ligament receptors. *J Bone Joint Surg* 1993, 75B: 433–36.

59. Lephart SM, Warner JP, Borsa PA, Kocher M, Fu FH. Proprioception in athletic individuals with unilateral shoulder instability. Paper presented at the Am Shoulder and Elbow Surgeons annual meeting, Williamsburg, VA, Oct 31–Nov 2, 1993.
60. Lephart SM, Borsa P, Fu FH, Warner JJP. Proprioception of the shoulder joint in normal, unstable, and postcapsulolabral reconstructed individuals. Paper presented at the Am Shoulder and Elbow Surgeons, 10th open meeting, New Orleans, Feb 27, 1994.
61. Lephart SM, Warner JPP, Borsa PA, Fu FH: Proprioception of the shoulder joint in healthy, unstable, and surgically repaired shoulders. *J Shoulder Elbow Surg* 1994, 3: 371–80.
62. Litt JC. The sprained ankle: Diagnosis and management of the lateral ligament injuries. *Aust Fam Phys* 1992, 21: 452–56.
63. Novotny GEK, Gommert-Novotny E. Silver impregnation of peripheral and central axons. *Stain Technology* 1988, 63: 1–14.
64. Meeuwsen HJ, Sawicki TM, Stelmach GE. Improved foot position sense as a result of repetitions in older adults. *J Gerontol* 1993, 48: 137–41.
65. Morisawa Y, Kawakami T, Uemura H, Yamamoto H. Mechanoreceptors in the coracoacromial ligament: A study of its aging process. Paper presented at the 3rd Scandinavian-Japanese Congress on Shoulder Surgery, Aarhus, Denmark, July 6–9, 1993.
66. Moseley HF, Övergaard B. The anterior capsular mechanism in recurrent anterior dislocation of the shoulder: Morphological and clinical studies with special reference to the glenoid labrum and the glenohumeral ligament. *J Bone Joint Surg* 1962, 44B: 913–27.
67. Murakami M, Kojima Y, Maeda T. Sensory nerve endings in the shoulder joint capsule of the monkey as sensors of dynamic stabilizing system. *Trans of comb meeting of ORS of USA, Japan, and Canada*, 31, 1991.
68. Payr E. Der heutige Stand der Gelenkchirurgie. *Arch Klin Chir* 1900, 148: 404–51.
69. Poore GV. Paralysis of the muscular and articular sensibility. In: *Selections from the clinical work of Dr. Duchenne.* London: New Sydenham Society, 1883, pp. 378–98.
70. Pope MH, Johnson RJ, Brown DW, Tighe C. The role of the musculature in injuries to the medial collateral ligament. *J Bone Joint Surg* 1970, 61A: 398.
71. Rhaades CE, Neff JR, Rengachary SS. Diagnosis of posttraumatic syringohydromyelia presenting as neuropathic joints. *Clin Orthop* 1983, 180: 182–87.
72. Resch H, Helweg G, zur Nedden D, Beck E. Double contrast computed tomography examination techniques of habitual and recurrent shoulder dislocations. *Europ J Radiol* 1988, 8: 441–45.
73. Richards RR, Delaney J. Syringomyelia presenting as shoulder instability. *J Shoulder Elbow Surg* 1992, 1: 155–61.
74. Robinson AP, Tearse DS, Koch B, Callaghan JJ, Brand RA. Mechanoreceptors in capsular and juxtalabral tissue of the human shoulder. Paper presented at the Am Shoulder and Elbow Surgeons, 10th open meeting, New Orleans, Feb 27, 1994.
75. Rockwood CA, Matsen FA. *The shoulder.* Philadelphia: Saunders, 1990, pp. 678–712.
76. Rowe CR. Acute and recurrent anterior dislocations of the shoulder. *Orthop Clin N Am* 1980, 11: 253–70.
77. Rowe CR, Zarins B. Recurrent transient subluxation of the shoulder. *J Bone Joint Surg* 1981, 63A: 863–72.
78. Rudinger N. *Die Gelenknerven des menschlichen Körpers.* Erlangen: Enke Verlag, 1857.
79. Saha AK. Anterior recurrent dislocation of the shoulder. *Acta Orthop Scand* 1967, 38: 479–93.
80. Saha AK. Dynamic stability of the glenohumeral joint. *Acta Orthop Scand* 1971, 42: 491–505.
81. Sainburg RL, Poizner H, Ghez C. Loss of proprioception produces deficits in interjoint coordination. *J Neurophysiol* 1993, 70: 2136–147.
82. Schlemm F. Über die Verstärkungsbänder am Schultergelenk. *Arch Anat* 1853, 45–48.
83. Schultz RA, Miller DC, Kerr CS, Micheli L. Mechanoreceptors in human cruciate ligaments. A histological study. *J Bone Joint Surg* 1984, 66A: 1072–1076.
84. Schutte MJ, Dabezies EJ, Zimny ML, Happel LT. Neural anatomy of the human anterior cruciate ligament. *J Bone Joint Surg* 1987, 69A: 243–47.
85. Schwartz RE, Torzilli PA, Warren RF. Capsular restraints to anterior-posterior motion of the shoulder. *Trans Orthop Res Soc* 1987, 12: 78.
86. Skinner HB, Barrack RL, Cook SD. Age-related decline in proprioception. *Clin Orthop* 1984, 184: 208–11.
87. Skinner HB, Barrack RL, Cook SD, Haddad RJ Jr. Joint position sense in total knee arthroplasty. *J Orthop Res* 1984, 1: 276–83.
88. Skinner HB, Wyatt MP, Hodgdon JA, Conard DW, Barrack RL. Effect of fatigue on joint position sense of the knee. *J Orthop Res* 1986: 112–18.
89. Skoglund S. Anatomical and physiological studies of the knee joint innervation in the cat. *Acta Physiol Scand* 1956, 124(36 Suppl.): 1–101.

90. Skoglund S.T. Joint receptors and kinesthesis. In: *Handbook of sensory physiology.* Vol. 2, New York: Springer-Verlag, 1973, pp. 111–36.
91. Solomonow M, Guanche C, Wink C, Knatt Th, Baratta R, Lu Y. Mechanoreceptors and reflex arc in the feline shoulder. *J Shoulder Elbow Surg* 1996, 5: 139–46.
92. Smith RL, Brunolli J. Shoulder kinesthesia after anterior glenohumeral joint dislocation. *Phys Ther* 1989, 69: 106–11.
93. Terry GC, Hammon D, France P, Norwood LA. The stabilizing function of the passive shoulder restraints. *Am J Sports Med* 1991, 19: 26–34.
94. Tibone JE, Fechter J, Kao JT. Evaluation of a proprioception pathway in patients with stable and unstable shoulders with somatosensory cortical evoked potentials. *J Shoulder Elbow Surg* 1997, 6: 440–43.
95. Townley CO. The capsular mechanism in recurrent dislocation of the shoulder. *J Bone Joint Surg* 1950, 32A: 370–80.
96. Tully JG, Latteri A. Paraplegia, syringomyelia tarda, and neuropathic arthrosis of the shoulder: A triad. *Clin Orthop* 1978, 134: 244–48.
97. Turkel SJ, Panio MW, Marshall JL, Girgis FG. Stabilizing mechanisms preventing anterior dislocation of the glenohumeral joint. *J Bone Joint Surg* 1981, 63A: 1208–217.
98. Vangsness T, Ennis M. Neural anatomy of the human glenoid labrum and shoulder ligaments. *Proceedings of the Am Academy of Orthopedic Surgeons*, Washington, DC, Feb 20–25, 1992, 205.
99. Warner JJ, Deng XH, Warren RF. Static capsuloligamentous restraints to superior-inferior translation of the glenohumeral joint. *Am J Sports Med* 1992, 20: 675–85.
100. Warren LF, Marshall JL. The supporting structures and layers on the medial side of the knee: An anatomical analysis. *J Bone Joint Surg* 1979, 61A: 56–62.
101. Wheeler JH, Ryan JB, Arciero AR, Molinari RN. Arthroscopic versus nonoperative treatment of acute shoulder dislocations in young athletes. *Arthroscopy* 1989, 5: 213–17.
102. Wrete M. The innervation of the shoulder joint in man. *Acta Anat* 1949, 7: 173–90.
103. Wyke BD. Structural and functional characteristics of articular receptor system. *Acta Chir Orthop Traumatol Cechoslovaca* 1973, 40: 489–97.

CHAPTER 24

Role of Shoulder Stabilization Relative to Restoration of Neuromuscular Control and Joint Kinematics

Roger G. Pollock, MD

Glenohumeral stability is achieved through a number of different mechanisms involving the articular geometry, dynamic (muscular) stabilizers, static capsuloligamentous tissues, and intraarticular forces (negative intraarticular pressure, surface forces of adhesion and cohesion). At mid ranges of motion, the capsular ligaments are relatively lax, and stability is maintained largely by the muscle forces of the rotator cuff, which compress the humeral head into the relatively concave glenoid ("concavity compression") (1). As end ranges of motion are approached the capsular stabilizers assume importance in providing stability for the joint. More recently, interest has focused on how these capsulolabral tissues may interact with the dynamic stabilizers (i.e., the rotator cuff and scapular muscles) (2, 3). Specifically, there has been more attention paid to the role of proprioceptive feedback from the ligaments to the muscles in contributing to glenohumeral stability (4–6). Loss or diminution of such proprioceptive feedback is now thought to be an important predisposing factor to glenohumeral instability.

It has also been recently shown that surgical stabilization may restore proprioception to the shoulder (7), but little is known about how this may occur. Glenohumeral kinematics has also been shown to be disturbed in individuals with glenohumeral instability (8, 9). The purpose of this section is to consider how shoulder stabilization facilitates the restoration of neuromuscular control and normal glenohumeral kinematics. In order to address these issues, it is necessary to review our current understanding of proprioception in the shoulder, normal and abnormal glenohumeral kinematics, structural damage in unstable shoulders, and techniques of shoulder stabilization, particularly labral repair and capsulorrhaphy.

Proprioception of the Shoulder

The existence of mechanocreceptors and free nerve endings in the glenohumeral ligaments has been reported by several authors (10, 11). Jerosch and associates found axonal structures varying in size from 0.2 μm to 70 μm in diameter within the glenohumeral ligaments. These authors also detected type II mechanoreceptors (Pacinian corpuscles) in the ligaments and suggested that these mechanoreceptors may control the stabilizing musculature (10, 11). Vangsness and associates found that the most abundant mechanoreceptors in the glenohumeral ligaments were classic Ruffini end organ receptors, but they also located Pacinian corpuscles in the capsular ligaments. The glenoid labrum had no mechanoreceptors, but occasional free nerve endings were seen in the surrounding connective tissue and in the peripheral half of the labrum (4). These authors speculate that injury to these afferent fibers from dislocation or from surgery may result in a diminished proprioceptive capacity and that such diminished proprioception may subsequently lead to further events of instability. Finally, the authors point out that their neural findings are descriptive and qualitative and that further work is necessary to quantify nerve ending densities in various regions of the ligaments.

Guanche and associates have demonstrated the existence of several ligamentomuscular reflex arcs in the feline glenohumeral joint (5, 12). In one report, they stimulated three branches of the axillary nerve, which terminates in the glenohumeral joint capsule. Stimulation of the anterior and inferior articular branches resulted in electromyographic activity in the biceps, subscapularis, supraspinatus, and infraspinatus muscles, while stimulation of the posterior articular branch elicited activity in the deltoid. Transection of these articular branches results in electrical silence in the rotator cuff on stimulation, demonstrating that these branches are an afferent type (5). In another study, these authors located another reflex arc in the feline shoulder involving afferent branches from the suprascapular and subscapular nerves. Stimulation of the suprascapular articular branches resulted in electromyographic activity in the biceps and infraspinatus, and stimulation of the subscapular articular branches caused activity in the biceps, supraspinatus, infraspinatus, and subscapularis muscles. The authors assume that these reflex arcs are spinal reflexes that are deployed automatically with stress to the capsule. They conclude that the existence of such ligamentomuscular reflex arcs in the glenohumeral joint suggests that the ligaments and muscles function synergistically in stabilizing the shoulder (12).

A number of clinical reports have also studied the perception of joint position and joint motion in the shoulder (7, 13–17). Smith and Brunolli compared kinesthesia in normal shoulders and those with a history of dislocation and found that kinesthetic deficits occur after glenohumeral dislocation. Proprioceptive differences, which are highly significant ($p < .001$), were measured in all three tests (accuracy of angular reproduction, threshold to sensation of movement, and end range reproduction) in the previously dislocated shoulders. Extremity dominance was not found to affect shoulder kinesthesia in this study. The authors suggested that increased laxity in joints as a result of trauma or stretching may result in damage to the joint capsule mechanoreceptors, resulting in diminished proprioception. Recurrence of dislocation may occur as a result of this diminished neuromuscular coordination (13).

Blasier and associates measured shoulder proprioception in a group of subjects without known shoulder pathology. They found that individuals with generalized joint laxity were less sensitive in detecting passive shoulder rotation than those with clinically "tight" joints. Proprioception for external rotation was significantly more sensitive than that for internal rotation, and detection of external rotation became more sensitive as the limit of external rotation was approached. They concluded that capsular tightening is one mechanism for shoulder proprioception (15).

Lephart and associates measured shoulder proprioception in 90 subjects who were divided into three groups: normal controls (n = 40), patients with anterior instability (n = 30), and patients who had undergone surgical reconstruction of the shoulder for recurrent, traumatic anterior shoulder instability (n = 20) (7). A specially designed proprioceptive testing device (see figure 24.1) was used to mea-

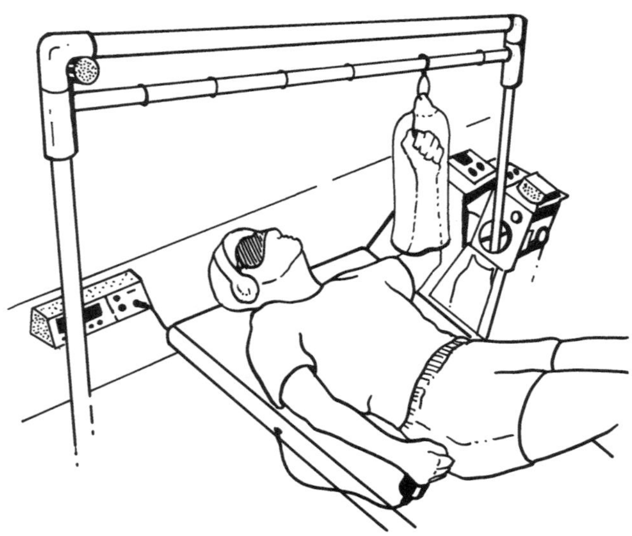

Figure 24.1 Proprioceptive testing device.

sure joint position sense (reproduction of passive positioning test) and kinesthesia (threshold to detection of passive motion test). The unstable shoulder demonstrated proprioceptive deficits for both tests compared to the normal contralateral shoulder in these individuals. No significant mean differences were seen between the shoulder that had undergone repair and the normal contralateral shoulders. Based on their findings, the authors conclude that injury to the capsuloligamentous structures of the glenohumeral joint disrupts the normal neuromuscular feedback mechanisms. These deficits in proprioception may contribute to ongoing instability of the shoulder but, interestingly, appear to be restorable through surgical reconstruction (6, 7).

In another recent report, Voight and associates found that shoulder proprioception is diminished in the presence of shoulder muscle fatigue (17). In that study, there was no relationship between arm dominance and shoulder proprioceptive ability. However, Allegruci and associates, studying the shoulders of healthy overhead-sport athletes, found that the dominant shoulder exhibited decreased kinesthesia compared to the nondominant shoulder, both at 0° and 75° of external rotation (16). Since the dominant arm exhibited greater external rotation, the authors point out that these kinesthetic differences may be related to these differences in range of motion (i.e., the capsule of the dominant arm is not as taut at 75° and thus the proprioceptive feedback via mechanoreceptors sensitive to stretch is not as great). They also suggest that repetitive microtrauma to the dominant shoulder in the overhead-sport athlete may lead to gradual, progressive damage to the proprioceptive mechanisms (6, 16).

Glenohumeral Kinematics

Differences in glenohumeral kinematics between stable and unstable shoulders have been demonstrated in several radiographic studies (8, 9). Poppen and Walker, studying abduction of the shoulder in the plane of the scapula, found that the center of rotation of the glenohumeral joint was located within 6 mm of the geometric center of the humeral ball for this motion. Humeral ball excursions of the face of the glenoid in the superoinferior plane between each 30° arc of motion averaged only 1 to 2 mm in normal subjects. However, patients with a history of prior glenohumeral dislocations had abnormal instant center values and high humeral ball excursions (8). Howell and associates, studying glenohumeral motion in the horizontal plane, found that there was precise centering of the humeral head in this plane of motion in normal shoulders, except with the arm in maximum extension and external rotation (9) In this position, the humeral head was posteriorly translated 4 mm with respect to the axis of the glenoid. In a majority of patients with anterior glenohumeral instability, abnormal anterior translations were seen in several of the tested positions. The authors concluded that these altered mechanics resulted from disruption of the anterior containing structures in some patients with anterior instability (9).

More recently, several groups of investigators have used newer forms of kinematic analysis and have even simulated the active role of the muscles in dynamic models (18–25). Kelkar and associates have reported on the use of stereophotogrammetry to study the effects of articular congruence, external rotation, and anterior capsular tightening on the kinematics and contact patterns of the glenohumeral joint during abduction (18–20). They demonstrated that kinematics analysis using subchondral bone data overestimates the actual translations of the center of the humeral head. The stereophotogrammetric technique allows precise study of the articulating surfaces of the joint, rather than the underlying subchondral bone surfaces. The ranges of translation of the humeral head during active abduction of the humerus in the scapular plane using simulated muscle forces were less than 3 mm for all joints in all three directions (anterior-posterior, lateral-medial, and inferior-superior). Incongruent joints were found to have larger anteroinferior translations than congruent joints, and testing in external rotation yielded higher translations than testing in neutral rotation (19).

Karduna and associates have recently performed a quantitative comparison of active and passive glenohumeral joint kinematics. Using a Polhemus 3 Space Fastrak device to perform kinematic measurements, they found that mean translations for all positions of elevation and rotation were greater for the passive case along both the superior-inferior and anterior-posterior axes. Mean active translations averaged only approximately 2 mm along both axes (22). In their study of glenohumeral joint kinematics during scapular plane abduction, Debski and associates used a dynamic shoulder testing apparatus with simulated deltoid and rotator cuff muscle forces. They, too, reported that only minimal humeral translations occurred in the anterior-posterior, medial-lateral, and superior-inferior directions during abduction in the scapular plane. Specifically, translation in the superior-inferior direction averaged less than two millimeters (23).

The effects of tightening the glenohumeral ligaments on joint kinematics have also been investigated (25). Janevic and associates placed cadaver shoulders in varying positions, which simulated the extremes of motion, and measured the resulting translations of the humeral head and the glenohumeral contact areas. They tested normal joints, shoulders with a Bankart lesion, those that had undergone Bankart repair with either a standard or an overtightened capsular reconstruction, and those that had undergone either a standard or overtightened capsular shift. They found that repairs that overtightened the capsule anteriorly caused the humeral head and joint contact to shift posteriorly (25).

Kelkar and associates compared glenohumeral kinematics and contact in the normal and anteriorly tightened states using the noninvasive stereophotogrammetric technique. They found no significant differences in the lateral-medial or inferior-superior directions, but the humeral head center in the tightened state was consistently posterior to its position in the normal state. This results in posteriorly shifted contact patterns on the glenoid. Moreover, the posterior contact shift was greatest in one of the most incongruent joints (where the glenoid cartilage radius of curvature was 2.5 mm larger than that of the humeral head) (21). Thus, it appears that overtightening of the capsular ligaments results in alterations in both kinematics and contact areas of the glenohumeral joint.

Anatomic Considerations in Glenohumeral Instability

Damage to the capsulolabral structures—detachment of the labrum from the anterior inferior glenoid rim, stretching out or redundancy of the anteroinferior capsular ligaments, or both of these lesions in combination—is thought to comprise the major pathoanatomy of anterior glenohumeral instability. Bankart cited detachment of the fibrocartilaginous glenoid labrum from the anterior glenoid margin as "the essential anatomical defect" in recurrent anterior dislocations (26, 27), and others have verified the high prevalence of this lesion in patients with anterior shoulder instability (28–30). However, it has also been recognized that a significant subset of patients with glenohumeral instability does not have a "Bankart lesion" but instead appears to have excessive capsular volume on the basis of lax or stretched glenohumeral ligaments (31–32). This pathological state may occur on the basis of major trauma or congenital (atraumatic) laxity. Moreover, it has been postulated in recent decades, by Neer and Jobe separately, that repetitive microtrauma to the glenohumeral joint capsule, such as is seen in high-demand overhead sport activities like pitching a baseball or swimming, may result in the gradual stretching out of these structures, resulting in "acquired instability" (31, 33). Whether on the basis of major trauma, congenital laxity, or repetitive microtrauma (or often on the basis of some combination of these etiological factors), capsulolabral pathology is implicated as a cause of recurrence in most cases of glenohumeral instability.

The dynamic stabilizers, chiefly the rotator cuff and scapular muscles, are crucial to providing stability for the glenohumeral joint, and abnormalities in their functioning have been cited as contributing to the development of instability. Glousman and associates performed electromyographic analyses of the shoulder during throwing and found that, in normal shoulders, the subscapularis functions in the late cocking stage, presumably to decelerate the external rotation of the shoulder. They observed a marked decrease in subscapularis activity in throwers with instability, as well as in the activity of other internal rotators of the shoulder. Moreover, they found decreased electromyographic activity of the serratus anterior in throwers with anterior instability. Decreased activity of this muscle diminishes protraction of the scapula at a time when the humerus is flexing forward and externally rotating, resulting in higher stresses to the anterior capsular restraints (34). Similarly, Cain and associates used a cadaver model to demonstrate that the posterior rotator cuff can reduce strain in the anterior structures of the shoulder by pulling the humeral head posteriorly during external rotation of the shoulder (35). Thus, while gross abnormalities in muscle appearance or structure are usually not present in patients with shoulder instability, subtle alterations in muscle firing patterns, perhaps resulting from alterations in the proprioceptive feedback loops previously discussed, may contribute to the development of acquired glenohumeral instability by failing to shield the capsular restraints from the high repetitive stresses that may ultimately result in stretching and incompetence of these tissues.

A number of biomechanical studies have demonstrated that different regions of the glenohumeral joint capsule act as the chief static restraint against anterior instability, depending on the joint position (36–41). In the lower range of abduction, the superior and middle glenohumeral ligaments are the most important capsular structures in providing static stability for the shoulder (36, 37). As the arm is progressively abducted and externally rotated, the inferior glenohumeral complex becomes the primary capsular restraint against inferior translation of the adducted shoulder. With progressive abduction, the inferior glenohumeral ligament assumes the role of primary static restraint against inferior instability (36, 37). Different regions of the capsule assume primacy as static restraints, depending on the arm position, but the various regions appear to act in concert and share the tension required to stabilize the shoulder, especially at extremes of motion (38).

Much attention recently has been focused on the inferior glenohumeral ligament complex, as this structure is the chief static restraint in the clinically important position of combined abduction and external rotation (i.e., the arm position in which most dislocations and subluxations occur) (42–47). Researchers found that the superior band was consistently the thickest region (averaging 2.8 mm) and thickness progressively decreased from anterosuperiorly to posteroinferiorly, with the posterior axillary region of the inferior glenohumeral ligament averaging only 1.7 mm in thickness (42). Regional differences were also seen in mechanical testing to failure in tension among the three regions of the inferior glenohumeral ligament, with the anterior pouch failing at a higher strain than the other regions. The average strain to failure for all of the bone-ligament-bone complexes tested was surprisingly high, 27%. Capsular rupture (midsubstance failure) was seen almost as frequently as glenoid insertion avulsion as the mode of inferior glenohumeral ligament failure. Moreover, even when the ligament failed at its glenoid insertion, significant capsular stretching was seen prior to ultimate failure (see figure 24.2) (42, 43).

Correlative studies of the biochemical composition, histological characteristics, biomechanical properties, and structural behavior of the inferior glenohumeral ligament have also been carried out (44). Proteoglycan content was highest in the superior band and decreased posteroinferiorly. The higher proteoglycan content in the superior band was thought to correlate with the higher viscoelasticity of this region of the ligament (44). For all three regions of the ligament, greater fiber interweaving was seen near the insertion sites, with more

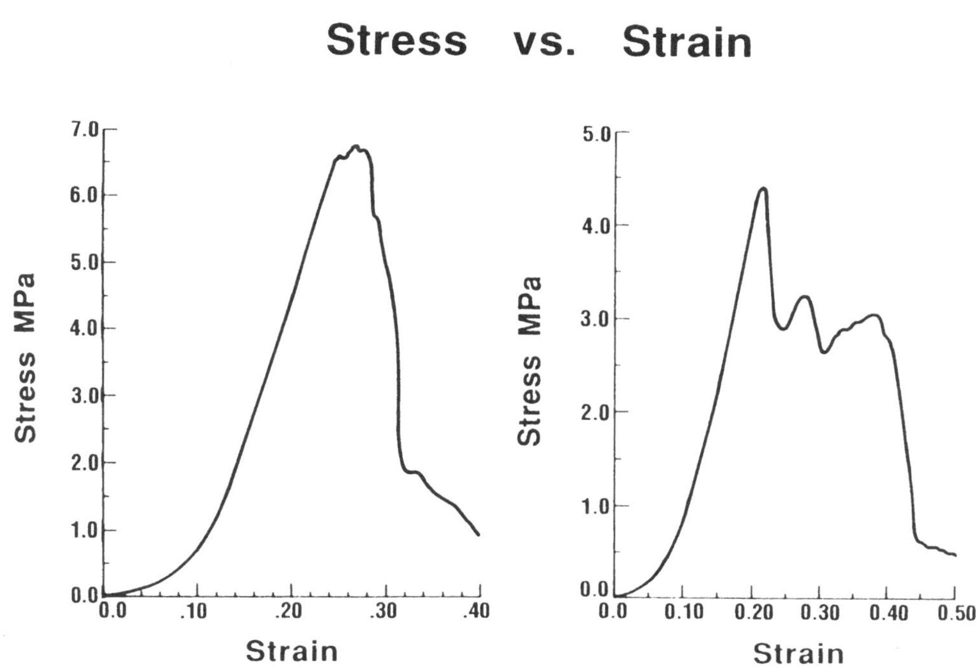

Figure 24.2 Left, typical tensile stress-strain curve for IGHL bone-ligament-bone specimens that failed at the glenoid insertion site. Right, typical stress-strain curve for specimens failing in ligament substance. Substantial strains to failure were seen with bone failure modes.

Reprinted with permission from Bigliani, L. et al: Tensile properties of the inferior glenohumeral ligament. *J Orthop Res* 1992; 10:187-197.

uniformly oriented fiber bundle patterns in the ligament midsubstance. Moreover, the anterior axillary pouch was found to have the most uniform fiber pattern and the most crimping, perhaps explaining its higher strain to failure than that of the other inferior glenohumeral ligament regions (44). Finally, the inferior glenohumeral ligament was found to have a more elastic behavior in its central portion within the ligament substance and more viscoelastic behavior near its glenoid and humeral insertions, also correlating well with the histological findings for the ligament (44).

Other studies on the anatomy and histology of the inferior glenohumeral ligament complex have added to the understanding of this important stabilizer. O'Brien and associates performed arthroscopic observations and histological analyses of the inferior glenohumeral ligament and reported that the inferior glenohumeral ligament supports the humeral head much like a hammock, with the different bands reciprocally tightening as the head is rotated in the abducted position. The ligament was found to insert at the humeral side in one of two distinct configurations: a collar-like attachment or a V-shaped insertion (45). Gohlke and associates performed histological analysis of the glenohumeral joint capsule and found a complex pattern of cross-linking in the superior capsule and a system of fiber bundles spirally crossing each other in the anterior-inferior capsule (46). Overall, the capsule is described as a three-dimensional structure in which the fiber bundles adapt themselves to the curvature of the spherical humeral head, with radial fibers that are linked together by circular elements (see figure 24.3). They conclude that the complicated structure of the joint capsule suggests that the capsular cylinder must be regarded as a functional entity, and capsular repairs should take into consideration the structure of the fiber bundles.

Further indirect evidence that permanent stretching or elongation of the inferior glenohumeral ligament is necessary to produce anterior shoulder dislocations was provided by a recent biomechanical study of a simulated Bankart lesion (48). In this study, Speer and associates compared glenohumeral joint translations before and after sectioning the glenoid insertion of the inferior glenohumeral ligament. The simulated Bankart lesion resulted in an increase in anterior and inferior translations at all positions of elevation, but these increases were quite small, with the maximum mean increase being only 3.4 mm. The authors concluded that detachment of the anterior portion of the inferior glenohumeral ligament from the glenoid rim does not account alone for the increased glenohumeral translation that is necessary to produce an anterior dislocation of the shoulder. The authors speculate that permanent stretching or elongation of the inferior glenohumeral ligament (i.e., additional capsular injury) may also be necessary for an anterior dislocation to occur (48).

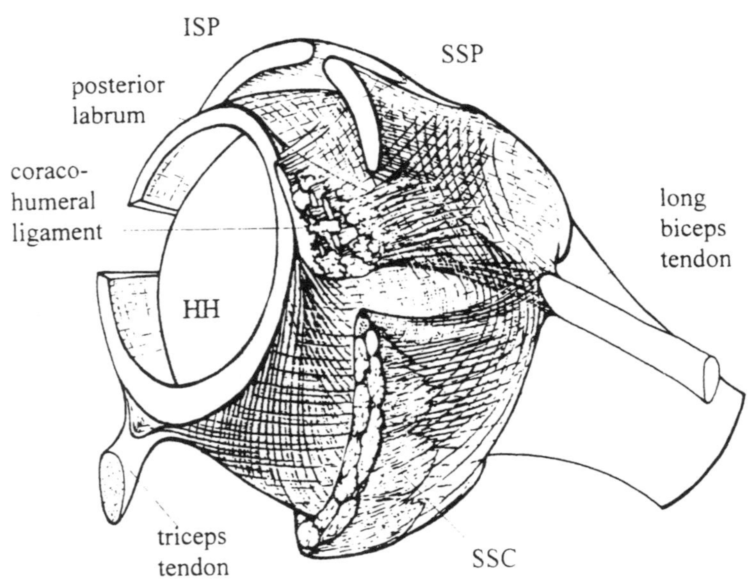

Figure 24.3 Schematic of the orientation of collagen fiber bundles in the capsule of the glenohumeral joint.
Reproduced with permission from Gohlke F., et al: The pattern of the collagen fiber bundles of the capsule of the glenohumeral joint. *J Shoulder Elbow Surg*, 1994; 3:111-128.

Repetitive microtrauma to the glenohumeral ligaments has also been cited as an etiologic factor in producing glenohumeral instability (31, 33), and recent biomechanical work has focused on this possible mechanism for ligament stretching (47). Pollock and associates have reported on the effects of repetitive subfailure strains on the mechanical behavior of the inferior glenohumeral ligament (47). They found that cycling to high levels of subfailure strains produced dramatic declines in the peak load response of the ligament. Moreover, for all three regions of the ligament there was a significant difference between the initial and posttesting lengths ($p = .0001$), with the ligaments measured to be, on average, 7.2% longer at the conclusion of testing (47). The authors concluded that the dramatic decreases in the load response of the ligaments and the significant elongations measured in this study suggest that structural microdamage has occurred under these cyclic loading conditions. This type of capsular stretching with repetitive subfailure loading may be a mechanism contributing to the development of acquired instability, especially in overhead-sport athletes, many of whom are found to have "capsular laxity" without labral avulsion at surgery.

Surgical Stabilization and Its Effects on Glenohumeral Joint Proprioception and Kinematics

Many different procedures have been employed to achieve stability in dislocating or subluxating shoulders. However, a number of these repairs have fallen into disfavor because they do not address the pathology in glenohumeral instability, distort the surrounding anatomy, or stabilize the shoulder by restricting motion (especially external rotation), resulting in restricted function and even in the development of early glenohumeral arthritis (49–54). Thus, the Putti-Platt repair, Magnuson-Stack repair, and Bristow procedure are presently less commonly performed than in previous decades. Currently, the most widely used repairs for glenohumeral instability are those that emphasize repair of the detached capsulolabral complex (inferior glenohumeral ligament and labrum) and capsulorrhaphy to reduce capsular volume (26, 29, 49, 55–59). These can be performed through open or arthroscopic techniques (60–63), though it has been suggested that capsular tensioning may be more difficult to achieve arthroscopically, perhaps accounting for the higher instability recurrence rates reported to date in most series of arthroscopic repair (64).

Capsulorrhaphy procedures can be performed using either a lateral (humeral side) (see figure 24.4) or medial (glenoid side) capsular incisio (32, 49, 55–57). These repairs allow a simultaneous repair of a detached anteroinferior labrum and a reduction in joint volume to restore effective function of the glenohumeral ligaments. The subscapularis is either split (to avoid detachment) or detached and repaired anatomically, but it is not shortened, thus allowing restoration of full motion. These repairs can address inferior or multidirectional elements of the instability, if they are present, allowing appropriate balancing and tensioning of the ligaments (32, 49, 55). When inferior or multidirectional instability is present, the lateral approach is favored, given the funnel-shaped geometry of the joint capsule with its broader attachment laterally, thus allowing more tissue to be shifted further on the lateral aspect of the joint (65). These procedures have resulted in effective stabilization in approximately 95% of patients in several large series and have allowed 75% to 80% of athletes to return to their sports at similar levels of competition (32, 55, 58).

The effects of capsulorrhaphy and labral repair on glenohumeral kinematics in a clinical population remain unknown. As previously discussed, Kelkar and associates have demonstrated kinematic abnormalities after overtightening of the anterior shoulder capsule, with posterior displacement of the humeral head center and posterior shifting of contact patterns on the glenoid resulting from the overtightening (21). However, they deliberately overtightened the capsule and did not seek to simulate an anatomic capsulorrhaphy, such as the anterior inferior capsular shift, which emphasizes a symmetric reduction of joint volume. Janevic and associates did investigate glenohumeral kinematics after performing several types of labral repair and capsulorrhaphy procedures on cadaver shoulders (25). They also demonstrated posterior shifts in the humeral head center and joint contact with anterior capsular tightening. However, the repairs were performed on cadaver specimens that likely had normal joint volume prior to tightening. This does not accurately simulate the clinical situation, where presumably the capsulolabral structures in the unstable shoulders are stretched or redundant prior to repair. To date, the kinematics after surgical reconstruction of pathologically unstable shoulders have not been studied, either in a clinical population or using a biomechanical cadaver model that simulates the ligamentous laxity, present prior to repair.

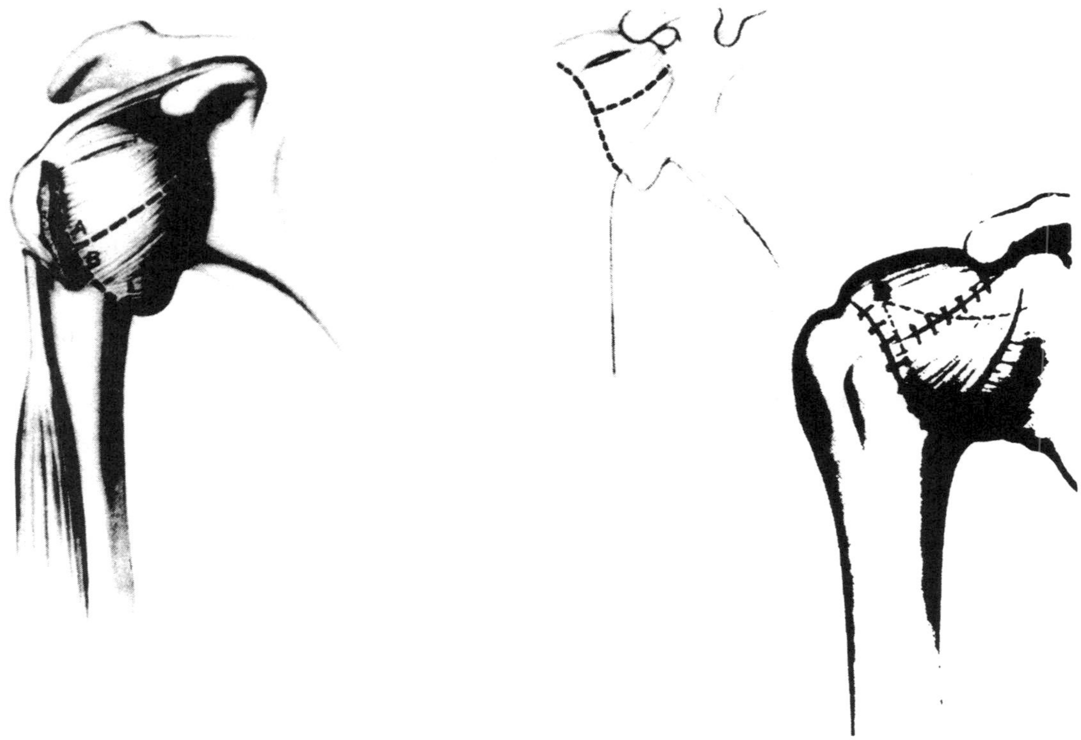

Figure 24.4 Schematic of the inferior capsular shift, a laterally-based (humeral side) capsulorrhaphy. The inferior flap (B) is shifted superiorly and the superior flap (A) is shifted inferiorly.
Reproduced with permission from Neer CS II and Foster CR: Inferior capsular shift for involuntary and multidirectional instability of the shoulder. *J Bone Joint Surg*, 1980; 62A:1 897-908.

Proprioceptive mechanisms involving the glenohumeral joint capsule may assist in stabilizing the shoulder, as reviewed earlier in this section. Lephart and associates have reported that deficits in proprioception are found in unstable shoulders but that proprioception appears to be able to be restored through surgical reconstruction (7). Injury to the capsuloligamentous structures—by detachment from the glenoid rim, by stretching these ligaments, or by a combination of these lesions—may result in an inability of the stretch receptors to recognize that an end range of motion, or "dangerous position," is being approached, which results in a failure to signal the dynamic stabilizers to fire and stabilize the joint. Thus, if the capsuloligamentous structures are pathologically lengthened, the normal neuromuscular feedback mechanisms may no longer be operative, predisposing the shoulder to instability. Restoration of appropriate length-tension relationships for the ligaments through surgical reconstruction may again allow these proprioceptive stretch receptors to become operative at appropriate arm positions, as suggested by the data of Lephart and associates.

The best type of capsular reconstruction for preserving proprioceptive structures and restoring proprioceptive function remains unknown. Guanche and associates have pointed out that the ideal surgical procedure would preserve as much neural supply to the capsule as possible. They suggest that capsular shift procedures should be performed from the humeral (or lateral) side to decrease the likelihood of damage to the nerve supply of the capsule (5). On the other hand, Gohlke and associates have suggested that medially based T-shifts are most suitable for restoring the capacitance of the capsule, since they least violate the fiber bundle structure of the capsule (46). Surgical implications will certainly become clearer as our knowledge about the histology and physiology of these neuromuscular feedback mechanisms in the shoulder becomes greater.

In summary, proprioceptive mechanisms appear to play a role in stabilizing the glenohumeral joint and may serve as a means for interplay between the static (ligamentous) stabilizers and the dynamic muscle restraints. A number of biomechanical and clinical studies have emphasized the importance of the inferior glenohumeral ligament as a shoulder stabilizer in the position of anterior dislocation, namely, combined abduction and external rotation, and have suggested that this structure may be stretched out or elongated in unstable shoulders. This elongation may result in an inability to sense and relay changes in shoulder position and motion, allowing recurrent episodes of instability and progressive damage to these structures. Finally, it appears that surgical stabilization may restore the proprioceptive function of the shoulder capsule, presumably by restoring the appropriate length-tension relationships of these ligaments.

References

1. Lippitt SB, Vanderhooft JE, Harris SL, et al: Glenohumeral stability from concavity compression: A quantitative analysis. *J Shoulder Elbow Surg* 1993, 2: 27–35.
2. Clark J, Sidles JA, Matsen FA: The relationship of the glenohumeral joint capsule to the rotator cuff. *Clin Orthop* 1990, 254: 29–34.
3. Warner JJP, Caborn DNM, Berger R, et al: Dynamic capsuloligamentous anatomy of the glenohumeral joint. *J Shoulder Elbow Surg* 1993, 2: 115–33.
4. Vangsness CT, Ennis M, Taylor JG, et al: Neural anatomy of the glenohumeral ligaments, labrum, and subacromial bursa. *Arthroscopy* 1995, 11: 180–84.
5. Guanche C, Knatt T, Solomonow M, et al: The synergistic action of the capsule and the shoulder muscles. *Am J Sport Med* 1995, 23: 301–306.
6. Warner JJP, Lephart S, Fu FH: Role of proprioception in pathoetiology of shoulder instability. *Clin Orthop* 1996, 330: 35–39.
7. Lephart SM, Warner JJP, Borsa PA, et al: Proprioception of the shoulder joint in healthy, unstable, and surgically repaired shoulders. *J Shoulder Elbow Surg* 1994, 3: 371–80.
8. Poppen NK, Walker PS: Normal and abnormal motion of the shoulder. *J Bone Joint Surg* 1976, 58A: 195–201.
9. Howell SM, Galinat BJ, Renzi AJ, et al: Normal and abnormal mechanics of the glenohumeral joint in the horizontal plane. *J Bone Joint Surg* 1988, 70A: 227–32.
10. Jerosch J, Steinbeck J, Clahsen H, et al: Function of the glenohumeral ligaments in active stabilization of the shoulder joint. *Knee Surg Sports Trauma Arthroscopy* 1993, 1: 152–58.
11. Jerosch J, Castro, WH, Grosse-Hackmann A, et al: Function of the glenohumeral ligaments in active protection of shoulder stability. *Zeitschrift für Orthopadie und Ihre Grenzgebiete* 1995, 133: 67–71.
12. Solomonow M, Guanche C, Wink C, et al: Mechanoreceptors and reflex arc in the feline shoulder. *J Shoulder Elbow Surg* 1996, 5: 139–46.
13. Smith RJ, Brunolli J: Shoulder kinesthesia after anterior glenohumeral joint dislocation. *Phys Ther* 1989, 69: 106–12.
14. Hall LA, McCloskey DI: Detection of movements imposed on finger, elbow, and shoulder joints. *J Physiol* 1983, 335: 519–33.
15. Blasier RB, Carpenter JE, Huston LJ: Shoulder proprioception: Effect of joint laxity, joint position, and direction of motion. *Orthop Rev* 1994, 23: 45–50.
16. Allegrucci M, Whitney SL, Lephart SM, et al: Shoulder kinesthesia in healthy unilateral athletes participating in upper extremity sports. *JOSPT* 1995, 21: 221–26.
17. Voight ML, Hardin JA, Blackburn TA, et al: The effects of muscle fatigue on and the relationship of arm dominance to shoulder proprioception. *JOSPT* 1996, 23: 348–52.
18. Kelkar R, Flatow EL, Bigliani LU, et al: A stereophotogrammetric method to determine the kinematics of the glenohumeral joint. *ASME Adv Bioeng* 1992, 22: 143–46.
19. Kelkar R, Flatow EL, Bigliani LU, et al: The effects of congruence and humeral head rotation on glenohumeral kinematics. *ASME Adv Bioeng* 1994, 28: 19–20.
20. Kelkar R, Newton PM, Armengol J, et al: Three-dimensional kinematics of the glenohumeral joint during abduction in the scapular plane. *Trans Orthop Res Soc* 1993, 18: 136.
21. Bigliani LU, Kelkar R, Flatow EL, et al: Glenohumeral stability: Biomechanical properties of passive and active stabilizers. *Clin Orthop* 1996, 330: 13–30.
22. Karduna AR, Williams GP, Iannotti JP: A quantitative comparison of active and passive glenohumeral joint kinematics. *Trans Orthop Res Soc* 1994, 19: 226.
23. Debski RE, Boardman ND, Thompson WD, et al: Measurement of muscle force and glenohumeral joint kinematics during scapular plane abduction. *ASME Adv Bioeng* 1994, 28: 107–108.
24. Wuelker N, Schmotzer H, Thren K, et al: Translation of the glenohumeral joint with simulated active elevation. *Clin Orthop* 1994, 93–200.
25. Janevic J, Craig EV, Hsu K-C, et al: Biomechanics of repair of anterior glenohumeral instability. *Trans Orthop Res Soc* 1992, 17: 495.

26. Bankart ASB: Recurrent of habitual dislocation of the shoulder joint. *Br Med J* 1923, 2: 1132–133.
27. Bankart ASB: The pathology and treatment of recurrent dislocation of the shoulder joint. *Br J Surg* 1938, 26: 23–29.
28. McLaughlin HL: Recurrent anterior dislocation of the shoulder: Morbid anatomy. *Am J Surg* 1960, 99: 628–32.
29. Thomas SC, Matsen FA II: An approach to the repair of avulsion of the glenohumeral ligaments in the management of traumatic anterior glenohumeral instability. *J Bone Joint Surg* 1989, 71A: 506–12.
30. Taylor DC, Arciero RA: Pathological changes associated with shoulder dislocation: Arthroscopic and physical examination findings in first-time traumatic anterior dislocations. *Am J Sports Med* 1997, 25: 306–11.
31. Neer CS II: *Shoulder Reconstruction.* Philadelphia: Saunders, 1990.
32. Bigliani LU, Kurzweil PR, Schwartzbach CC, et al: Inferior capsular shift procedure for anterior inferior shoulder instability in athletes. *Am J Sports Med* 1994, 22: 578–84.
33. Jobe FW, Tibone JE, Jobe CM, et al: The shoulder in sports. In Rockwood CA Jr, Matsen FA, II, eds. *The Shoulder.* Philadelphia: Saunders, 1990.
34. Glousman R, Jobe FW, Tibone JE, et al: Dynamic electromyographic analysis of the throwing shoulder with glenohumeral instability. *J Bone Joint Surg* 1988, 70A: 220–26.
35. Cain PR, Mutschler TA, Fu FH, et al: Anterior stability of the glenohumeral joint: A dynamic model. *Am J Sports Med* 1987, 15: 144–48.
36. Turkel SJ, Panio MW, Marshall JL, et al: Stabilizing mechanisms preventing anterior dislocation of the glenohumeral joint. *J Bone Joint Surg* 1981, 63A: 1208–217.
37. Ovesen J, Nielsen S: Stability of the shoulder joint: Cadaver study of stabilizing structures. *Acta Orthop Scand* 1985, 56: 149–51.
38. Terry GC, Hammon D, France P, et al: The stabilizing function of passive shoulder restraints. *Am J Sports Med* 1991, 19: 26–34.
39. Schwartz RE, Torzilli PA, Warren RF: Capsular restraints to anterior-posterior motion of the shoulder. *Trans Orthop Res Soc* 1987, 12: 78.
40. Curl LA, Warren R: Glenohumeral joint stability: Selective cutting studies on the static capsular restraints. *Clin Orthop* 1996, 330: 54–65.
41. Warner JJP, Deng X-H, Warren RF, et al: Static capsuloligamentous restraints to superior-inferior translation of the glenohumeral joint. *Am J Sports Med* 1992, 20: 675–85.
42. Pollock RG, Soslowsky LJ, Bigliani LU, et al: The mechanical properties of the inferior glenohumeral ligament. *Trans Orthop Res Soc* 1990, 15: 510.
43. Bigliani LU, Pollock RG, Soslowsky LJ, et al: The tensile properties of the inferior glenohumeral ligament. *J Orthop Res* 1992, 10: 187–97.
44. Ticker JB, Flatow EL, Pawluk RJ, et al: The inferior glenohumeral ligament: A correlative biomechanical and histological investigation. *Trans Orthop Res Soc* 1993, 18: 313.
45. O'Brien SJ, Neves MC, Arnoczky SP, et al: The anatomy and histology of the inferior glenohumeral ligament complex of the shoulder. *Am J Sports Med* 1990, 18: 449–56.
46. Gohlke F, Essigkrug B, Schmitz F: The pattern of the collagen fiber bundles of the capsule of the glenohumeral joint. *J Shoulder Elbow Surg* 1994, 3: 111–28.
47. Pollock RG, Bucchieri JS, Wang VM, et al: Subfailure repetitive loading of the inferior glenohumeral ligament affects it mechanical properties. *Trans Orthop Res Soc* 1997, 22: 164.
48. Speer KP, Deng X, Borrero S, et al: Biomechanical evaluation of a simulated Bankart lesion. *J Bone Joint Surg* 1994, 76: 1819–826.
49. Neer CS II, Foster CR: Inferior capsular shift for involuntary inferior and multidirectional instability of the shoulder: A preliminary report. *J Bone Joint Surg* 1980, 62A: 897–908.
50. Hawkins RH, Hawkins RJ: Failed anterior reconstruction for shoulder instability. *J Bone Joint Surg* 1985, 67: 709–14.
51. Hawkins RJ, Angelo RL: Glenohumeral osteoarthrosis. *J Bone Joint Surg* 1990, 72A: 1193–197.
52. Lusardi DA, Wirth MA, Wurtz D, et al: Loss of external rotation following anterior capsulorrhaphy of the shoulder. *J Bone Joint Surg* 1993, 75A: 1185–192.
53. Bigliani LU, Weinstein DM, Glasgow MT, et al: Glenohumeral arthroplasty for arthritis after instability surgery. *J Shoulder and Elbow Surg* 1995, 4: 87–94.
54. Young DC, Rockwood CA Jr: Complications of a failed Bristow procedure and their management. *J Bone Joint Surg* 1991, 969–81.
55. Altchek DW, Warren RF, Skyhar MJ, et al: T-plasty modification of the Bankart procedure for multidirectional instability of the anterior and inferior types. *J Bone Joint Surg* 1991, 73A: 105–12.
56. Jobe FW, Giangarra CE, Kvitne RS, et al: Anterior capsulolabral reconstruction of the shoul-

der in athletes in overhand sports. *Am J Sports Med* 1991, 19: 428–34.
57. Warner JJP, Johnson D, Miller M, et al: Techniques for selecting capsular tightness in repair of anterior-inferior shoulder instability. *J Shoulder Elbow Surg* 1995, 4: 352–64.
58. Montgomery WH, Jobe FW: Functional outcomes in athletes after modified anterior capsulolabral reconstruction. *Am J Sports Med* 1994, 22: 352–58.
59. Rowe CR, Patel D, Southmayd WW: The Bankart procedure: A long-term end-result study. *J Bone joint Surg* 1978, 60A: 1–16.
60. Morgan CD, Bodenstab AB: Arthroscopic Bankart suture repair: Technique and early results. *Arthroscopy* 1987, 3: 111–22.
61. Arciero RA, Wheeler JH, Ryan JB, et al: Arthroscopic Bankart repair versus non-operative treatment for acute, initial anterior shoulder dislocation. *Am J Sports Med* 1994, 22: 589–94.
62. Green MR, Christiansen KP: Arthroscopic versus open Bankart procedures: A comparison of early morbidity and complications. *Arthroscopy* 1993, 9: 371–74.
63. Caspari RB, Savoie FH: Arthroscopic reconstruction of the shoulder: The Bankart repair. In McGinty JB ed. *Operative Arthroscopy.* New York: Raven Press, 1991.
64. Grana WA, Buckley PD, Yates CK: Arthroscopic Bankart suture repair. *Am J Sports Med*, 1993, 21: 348–53.
65. Pollock RG, Bigliani LU: Lateral capsular shift for shoulder instability. *Sports Med Arthroscopy Rev* 1993, 1: 217–26.

SECTION 3

Special Issues Related to Proprioception and Neuromuscular Control

Section Leaders: Peter J. Fowler, MD, FRCSC, and Per A. Renström, MD, PhD

Section Participants: James A. Ashton-Miller, PhD, Mary Lloyd Ireland, MD,
John Albright, MD, C. Buz Swanik, PhD, ATC, Jon J.P. Warner, MD

In this section the authors address selected issues related to the influence of the sensorimotor system on injury prevention, special populations, orthopedic management approaches, and the effect of bracing and orthoses. The authors provide paradigms that have been tested related to these issues and set forth a number of plausible hypotheses in need of testing as they relate to the sensorimotor system.

Ashton-Miller presents prophylactic elements of the proprioceptive mechanism using the ankle model. Ireland then discusses the incidence of knee injuries in the female athlete and the potential influence of the sensorimotor control system on these injuries. Renström and associates discuss the stability role of orthoses on proprioception and neuromuscular control, followed by a discussion by Lo and Fowler on specific surgical considerations and their influence on proprioception. Lastly Swanik, Giraldo and their associates discuss the effects that aging and degenerative arthritis have on the sensorimotor system as well as the potential influences on the processes as a result of their manifestation.

Contemporary research related to the sensorimotor system has predominantly focused on the effects of acute injury to the primary restraint mechanisms of the knee, ankle, and shoulder. However, this group has identified many of the nontraditional considerations related to risk factors, prophylaxis, disease, and intervention. The authors have identified the following directions for future research on these special issues as they relate to proprioception and neuromuscular control.

Directions for Future Research

1. Develop paradigms to systematically investigate sensorimotor risk factors influencing joint pathology.
2. Describe gender specific anatomical and sensorimotor variables placing the female in positions known to induce excessive loads to the knee joint (position of no return).
3. Determine if there are gender-by-fatigue interactions related to ACL injury.
4. Investigate the influence of hormonal fluctuation on risk of knee joint ligament injury in females.
5. Study issues of muscle firing sequence as it relates to external loading of the knee joint. This is of particular concern as it relates to gender discrepancies.
6. Design prospective investigations to assess the effects of prophylactic orthoses and taping. Differentiate between the mechanical restraint characteristics of these devices and their effects on the sensorimotor system.
7. Determine the effect of surgical intervention on joint afferents.
8. Determine the role degenerative change plays relative to both joint afference and the effect of associated pain on these mechanisms.
9. Determine if deficits in proprioception predispose the joint to more rapid degenerative changes.
10. Determine if the remnants of articular trauma (i.e., an ACL stump) have any viable proprioceptive qualities warranting their preservation during surgical reconstruction.

CHAPTER 25

Proprioceptive Thresholds at the Ankle: Implications for the Prevention of Ligament Injury

James A. Ashton-Miller, PhD

Introduction

The ankle is one of the most frequently injured joints in athletics (35), usually upon ground contact (9) when landing with the foot inverted and plantar flexed (11, 12). Injuries range from mild sprains to severe sprains and, less commonly, fractures. Once injury threatens, both sensory and motor subsystems contribute to a reactive avoidance strategy. If time permits, the afferent subsystem can attempt to signal the onset of tissue strain rates associated with an impending sprain, which, if allowed to continue for too long, are recognized centrally as being likely to lead to failure of muscles and ligaments at the ankle joint. An effective motor strategy must then be executed, often in time-critical circumstances, to prevent the accumulated strain in the relevant tissues from reaching injurious levels. This chapter will focus on the sensory subsystem performance. Under what conditions can afferent mechanisms give adequate warning of an impending ankle sprain? And how adequate are standard tests of afferent or proprioceptive function for assessing afferent function under time-critical situations? I shall argue in this chapter that the classic tests of joint position sense involving memory are probably poor predictors of afferent performance under emergent time-critical circumstances, because the associated cortical time delays likely make them irrelevant. On the other hand, proprioceptive tests identifying the threshold for sensing joint movement are relevant to understanding a failure of the neuromuscular system to protect the intact ankle.

We first review several studies of ankle proprioception performed in our laboratories (13, 32, 34). These studies employed a number of psychophysical and statistical procedures to improve methods for estimating the threshold for detecting joint rotation. Specifically, we consider the effects of joint rotation direction, angle, and speed on the threshold for sensing foot rotations when standing and bearing weight on the limb. In addition, the effects of age, gender, and disease on the threshold for detecting joint rotation are considered in terms of mechanisms for preventing soft tissue injury in ankle inversion.

Historical Perspective

The term "proprioception" was introduced by Sir Charles Sherrington in 1906 to describe awareness of body segment position and orientation by combining the Latin words (re)ception (the act of receiving) and proprius (one's own) (28). By 1889 Goldscheider (14) already had systematically measured and compared the smallest joint rotations that could be detected at nine different joints in the body. As a result of 4,000 measurements made at a constant velocity (0.3°/s), he reported that the ankle exhibited the largest threshold (1.2°) while the shoulder exhibited the smallest threshold (0.2°) of the joints studied. As can happen in science, his landmark study has largely been forgotten, and subsequent generations have reported their own results in ignorance of his insights. See Gilsing and associates (13) for a review.

Since a large body of literature describes the afferent receptors and mechanisms subserving proprioception (for review, see chapter 1, Johansson, Pederson, Bergenheim and Djupsjöbacka), as well as the role of proprioception in the control of body posture, movements, and balance (see chapter 4, Riemann & Guskiewicz), we shall not dwell on that topic here.

Gaining Insights from Proprioceptive Impairments

Physicians have long known that individuals with chronic central or peripheral proprioceptive impairments are more prone to exhibit articular pathology. Examples include Charcot changes occurring in the upper or lower extremities due to central nervous system deficits over several levels of the spinal cord by syringeomyelia and changes in the foot or ankle due to diabetic neuropathy. The role of proprioceptive impairments in determining whether or not soft tissue injuries occur at a joint, however, has not been established. This is true despite considerable research seeking to establish a role for proprioceptive deficits in reinjury of a joint as a result of soft tissue injuries to the ACL or lateral ankle complex (see, for example, reviews in section two).

In recent years my colleagues and I have been interested in why patients with peripheral neuropathy (PN) exhibit a 23-fold increased risk of falls and 6-fold increased risk of fracture (25) when compared with healthy controls, and why PN patients have significantly poorer unipedal balance than normal (24). As part of our investigations of the magnitude of the sensory deficits underlying these striking mobility impairments, we measured the effect of PN on ankle proprioception thresholds (34). That study offers an opportunity to review how much a known neural deficit can affect thresholds for detecting joint movement. The findings are discussed in terms of how they adversely affect the "early warning" of impending ankle inversion available to the central nervous system.

Limitations of Current Methods for Quantifying Proprioception

One of the most widely used methods for testing proprioception involves quantifying joint position sense. This is the accuracy and reliability with which a given joint angle or limb configuration can be reproduced in a subsequent trial or with respect to matching the angle at the contralateral joint (for example, see Perrin and Schultz, chapter 31). This "joint position sense" should be differentiated from another measure of proprioception: the threshold for detecting joint rotation (see below). Because tests of joint position sense usually take several seconds to complete per trial, the test results really only have validity for slow movements made over several seconds. In addition, because they usually pertain to the nonweight-bearing limb, these test results can only have relevance for considering slow nonvisually guided positioning of a limb in the air. In the current sport injury literature this fact is almost universally ignored. These tests, therefore, may have little relevance for estimating the thresholds for detecting limb movement under weight-bearing or weight acceptance conditions. Furthermore, they have little relevance for understanding the causes of ankle, or even knee, injury in time-critical situations because the weight acceptance phase when landing from a jump takes less than 1/20 s, nearly a hundred times faster than the typical joint position sense trial takes to complete. There are, moreover, other problems with these tests of one proprioceptive modality.

These problems include the failure to include an adequate number of trials to assess the probability associated with detection of a movement, failure to standardize limb movement velocities, failure to estimate the reliability with which a given threshold rotation can be detected, and a failure to control for the state of arousal, mental fatigue, or external factors such as distractions or cues that can alter accuracy rates. Nonetheless, if such factors are taken into consideration, tests of nonweight-bearing joint position sense might contain useful information for considering specific types of motions, such as the lower extremity in its swing phase, and the upper extremities during nonweight-bearing activities. It would, however, be better to test the ability to discriminate differences in arm configurations or velocities directly, as has indeed been done recently using an elegant forced choice paradigm (19).

An example of the importance of nonweight-bearing proprioception in the lower extremity is in its involvement in reliably gauging the "carrying angle" of the swing foot in terms of the angles of ankle dorsiflexion and inversion during the swing phase of locomotion. An unintentional decrease in dorsiflexion or increase in inversion during midstride, such as can happen in the patient with drop foot, reduces foot-ground clearance, thereby increasing the probability of a trip or stumble. Such a stumble can lead to injurious inversion if weight is placed too quickly upon the limb as the foot is rolled over the point of ground contact by the momentum of the leg and body. A simple calculation will illustrate just how important reliable knowledge of swing foot carrying angles can be.

My colleagues and I have shown that during level gait the usual average (*SD*) foot-ground clearance in healthy individuals in the range 20 through 70 yrs is 20.2 (7.7) mm (5). If the forefoot extends 20 cm anterior to the ankle joint, then simple geometry shows that an unrecognized decrease of 1° in the angle of ankle dorsiflexion will reduce foot clearance by approximately 4 mm or 20%. Similarly, an unrecognized 1° increase in the angle of inversion would further decrease foot clearance by 2 mm. Thus, a 1° decrease in dorsiflexion and increase in inversion would reduce average ground clearance by about 30%. We know that ground clearance in normal locomotion is usually sufficient to reduce the probability of tripping over a 1-inch-high object on the floor to 1% (mean foot clearance minus 3*SD*) (5) or about 1 in every 100 times one steps over a 1″ threshold. Unintentionally reducing ground clearance from 20 to 14 mm due to a 1° change in foot carrying angles would increase the risk of tripping to about 6% (mean "reduced" clearance minus 2*SD*) or just over 1 in 20 strides over a threshold. It should not be surprising, then, that a proprioceptive impairment at the ankle can be expected to markedly increase the likelihood of stumbles and trips.

Newer Methods for Measuring the Detection of Joint Rotation

In a time-critical situation the most appropriate measure of proprioceptive signaling would appear to involve the original Goldscheider approach of measuring the threshold for detecting the rotation of a joint by an external (turning) moment. In what follows I describe several recent studies of this type.

Methods for Measuring Thresholds for Detecting Ankle Rotation in the Frontal Plane

Eighteen healthy young subjects (mean age (*SD*) 23 (3) yrs) and 18 healthy older subjects (mean age (*SD*) 70 (3) yrs) were studied while standing with a foot placed in a custom-built servomotor-driven cradle (see figure 25.1) (13). A randomized quadruple staircase method and probit analysis were developed and used to improve the measurement of the magnitude of the thresholds for sensation of ankle inversion and eversion (see figure 25.2) (13). Studies were performed in 8 blocks of 25 trials, 5 of which were dummy control trials (in which no movement oc-

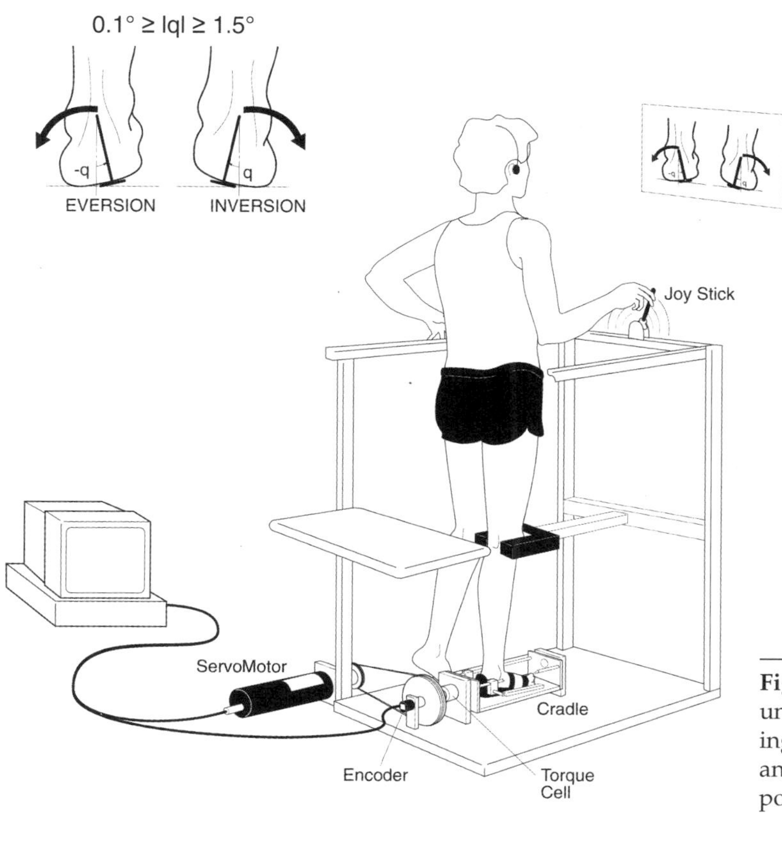

Figure 25.1 Schematic drawing of a subject undergoing a unipedal stance test. Audio warning cues are delivered via the headphones. If an ankle rotation is detected, its direction is reported using the joystick.

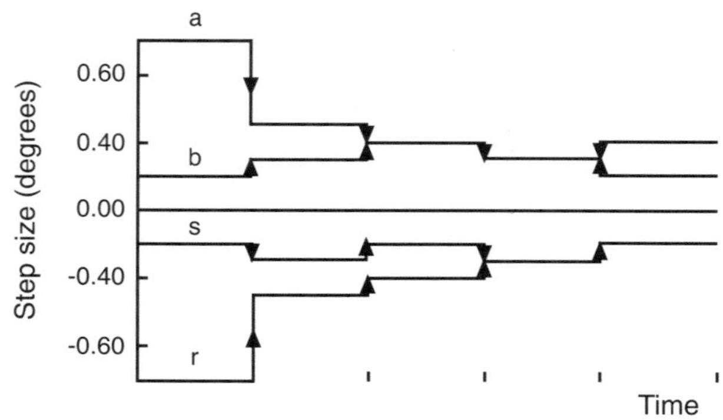

Step Number	Step ID	Step Angle Change (°)	Absolute Angle (°)	Response Correct?	Current Inversion Threshold (°)	Current Eversion Threshold (°)
1	c(4)	0.0*	0.0*	N		
2	r(2)	–1.0	–1.0	Y		
3	b(1)	0.2	–0.8	N		
4	s(3)	–0.2	–1.0	N		
5	a(0)	1.0	0.0	Y		
6	a(0)	0.5	0.5	Y	0.5	
7	r(2)	–0.5	0.0	Y		–0.5
8	b(1)	0.3	0.3	N		
9	s(3)	–0.3	0.0	Y		–0.3⁺
10	b(1)	0.4	0.4	Y	0.4	
11	a(0)	0.4	0.8	Y		
12	r(2)	–0.4	0.4	Y		
13	b(1)	0.3	0.7	N		
14	c(4)	0.0*	0.7	N		
15	b(1)	0.4	1.1	Y		
16	a(0)	0.3	1.4	Y	0.3⁺	
17	c(4)	0.0*	1.4	N		
18	a(0)	0.2	1.6	N		
19	r(2)	–0.3	1.3	Y		
20	c(4)	0.0*	1.3	N		
21	s(3)	–0.2	1.1	N		
22	r(2)	–0.2	0.9	N		
23	c(4)	0.0*	0.9	N		
24	s(3)	–0.3	0.6	Y		
25	s(3)	–0.2	0.4	N		

*Denotes dummy trial; ⁺denotes minimum angle found in this trial block.

Figure 25.2 The schematic illustration shows an actual example (single block of 25 trials) of the quadruple staircase method as presented to one subject. Correct (Y) and incorrect (N) responses are shown in the table.

curred so that the rate at which test subjects were guessing could be quantified). To estimate the effect of weight bearing, in half the trials the subject was tested while standing bipedally, while in the other half of trials the subject stood in unipedal stance.

Two different estimates of the detection threshold were made. The lower threshold (TH_{min}) was defined as the absolute smallest foot rotation ever discriminated correctly in inversion or eversion. Descriptive statistics for TH_{min} were then calculated by group and test condition. Although the values of TH_{min} represent the smallest rotation detectable under that test condition, the reliability with which that detection was made remains unspecified, as in earlier studies. But unless the reliability of detecting a threshold rotation is known, the functional interpretation of that threshold can be problematic. We therefore developed for the first time in proprioception testing a complementary definition of detection threshold that incorporates the probability of detecting that rotation. These thresholds were estimated using probit analyses. In such analyses the estimated probit (inverse normal cumulative probability density function) of the probability of detection is a linear function of the angle change. Then we defined TH_{75} as that change required for which an estimated probability of detection was 0.75 (or 75%). Values were then compared for both inversion and eversion across group (young, older subjects) and condition (inversion, eversion, unipedal, bipedal stance) using analysis of variance (ANOVA).

To quantify how much the subjects tried to guess in the test, we performed a binomial test on the results of the dummy trials. To quantify the effect of varying the rate of rotation of the ankle, 5 young subjects were tested 1 wk later at both 200°/s and 2°/s.

Methods for Measuring Rotation Thresholds in the Sagittal Plane

Because inversion and plantarflexion movements are commonly associated with inversion injuries (see introduction above), it may be fruitful to compare results from the frontal plane tests discussed above with sagittal plane tests of movement detection thresholds. Twelve healthy young females (mean age (*SD*) 22 (2) yrs) and 12 healthy older females (mean age (*SD*) 70 (4) yrs) were studied (32). Subjects stood bipedally with one foot placed on a servomotor-driven platform. The foot was positioned such that a line through the medial and lateral malleoli was parallel with the axis of platform rotation, which lay 10 cm above the platform surface and approximately collinear with the center of rotation of the ankle joint in the sagittal plane.

Subjects were tested using platform angular speeds of 0.1°/s (slow), 0.5°/s (medium) and 2.5°/s (fast) to angles of 0.05°, 0.1°, 0.2°, 0.4°, and 0.8° in both dorsiflexion and plantarflexion. Subjects performed 5 trials at each velocity-angle combination and 30 dummy trials in which no rotation occurred, for a total of 180 trials. The protocol was presented in 5 blocks of 36 initially randomized, fixed-order trials. Each block was performed as 2 sets of 18 trials with a 1 min rest between sets.

A subject's ability to detect platform rotation was quantified by the number of trials in which either the occurrence of rotation or its direction was correctly detected. In this more recent paper slightly different outcome measures were employed than in the Gilsing and associate study (13). A rotation success rate (SRR) was defined with regard to whether or not the occurrence of any rotation was correctly detected. A direction success rate (SRD) was correspondingly defined as the ratio of trials in which the direction of the rotation was correctly identified to the number of nonzero angle trials. SRR and SRD were determined for each subject for each speed-angle combination and expressed in percent of the total number of trials conducted for that condition. Repeated measures analysis of variance (rm-ANOVA) was used to determine the effects of age, angle, direction, and speed on SRR and SRD. In tests of these primary hypotheses, p values less than .05 were considered statistically significant.

Cumulative success rates for each speed-angle combination were determined separately for young subjects and older subjects. At each velocity, and separately for young and old, nonlinear logistic regression was used to relate success rate to angle. The identified regression equations were used to estimate the platform rotation angle required to achieve a nominal 75% success rate at a given velocity (13). We selected that criterion because we have earlier shown that statistical estimates of the detection threshold, which are commonly used in signal detection theory and psychophysical research (21, 22), are consistent (13) and because estimates of the 100% threshold are too sensitive to small fluctuations in slope of the regression function in that region.

Measuring the Effect of Peripheral Neuropathy on Detection Thresholds

Using the methods described above, my colleagues and I quantified the effect of peripheral neuropathy (PN) on ankle inversion and eversion thresholds (34). The performance of 7 geriatric patients with PN (mean age (*SD*) 66.7 (6.0) yrs) with electrodiagnostically documented PN were compared with 7 age- and gender-matched controls with electrodiagnostically confirmed normal nerve function. The average sural, tibial, and peroneal nerve conduction amplitudes in the PN subjects were reduced to 16%, 15%, and 24% of the control values, respectively.

Results: Age Effects

The results of over 3,600 trials show that the mean (*SD*) threshold for detecting inversion with a probability of 75% was 0.09° (0.09°) in the younger subjects, a value that was significantly different from the 0.39° (0.44°) found in the older subjects. The corresponding values for eversion were 0.32° (0.15°) and 0.49° (0.30°) in the younger and older subjects, respectively. The TH_{min} in inversion ranged from 0.1° to 0.14° in both unipedal and bipedal stance for the four groups tested.

Results: Effect of Rotation Direction

Across all subjects and trials the threshold in eversion was significantly (80%) larger than that in inversion.

Results: Effect of Gender

Few meaningful gender effects were found.

Results: Rate Effects

When the speed of a 0.1° inversion rotation stimulus was increased from 2°/s to 200°/s the probability of detecting motion increased from 56% to 80%.

Results: Joint Position Sense

The mean (*SD*) absolute angular error in rotating the cradle to the horizontal was 1.2° (0.9°) for the young and 1.6° (1.3°) for the older subjects.

Results: Dorsiflexion and Plantarflexion Thresholds

The results show that humans consistently sensed platform rotations of less than 1° in both dorsiflexion and plantarflexion during upright bipedal stance. Age ($p < .0001$), speed ($p < .0001$) and direction ($p < .05$) were found to have significant effects on the reliability for detecting both foot rotation and direction (rm-ANOVA).

Effect of Age

The young subjects consistently had greater rotation success rates (SRRs) and direction success rates (SRDs) than older subjects at every speed-angle combination tested. For example, SRDs of the young subjects were greater than 78% for all of the 2.5°/s rotations, but they were as low as 30% for the older subjects at this speed.

The dummy "no movement" control trials were correctly identified by the young subjects with a 97% success rate, a 21% higher success rate than that of the older subjects. This is additional evidence that age affects the consistency with which foot rotations can be sensed.

Nonlinear regression models showed that the young subject thresholds for sensing the direction of platform rotation with a probability of 75% in dorsiflexion were 0.04°, 0.09°, and 0.41° at the fast, moderate, and slow velocities, respectively; dorsiflexion threshold values for older subjects were 2.8 to 4 times larger. The corresponding young subject values in plantarflexion were 0.03°, 0.16°, and 0.43°, with older subjects having 3.2 to 4.3 times larger values than the younger subjects.

Effect of Speed

Success rates generally improved with increasing angular speed for a given angle. For example, thresholds for detecting plantarflexion rotation for young subjects were 0.43° at the 0.1°/s speed, but less than 0.05° at the 2.5°/s speed. Similarly, while older subjects did not achieve a 75% SRD at the 0.1°/s speed for any of the angles presented, only 0.13° of plantarflexion rotation was required to achieve a 75% SRD at the 0.1°/s speed. For the young subjects a greater than 10-fold increase was observed in the angular threshold on decreasing the speed of rotation from 2.5 to 0.1°/s. For the older subjects a greater than 3-fold increase in angular threshold was observed on decreasing the speed from 2.5 to 0.5°/s; older subjects did not achieve a 75% SRD at the 0.1°/s speed for any of the angles presented.

Effect of Rotation Direction

The SRDs were significantly different in dorsiflexion and plantarflexion ($p < .05$, ANOVA) with rotation directions generally being detected with slightly greater reliability in dorsiflexion than in plantarflexion.

Comparison of SRD and SRR

SRD values ranged up to 60% lower than the corresponding SRR values while following similar trends with respect to speed and angle effects. Therefore, ankle rotation alone was detected with considerably more reliability than when the direction of that rotation also had to be identified.

Effect of Peripheral Neuropathy on Frontal Plane Thresholds

Mild to moderate primary axonal peripheral neuropathy reduced the average sural, tibial, and peroneal nerve conduction amplitudes to 16%, 15%, and 24% of control values, respectively, which significantly and thereby adversely affected the threshold for reliably detecting foot rotations. Across all test conditions, the PN group had a 4.6-fold larger ($p = .0026$) threshold (mean 1.37°) (*SD* 1.74°) for perceiving the presence and direction of an ankle rotation with 75% probability of success than did the matched control group (mean 0.3°) (*SD* 0.17°) with normal nerve function. Inversion acuity was approximately twice that in eversion in both groups. The PN groups demonstrated better proprioceptive acuity in unipedal stance than in bipedal stance, whereas there was no such difference in the healthy controls.

Discussion

The results show that the threshold for consistently and reliably detecting rotation of the foot under weight-bearing conditions is, at best, hundredths of a degree and, at worst, a few tenths of a degree, even in healthy older subjects. No meaningful effects due to gender were found at the ankle. Because such values are an order of magnitude smaller than those found in the nonweight-bearing extremity (3, 15), we can conclude that the results of nonweight-bearing proprioception tests cannot reliably be extrapolated to indicate weight-bearing results. Other recent studies have also reported significantly lower thresholds for detecting movement in the weight-bearing lower extremity than in the nonweight-bearing extremity. In the sagittal plane, for example, Fitzpatrick and McCloskey (10) demonstrated that young adults were capable of detecting less than 0.2° angular perturbations of standing sway using their ankle afference. These findings are corroborated by those of Gilsing and associates (13), who demonstrated a threshold of 0.06° for detecting ankle inversion with a 75% rate of success while weight bearing.

An important finding was that the threshold of detecting ankle rotation is rate dependent, decreasing 10-fold when foot rotation speed was increased from 0.1°/s to 2.5°/s (32); however, only a small difference was found in detection probability when the speed was further increased to 200°/s (13). This rate sensitivity is consistent with findings of others (e.g., 7, 16, 21, 22, 29); it is also characteristic of most sensory receptors, since receptor adaptation facilitates the perception of the rate of change of a stimulus as well as the absolute sensation itself. So, faster movements lead to earlier warning of joint rotation than do slow rotations, because we know that less rotation is required to trigger the sensation of ankle rotation.

Implications for Inversion Injuries

It seems reasonable to assume that as the rate of increase and magnitude of the loads acting on the musculoskeletal system increase, so the risk for injury also increases. This is not only because of rising tissue stresses and strains, but also because of fixed delays within the neuromuscular system assigned to protect those very structures. The large and rapidly increasing ground reaction forces acting on the foot landing from a jump, for example, place considerable demands on the foot and ankle neuromusculoskeletal system. Thus, when landing on a hard surface following a jump, say, the ground reaction force can increase from zero to several times body weight in as little as 50 ms (9). In fact, my colleagues and I have found ankle inversion rotation reaching 17° in an average of 39 ms, and sometimes in as little as 17 ms (17), under some circumstances when landing on a hard, stiff surface, in other words long before the ground reaction force has peaked. Such rapid rises in ground reaction force and inversion of the foot must lead to a time-critical situation for the neuromuscular systems responsible for injury avoidance. We shall see that for every set of initial biomechanical conditions on landing, there is a temporal "window of opportunity" within which motor strategies must be completed for successful recovery and outside which recovery is not possible. What are the factors affecting that temporal window?

In what follows we shall consider the scenario in which one is unlucky enough to land unwittingly on an unyielding prominence several cm high under the medial foot. The resulting increase in inversion moment will cause foot inversion to occur in approximately 50 ms due to the large external moment about the subtalar joint, the low rotational inertia of the foot, and the low muscular stiffness acting about the subtalar joint (1). If the foot rotates 17° from neutral to full inversion (18) in that 50 ms (17), at what would amount to an average speed of 340°/s (or 17°/.050 s; peak speeds can be much higher), then we can infer from the above rotation threshold studies that the inversion is probably already signaled as having commenced after 0.1° (13, 34) or after 0.3 ms. Even with the fastest monosynaptic reflexes (the 20 ms afferent latency for the fastest axons to transmit the information at 50 m/s from the periphery to the spinal cord and the corresponding 20 ms efferent latency back to a muscle) there would not be enough time to execute and complete an appropriate injury avoidance strategy within the 20 ms available temporal window of opportunity. This is true even if onset of myoelectric activity (EMG) were to be observed in the effector muscles within that time, because the onset of myolectric activity does not signal that the muscle has usefully increased its level of contractile force (31, 33). Unfortunately, many papers published in the literature, either implicitly or explicitly, make the erroneous assumption that onset of myoelectric activity signals a biomechanically significant change in the muscle contractile force.

We know that healthy young ankle muscle averages 94 ms to develop even half its maximal contractile force after the force rises above threshold (33), so even a monosynaptic reflex simply does not have sufficient time to develop the muscular moment required to decelerate the ankle inversion before injury occurs to the lateral ligaments at full inversion. And if a monosynaptic reflex is too slow then, by definition, any polysynaptic reflex or longer loop reflex taking 120 ms (8) or longer must be too slow to protect the ankle. Of course that response does not include cognitive processing. If conduction latencies delay arrival of peripheral afferent information at the cortex by 60 ms, and cortical processing takes from 25–70 ms, then the individual can perceive the onset of inversion after 85 to 130 ms. Given a 60 ms efferent conduction latency from the cortex back to the periphery, the earliest the individual can begin to volitionally start changing muscle force in the weight-bearing extremity is 120 ms, and more likely 145–190 ms (4), after the onset of inversion. This again is too slow to be useful in triggering a suitable muscular reaction at the ankle. Thus if the inversion moment leads to the subtalar joint reaching maximum inversion rotation within 40 ms then the monosynaptic reflexes will likely be ineffective, within 120 ms the polysynaptic reflexes will likely be ineffective, and within 145 ms volitional mechanisms will likely be ineffective to reliably prevent ankle injury, even if the response is triggered at the onset of the inversion moment. Under the most challenging conditions, then, if the neuromuscular system waits to determine whether the inversion will exceed a critical rotation value, any ensuing motor response is further delayed by the duration of that decision-making process.

When impact occurs with a more compliant surface the potentially injurious moment peaks in several hundred ms (150 to 250 ms). This occurs, for example, at heel contact when walking or running on a softer surface. Now, possibilities exist for afferent systems to signal impending injurious strains and cortical reflexes within the time frame needed to prevent ankle injury. And if the injurious moment is reached in longer than 250 ms, as in pushing, pulling, or lifting tasks, then at 68°/s (calculated from a 17° sweep in 0.25 s), the onset of inversion (0.1°) should be signaled by the receptors after 6 ms, leaving sufficient time for volitional responses to start being involved in helping to avoid such an injury. So in answer to the questions posed in the introduction, at the highest loading rates the nociceptive-mediated warning will simply fail to reach the central nervous system in time for it to be able to prevent injury via motor strategies, and injury may be a foregone conclusion. But under more moderate loading rates (peaking in 50–250 ms) there is a "gray zone," a temporal window of opportunity within which an appropriate motor response may be executable depending upon several biomechanical and neuromuscular factors. And under the lowest rates (peaking in > 250 ms), we shall assume injury should be preventable as long as the magnitude of the external load is not excessive, because more than sufficient time is available to execute the necessary motor program. These speculations remain to be tested experimentally.

One obvious biomechanical consideration concerning the warning time for impending injurious inversion in the above example is the effect of the initial angle of inversion at ground contact. Its importance seems to me to be underrecognized. Essentially the greater the initial angle of inversion at impact, the less time available before the extreme range of motion of the ankle is reached in inversion. If, for example, the ankle is already inverted 15° when the ground reaction force begins its rise over 500 ms, then even at the moderate inversion rate of 34°/s, it will reach 17° at the end of range of motion constraint in 59 ms. In such a case, the unfavorable initial angle of inversion at impact has therefore turned what should have been be a moderate challenge to the ankle musculoskeletal protective system into a time-critical provocation; there is now little that can be done reactively to prevent injury within the temporal window available.

As indicated, more work is needed in determining how the various factors such as ground surface compliance and damping, lower extremity joint angles, and muscle stiffness and damping affect the rate of inversion moment increase and how the various involuntary and volitional response strategies and neuropsychological factors, such as attention division (6, 20), cognitive tasks (26), and arousal state interact to detect and avoid soft tissue injuries at the ankle. Despite this, and despite not knowing the relative contributions of the sensory, motor, and educational training involved, we do know enough to train individuals to reduce their risk for ankle injuries, given that a recent Norwegian intervention reduced the rate of ankle injuries by almost half (2).

The effects of physical or mental fatigue on the thresholds for detecting ankle rotation are unknown. It is known that fatiguing shoulder muscle contractions significantly and adversely affect the ability to detect differences in shoulder velocity (19). Similarly, joint position sense is adversely affected by muscle fatigue (27, 30), although the roles of peripheral and central factors need still to be clarified. So, although one might reasonably hypothesize that muscle fatigue might adversely affect the ability to detect ankle movement, such a hypothesis remains to be tested directly using modern psychophysical methods.

Finally, if the healthy individual is placed at a disadvantage under rapid loading rates, then an individual with peripheral neuropathy must surely be at an even greater disadvantage because a significantly greater rotation has to occur before he or she can reliably detect it (29, 34). Based on the Gilsing and coworkers (13) results the normative (mean + 2*SD*) values for healthy young and older individuals to sense inversion of the foot were 0.27° and 1.27°, respectively, meaning that 95% of similarly aged healthy individuals would reliably sense inversion rotation of these magnitudes. In the example cited in the preceding paragraph, while all of the healthy subjects would sense the additional 2° of inversion although few could act appropriately on it, many PN subjects would not even detect it and so would not even react, because they have no early warning of impending injury. In this case it is the PN patients with thresholds in the range between 2° and to the "+ 2*SD*" population value of 4.8° that would never implement a reactive injury avoidance. Epidemiologists have yet to quantify the rate of ankle injuries in patients with mild to moderate peripheral neuropathy, but one might predict that it should be significantly higher than in healthy controls, at least until patients develop insight into their condition. Through educational interventions physicians and therapists can alert these patients to their known increased risk for fractures (23), and it may be worth alerting them to their increased risk for ankle inversion injury postulated in this paper.

Conclusions

Recent psychophysical test methods offer more reliable means to test ankle rotation detection thresholds in the adult than current clinical tests of proprioception.

1. The healthy young adult can reliably detect inversion rotations of less than a tenth of a degree while an older adult can detect rotations of less than one-half a degree.
2. Age does systematically degrade the thresholds for detecting ankle rotations but only to a minor degree.
3. Gender does not significantly affect the thresholds for detecting ankle rotation.
4. Peripheral neuropathy leads to a 4.6-fold increase in detection threshold for movement at the ankle, thereby decreasing the available warning time prior to an inversion injury.
5. The threshold for the reliable detection of foot rotation is 10 times smaller under weight-bearing than under nonweight-bearing conditions.
6. The threshold for sensing inversion was 80% (significantly) smaller than that in eversion.
7. The probit and logistic regression analyses show that the smaller the foot rotation, the less reliably it will be sensed.
8. Up to speeds of 2.5°/s, the more rapid the foot rotation, the more reliably it will be sensed.
9. Ankle rotation detection thresholds were similar in the frontal and sagittal planes.
10. Under certain ground contact conditions, a large inversion angle at footstrike may predispose an individual to injury because inherent latencies will compromise the ability of the afferent system to provide adequate warning of an impending inversion injury, even at moderate rates of external inversion moment increase.
11. Due the considerable time it takes a muscle to develop substantial tension after the onset of peroneal myoelectric activity, peroneal reaction times based on myoelectric latencies are not reliable indicators of whether or not those muscles can prevent an inversion injury under time-critical conditions.
12. Theoretical considerations of the neural conduction delays following ground recontact from a jump lead to the following conclusions:

    - Under the most rapid loading (when the level of injurious inversion moment is reached in less than 40 ms), the sensory afferents will fail to warn the central nervous system in time for it to be able to ameliorate the risk of impending ankle ligament injury.
    - At more moderate loading rates (tissue strain reaching the injury threshold between 120 and 250 ms), sensory afferents can allow long loop reflexes to ameliorate ankle injury risk under many conditions. Reliability of response will increase with available response time.
    - At moderate loading rates, the greater the angle of inversion at ground recontact, the less time afferent mechanisms have to warn of the impending ankle soft tissue injury.
    - At slow loading rates (tissue strain reaching injury threshold after 250 ms) both reflexes and proprioception should reliably warn of impending ankle injury in time to allow effective countermeasures to be implemented.

References

1. Ashton-Miller, J.A., R.A. Ottaviani, C. Hutchinson, and E.M. Wojtys. What best protects the inverted weight-bearing ankle against further inversion? Evertor muscle strength compares favorably with shoe height, athletic tape, and three orthoses. *Am. J. Sports Med.*, 1996. 24: 800–809.

2. Bahr, R., O. Lian, and I.A. Bahr. A twofold reduction in the incidence of acute ankle sprains in volleyball after the introduction of an injury prevention program: A prospective cohort study. *Scan. J. Med. & Sci. in Sports,* 1997. 7: 172–77.
3. Berenberg, R.A., J.M. Shefner, and J.J. Sabol. Quantitative assessment of position sense at the ankle: A functional approach. *Neurology,* 1987. 37: 89–93.
4. Card, S.K., and T.P. Moran. The model human processor (ch. 45). In *Handbook of human perception and performance,* K. Boff, L. Kufman, and J. Thomas, editors. 1986, New York: Wiley, 45–136.
5. Chen, H.-C., J.A. Ashton-Miller, N.B. Alexander, and A.B. Schultz. Stepping over obstacles: Gait patterns of healthy young and old adults. *J. Gerontol.: Med. Sci.,* 1991. 46: 196–203.
6. Chen, H.-C., A.B. Schultz, J.A. Ashton-Miller, B.J. Giordani, et al. Stepping over obstacles: Dividing attention impairs performance of old more than young adults. *J. Gerontol.: Med. Sci.,* 1996. 51A: M116–22.
7. Clark, F.J., R.C. Burgess, J.W. Chapin, and W.T. Lipscomb. Role of the intramuscular receptors in the awareness of joint position. *J. Neurophysiol.,* 1985. 54: 1529–540.
8. Dewhurst, D.J. Neuromuscular control system. *I.E.E.E. Trans. Biomed. Engin.,* 1967. 14: 167–71.
9. Dufek, J.S. and B.T. Bates. Biomechanical factors associated with injury during landing during sports. *Sports Med.,* 1991. 12: 326–37.
10. Fitzpatrick, R. and D.I. McCloskey. Stable human standing with lower-limb muscle afferents providing the only sensory input. J. *Physiol.,* 1994. 80: 395–403.
11. Garrick, J.G. The frequency of injury, mechanism of injury, and epidemiology of ankle sprains. *Am. J. Sports Med.,* 1977. 5: 241–42.
12. Garrick, J.G. and R.K. Requa. The epidemiology of foot and ankle injuries in sports. *Clin. Sports Med.,* 1988. 7: 29–36.
13. Gilsing, M.G., C.G. Van den Bosch, S.-G. Lee, J.A. Ashton-Miller, et al. Effects of age on the reliability of detecting ankle inversion and eversion. *Age and Aging,* 1995. 24: 58–66.
14. Goldscheider, A. Untersuchungen über den Muskelsinn. *Arch. Anat. Physiol.,* 1889. 3: 369–502.
15. Gurfunkel, V.S., M.I. Lipshits, and K.E. Popov. Threshold of kinesthetic sensation in the vertical position. *Hum. Physiol.,* 1982. 8: 439–45.
16. Kokmen, E., R.W. Bossmeyer, and W.J. Williams. Quantitative evaluation of joint motion sensation in an aging population. *J. Gerontol.,* 1978. 33: 62–67.
17. Milia, M., M.J. Siskoskey, Y.-X. Wang, J.P. Boylan, et al. The role of the ankle evertor muscles in preventing inversion during a one-footed landing on a hard surface: An experimental study in healthy young males. Paper presented at the annual meeting of American Orthopaedic Society for Sports Medicine. 1998. Vancouver, B.C.
18. Ottaviani, R.A., J.A. Ashton-Miller, S.U. Kothari, and E.M. Wojtys. Basketball shoe height and the maximal muscular resistance to applied ankle inversion and eversion movements. *Am. J. Sports Med.,* 1995. 23: 418–23.
19. Pedersen, J., J. Lonn, Hellstrom, M. Djupsjobacka, and H. Johansson. Alterations in movement sense acuity in the human shoulder during muscle fatigue. Submitted for publication, 1997.
20. Persad, C.C., B.J. Giordani, H.-C. Chen, J.A. Ashton-Miller, et al. Neuropsychological predictors of complex obstacle avoidance in healthy older adults. *J. Gerontol.: Psychol. Sci.,* 1995. 50: P272–77.
21. Refshauge, K.M., R. Chan, J.L. Taylor, and D.I. McCloskey. Detection of movements imposed on human hip, knee, ankle, and toe joints. *J. Physiol.,* 1995. 488: 231–41.
22. Refshauge, K.M. and R.C. Fitzpatrick. Perception of movement at the human ankle: Effects of leg position. *J. Physiol.,* 1995. 488: 231–41.
23. Richardson, J.K. and J.A. Ashton-Miller. Peripheral neuropathy: An oft-overlooked cause of falls in the elderly. *Post Grad. Med.,* 1996. 99: 161–72.
24. Richardson, J.K., J.A. Ashton-Miller, S.-G. Lee, and K. Jakobs. Moderate peripheral neuropathy impairs weight transfer and unipedal balance in the elderly. *Arch. Phys. Med. Rehab.,* 1996. 77: 1152–156.
25. Richardson, J.K., C. Ching, and E.A. Hurvitz. The relationship between electromyographically documented peripheral neuropathy and falls. *J. Am. Ger. Soc.,* 1992. 40: 1008–1012.
26. Schumway-Cook, A., M. Woollacott, K.A. Kerns, and M. Baldwin. The effects of two types of cognitive tasks on postural stability in older adults with and without a history of falls. *J. Ger.: Med. Sci.,* 1997. 52A: M232–40.
27. Sharpe, M.H. and T.S. Miles. Position sense at the elbow after fatiguing contractions. *Exp. Brain Res.,* 1993. 94: 179–82.
28. Sherrington, C.S. *The integrative action of the nervous system.* 1947, New Haven: Yale University Press. (Original work published 1906).
29. Simoneau, G.G., J.A. Derr, J.S. Ulbrecht, M.B. Becker, and P.R. Cavanagh. Diabetic sensory neuropathy: Effect on ankle joint movement perception. *Arch. Phys. Med. Rehab.,* 1996. 77: 453–60.
30. Skinner, H.B., M.P. Wyatt, J.A. Hodgdon, D.W. Conard, and R.L. Barrack. Effect of fatigue on

joint position sense of the knee. *J. Orthop. Res.*, 1986. 4: 112–18.

31. Thelen, D.G., J.A. Ashton-Miller, A.B. Schultz, and N.B. Alexander. Do neural factors underlie age differences in rapid ankle torque development? *J. Am. Ger. Soc.*, 1996. 44: 804–808.
32. Thelen, D.G., C. Brockmiller, J.A. Ashton-Miller, A.B. Schultz, and N.A. Alexander. Thresholds for sensing ankle dorsi- and/or plantarflexor rotation during upright stance: Effects of age and velocity. *J. Gerontol.: Med. Sci.*, 1998. 53A: M33–38.
33. Thelen, D.G., A.B. Schultz, N.B. Alexander, and J.A. Ashton-Miller. Effects of age on rapid ankle torque development. *J. Gerontol.: Med. Sci.*, 1996. 51A: M226–32.
34. van den Bosch, C., M. Gilsing, S.-G. Lee, J.K. Richardson, and J.A. Ashton-Miller. Peripheral neuropathy: Effect on ankle inversion and eversion detection thresholds. *Arch. Phys. Med. Rehab.*, 1995. 76: 850–56.
35. Yeung, M.S., K.M. Chan, C.H. So, and W.Y. Yuan. An epidemiological survey on ankle sprain. *Br. J. Sports Med.*, 1994. 28: 112–16.

CHAPTER 26

Proprioception and Neuromuscular Control Related to the Female Athlete

Mary Lloyd Ireland, MD

An alarmingly high incidence of noncontact anterior cruciate ligament (ACL) tears has been observed in females compared to males in sports. The higher risk sports are basketball (1–11) soccer (1), and gymnastics (12, 13). Rates of ACL tears are three to four times greater in the female. Epidemiological studies comparing males and females document this increased rate (12, 14–18).

In the U.S. military, the rates of injuries such as stress fractures have equalized for females and males over the past 10 years (19, 20). The concern is that this injury rate for women is not decreasing in organized sports, particularly high school and college basketball and soccer. In Europe, similar rates occur for team handball and skiing (1). The National Collegiate Athletic Association (NCAA) surveys 18% of all colleges in sixteen sports. This survey is published as the injury surveillance system (13). Rates of injury of the ACL and meniscus are shown in table 26.1. These rates are reported based on number of injuries per 1,000 athletic exposures and averaged over a 3 yr period. Women's gymnastics, women's basketball, and women's soccer lead categories for ACL injury and meniscal injury. Rates of ACL injuries are women's gymnastics, 0 .41; women's basketball, 0.33, compared to men's basketball, 0.11; and women's soccer, 0.32, compared with men's soccer, 0.12. Meniscal injuries are highest in men's wrestling; however, women's soccer, women's basketball, women's gymnastics, and spring football are almost tied for the next highest rate following wrestling. Over the years no trend or statistically significant change in knee injury rates has occurred.

As basic scientists and clinicians, we must assess the risk—then, prioritize factors, develop an equation, and reduce it. In the 1988 Olympic Trials for the United States, which was prior to the men's preselected professional athletes' involvement, 80 males and 64 females tried out for the U.S. basketball teams. A significantly increased rate of knee injury and ACL tear was seen in the females (see table 26.2) (5, 21). Of the 64 females participating in the trials, 34 (53%) had previous knee injuries, and of the 80 males, 11 (13.7%) had previous knee injuries (statistically significant, $p < .0001$). The numbers of ACL injuries were 13 in the females and 3 in the males. Six males underwent 6 surgical procedures, 3 of which were ACL reconstructions. Twenty of the female athletes underwent 25 procedures, 8 of which were ACL reconstructions.

The increase in patellofemoral problems from miserable malalignment, patellar instability, is well known in the female athlete. Alignment, generalized physiologic laxity, excessive valgus, vastus medialis obliquus dysplasia, and quadriceps weakness are contributing factors. The normal alignment of the lower extremity is shown in figure 26.1, and miserable malalignment syndrome is shown in figure 26.2 (22). Comparisons between knees for

Table 26.1 NCAA Injury rates: ACL, Meniscus*

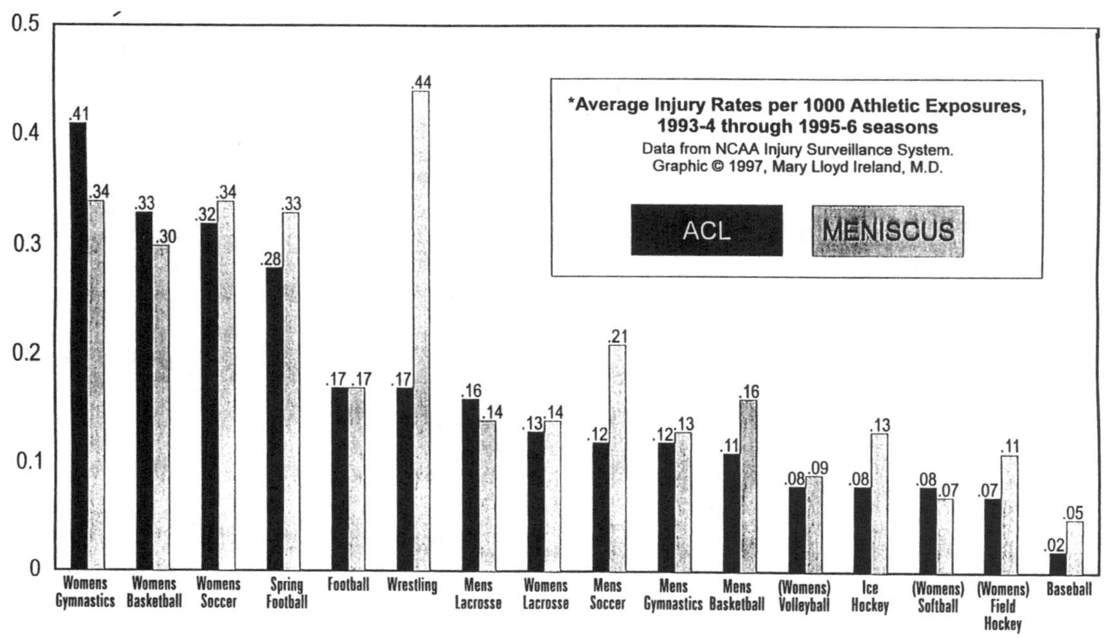

Table 26.2 Injuries Sustained During 1988 Olympic Basketball Trial

Parameter	Males	Females	Total
Number of participants	80	64	144
Athletes with knee injuries	11*	34	45
ACL injuries	3	13	16
Number of athletes requiring surgery	6**	20	26
Number of procedures	6	25	31
Type of procedure			
Arthroscopy	3	17	20
ACL Reconstruction	3	8	11

Abbreviations and symbols: ACL = anterior cruciate ligament; *,** indicate a statistically significant difference between male and female athletes (* = $p < 0.0001$; ** $p < 0.0007$).

Reprinted by permission from the Adis International Limited: Hutchinson MR, Ireland ML. Knee injuries in female athletes. *Sports Med*, 19(4):288-302, 1995.

normal alignment can be made from neuromuscular function, and dysfunction can be determined from anterior knee pain and ACL injuries. Inhibition of the neuromuscular control of the lower extremity occurs in both malalignment and dysfunction.

When comparing males and females for risk of ACL, multiple intrinsic or nonchangeable factors are observed. The male athlete is more muscle dominant, has greater knee varus, less flexibility, wider notch and hence larger ligament, and internal rotation of the tibia (36) (see figure 26.3). The female athlete is more ligament dominant and has less muscular development, generalized laxity, greater knee valgus, smaller notch and hence smaller ligament. Tibial external rotation and foot pronation is commonly seen (see figure 26.4).

Factors contributing to ACL injury can be divided into intrinsic (not controllable)—physiological rotatory laxity, size of ACL, valgus alignment, hyperextension, proprioception, neuromuscular firing order, and hormonal influences, extrinsic (potentially controllable)—strength, conditioning, shoes, motivation, deceleration forces during injury, and

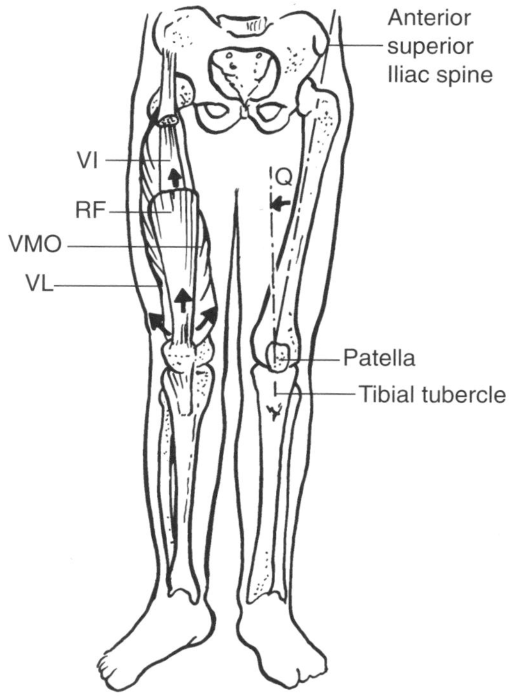

Figure 26.1 Normal alignment with normal Q angle (measured from anterosuperior iliac spine central portion of the patella) from patella to tibial tubercle of less than 15° and normal musculature of developed vastus medialis obliquus create forces that centralize the patella, which results in normal patellofemoral tracking. (Reprinted with permission: Fu FH, Stone DA (eds). *Sports Injuries: Mechanisms, Prevention, Treatment*. Williams & Wilkins, 1994.)

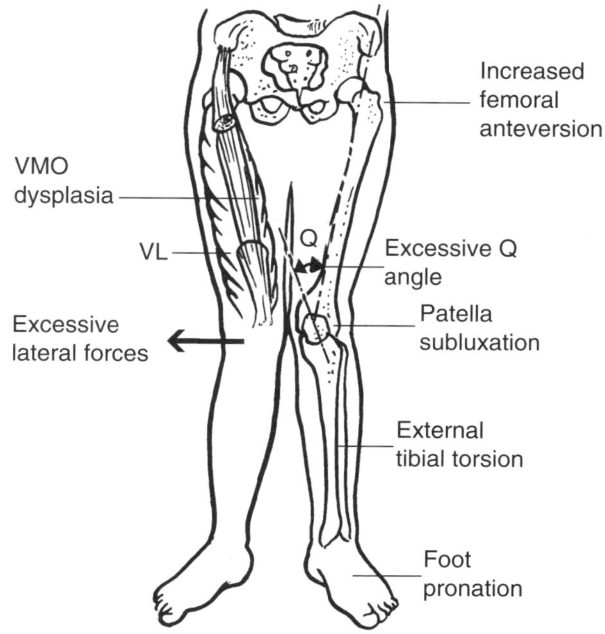

Figure 26.2 Miserable malalignment syndrome consists of increased femoral anteversion, excessive Q angle, external tibial torsion, and foot pronation. These factors cause lateral patellar subluxation. This miserable malalignment syndrome is frequently seen in females. (Reprinted with permission: Fu FH, Stone DA (eds). *Sports Injuries: Mechanisms, Prevention, Treatment*. Williams & Wilkins, 1994.)

a combination of both (partially controllable)—skill and coordination (24) (see table 26.3). The alignment, ligament dominance, and physiological rotatory laxity put the female in a high-risk position for noncontact ACL injuries.

Notch stenosis has been addressed. The notch forms in relation to the size of the ACL, that is, small ligament, small notch. The ACL is not actually amputated by a stenotic notch. Notch measurements may be reported as absolute width or ratios. Notch ratios of the width of the notch to the distal femur have been reported (24–26). Ratio versus absolute width has been discussed. The size < 15 mm is felt to place the knee at higher risk for ACL injury (27).

Basketball was the sport of injury in 40% of the ACL reconstructions that I have performed. It is the No. 1 sport of ACL injury at Kentucky Sports Medicine. Reviewing 5 years of data for reconstruction in basketball athletes, we found that 59% were age 15–18, and 67% of males were older than age 22 (38). In basketball, noncontact mechanisms were responsible in 82% of injuries in females and 87% in males. ACL injuries occurred during games in 59% of the females and 87% of males. Factors that make the female more vulnerable during her teen years include recent growth phase with change of center of gravity, leg length and valgus alignment, relative weakness, hormonal effects, particularly estrogen, smaller size of the ligament with smaller notch, and less neuromuscular control. Hormonal cyclic influences occur, but their degree of expression and significance are still under investigation. Estrogen receptors are present in the ACL (29). However, the question of receptor activity and effects remains. Estrogen and other hormones influence many tissues. The relation of the hormone cycle to ACL tears has been presented, and the ACL tears did not tend to occur at a high-estrogen level time (30).

Developmental factors cannot be overlooked. The young female participating in athletics in the '90s may not have been as active as her male counterpart during the time of free play, jumping, running, and

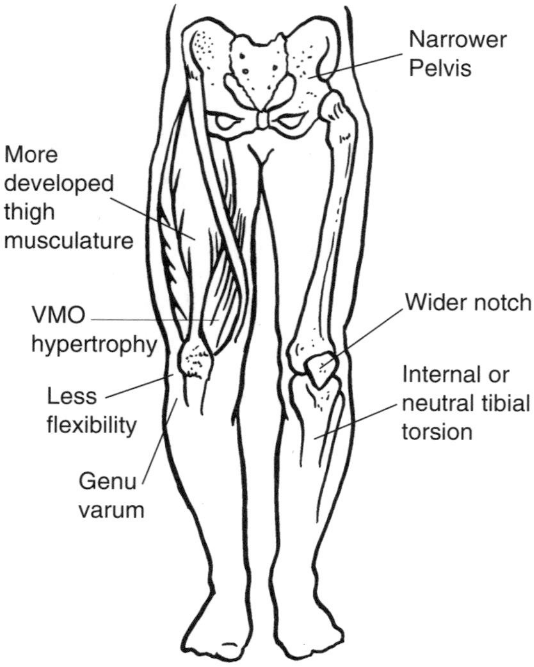

Figure 26.3 Male lower extremity alignment, showing narrower pelvis, more developed thigh musculature, VMO hypertrophy, less flexibility, neutral genu varum, a wider femoral notch, and internal or neutral tibial torsion. (Reprinted with permission: Fu FH, Stone DA (eds). *Sports Injuries: Mechanisms, Prevention, Treatmen*t, Williams & Wilkins, 1994.)

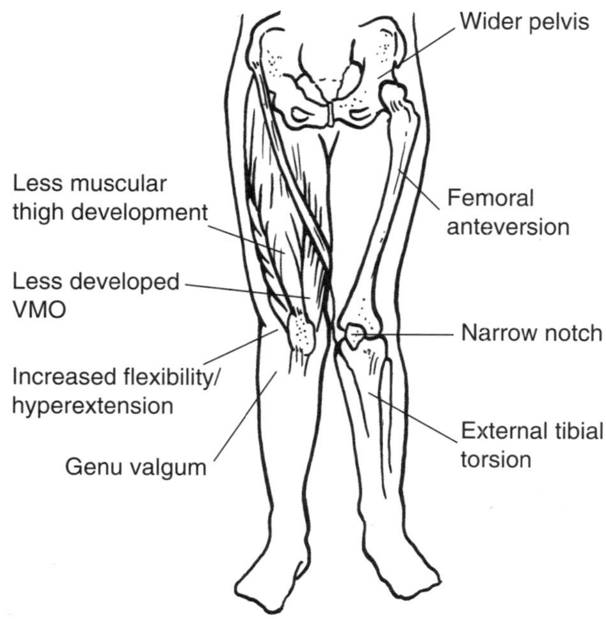

Figure 26.4 Lower extremity anatomic alignment in the female, showing wider pelvis, femoral anteversion, internal rotation, narrower femoral notch, genu valgum, less muscular development, increased flexibility, hyperextension, external tibial torsion, and pronated foot. (Reprinted with permission: Fu FH, Stone DA (eds). *Sports Injuries: Mechanisms, Prevention, Treatment*, Williams & Wilkins, 1994.)

Table 26.3 Mechanism of Injury: Contributory Factors

Intrinsic (not controllable)
- physiological rotatory laxity
- size of ACL
- valgus alignment
- hyperextension
- proprioception
- neuromuscular firing order
- hormonal influences

Extrinsic (potentially controllable)
- strength
- conditioning
- shoes
- motivation
- deceleration forces during injury

Both (partially controllable)
- skill
- coordination

cutting when the ACL and proprioception develop. A more sedentary lifestyle—sitting, being driven to practices, and sitting in front of the computer—is the trend for the '90s. In previous decades, free play walking and running was the rule. Potential changes in strength, size, and attachments of the ACL may have evolved. Are we missing the window of opportunity, the patterns of protective landing behavior, and potentially increased ACL size and strength?

Excellent ongoing research is being done comparing neuromuscular patterns in average and elite athletes (31). Delay in hamstring activity and early quadriceps firing in elite athletes has been shown, which places the ACL at risk.

Fatigue plays a role in injury patterns (32, 33). Fatigue has also been shown to influence neuromuscular performance and affect anterior tibial translation (34). Comparing the uninjured with the injured knee in basketball and volleyball female athletes, no significant differences were found in the orthopedic knee exam or KT-1000 test. We have performed studies assessing how fatigue causes changes in muscle activity and knee flexion angles in women volleyball and basketball athletes doing maneuvers involving running and rapid stopping (32). In the fatigued state, we found that there was later recruitment of rectus femoris, vastus lateralis, biceps femoris, and medial hamstrings and earlier maximal knee flexion.

Studies are underway in the lab for sport specific side cutting, rapid deceleration, and other activities, measuring joint kinematics and EMG of the musculature including back, hip, quadriceps, hamstring, calf, plantar, and dorsiflexors. Research and proprioception activation patterns of hamstrings have been reported (35–37). Reflex inhibition of quadriceps femoris occurs in certain groups' activity following injury or reconstruction. (38) The effects of back or hip injury on lower extremity proprioception cannot be overlooked. Specific research has been done on the effect of ankle sprains on proprioception of the ankle (39). Proximal control is key to injury prevention. Distal deceleration and improved proprioception sense in the entire lower extremity can be learned. It is felt that proprioception sense can be improved with sport and balance specific training programs in six to eight weeks (40).

Mechanoreceptors have been demonstrated in the ACL (41–43). After an ACL reconstruction, there is evidence of development of neural elements (28). Is there some basic deficit of control or position sense inherent in the individual who tears the ACL? There are people who cope very well without an ACL and others who do not cope well. Determining the factors that allow some people to cope well and doing specific training to make everyone able to cope with an ACL injury needs to be done.

Following an ACL injury, the nonreconstructed ACL is the one more likely to be injured (28). Proposed reasons why the opposite is torn include the following: the reconstructed ACL is larger; the importance and illustration of proprioception is emphasized on the reconstructed knee and landing patterns may increase stress on the uninjured knee; general proprioceptive deficits or neuromuscular dyssynchrony affect the uninjured ACL.

Observation of mechanisms of injury, particularly in basketball and gymnastics has been done (44). Analysis of the videotaped injuries of 40 individuals showed that their positions were varied (45), but varus thrust was most common and tibial rotation was involved.

In the most common noncontact ACL-tear mechanism and body position that I have observed, the body is falling forward, rotating to the opposite side, the hip is internally rotated and adducted, the knee is in valgus, the foot is usually fixed and pronated, resulting in external rotation of the tibia (see figure 26.5). With further analysis and additional videos of injuries, this position of no return can be determined. Hopefully, sport specific training may be possible to prevent progression to this position of no return. The ACL-injury cycle of the twisting falling-tree position must be interrupted (see figure 26.6). The athlete's position and muscle action must be antagonistic to the injury position. Important factors that reduce risk include improved body position, proximal control, improved muscle activity, timing, improved strength, distal segment changes of foot movements, and proximal segment control (see table 26.4). Muscle activity that would be most beneficial in responding to break the injury cycle, similar to the avoidance of painful stimulus, is to fire the back extensors, hip abductors, external rotator extensors, knee flexors, ankle invertors, and plantar flexors. To improve the distal segment foot movements the athlete should get more weight posterior, get back on the heels, increase the squeaking of shoes to surface, use two-footed landings and

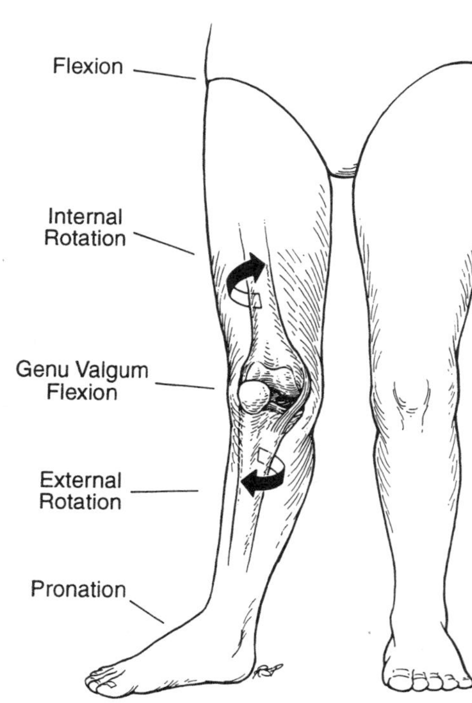

Figure 26.5 Based on videotape analysis, this diagram shows the position of no return for the ACL. The lower extremity position is one of body-forward flexion, hip adduction, internal rotation, 20-30° knee flexion, external rotation of the tibia, and forefoot pronation. The knee will buckle; the patient is usually falling forward and toward the opposite side in a rapid distal deceleration mechanism.

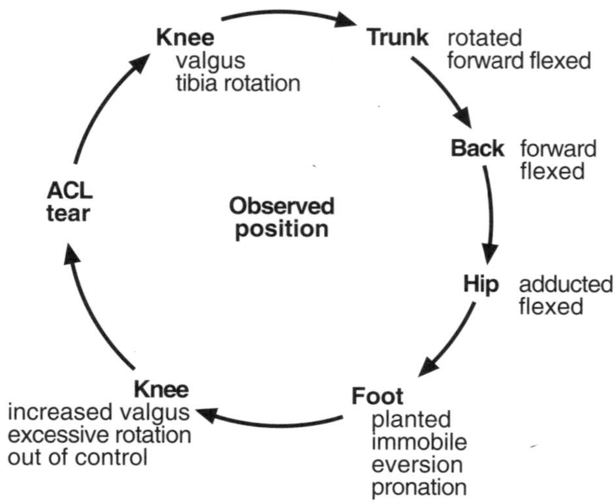

Figure 26.6 The observed body position of trunk, back, hip, knee, and foot of the noncontact ACL injury. To prevent injury, the cycle must be broken. This can be with a trained timing and neuromuscular response.

Table 26.4 Important Factors to Reduce Risk

- Improved position
- Muscle activity timing and strength
  Back extensors
  Hip abductors/ER/extensor
  Knee flexors
  Ankle inversion/plantarflexion
- Distal segmental foot movements
  More force back on heels
  Increase squeaking
  Two-footed landings
  Less fixed foot
  Improve shoe fit
  Reduce friction, shoe to floor
- Proximal segment
  Trunk balance and control
  Hip abduction/ER

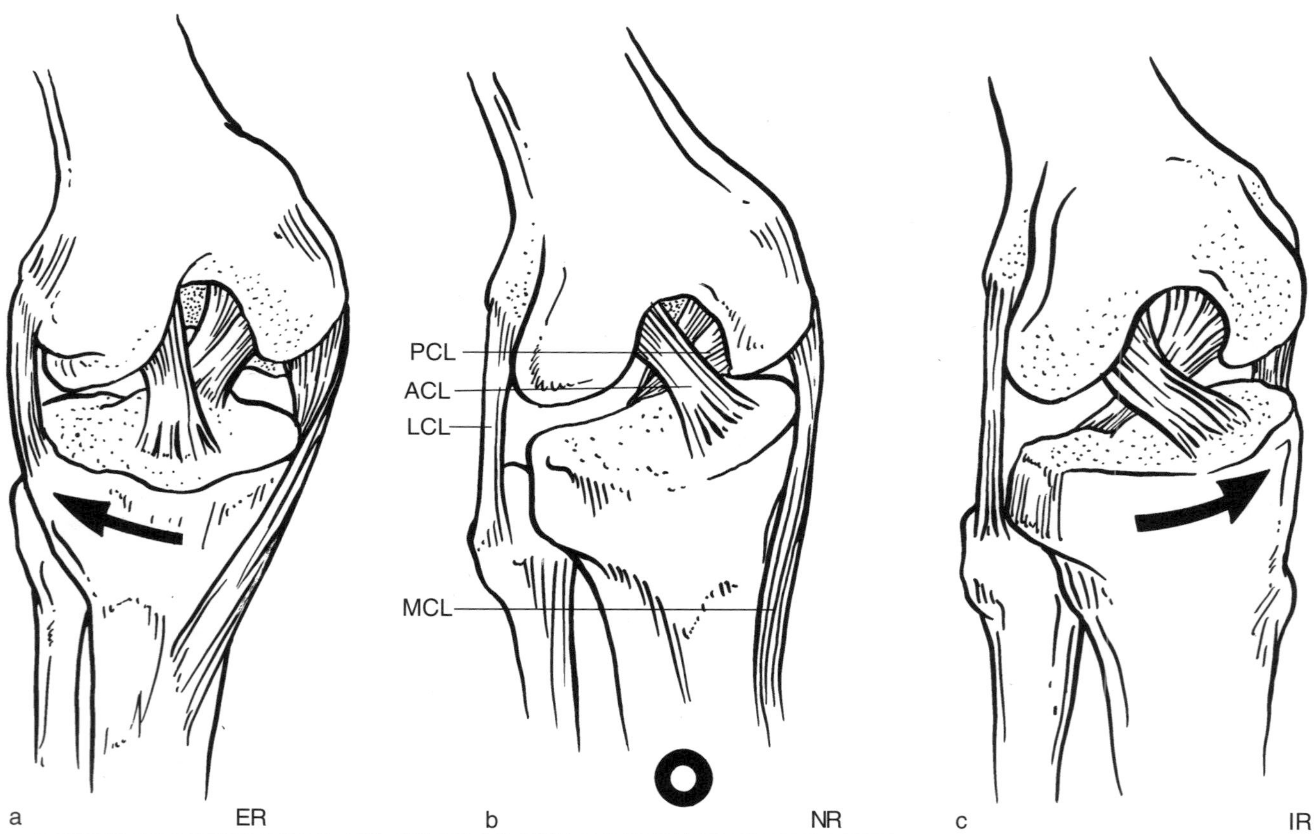

Figure 26.7 The synergistic functions of the collateral ligaments and cruciates are shown. (*a*) In external rotation the collateral ligaments tighten and cruciates relax. (*b*) In neutral, no ligaments are under unusual tension. (*c*) The cruciate ligaments tighten in internal rotation while the collateral ligaments are more vertical and lax. (Reprinted with permission: Muller W. *The Knee: Form, Function, and Ligament Reconstruction*. New York: Springer-Verlag, 1983.)

fewer fixed foot landings, improve shoe fit, and reduce the friction ratio of shoe to floor. Proximal segment improvements include balance and control and hip abduction external rotation.

In basketball and gymnastics injuries, the foot has been observed in a position of pronation and external rotation. This would indicate that the femur internally rotates on the tibia. In the valgus knee with some movement at the foot, the ACL will be loaded prior to the medial collateral ligament. Anatomically, the cruciate ligaments should be coiled on each other and tighter in internal rotation, while the lateral ligaments are then more vertical and relaxed (46) (see figure 26.7, *a–c*). In external rotation, the collateral ligaments are tighter. However, when we look at the position of injury, there are other forces involved, namely, forces anterior on the tibia and a fixed external rotation of the foot from the ground. The rotational component is therefore very important, but the ACL must be loaded in this position as injury occurs. Further studies need to be done: on tension, using cadavers and varying degrees of rotation; on valgus at the knee, with strain gauges in the collateral ligaments; on the ACL and PCL, correlating mechanism of injury to greatest strain. From this basic research, we can base teaching the avoidance of high-risk positions and muscle retraining programs.

The goal is to avoid the position of no return. When one sees an injury approaching, an intracranial alarm should sound to prepare for point of no return. Prevention programs have been outlined (14), and further programs are needed. Prevention programs in football and skiing have been published (47).

After an athlete has had an ACL reconstruction of one injured knee, it is necessary to begin studies looking at timing of muscular activity during sport specific drills, looking at joint angles and forces; and EMG measurements for timing of onset of activity studies are necessary. Attempting to keep the individual out of this point of no return ("falling-tree position") should be investigated. In the same frame as Pavlov's experiments, a virtual reality situation of avoiding that position should be demonstrated and practiced, until the athlete has an acquired position sense. Avoid painful stimuli! Sport specific programs on the prevention of getting into these positions of no return and a virtual reality video, shadowboxing types of sport specific programs, can be developed. Ongoing research will require funding, multiple center involvement, and longitudinal studies. Prevention and protection of the uninjured knee should be the goal (48). Further basic research, determining gender differences, and emphasizing those factors that can be changed are necessary. Now is the time to organize and begin these efforts.

References

1. Arendt E, Dick R. Knee injury patterns among men and women in collegiate basketball and soccer: NCAA data and review of literature. *Am J Sports Med* 1995; 23(6): 694–701.
2. Gomez E, DeLee JC, Farney WC. Incidence of injury in Texas girls high school basketball. *Am J Sports Med* 1996; 24(5): 684–87.
3. DeLee JC, Farney WC. Incidence of injury in Texas high school football. *Am J Sports Med* 1992; 20(5): 575–80.
4. Gray J, et al. A survey of injuries to the anterior cruciate ligament of the knee in female basketball players. *Int J of Sports Med* 1985; 6: 314–16.
5. Ireland ML, Wall C. Epidemiology and comparison of knee injuries in elite male and female United States basketball athletes. *Med Sci Sports Exer* [Abstract] 1990; 14.
6. Malone TR, et al. Relationship of gender to anterior cruciate ligament injuries in intercollegiate basketball participants. *J Sou Orth Ass* 1993; 2(1): 36–39.
7. Zelisko JA, Noble HB, Porter M. A comparison of men's and women's professional basketball injuries. *Am J Sports Med* 1982; 10: 297–99.
8. Zillmer DA, Powell JW, Albright JP. Gender specific injury patterns in high school varsity basketball. *J Women's Health* 1992; 1(1): 69–76.
9. Harrer MF, Berson L, Hosea TM, Leddy TP. Lower extremity injuries: Females vs. males in the sport of basketball. The AOSSM 22d annual meeting [Abstract], Lake Buena Vista, FL, June 16–20, 1996.
10. Oliphant JG, Drawbert JP. Gender differences in anterior cruciate ligament injury rates in Wisconsin intercollegiate basketball. *J Ath Training* 1996; 31(3): 245–47.
11. Whiteside PA. Men's and women's injuries in comparable sports. *Phys Sportsmed* 1980; 8(3): 130–40.
12. Garrick JG, Requa RK. Girl's sports injuries in high school athletics. *JAMA* 1978; 239: 2245–248.
13. National Collegiate Athletic Association. *NCAA injury surveillance system.* Overland Park, KS: NCAA, 1990–1996.
14. Andrish JT. Knee injuries in gymnastics. *Clin Sports Med* 1985; 4: 111–22.
15. Clarke K, Buckley W. Women's injuries in colle-

giate sports. *Am J Sports Med* 1990; 8(3): 187–91.
16. DeHaven KE, Linter DM. Athletic injuries: Comparison by age, sport, and gender. *Am J Sports Med* 1986; 14: 218–24.
17. Gillette J. When and where women are injured in sports. *Phys Sportsmed* 1975; 2: 61–63.
18. Kowal DM. Nature and causes of injuries in women resulting from an endurance training program. *Am J Sports Med* 1980; 8: 265–69.
19. Cox JS, Lenz HW. Women midshipmen in sports. *Am J Sports Med* 1984; 12: 241–43.
20. Good JE, Klein KM. Women in the military academies: US Navy (part 1 of 3). *Phys Sportsmed* 1989; 17: 99–106.
21. Hutchinson MR, Ireland ML. Knee injuries in female athletes. *Sports Med* 1995; 19(4): 288–302.
22. Ireland ML. Special concerns of the female athlete. In: Fu FH, Stone DA, eds. *Sports injuries: Mechanism, prevention, and treatment,* 2nd ed. Baltimore: Williams & Wilkins, 1994.
23. Ireland ML, Gaudette M, Crook S. ACL injuries in the female athlete. *J Sport Rehab* 1997; 6(2): 97–110.
24. Souryal TO, Freeman TR. Intercondylar notch size and anterior cruciate ligament injuries in athletes: A prospective study. *Am J Sports Med* 1993; 21(4): 535–39.
25. Souryal TO, Moore HA, Evans JP. Bilaterality in anterior cruciate ligament injuries: Associated intercondylar notch stenosis. *Am J Sports Med* 1980; 8(3): 449–54.
26. LaPrade RF, Burnett QM. Femoral intercondylar notch stenosis and correlation to anterior cruciate ligament injuries: A prospective study. *Am J Sports Med* 1994; 22(2): 198–203.
27. Shelbourne KD, Davis TJ. A prospective study determining the relationship of the intercondylar notch width of the femur and the incidence of anterior cruciate ligament tears. American Orthopaedic Society for Sports Medicine, 23rd annual meeting, Sun Valley, Idaho, June 22–25, 1997, *Book of abstracts and outlines,* 807.
28. Ireland ML. [Kentucky Sports Medicine experience: ACL.] Lexington, KT. Unpublished data, 1991–1995.
29. Lie SH, Yu W, Hatch J, Panossian V, Finerman GAM. Estrogen affects the cellular metabolism of the female anterior cruciate ligament: A potential explanation for female athletic injury. The AOSSM 23d annual meeting [Abstract], Sun Valley, Idaho, June 22–25, 1997.
30. Wojtys EM, Huston LJ, Lindenfeld TN, Hewett TE. Correlation between the menstrual cycle and ACL injuries in female athletes. The AOSSM 23d annual meeting [Abstract], Sun Valley, Idaho, June 22–25, 1997.
31. Huston LJ, Wojtys EM. Neuromuscular performance characteristics in elite female athletes. *Am J Sports Med* 1996; 24(4): 427–36.
32. Nyland JA, Shapiro R, Stine RL, Horn TS, Ireland ML. Relationship of fatigued reaction forces, lower extremity kinematics, and muscle activation. *JOSPT* 20(3): 132–37.
33. Wojtys EM, Wylie BB, Huston LJ. The effects of muscle fatigue on neuromuscular function and anterior tibial translation in healthy knees. *Am J Sports Med* 1996; 24(5): 615–21.
34. Wojtys EM, Bradford BW, Huston LJ. The effects of muscle fatigue on neuromuscular function and anterior tibial translation in healthy knees. *Am J Sports Med* 1996; 24(5): 615–21.
35. Corrigan JP, Cashman WF, Brady MP. Proprioception in the cruciate ligament deficient knee. *J Bone Joint Surg* 1992; 174B(2): 247–50.
36. Osternig LR, Caster BL, James R. Contralateral hamstring (biceps femoris) coactivation patterns and anterior cruciate ligament dysfunction. *Am J Sports Med* 1995; 805–808.
37. Lund-Hanssen H, Gannon J, Engebretsen L, Holen K, Hammer S. Isokinetic muscle performance in healthy female handball players and players with a unilateral anterior cruciate ligament reconstruction. *Scand J Med Sci Sports* 1996; 6: 172–75.
38. Snyder-Mackler L, De Luca PF, Williams PR, Eastlack ME, Bartolozzi AR. Reflex inhibition of quadriceps femoris muscle after injury or reconstruction of the anterior cruciate ligament. *J Bone Joint Surg* 1994; 76A(4): 555–60.
39. Leanderson J, Ericksson E, Nilsson C, Wykman A. Proprioception in classical ballet dancers: A prospective study of the influence of an ankle sprain on proprioception in the ankle joint. *Am J Sports Med* 1996; 24(3): 370–74.
40. ACL Study Group: Round Table, Nevis, West Indies, April 27–May 3, 1996.
41. Schultz RA, Miller DC, Kerr CS, Micheli L. Mechanoreceptors in human cruciate ligaments: A histological study. *J Bone Joint Surg* 1984; 66A(7): 1072–1076.
42. Schutte MJ, Dabezies EJ, Zimny ML, Happel LT. Neural anatomy of the human anterior cruciate ligament. *J Bone Joint Surg* 1987; 69A(2): 243–47.
43. Kennedy JC, Alexander IJ, Hayes KC. Nerve supply of the human knee and its functional importance. *Am J Sports Med* 1982; 10(6): 329–35.

44. Ireland ML. Anterior cruciate ligament injuries in young female athletes. *Your Patient and Fitness* 1996; 10(5): 26–30.
45. Boden BP, Garrett WE Jr. Mechanisms of injuries to the anterior cruciate ligament. *Med Sci Sports Exer Suppl* [Abstract], May 1996; 28(5): S26.
46. Muller W. *The knee: Form, function, and ligament reconstruction.* New York: Springer-Verlag, 1983.
47. Ryder SH, Johnson RJ, Beynnon BD, Ettlinger CF. Prevention of ACL injuries. *J Sport Rehab* 1997; 6(2): 80–96.
48. Griffis ND, Vequist SW, Yearout KM, et al. Injury prevention of the anterior cruciate ligament. In: *AOSSM meeting abstracts, symposia, and instructional courses* [Abstract], 15th annual meeting, June 19–22, 1989.

CHAPTER 27

Influence of Knee and Ankle Support on Proprioception and Neuromuscular Control

Per A. Renström, MD, PhD
Lars Konradsen, MD
Bruce D. Beynnon, PhD

Introduction

The interest in bracing has primarily been focused on the prevention of ligament injury, prevention of intraarticular injury, and on rapid return to sports after either operative or nonoperative treatment programs.

The sports medicine committee of the American Academy of Orthopedic Surgeons has classified knee braces as rehabilitative, prophylactic, and functional. (12) Rehabilitation braces are designed to allow for early and protected motion of an injured joint. Prophylactic braces are those designed to prevent or reduce the incidence and severity of injuries during contact sports. Functional braces are designed to provide stability to a joint that suffers from instability, usually due to insufficiency of ligamentous structures. These braces are prescribed to patients with ligamentous deficiency in the hope that the brace will prevent re-injury. The division of knee braces into three types is based on their different applications, but they do have different designs. Ankle braces also fall into these three applications, but there is usually no major difference in design between application groups. However, from a biomechanical perspective, all brace types are designed with the common objective of providing the joint with normal kinematics while limiting abnormal kinematics that may damage the joint.

During the last decade a proprioceptive mechanism behind the effect of bracing has been investigated with increasing interest. This chapter deals first with the question of whether bracing has a prophylactic and re-injury protecting effect. Research on the mechanical effect models is briefly discussed. The prevailing theory on the mechanism of effect of braces on proprioception is presented; and finally studies on the effect of knee and ankle braces on proprioception are reviewed.

Clinical Effect of Bracing

The only kinds of research that can answer whether or not bracing reduces the rate of certain injuries are well-prepared clinical studies. For the knee, Sitler and coworkers (50) found that a prophylactic brace reduced the number of ACL and MCL injuries in athletes. Qualitative studies of functional knee bracing have demonstrated that a majority of the patients are satisfied and feel it to be of some value. (15, 58) Noyes and associates (43) found that 78% of ACL-deficient patients who wore functional knee braces felt that the brace decreased their symptoms, and 60% of the patients were able to increase their level of activity by one grade.

For the ankle, taping and bracing have been used prophylactically in healthy subjects who are at risk of injury and functionally for chronically unstable ankles to protect against recurrent sprains. Garrick and Requa (22) studied 2,562 participants in intramural basketball and found a decreased incidence of ankle sprains with the use of tape. The decrease was particularly evident in those with previous injuries, reducing their likelihood of re-injury by two-thirds. Clinical studies examining the effect of injury prevention with ankle bracing have shown similar beneficial effects. (22, 38, 39, 48, 51, 55, 56)

Modeling the Effect of Bracing

While clinical studies can answer the question of whether or not bracing can reduce the frequency of a specific injury, modeling can give an idea of how a given brace may exert its protective effect.

Biomechanical Modeling

To mechanically protect ligaments and articular surfaces the brace must directly control relative bony kinematics through attachments to a compliant musculature interface, which changes surface dimensions as an athlete contracts, relaxes, or moves the lower limb. Control must be present to the extent that abnormal joint kinematics and associated loading are prevented.

There is little objective evidence that demonstrates that any brace design has indeed the ability to mechanically protect joint ligaments from harmful strains or loads of the magnitude seen in injury situations. (9) It must, however, be emphasized that all modeling is done in restricted situations with loads and speeds far less than real-life injury situations. Researchers often draw conclusions to clinical situations by extrapolating data outside the scope of the studies.

For the knee, Paulos and associates (44) used a cadaver model to investigate the effectiveness of prophylactic knee bracing. Both static and dynamic tests revealed that prophylactic bracing did not have an effect on limiting ligament failure or the static stiffness of the knee. With a Hall effect strain transducer Erickson and coworkers (17) characterized intraligamentous strain biomechanics of the ACL along with the anterior and posterior portions of the medial collateral ligaments. This study revealed that the brace was capable of decreasing the strain along the posterior portion of the MCL, but only at 0° of knee flexion. At 30° of flexion the ligaments did not exhibit a significant reduction in strain in comparison to the unbraced condition. Similar findings were reported by Baker and associates. (5)

Hoffman and associates (27) evaluated six different rehabilitation braces by loading the tibia of cadaveric knees in valgus, anterior, and rotational directions. All of the braces were found to provide some stability. However, none of the braces could restore the joint stability afforded by intact ligaments. Finally, studies of functional bracing in ACL-deficient subjects have shown that the brace may reduce instrumented laxity or ACL strain in low-load situations, but in the presence of high anterior shear loads, the braces could not restore normal laxity. (7, 8, 10, 15, 59)

For the ankle the mechanical effect of bracing and taping is expected to be a reduction of the maximal range of inversion motion, an increase in rotational stiffness, and an increase in maximal resistance to movement past the anatomical limits of subtalar inversion. There is substantial evidence that the effect of tape on these parameters is lost after a short period of physical activity. (3, 12, 21, 35, 46) The ankle brace retains its mechanical effect during exercise, but this effect has only been tested at torque levels well below those seen in injury situations. (49) As shown by Ashton-Miller and coworkers (4) the evertor muscles are capable of producing 3–4 times as much resistance to inversion as the brace.

Faced with the seemingly contrary results of mechanical and clinical studies, it has been suggested that the true benefit of functional bracing may not be biomechanical reinforcement but, rather, proprioceptive enhancement.

Proprioceptive Modeling

The proprioceptive effect of bracing can be classified as either prophylactic or functional. A prophylactic effect implies that proprioception or neuromuscular control of the uninjured subject can be enhanced by the application of an external support. It may be that not all uninjured subjects will show this effect; an effect may be present only in a subgroup of individuals who present an inherent suboptimal level of proprioception or neuromuscular control. The application of a brace may then normalize their proprioceptive values. (45)

A functional effect suggests that the brace may normalize or improve proprioception of the chronically injured individual. This implies that the injury has resulted in a proprioceptive deficit or loss of neuromuscular control that can be changed. As discussed in other chapters, this question still has to be answered.

Mechanism of Proprioceptive Enhancement

There is evidence that afferent receptors are present in the skin, muscle, ligaments, and joint capsule and that these contribute to the proprioceptive input of both the knee and ankle. (14, 28, 32, 41) The primary position sense or movement receptors in the joint capsule and ligaments are located deep within the soft tissues and therefore may not be affected by an external ankle or knee support even if the support is an elastic bandage or tape with full contact of the skin. With the goal of preventing abnormal kinematics, the connection between the brace and soft tissues surrounding the lower limb is kept as rigid as possible. (9) This allows for massive stimulation of the skin and subcutaneous structures and increased pressure on the underlying musculature. (54) Plausible receptors to be involved include free nerve endings and hair end organs that react strongly to new stimuli and adapt quickly. (45) In deeper subcutaneous levels Ruffini organs show tonic and slow adapting responses that can provide dynamic and static input. (26) The afferent signals from the cutaneous receptors may themselves provide proprioceptive information or they may facilitate proprioception and neuromuscular control by increasing relevant sensitive or motorneuron excitability. (42).

Proprioceptive Effect of Knee Bracing

Three principle methods exist for objectively quantifying knee joint proprioception and neuromuscular control: (1) Joint position sense measures the ability to reproduce a joint position previously set by active or passive positioning. (2) Joint kinesthesia measures the threshold to detection of passive motion or the ability to detect a change in joint position. (3) The latency of muscle reflex reaction to sudden perturbation measures a combination of proprioception and neuromuscular control.

Knee Joint Position Sense: Proprioceptive Effect of Bracing on Knee-Healthy Subjects

Perlau and associates (45) tested 54 knee-healthy subjects before application of an elastic bandage, immediately after application, one hour after application, and after removal of the bandage. Subjects were seated blindfolded with the knee strapped in a Kin Com. The knee index angles were reached passively and were reproduced passively with the examiner moving the leg and the subject indicating when the index angle was reproduced. Error of angle replication was expressed as the absolute value of the error. It was found that application of the elastic bandage improved the ability of an individual to replicate knee joint position by 1° (from 4° to 3°; $p < .05$), and this benefit was lost after removal of the bandage. The magnitude of improvement was greatest in the group that, prior to bandage application, showed a replication error outside the normal confidence interval. McNair and associates (40) required subjects to reproduce with the contralateral knee a pattern of passively induced flexions and extensions of the target knee. The magnitude of error in tracking was established by determining the difference between the active and passively moving limbs and calculating the root mean square value. An 11% improvement in error was seen when normal subjects wore a knee sleeve.

Knee Joint Position Sense: Proprioceptive Effect of Knee Bracing on Injured Subjects

Barrett and coworkers (6) used a technique where the subject's leg was strapped to a Thomas splint. The index angle was set passively and replicated by the subject using a visual analogue of the leg. Subjects with poor joint position sense as a result of osteoarthrosis or knee replacement had an improved error of angle replication of 40% ($p < .01$) with the application of an elastic bandage. Jerosch and Bischof (29) performed two studies where subjects replicated passively set knee flexion angles using a manual goniometer and using an approach similar to that described by Barrett and coworkers. (6) In one study, where the group of subjects had meniscal injuries, no effect of an elastic bandage could be found. In another study, a group of subjects with posttraumatic patella dislocation showed a 33% decrease in absolute replication error after bandage application. The reason for this difference is unclear. Jerosch and Bischof suggest that in the case of meniscal injury, the rupture to the meniscus did not alter an appreciable proportion of the proprioceptors about the knee joint. Instead, the pain stimulus from the torn meniscus provided distracting input that interfered with the intact receptors. This could explain why the increased cutaneous stimulation from the bandage had no effect on the error of angle replication and that resection of the torn meniscus in itself reduced replication error by removing the proprioceptive disturbance. (29)

Knee Bracing and Kinesthesia

A literature review revealed no information on the effect of knee bracing on kinesthesia. In a recent study we have looked at the effect of braces and knee sleeves on knee kinesthesia (Beynnon, et al., 1997; unpublished). Twenty unilaterally ACL-deficient subjects were tested with and without braces using a validated movement threshold technique. The threshold for movement detection was found to be significantly increased in ACL-deficient knees when compared to the contralateral control knees (from an average value of 1.2° to 1.5°). With the application of a brace to the ACL-deficient knee the average movement threshold was found to be 1.3° and similar to the unbraced condition.

Knee Bracing and Muscle Latency Reflexes

Several studies suggest that complex changes in muscle activation patterns and higher central nervous system strategies are seen in patients with a torn ACL. Solomonow (52) found that during knee extension and flexion a subluxation of the tibia took place at about 50° degrees of flexion, during which the torque was drastically reduced and EMG recordings from the quadriceps muscle decreased while the hamstring EMG response increased significantly. The same pattern was found by Erickson and coworkers. (17) Lass and associates (36) have described early onset, early peak, and longer activation time of the gastrocnemius muscles during gait in chronic ACL-deficient individuals with good functional results, when compared to a group with poor results. The hamstring muscles have shown an increased level of EMG activity while the quadriceps showed decreased activity during the stance phase for the ACL-deficient knee when performing side step cuts on the leg. (11)

The effect of bracing on muscle performance was first studied by Branch. (11) Ten subjects with unilateral isolated ACL-deficient knees and five controls performed side step cutting maneuvers without a brace, with a shell-dominant, and with a strap-dominant brace. In the stance phase, ACL-deficient subjects showed less quadriceps and gastrocnemius activity than controls. When braced, ACL-deficient legs demonstrated a further reduction of 18% in quadriceps activity and 14% in peak activity compared to the unbraced situation. The hamstrings showed a concomitant decrease of 18% in activity. No timing differences were noted between braced and unbraced conditions. It was concluded that bracing did not alter the relative EMG activity nor did it change firing patterns compared to the unbraced situation. Gottlieb and associates (25) used a perturbation technique where the foot of the standing subject was anteriorly translated 15 cm over 1 s. Middle loop latency was measured for the biceps femoris, vastus lateralis, and semitendinosus. No difference in latencies could be found for the ACL-deficient subjects between braced and unbraced conditions.

Wojtys and associates produced sudden anterior translation of the tibia with the knee under partial weight bearing (30 lbs). Five subjects were tested with and without six different braces. Bracing decreased anterior tibial translation by 34% of the unbraced condition without the stabilizing contractions of the hamstring, quadriceps, and gastrocnemius muscles. With partial weight bearing combined with lower limb muscle activation and bracing, anterior tibial translation was decreased 77% in comparison to the unbraced condition. Some improvement in spinal level muscle latency was seen with brace use. At the voluntary level most braces consistently appeared to delay hamstring activation. The implication of this finding (good or bad) is unknown.

Proprioceptive Effect of Ankle Bracing

In comparison to the proprioceptive studies done on knees, proprioceptive studies on the ankle have applied the method of testing single-limb postural stability as a common technique. It is a problem with this technique that it measures complex proprioceptive functions including afferent information from the vestibular system and from vision as well as efferent motor skills. When studying the same individuals within a short time frame and changing only the parameter braced/nonbraced, comparisons on the afferent effect of bracing can be done.

Postural Sway: Proprioceptive Effect of Ankle Bracing in Ankle-Healthy Subjects

In a group of 15 healthy uninjured subjects Feuerbach and Grabiner (18) measured postural sway as medial-lateral and anterior-posterior center of force position and amplitude, and sway frequency. This was performed with a static support surface and with a surface that could undergo sudden translation or rotation perturbations. They found that the application of an Aircast brace (Aircast Inc., Summit, NJ) resulted in a reduction of one or both measurements. In the most frequently used testing condition, with the subject standing on a stable support surface, both the sway amplitude and the sway frequency measured in the medial-lateral plane were significantly reduced with the application of the brace (12% reduction).

Calmels and coworkers (13) found that an elastic stocking reduced anterior-posterior sway but not medial-lateral sway in 34 healthy subjects.

Proprioceptive Effect of Ankle Bracing in Injured Subjects

Tropp (56) tested 38 soccer players with a history of functional instability with and without stirrup and horseshoe taping. The subjects performed single-limb stance on a half-cylindrical support surface mounted on a force platform. They were required to balance for 60 s. From the center of force values an ellipse was constructed that encompassed 61% of the force values. The area of this ellipse was considered a measure of postural sway. No difference in sway ellipse area could be found between taped and nontaped conditions. Using a different approach, Jerosch and associates (30) tested 16 subjects with functionally unstable ankles and with no new sprain 3 mo prior to testing and compared the influence of 3 types of external ankle support on postural control. Subjects maintained balance on a soft surface for 1 min with their eyes open and 1 min with their eyes closed. The number of touchdowns was considered a measure of postural stability. Taping did not change the number of touchdowns; however, the lace-on and stirrup braces significantly reduced the number of touchdowns required to maintain an upright posture.

Leanderson (37) showed that taping unilaterally in functionally unstable soccer players reduced postural sway during single-limb stance on a perturbation platform. Postural sway was measured as maximal sway amplitude in the lateral plane. Sway was reduced immediately after application of the tape. This effect was still present after exercise. In the study, untaped controls also demonstrated a decrease in the magnitude of sway after exercise.

Fridén and coworkers (20) braced acutely injured ankles (injury 3–8 days old) in 14 subjects. Before the application of an ankle brace average speed of sway was significantly greater on the injured side compared to the uninjured side (16% difference, $p < .05$). With the application of a brace the significant difference was no longer present (5% difference, n.s.).

In summary most studies have found that bracing improves postural stability; however, the effect of taping on postural stability remains unclear.

Bracing and the Peroneal Muscle Reflex Latency to Sudden Ankle Inversion

In a study by Karlsson and Andreasson, (31) 20 subjects with unilateral mechanical ankle instability were subjected to a sudden ankle inversion. Subjects stood with the body weight evenly distributed on both feet. The feet were strapped onto two platforms that could rotate suddenly in the frontal plane. The time from the beginning of rotation to the first measurable activity in the peroneal muscles was designated the peroneal muscle latency. Chronically unstable ankles showed peroneal reaction latencies of mean 85 ms while the healthy contralateral ankles showed latencies of mean 70 ms. Application of tape reduced reflex latency significantly to an average of 73 ms. Using a similar approach to study subjects with functionally unstable ankles the same result was not found by Konradsen and coworkers (33) or by Daanen and associates. (16)

In a study by Sprigings and coworkers (53) the number of spike counts on the peroneal EMG in response to sudden inversion was used as a measure to quantify the magnitude of the peroneal response to sudden inversion. A difference between taped and nontaped situations was not seen.

Joint Position Sense: Proprioceptive Effect of Ankle Bracing in Ankle-Healthy Subjects

Feuerbach and associates (19) measured ankle joint position sense in 12 ankle-healthy subjects with the outcome measures of absolute and variable angle replication error. The absolute error was the absolute value of the replication error, and the variable error was the standard deviation of the replication errors of a full trial. The experimenter manually moved the right foot at approximately 30°/s to a reference position. The position was held for 5 s. The foot was then passively returned to neutral and the subject then tried to reproduce the foot placement. Foot position was measured using a 3-D tracking system of light markers. Both the absolute and variable errors were reduced significantly with the application of an orthosis ($p < .05$).

Joint Position Sense: Proprioceptive Effect of Ankle Bracing in Injured Subjects

Jerosch and associates (30) compared the influence of three stabilization devices (Mikros, Aircast, and tape) on the absolute angle reproduction error in 16 functionally unstable subjects. They found that all three stabilizers produced lower absolute error values (1.46°, 1.62°, and 1.84°, respectively) when compared to unbraced values (2.36°). Comparing taped and untaped situations in 11 functionally unstable subjects who regularly used tape in sporting situations, we found a trend ($p = .07$) towards a reduction in absolute angle replication error (Konradsen, et al., 1998 unpublished).

Using a paradigm where subjects quantified different degrees of rotation of the ankle during full weight bearing, Robbins and coworkers (47) found a decrease in position error after application of tape. They revealed a detrimental effect on position sense of athletic footwear. Compared to barefoot data, the magnitude of foot position error was 207% with athletic footwear when untaped, but only 158% when taped. They concluded that ankle taping partly corrected impaired proprioception caused by the athletic footwear.

Ankle Bracing and Neuromuscular Control During Ambulation

Few studies have looked at the effect of external ankle support on the firing pattern of the peroneal muscles during walking and running. In a study of four mechanically unstable subjects, Glick and associates (24) found that tape increased the length of the swing-phase activity of the peroneus brevis and longus muscles prior to heel strike during running. This would imply that tape stimulated the muscles to be preactivated and may have made them capable of resisting sudden ankle inversion situations. Using a rigid brace that could hold the ankle in a neutral position during walking and running, Konradsen and coworkers (34) measured peroneal muscle activity during the last 300 ms of the swing phase. As found by van Linge, (57) a substantial number of steps were without swing-phase peroneal muscle activity. The frequency of a peroneal muscle signal measured over 100 gait cycles when subjects were walking briskly, jogging, or running at an even pace was recorded. A decreased frequency of preheel strike muscle activity was seen after application of a brace.

Geyer and coworkers (23) studied surface electromyography and 3-dimensional motion analysis of three standard ballet positions in 6 ballet dancers. Application of tape that did not afford any greater mechanical stability led to increased peroneus longus activity in the stable subject while decreased activity was seen in unstable dancers. Stability of the three positions was improved by taping.

Neurophysiological Effect of Ankle Bracing

Nishikawa and Grabiner (42) found that a 4° medium speed toes-up tilt with an external ankle brace increased the amplitude of the short latency EMG reflex response of the peroneus longus by 25%. In a parallel study, the peroneus longus H-reflex amplitude when the peroneal nerve was stimulated was found to be larger in a braced condition. Both experiments suggest that an external ankle support can increase motoneuron excitability.

Conclusion

Clinical studies suggest that knee and ankle bracing has a prophylactic and re-injury protecting effect in the clinical setting. Mechanical studies of the mechanism of protection suggest that braces cannot protect the joint ligaments and articular surfaces from harmful strains or loads. As a model of brace function a primarily proprioceptive effect of bracing has been proposed.

In theory it is believed that the massive stimulation of the skin and subcutaneous structures exerted by the brace on the brace/skin interface will stimulate afferent skin receptors. The afferent signals from the cutaneous receptors may themselves provide proprioceptive information or may facilitate joint proprioception by increasing relevant sensitive or motoneuron excitability.

Knee braces have shown a potential enhancing effect on proprioception in healthy subjects, using joint position sense as the proprioceptive measurement. An effect on reducing proprioceptive deficiencies in injured knees (a functional effect) has also been shown using the same outcome measure. However, a similar number of studies could not show this effect. Kinesthesia and reflex muscle reactions do not seem to be affected by brace application either in the normal subjects or in proprioceptive deficient individuals.

For ankle braces a decreased magnitude of postural sway and a reduced error of joint position assessment has been found in healthy subjects. In groups of functionally unstable subjects, ankle braces improved proprioception as measured by postural sway, peroneal muscle reflex latency, and joint position sense. However, the number of studies showing a positive effect of ankle bracing are balanced by studies unable to show an effect on proprioception.

It must be concluded that to date it is still unclear whether knee and ankle braces have an effect on proprioceptive functions. This is true both for the claim that bracing improves proprioception in healthy subjects (a prophylactic effect) and for the claim that bracing reestablishes normal proprioceptive values in proprioceptive deficient individuals.

References

1. AAOS. Knee braces. *AAOS Seminar Report* 1984; 17.
2. AAOS. The use of knee braces. *AAOS Bulletin* 1988; 17.
3. Andreasson G, Reese D, Renström PA. *Subjective experience of medical tape used to prevent athletic ankle injuries.* Gothenburg, Sweden: Chalmers University of Technology, 1985.
4. Ashton-Miller JA, Ottaviani RA, Hutchinson C, Wojtys EM. What best protects the inverted weight-bearing ankle against further inversion. *Am J Sports Med* 1996; 24(6): 800–809.
5. Baker B, Van Hanswyk E, Bogosian S, Werner F, Murphy D. A biomechanical study of the static stabilizing effect of knee braces on medial stability. *Am J Sports Med* 1987; 15: 566.
6. Barrett D, Cobb A, Bentley G. Joint proprioception in normal, osteoarthritic, and replaced knees. *J Bone Joint Surg* [Br] 1991; 73B: 53–56.
7. Bassett GS, Fleming BW. The Lenox Hill brace in anterolateral rotatory instability. *Am J Sports Med* 1983; 11: 345.
8. Beck C, Drez D, Young J, Cannon DW, Stone ML. Instrumented testing of functional knee braces. *Am J Sports Med* 1986; 14:253.
9. Beynnon BRP. The effect of bracing and taping in sports. *Ann Chir Gyn* 1991; 80: 230–38.
10. Beynnon BD, Johnson RJ, Fleming BC, et al. The effect of functional knee bracing on the anterior cruciate ligament in the weight-bearing and nonweight-bearing knee. *Am J Sports Med* 1997; 25(3): 353–59.
11. Branch T. Dynamic EMG analysis of anterior cruciate-deficient legs with and without bracing during cutting. *Am J Sports Med* 1989; 17: 35–41.
12. Bunch RP, Bednarski K, Holland D, Macinanti R. Ankle joint support: A comparative of reusable lace-on braces with taping and wrapping. *Phys Sports Med* 1985; 13(5): 59.
13. Calmels P, Escafit M, Domenach M, et al. Posturographic evaluation of the proprioceptive effect of ankle orthoses in healthy volunteers. *Int Disabil Studies* 1991; 13: 42–45.
14. Clark FJ, Burgess RC, Chapin JW, et al. Role of intramuscular receptors in the awareness of limb position. *J Neurophysiol* 1985; 54: 1529–540.
15. Colville MR, Lee CL, Ciullo JV. The Lenox Hill brace: An evaluation of effectiveness in treating knee instability. *Am J Sports Med* 1986; 14: 257.
16. Daanen HAM, Deegenaars WC, Fraterman H, DeGraaf WA, Rozing PM. Muscular response to sudden ankle inversion: Differences between a taped, braced, and bare ankle. *Electromyograph Kinesiol* 1991; 107–10.
17. Erickson AE, Yasuda K, Beynnon B, Johnson RJ, Pope MH. A dynamic evaluation of the effectiveness of prophylactic knee braces. Paper presented at the 37th ORS.
18. Feuerbach JW, Grabiner MD. Effect of the aircast on unilateral postural control: Amplitude and frequency variables. *JOSPT* 1993; 17(3): 149–54.
19. Feuerbach JW, Grabiner MD, Koh TJ, Weiker GG. Effect of an ankle orthosis and ankle ligament anesthesia on ankle joint proprioception. *Am J Sports Med* 1994; 22(2): 223–29.
20. Friden T, Zätterström R, Lindstrand A, Moritz U. A stabilometric technique for evaluation of lower limb instabilities. *Am J Sports Med* 1989; 17(1): 118–22.
21. Fumich RM, Ellison AE, Guerin GJ, Grace PD. The measured effect of taping on combined foot and ankle motion before and after exercise. *Am J Sports Med* 1981; 9(3): 165–70.
22. Garrick JG, Requa RK. Role of external ankle support in the prevention of ankle sprains. *Med Sci Sports* 1973; 5: 200–203.
23. Geyer M, Bergmann C, Siebert WE. [Overuse syndrome in ballet: Study of the effect of a tape bandage of the upper ankle joint with motion analysis]. *Sportverletz Sportschaden* 1993; 7(2): 78–83.
24. Glick JM, Gordon RB, Nashimoto D. The prevention and treatment of ankle injuries. *Am J Sports Med* 1976; 4:136-41.
25. Gottlieb DJ, Westmoreland K, Elmquist LG, Renström PA, Beynnon BD. The effect of func-

tional knee bracing on the latency of reflex muscle contraction in normal and ACL-deficient limbs. Paper presented at the ORS.
26. Guyton AC. Somatic sensations: The mechanoreceptive sensations. In *Textbook of Medical Physiology*, 7th ed. Philadelphia: Saunders, 1986; 588–89.
27. Hoffmann AA, Wyatt RWB, Bourne MH, Daniels AU. Knee stability in orthotic knee braces. *Am J Sports Med* 1984; 12: 371.
28. Horch KW, Clark FJ, Burgess PR. Awareness of knee joint angle under static conditions. *J Neurophysiol* 1975; 38: 1436–447.
29. Jerosch J, Bischof M. Proprioceptive capabilities of the ankle in stable and unstable joints. *Sports Exer Inj* 1996; 2: 167–71.
30. Jerosch J, Hoffstetter I, Bork H, Bischof M. The influence of orthoses on the proprioception of the ankle joint. *Knee Surg Sports Traumatol Arthroscopy* 1995; 3(1): 39–46.
31. Karlsson J, Andreasson GO. The effect of external ankle support in chronic lateral ankle joint instability: An electromyographic study. *Am J Sports Med* 1992; 20(3): 257–61.
32. Kennedy JC, Alexander IJ, Hayes KC. Nerve supply of the human knee and its functional importance. *Am J Sports Med* 1982; 10: 329–35.
33. Konradsen L, Ravn JB. Ankle instability caused by prolonged peroneal reaction time. *Acta Orthop Scand* 1990; 61(5): 388–90.
34. Konradsen L, Ravn JB, Sørensen AI. Proprioception at the ankle: The effect of anaesthetic blockade of ligament receptors. *J Bone Joint Surg* [Br] 1993; 75(3): 433–36.
35. Larsen E. Taping the ankle for chronic instability. *Acta Orthop Scand* 1984; 55(5): 551–53.
36. Lass P, Kaalund S, leFevre S, et al. Muscle coordination following rupture of the anterior cruciate ligament: Electromyographic studies of 14 patients. *Acta Orthop Scand* 1991; 62: 9–14.
37. Leanderson J. *Ankle sprain: Subjective and objective measures of functional impairment and treatment*. Stockholm: University of Stockholm, 1996.
38. Lepp TM, Teal SW. The effectiveness of a semirigid orthosis as a prophylaxis for ankle injuries: A retrospective study. *Athl Train* 1991; 26: 158.
39. Lindenberger U, Reese D, Andreasson G, Renström P. *The effect of prophylactic taping of ankles*. Gothenburg, Sweden: Chalmers Technical University, 1985.
40. McNair P, Stanley S, Strauss G. Knee bracing: Effects on proprioception. *Arch Phys Med Rehabil* 1996; 77: 287–89.
41. Miyatsu M, Atsuta Y, Watakabe M. The physiology of mechanoreceptors in the anterior cruciate ligament. *J Bone Joint Surg* 1993; 75B: 653–57.
42. Nishikawa T, Grabiner MD. Ankle braces influence the reflex amplitude of muscle in response to stretch. Paper presented at the 42nd annual meeting of the Orthopaedic Research Society, 1996.
43. Noyes FR, Mangine RE, Barber S. Early knee motion after open and arthroscopic ACL reconstruction. *Am J Sports Med* 1987; 15: 149.
44. Paulos LE, France PE, Rosenberg TD, Jayarman G, Abbott PJ, Jaen J. The biomechanics of lateral knee bracing. Parts I & II: Response of the valgus restraints to loading. *Am J Sports Med* 1987; 15: 419.
45. Perlau R, Frank C, Fick G. The effect of elastic bandages on human knee proprioception in the uninjured population. *Am J Sports Med* 1995; 23(2): 251–55.
46. Rarick GL, Bigley G, Karst R. The measurable support of the ankle joint by conventional methods of taping. *J Bone Joint Surg* 1962; 44A: 1183–190.
47. Robbins S, Waked E, Rappel R. Ankle taping improves proprioception before and after exercise in young men. *Br J Sports Med* 1995; 29: 242–47.
48. Rovere GD, Clarke TJ, Yates CS. Retrospective comparison of taping and ankle stabilizers in preventing ankle injuries. *Am J Sports Med* 1988; 16: 228–33.
49. Shapiro MS, Kabo JM, Mitchell PW, Loren G, Tsenter M. Ankle sprain prophylaxis: An analysis of the stabilizing effects of braces and tape. *Am J Sports Med* 1994; 22(1): 78–82.
50. Sitler M, Ryan J, Hopkinson W, et al. The efficacy of a prophylactic knee brace to reduce knee injuries in football. *Am J Sports Med* 1990; 18(3): 310.
51. Sitler M, Ryan J, Wheeler B, et al. The efficacy of a semirigid ankle stabilizer to reduce acute ankle injuries in basketball: A randomized clinical study at West Point. *Am J Sports Med* 1994; 22(4): 454–61.
52. Solomonow MB. The synergistic action of the anterior cruciate ligament and thigh muscles in maintaining joint stability. *Am J Sports Med* 1987; 15: 207–13.
53. Sprigings EJ, Pelton JD, Brandell BR. An EMG analysis of the effectiveness of external ankle support during sudden ankle inversion. *Canadien J Sports Sci* 1981; 6(2): 72–75.

54. Styf JR, Lundin O, Gershuni DH. Effects of a functional knee brace on leg muscle function. *Am J Sports Med* 1994; 22(6): 830–34.
55. Surve I, Schwellnus MP, Noakes T, Lombard C. A fivefold reduction in the incidence of recurrent ankle sprains in soccer players using the Sport-Stirrup orthosis. *Am J Sports Med* 1994; 22(5): 601–606.
56. Tropp H. *Functional instability of the ankle joint.* Linköping, Sweden: Linköping University, 1985.
57. Van Linge B. Activity of the peroneal muscles, the maintenance of balance, and prevention of inversion injury of the ankle: An electromyographic and kinematic study. *Acta Orthop Scand* 1988; 59(Suppl 227): 67–68.
58. Wellington P, Strother G. The Lenox Hill derotation brace in chronic posttraumatic instability of the knee. *Injury* 1984; 15: 242.
59. Wojtys EM, Goldstein SA, Redfern M, Trier E, Matthews LS. A biomechanical evaluation of the Lenox Hill knee brace. *Clin Orthop* 1987; 220: 179.
60. Wojtys EM, Kothari SU, Huston LJ. Anterior cruciate ligament functional brace use in sports. *Am J Sports Med* 1996; 24(4): 539–46.

CHAPTER 28

Surgical Considerations Related to Proprioception and Neuromuscular Control

Ian K.Y. Lo, MD
Peter J. Fowler, MD, FRCSC

Introduction

Neuromuscular control, and in particular proprioception, has gained increasing attention over the last 20 years. Its role in preventing injury, disability, and rehabilitation following injury has been documented by numerous investigators. As early as 1944, Abbott and coworkers (1) proposed that ligaments within the knee possessed a rich sensory innervation, which allowed impulses to be transmitted through the central nervous system and relayed to adjacent muscles, allowing for normal, smooth, and coordinated motion of a joint. They further postulated that abnormal impulses resulting from stretched ligaments might lead to muscular contraction, protecting the knee from further injury.

More recently, Kennedy and associates (67) revisited the neuroanatomy of the human knee. They noted a constant nerve supply (posterior articular nerve and a terminal branch of the obturator nerve) to the knee and demonstrated, by silver staining techniques, mechanoreceptors in the soft tissues of the knee including the anterior cruciate ligament. The Kennedy group hypothesized that injuries to the knee resulted in ligamentous laxity and failure to provide adequate neurological feedback to the knee. This subsequently predisposed the knee to secondary re-injury and further ligamentous laxity initiating the vicious cycle of injury, laxity, poor feedback, and re-injury. Since this classic article, numerous investigators have reported on the neurosensory significance of injuries to the knee (8, 11, 12, 15, 18, 21, 25, 27, 30, 31, 34, 35, 39, 46, 63, 67, 68, 78, 81, 83, 84, 86, 87, 89, 97, 98, 101, 110, 114, 117, 123, 130), shoulder (4, 24, 47, 71–76, 112, 122, 125, 126), and ankle (37, 41, 43, 96, 118–120, 128).

The purpose of this paper is not to review the current knowledge of proprioception and neuromuscular control but to apply what is known in these areas clinically and in particular to the surgeon's daily practice. While much has been published on proprioception, little research has focused on the effects of surgery. Most studies have involved patients after ACL reconstruction (11, 12, 15, 17, 30, 34, 35, 48, 72, 84, 89), knee (9, 16, 18, 28, 105, 106, 109, 121) or hip (53, 65) arthroplasty, and reconstruction of the glenohumeral joint (24, 36, 74). However, the exact clinical implications of statistically significant differences observed in the laboratory are controversial. The most sensitive test of joint proprioception is the threshold to detection of passive motion performed at an angular velocity of less than 1°/s (129). Considering that during the acceleration phase a professional pitcher's elbow may reach an angular velocity of 4,600°/s (93), these laboratory conditions and results are of questionable clinical significance. Despite this, the role of proprioception in the initiation, propagation, and rehabilitation of injuries continues to be elucidated. The influence of proprioception in the surgeon's clinical practice may be discussed under preoperative, intraoperative and postoperative considerations.

Preoperative Considerations

As with all medical conditions, prevention is ideal. Studies on the highly trained athlete have indicated that extensive training may improve proprioceptive ability (11, 13, 14). Conversely, muscular contraction to the point of fatigue was found to transiently decrease joint position sense (110). This proprioceptive deficit may be secondary to the effect of fatigue on muscle receptors or due to a temporary increase in laxity of the knee joint (111). These results suggest that patients who are fatigued may have altered proprioceptive abilities, and, in addition, the fatigued muscles have an impaired ability to stabilize the joint. Therefore, these patients may be more prone to injury (40).

Whether proprioceptive training may prevent injury has recently been investigated. Several studies have documented increased postural sway in subjects with ankle sprains and functional instability (43, 118–120). Furthermore, soccer players with poor postural sway were found to have a higher incidence of subsequent ankle injury (118). Following proprioceptive training on an ankle disk, improvements in postural sway were demonstrated in patients with functional ankle instability and subjective complaints of ankle "giving way" were also reduced (43, 118).

Caraffa and associates (27) studied 600 semiprofessional and amateur soccer players, half of whom underwent a specialized proprioceptive training regimen during the pre- and active soccer season and the other half of whom trained "normally." After a follow-up period of 3 yrs, the number of ACL injuries in the proprioceptively trained group was dramatically less (0.15 injuries per team/season) than the group who had trained normally (1.15 injuries per team/season). These studies suggest that proprioceptive training may play a very important role in the prevention of injury, although further investigation is necessary.

Following trauma, proprioceptive defects have been noted in ligament injuries involving the ankle (37, 41, 43, 96, 118–120, 128), knee (8, 11, 12, 15, 18, 21, 25, 27, 30, 31, 34, 35, 39, 46, 63, 67, 68, 78, 81, 83, 84, 86, 87, 89, 97, 98, 101, 110, 114, 117, 123, 130), and shoulder (4, 24, 47, 71–76, 112, 122, 125, 126) as well as in osteoarthritis of the knee (16, 18, 109, 127). Whether the deficits are the cause or effect of injury remains controversial. It has been postulated that recurrent ankle instability damages the afferent nerve fibers in ruptured ankle ligaments leading to proprioceptive loss (37, 41, 46). This further leads to disorganized muscular stabilization and functional instability of the ankle (41). Studies on the shoulder have also suggested that the injury precedes proprioceptive deficits (71, 74, 75, 101). Secondary instability results, due to poor muscular coordination of the dynamic stabilizers of the shoulder. This may then propagate the vicious cycle, as proposed by Kennedy and coworkers (67) for the knee, of injury, ligamentous laxity, poor neurological feedback, and subsequent re-injury. Studies by O'Connor and associates (86, 87) have demonstrated that ACL transection when combined with neurectomy resulted in increased arthrosis when compared to ACL disruption alone. Isolated neurectomy, however, did not cause degeneration of the knee, suggesting that sensory neuropathy alone is not sufficient to cause degeneration of a stable joint.

Following injury, not every patient requires surgery to improve neuromuscular control or to obtain clinical function. Many injuries are associated with effusions, which in the knee is known to inhibit quadriceps contraction (39, 67). More recently, in our laboratory simulated ankle effusions produced altered gastrosoleus muscle complex facilitation (as assessed by the Hoffmann reflex and M response) and increased resistance to passive motion (96). Slowly adapting mechanoreceptors likely mediate this reflex, and therefore inhibition may be maintained indefinitely in the presence of a persistent stimulus (effusion). This may lead to muscle atrophy, functional impairment, or slowed rehabilitation, supporting the treatment of effusion either by aspiration, application of compression, or through joint motion (11).

Simple bracing techniques have also been shown to improve proprioceptive ability. Barrett and associates (18), Lephart and associates (72), and McNair and associates (81), using a neoprene sleeve, and Perlau and coworkers (94), using an elastic bandage, demonstrated improved threshold detection of passive motion and reproduction of passive motion following brace application. Although bracing likely improved conscious appreciation of joint position through input from the skin and subcutaneous tissue, studies have not substantiated whether stabilizing reflexes can originate from the stimulation of mechanoreceptors from these origins (11). More dynamic tests during cutting maneuvers in the ACL-deficient knee have shown decreased activity of the gastrocnemius and quadriceps muscle groups and increased activity of the hamstrings during stance phase (25). This did not change with the application of a brace, suggesting that bracing did not enhance proprioceptive input enough to significantly alter stabilizing muscle groups. However, the apparent conscious improvement in proprioception may explain the increased sense of security many patients feel with the addition of a brace or a simple sleeve.

Proprioceptive training following injury may also be beneficial (73). As reported by Freeman and associates (41) and others (43, 118–120, 128), proprioceptive training through stabilometry or training on an unstable board significantly reduced episodes of giving way in functional instability of the ankle. Further, Ihara and Nakayama (61) reported on the effects of "dynamic joint control" training on the hamstring reaction time in ACL-deficient knees. Patients underwent a program of training on unstable boards and were trained to react to suddenly applied forces. Following a training period of 3 mo, hamstring reaction times were significantly improved when compared to controls, and there was a subjective improvement in giving way episodes.

More recently, Beard and coworkers (19) validated this training regimen, prospectively randomizing 50 anterior cruciate ligament-deficient patients to two different physiotherapy programs. The traditional program emphasized open chain lower-limb strengthening with graduated weight-resisted exercises while the proprioceptive regimen was similar to that reported by Ihara and Nakayama (61). Following 3 mo of rehabilitation, the proprioceptively trained group had improved reflex hamstring contraction latency and Lysholm Gillquist scores when compared to the traditional group. As also demonstrated by Tibone and Antich (117), the investigators found no correlation between isometric muscle strength and hamstring reaction time, implying that simple muscle strengthening did not have the beneficial effects of dynamic training. These effects have been studied by Walla and associates (123), who demonstrated that in patients who were able to successfully avoid ACL surgery, 95% obtained "reflex level" hamstring control.

Zätterström and associates (130) reported on the effects of coordination, postural reaction, and endurance training of trunk and leg musculature using closed chain exercises in chronic ACL insufficiency. They noted improvements in body sway, on the injured knee, to normal values at 12 mo, which persisted at the 36 mo follow-up. Therefore following injury, it is recommended that some form of proprioceptive training be incorporated within rehabilitation programs to promote functional and dynamic joint stability (73).

Choosing the surgical patient following ACL injury is difficult and may be based on a number of factors (symptoms, physical examination, KT-1000, level of activity, associated pathology); most frequently the deciding factor is the failure of conservative management to return the patient to the desired level of function. This, however, is based on the patient's own evaluation and no good objective test exists. To address this, Beard and coworkers (20) evaluated proprioception after ACL rupture by measuring the latency of the ACL-hamstring reflex. They demonstrated that this reflex was significantly prolonged following ACL ruptures and that there was a direct correlation between prolongation of this reflex and the functional instability that patients experienced. Other researchers have found that proprioceptive measures correlate better with patient satisfaction after ACL disruptions than do knee scores, stability testing, and the ability to return to sports (15,17). Thus proprioceptive measures may be useful as an indication for surgery (20).

Intraoperative Considerations

Several investigators have reported improved proprioception following anterior cruciate ligament reconstruction (11, 12, 15, 17, 30, 34, 35, 48, 72, 84, 89), knee (9, 16, 18, 28, 105, 106, 109, 121) and hip (53, 65) arthroplasty, and shoulder stabilization (23, 36, 74). However, the exact mechanism of this enhancement or the way in which we affect proprioception intraoperatively is not known. All aspects of surgery, at least theoretically, may affect proprioception to a greater or lesser degree. We will attempt to summarize these aspects, as they have been identified by Safran and coworkers (100).

It has been suggested that repair or reconstruction of an acute ACL tear is the golden opportunity to restore normal function (45, 88, 90, 91). Surgical timing for early shoulder instability has also been shown to be important, especially when considering arthroscopic stabilization (10, 36, 50). Its role in the enhancement of proprioception is less clear. Denti and associates (34) have demonstrated that at 1–2 mo following injury ACL stumps continue to demonstrate numerous mechanoreceptors. However, at 6 mo or greater following injury there was a significant atrophy or absence of these mechanoreceptors, suggesting a time-dependent course of receptor atrophy. Thus it may be postulated that with early repair of the ACL, restoration of ligament tension, and maintenance of receptor stimuli, receptor atrophy may be impeded or reversed. However, the results of ACL repair alone are disappointing and the repair therefore likely requires augmentation (7, 45, 49, 55, 60, 85, 107, 115).

Time from injury may also be a factor in anterior glenohumeral instability. Studies by Lephart and associates (74, 75) have demonstrated that in patients with unidirectional, recurrent instability significant proprioceptive deficits were noted in the injured shoulder when compared to the uninjured shoulder. However, a recent study at our institution revealed that in patients with initial, acute, traumatic, anterior dislocations, no significant deficit was demonstrated (36). Although this may be related to the number of dislocations suffered with secondary laxity of the capsulolabral complex, a time-dependent loss of mechanoreceptors may also play a role.

The choice of surgical approach may also affect proprioceptive sensation. It is well known that surrounding joint structures (capsule, ligaments, fat pad, synovium, perimeniscal tissue) of the knee (3, 11, 12, 22, 29, 33, 34, 42, 51, 52, 54, 56, 57, 66–69, 83, 97, 102–104) and, more recently, of the shoulder (glenohumeral ligaments, coracoclavicular, coracoacromial ligaments, labrum, subacromial bursae) are well innervated (121). Although the contribution of each to proprioception is controversial, likely all play some role in joint sensibility (51). Thus minimizing the amount of damage caused by surgical dissection and technique may retain their neurosensory function. Once damage to the nerves or mechanoreceptors occurs, their innate ability to recover is unclear.

Although the arthroscopic reconstruction of ankle, knee, and shoulder was popularized for other reasons, the minimization of soft tissue trauma and preservation of nerve and mechanoreceptors may serendipitously enhance proprioception. There are no comparative studies evaluating proprioception in open or arthroscopic techniques. As previously stated, patients with unilateral, recurrent, anterior glenohumeral instability have significant deficits in proprioceptive sensibility when compared to the opposite uninvolved side (71, 74, 75, 112). Further, Lephart and associates (74) have demonstrated that patients who underwent open capsulolabral reconstruction had no significant differences in kinesthetic or position sense when comparing the involved to the uninvolved side.

A recent study at our institution evaluated the effect of early arthroscopic stabilization compared to immobilization and rehabilitation on proprioception of the shoulder after primary traumatic anterior dislocation. Twenty-four patients were evaluated (13 nonoperative, 11 operative) and again no significant differences in proprioceptive sensibility were noted between the involved and uninvolved limbs in patients who had undergone arthroscopic stabilization (36). However, no significant differences were found either between the injured and uninjured sides of patients who were treated with immobilization or between the two groups (nonoperative versus operative). Although this may be explained by differences in surgical technique (the ability to restore capsulolabral tension), other confounding variables may explain these differences, including patient population (primary anterior dislocators versus recurrent dislocators), sample size, rehabilitation protocols, and testing conditions.

Similarly, minimizing damage during graft harvest may be a consideration. The use of allografts or artificial ligaments theoretically should cause less disruption of neurosensory function. However, Denti and associates (34) recently evaluated three different types of ACL reconstruction in sheep. They demonstrated histologically mechanoreceptors in the grafts of sheep that had undergone patellar tendon reconstruction or patellar tendon reconstruction with LAD augmentation. However, those sheep that were reconstructed with artificial ligaments (Leeds-Keio) had no demonstrable mechanoreceptors, and therefore their use is not recommended, especially when considering their inferior clinical results (6, 93, 131). Oeffinger and coworkers (89) recently reported on 15 patients who underwent ACL reconstruction, 7 with patellar tendon autograft and 8 with patellar tendon allograft. The patients who underwent autograft reconstruction had a greater degree of proprioceptive deficit as measured by muscular contraction latency following the application of a simulated anteriorly directed force. The increased dissection necessary to harvest the patellar tendon autograft may contribute to the proprioceptive deficiencies. Other factors should be considered when using allografts, including disease transmission, immunologic response, biomechanical properties, and cost (82).

Several investigators (34, 48, 121) have demonstrated repopulating of mechanoreceptors in various animal models (canine, sheep, goat) following reconstruction with soft tissue grafts. Goertzen and coworkers (48) histologically evaluated ACL allograft reconstruction in foxhounds. At 3 mo no mechanoreceptors were identified; however at 6 mo, free nerve endings were seen and, furthermore, at

12 mo with Golgi tendonlike receptors. The two most popular grafts in human ACL reconstruction are the central third patellar tendon and the hamstring tendon autografts. Recent prospective trials by Marder and associates (80) and Aglietti and associates (2), however, have failed to demonstrate any statistically significant differences in knee stability and functional outcome. Similarly, recent studies at our institution have demonstrated that the nerve population and density of these two grafts are similar, suggesting that similar deficits would occur with graft harvest (5).

The preservation of native mechanoreceptors may also be worthwhile. Following injury to the ACL, in many cases, residual or remnant ACL tissue remains (77). In fact, many of these ACL remnants continue to be attached to the intraarticular environment, whether attached by scarring to the PCL or the intercondylar notch. Recent studies by Crain and coworkers (32) and Lo and associates (77) have demonstrated the morphology of ACL scars and their ability to provide some stabilization of the knee joint (implying that the scar does take some load). Thus, as postulated above and demonstrated by Denti and coworkers (34), many of these ACL scars may contain native nerves and mechanoreceptors. It is common protocol to debride the ACL remnant from its insertion sites, and, in fact, its preservation has been implicated in the development of Cyclops lesions (62). However, since the majority of mechanoreceptors have been identified at the insertions of ligaments and, in particular, the tibial insertion (57, 66, 103, 104), the preservation of this tissue may have neurosensory advantages.

ACL remnants may be sewn to the graft material to maintain its tension and impede or reverse mechanoreceptor atrophy. Alternatively, these stumps may provide a source of mechanoreceptors for graft repopulation and may also provide enhanced proprioceptive feedback to the reconstructed graft. Tsujimoto and coworkers (121), in the goat model, studied the effects of excision of the ACL remnant with patellar tendon autograft reconstruction, compared to ACL repair with patellar tendon augmentation. The investigators identified mechanoreceptors in both groups; however, more mechanoreceptors were demonstrated in goats where the ACL remnant was preserved.

Similarly, minimizing the amount of resection and dissection in arthroplasty surgery may minimize damage to neuroreceptors and preserve proprioception. Retention of the cruciate ligament, particularly the posterior cruciate ligament, has been hypothesized to contribute to a more normal gait and improved stair climbing (9). However, the results of several studies are contradictory. Barrett and coworkers (18) examined proprioception in normal, osteoarthritic, and replaced knees. They demonstrated that knee replacement improved joint position sense; however, semiconstrained implants (posterior stabilized implants) tended towards a greater effect than hinged replacements. They postulated that the increased dissection and surgical removal of the joint capsule and ligaments around hinged implants led to proprioceptive deficits.

The results of unicondylar, posterior cruciate retaining and posterior stabilized prosthesis, however, have not shown similar results (106). Presumably, the unicondylar implant, which preserves the anterior and posterior cruciate ligaments, and the posterior cruciate retaining prosthesis should perform better than the posterior stabilized prostheses. However, Simmons and associates (106) demonstrated no significant differences in threshold to detection of passive movement in any of the three groups, suggesting that retaining the anterior or posterior cruciate ligaments did not preserve proprioceptive function. Other investigators (28, 38, 105) have confirmed these findings when comparing posterior cruciate retaining and sacrificing prostheses.

Although the proprioceptive input from the cruciate ligaments is well documented, these seemingly contradictory results may be secondary to the decreased contribution of the cruciate ligaments to proprioception in an elderly population (3, 103). Proprioception has been shown to decrease with advancing age (18, 95, 108, 111) and to a greater extent in patients with osteoarthritis (18, 105, 106). Further, histological evaluations of the cruciate ligaments have revealed fewer mechanoreceptors in ligaments procured during arthroplasty surgery and in the presence of osteoarthritis (3, 103). In fact, the proprioceptive loss appears to occur early in the degenerative process(18, 108). This may explain the lack of any significant difference in these studies.

Simmons and coworkers (105) in a separate study, in fact, demonstrated the opposite. In patients with severe osteoarthritis, those patients with cruciate-substituting arthroplasties performed significantly better than those with cruciate-retaining prostheses. The authors proposed that the ability of a posterior cruciate-substituting prosthesis to more effectively restore the balance and tension of the capsuloligamentous structures, especially in a severe osteoarthritic, may explain these discrepancies.

Surgical procedures that "retension" the soft tissues may enhance proprioceptive function. Since mechanoreceptors are mechanically sensitive, they must be mechanically loaded to be stimulated. However, if adjacent soft tissues are lax, the tension developed may be insufficient to stimulate mechanoreceptors. Proprioceptive ability of the knee has been shown to be decreased in patients with hypermobility syndrome or ligamentous laxity (13, 58), and it has be postulated that this reduced sensory feedback may accelerate degenerative joint disease commonly seen in this patient population (58). Preliminary results at our institution have demonstrated decreased proprioceptive abilities in patients with symptomatic multidirectional instability of the shoulder when compared to the normal population (99). Recent studies by Lephart and associates (71, 74, 75) and Smith and Brunoli (112) have also evaluated the proprioceptive ability of the shoulder. Patients with unilateral, unidirectional, recurrent anterior instability had proprioceptive deficits when compared to the opposite uninjured side. Further, patients who underwent capsular shift procedures that tighten and "retension" the capsulolabral structures had proprioceptive abilities that matched the normal, uninjured side.

The tensioning of soft tissues in joint arthroplasty is also important. Much of the reduction of proprioceptive ability that occurs in degenerative conditions is felt to be due to deformity and angulation, resulting in altered laxity of the joint capsule and ligaments. Total knee arthroplasty does improve proprioceptive ability, although not to the level of age-matched controls (18). This enhancement may be secondary to retensioning and balancing of the remaining soft tissues. Recent evidence has suggested that this may be a more important factor than the preservation of mechanoreceptors by the retention of cruciate ligaments (posterior or anterior) (105).

Postoperative Considerations

Following surgery, the effects of joint effusion and muscle fatigue must again be considered. In addition, postoperative rehabilitation emphasizing proprioceptive training may improve clinical results. As demonstrated by Ihara and Nakayama (61) and Beard and associates (19), "dynamic joint control" training may improve the hamstring reflex arc and theoretically may protect an ACL graft from secondary injury. Few studies, however, have specifically evaluated proprioceptive training following anterior cruciate ligament reconstruction.

Pincivero and coworkers (98) recently reported on the preliminary results of 10 patients who underwent dynamic balance training on a kinesthetic ability trainer (KAT 2000) following ACL reconstruction. After completion of a 4 wk program patients demonstrated significantly improved dynamic balance scores and reproduction of passive motion (in flexion). A larger series by Losse and associates (78) randomized 24 patients to a standard postoperative rehabilitation program or a neurosensory specific rehabilitation program. The neurosensory program included beginning single leg support exercises on postoperative day 2 and using a balance training system (KAT 2000) at 2 wks. The investigators reported that the neurosensory program significantly improved double- and single-leg static balance of the involved leg. Functional ratings and activity were also greater at 3 mo evaluation. Although the authors concluded that early and aggressive neurosensory rehabilitation is important, the study was confounded due to the fact that the system used for kinesthetic evaluation was also the system on which the neurosensory group trained. Therefore, objective improvements in fact may be due to familiarity with exercises and the testing apparatus rather than the true enhancement in proprioceptive abilities.

Overall, rehabilitation following surgery should emphasize hamstring strengthening and enhancement of the hamstring reflex contraction to promote both stability and protection of the ACL graft. Closed kinetic chain exercises have been shown to be more effective than open kinetic chain regimens in increasing hamstring cocontractions, as well as decreasing the shear forces across the graft (79). Further, Bynum and coworkers (26), in a prospective randomized study, demonstrated that closed kinetic chain programs decreased the incidence of patellofemoral symptoms as well as decreasing the stress on the ACL graft, as reflected by a significantly lower displacement on KT-1000 measurement. Thus, currently most regimens should include isometric strengthening of the hamstring, gastrocnemius, and quadriceps and also dynamic reflex training and functional hamstring cocontraction. This may be achieved through stabilometry training, visual feedback, or other muscle training techniques emphasizing performance-based, weight-bearing, closed kinetic chain exercises.

Similarly, shoulder rehabilitation exercises emphasizing proprioceptive training may reduce recurrent instability by enhancing the dynamic stabilizers to support the surgically corrected restraints (73).

Conclusions and Future Directions

It is now apparent that proprioceptive issues influence the way in which surgeons practice. Such considerations must be made during each phase of treatment (whether operative or nonoperative) and can help guide treatment decisions (20). However, much of the research continues to be in its infancy and further studies are required. Clearly lacking are studies that have prospectively evaluated patients pre- and postoperatively or over an extended follow-up period. In addition, the effects of various treatment approaches should be evaluated in a randomized fashion (acute versus chronic reconstruction, arthroscopic versus open procedures, preservation versus resection of ACL remnants, ACL- and PCL-retaining versus ACL- and PCL-substituting prostheses, traditional versus neurosensory postoperative rehabilitation). Further, continued work on the basic science of mechanoreceptor repopulation, enhancement, and ultimate function are needed. Most importantly, further evaluation and development is needed on measurement tools and on the clinical implications of statistically significant differences observed in the laboratory under nonphysiological conditions.

References

1. Abbott LC, Saunders JB, Dec M, et al. Injuries to the ligaments of the knee joint. *JBJS* 26: 305–21, 1944.
2. Aglietti P, Buzzi F, Zaccherotti G, DeBlase P. Patellar tendon versus doubled semitendinosus and gracilis tendons for anterior cruciate ligament reconstruction. *AJSM* 22: 211–218, 1994.
3. Alexiades M, Scuderi G, Vigorita V, Scott WN. A histological study of the posterior cruciate ligament in the arthritic knee. *Am J Knee Surg* 2: 153, 1989.
4. Allegrucci M, Whitney SL, Lephart SM, Irrgang JJ, Fu FH. Shoulder kinesthesia in healthy unilateral athletes participating in upper extremity sports. *J Orthop Sports Phy Therapy* 21(4): 220–26, 1995.
5. Amendola A. Histological study of the posterior cruciate ligament in the arthritic knee. *Am J Knee Surg* 2: 153, 1989.
6. Anderson HN, Bruun C, Sondergard-Petersen PE. Reconstruction of chronic insufficient anterior cruciate ligament in the knee using a synthetic Dacron prosthesis: A prospective study of 57 cases. *Am J Sports Med* 20(l): 20–23, 1992.
7. Andersson C, Odensten M, Good L, Gillquist J. Surgical or nonsurgical treatment of acute rupture of the anterior cruciate ligament. *JBJS* 71A(7): 965–74, 1989.
8. Andriacchi TP, Birac D. Functional testing in the anterior cruciate ligament-deficient knee. *Clin Orthop* 288: 40–47, 1993.
9. Andriacchi TP, Galante JP, Fermier RW. Influence of total knee replacement design on walking and stair climbing. *JBJS* 64A: 1328–335, 1982.
10. Arciero RA, Wheeler JH, Ryan JBI, et al. Arthroscopic Bankart repair versus nonoperative treatment for acute initial anterior shoulder dislocations. *AJSM* 22: 589–94, 1994.
11. Barrack RL, Lund PJ, Skinner HB. Knee joint proprioception revisited. *J Sport Rehab* 3(1): 18–42, 1994.
12. Barrack RL, Skinner HB. The sensory function of knee ligaments. In Daniel D (ed), *Knee Ligaments: Structure, Function, Injury, and Repair.* New York: Raven Press, 95–114, 1990.
13. Barrack RL, Skinner HB, Brunet ME, Cook SD. Joint laxity and proprioception in the knee. *Phys Sportsmed* 11(6): 130–35, 1983.
14. Barrack RL, Skinner HB, Brunet ME, Cook SD. Joint kinesthesia in the highly trained knee. *J Sport Med Phys Fitness* 24: 18–20, 1983.
15. Barrack RL, Skinner HB, Buckley SL. Proprioception in the anterior cruciate-deficient knee. *AJSM* 17(1): 1–6, 1989.
16. Barrack RL, Skinner HB, Cook SD, Haddad RJ Jr. Effect of articular disease and total knee arthroplasty on knee joint-position sense. *J Neurophysiol* 50(3): 684–87, 1983.
17. Barrett DS. Proprioception and function after anterior cruciate reconstruction. *JBJS* 73B(5): 833–37, 1991.
18. Barrett DS, Cobb AG, Bentley G. Joint proprioception in normal, osteoarthritic, and replaced knees. *JBJS* 73B (1): 53–56, 1991.
19. Beard DJ, Dodd CA, Trundle HR, Simpson AHRW. Proprioception enhancement for anterior cruciate ligament deficiency: A prospective randomized trial of two physiotherapy regimes. *JBJS* [Br] 76B: 654–59, 1994.
20. Beard DJ, Kybert PJ, Fergusson CM, Dodd CAF. Proprioception after rupture of the anterior cruciate ligament: An objective indication of the need for surgery? *JBJS* 75B(2): 311–15, 1993.
21. Berchuck M, Andriacchi TP, Bach BR, Reider B. Gait adaptation by patients who have a deficient anterior cruciate ligament. *JBJS* 72A: 871–77, 1990.
22. Biedert RM, Stauffer E, Freiderich NF. Occurrence of free nerve ending in the soft tissue of

the knee joint: A histological investigation. *AJSM* 20(4): 430–33, 1992.
23. Blasier RB, Carpenter JE, Huston LJ. Shoulder proprioception: Effect of joint laxity, joint position, and direction of motion. *Orthop Rev*: 45–50, 1994.
24. Borsa PA, Lephart SM, Kocher MS, Lephart SP. Functional assessment and rehabilitation for glenohumeral instability. *J Sport Rehab* 3(1): 84–104, 1994.
25. Branch TP, Hunter R, Donath M. Dynamic EMG analysis of anterior cruciate-deficient legs with and without bracing during cutting. *AJSM* 17(l): 35–41, 1989.
26. Bynum EB, Barrack RL, Sedey PW, Ridgeway RK, Alexander AH. The sport cord—its use in accelerated anterior cruciate ligament rehabilitation: A prospective randomized study comparing open and closed kinetic chain exercises. Paper presented at the annual meeting of the American Orthopaedic Association, Coronado, CA, June 1993.
27. Caraffa A, Cerulli G, Projetti M, Aisa G, Rizzo A. Prevention of anterior cruciate ligament injuries in soccer: A prospective controlled study of proprioceptive training. *Knee Surg Sports Traumatol Arthroscopy* 4: 19–21, 1996.
28. Cash RM, Gonzalez MH, Garst J, Barmada R, Stem SH. Proprioception after arthroplasty: Role of the posterior cruciate ligament. *Clin Orthop* 331: 172–78, 1996.
29. Clark FJ, Burgess PR. Slowly adapting receptors in cat knee joint: Can they signal joint angle? *J Neurophysiol* 38: 1448–463, 1975.
30. Co FH, Skinner HB, Cannon WD. Proprioception of the knee following ACL reconstruction and it relation to heel strike impulse. *J Orthop Res* 11: 696–704, 1993.
31. Corrigan JP, Cashman WF, Brady ND. Proprioception in the cruciate-deficient knee. *JBJS* [Br] 74B: 247–50, 1992.
32. Crain EH, Fithian DC, Daniel DM. Variation in ACL scar pattern: Does this contribute to anterior stability in ACL-deficient knees? Paper presented at the annual meeting of the Arthroscopy Association of North America, San Diego, 1997.
33. Cross MJ, McCloskey DI. Position sense following surgical removal of joints in man. *Brain Res* 55: 443–45, 1973.
34. Denti M, Monteleone M, Berardi A, Panni AS. Anterior cruciate ligament mechanoreceptors: Histological studies on lesions and reconstruction. *Clin Orthop* 38: 29–32, 1994.
35. Dvir A, Koren E, Halperin N. Knee joint position sense following reconstruction of the anterior cruciate ligament. *J Orthop Phys Ther* 10(4): 117–20, 1988.
36. Edmonds G, Kirkley A, Fowler PJ. The effect of early arthroscopic stabilization compared to immobilization and rehabilitation on proprioception of the shoulder after primary traumatic anterior dislocation. Paper presented at the annual meeting of the Canadian Orthopaedic Association, Hamilton, 1997.
37. Evans GA, Hardcastle P, Frenyo AD. Acute rupture of the lateral ligament of the ankle. *JBJS* 66B: 209–12, 1984.
38. Faris PM, Jiang CC, Otis JC, Manouel M. Proprioceptive input of the posterior cruciate ligament in knee prostheses. *Trans Orthop Res Soc* 13: 353, 1988.
39. Fahrer H, Rentsch HU, Gerber NJ, Beyeler C, Hess CW, Gruning B. Knee effusion and reflex inhibition of the quadriceps: A bar to effective retraining. *JBJS* 70B: 635–38, 1988.
40. Feagin JA Jr. The syndrome of torn anterior cruciate ligament. *Orthop Clin North Am* 10: 81–90, 1979.
41. Freeman MAR, Dan MRE, Hanham IWF. The etiology and prevention of functional instability of the foot. *JBJS* 47B: 678–85, 1965.
42. Gardner E. The innervation of the knee joint. *Anat Rec* 101: 109–30, 1948.
43. Gauffin H, Tropp H, Odenrick P. Effect of ankle disk training on postural control in patients with functional instability of the ankle. *Int J Sports Med* 9: 141–44, 1988.
44. Geiger DF, Hurley JA, Tovey JA, Roa JP. Results of arthroscopic versus open Bankart suture repair. *Orthop Trans* 17: 307, 1992.
45. Gillquist J. Repair and reconstruction of the ACL: Is it good enough? *Arthroscopy* 9(l): 68–71, 1993.
46. Glencross D, Thornton E. Position sense following joint injury. *AJSM* 21: 23–27, 1981.
47. Glousman R, Jobe F, Tibone J, Moynes D, Antonelli D, Perry J. Dynamic electromyographic analysis of the throwing shoulder with glenohumeral instability. *JBJS* 70A: 220–26, 1988.
48. Goertzen M, Gruber J, Delmann A, Clahsen H, Schulity KP. Neurohistological finding after experimental anterior cruciate ligament allograft transplantation. *Arch Orthop Trauma Surg* 111: 126–29, 1992.
49. Golleon DL, Warren RF, Wickiewica TL. Acute repairs of the anterior cruciate ligaments: Past and present. *Orthop Clin North Am* 169(1): 111–25, 1985.
50. Green MR, Christensen KP. Arthroscopic versus open Bankart procedures: A comparison of early morbidity and complications. *Arthroscopy* 9(4): 371–74, 1993.

51. Grigg P. Peripheral neural mechanisms in proprioception. *J Sport Rehab* 3(l): 2–17, 1994.
52. Grigg P. Mechanical factors influencing response of joint afferent neurons from cat knees. *J Neurophysiol* 38: 1473, 1975.
53. Grigg P, Finerman GAM, Riley LH. Joint-position sense after total hip replacement. *JBJS* 56: 1016–1025, 1973.
54. Grigg P, Hoffman AH, Fogarty KE. Properties of Golgi-Mazzoni afferents in cat knee joint capsule as revealed by mechanical studies of isolated joint capsule. *J Neurophysiol* 47: 31, 1982.
55. Grontredt T, Engebretsen L, Benum P, et al. Prospective randomized study of three operations for acute rupture of the anterior cruciate ligament. *JBJS* 78A(2): 159–68, 1996.
56. Halata Z. The ultrastructure of the sensory nerve endings in the articular capsule of the knee joint of the domestic cat (Ruffini corpuscles and Pacinian corpuscles). *J Anat* 124: 717–29, 1977.
57. Halata Z, Haus J. The ultrastructure of sensory nerve endings in human anterior cruciate ligament. *Anat Embryol* 179: 415–21, 1989.
58. Hall MG, Ferrell WR, Sturrock RD, Hamblen DL, Baxendale RH. The effect of the hypermobility syndrome on knee joint proprioception. *Br J Rheum* 34: 121–25, 1995.
59. Harter RA, Osternig LR, Singer KM, James SL, Larson RL, Jones DC. Long-term evaluation of knee stability and function following surgical reconstruction for anterior cruciate ligament insufficiency. *AJSM* 16(5): 434–43, 1988.
60. Holmes PF, James SJ, Larson RL, Singer KM, Jones DC. Retrospective direct comparison of three intraarticular anterior cruciate ligament reconstructions. *AJSM* 19(6): 595–600, 1991.
61. Ihara H, Nakayama A. Dynamic joint control training for knee ligament injuries. *AJSM* 14: 309–15, 1986.
62. Jackson DW, Schaefer RK. Cyclops syndrome: Loss of extension following intraarticular anterior cruciate ligament reconstructions. *Arthroscopy* 6(3): 171–78, 1990.
63. Kålund S, Sinkjær T, Arendt-Nielsen L, Simonsen O. Altered timing of hamstring muscle action in anterior cruciate ligament-deficient patients. *AJSM* 18(3): 245–48, 1990.
64. Kaplan FS, Nixon JE, Reitz M, Rindfleish L, Tucker J. Age-related changes in proprioception and sensation of joint position. *Acta Orthop Scand* 56: 72–74, 1985.
65. Karanjia PN, Ferguson JH. Passive joint position sense after total hip replacement surgery. *Ann Neurol* 13: 654–57, 1983.
66. Katonis PG, Assimakopoulos AP. Agapitos MV, Exarchou EI. Mechanoreceptors in the posterior cruciate ligament: Histological study on cadaver knees. *Acta Orthop Scand* 62: 276–78, 1991.
67. Kennedy JC, Alexander IJ, Hayes KC. Nerve supply of the human knee and its functional importance. *AJSM* 10: 329–35, 1982.
68. Krauspe R, Schmidt M, Schaible HG. Sensory innervation of the anterior cruciate ligament: An electrophysiological study of the response properties of single identified mechanoreceptors in the cat. *JBJS* 74A(3): 390–97, 1992.
69. Krenn V, Hofmann S, Engel A. First description of mechanoreceptors in the corpus adiposum infrapatellare of man. *Acta Anat* 137: 187–88, 1990.
70. Lephart SM, Fu FH, Warner JP. Normal shoulder proprioception measurements in college age individuals. Paper presented at the annual meeting of the American Orthopaedic Society for Sports Medicine, San Diego, CA, 1992.
71. Lephart SM, Fu FH, Warner JP. Proprioception in the unstable shoulder. Paper presented at the Combined Congress of the International Arthroscopy Association and the International Society of the Knee, Copenhagen, Denmark, 1993.
72. Lephart SM, Kocher MA, Fu FH, Borsa PA, Hamer CD. Proprioception following ACL reconstruction. *J Sport Rhab* 1: 188–96, 1992.
73. Lephart SM, Pincivero DM, Giraldo JL, Fu FH. Proprioception in the management and rehabilitation of athletic injuries. *AJSM* 25(1): 130–37, 1997.
74. Lephart SM, Warner JJP, Borsa PA, Fu FH. Proprioception of the shoulder in normal, unstable and postsurgical individuals. *J Shoulder Elbow Surg* 3: 371–80, 1994.
75. Lephart SM, Warner JP, Borsa PA, Reddy JG, Fu FH. Proprioception and kinesthesia in the unstable shoulder. *Transactions of the annual meeting of the American Orthopaedic Society of Sports Medicine*, Sun Valley, CA, 1993.
76. Limbird TJ, Shiavi R, Frazer M, Borra H. EMG profiles of knee joint musculature during walking: Changes induced by anterior cruciate ligament deficiency. *J Orthop Res* 6: 630–38, 1988.
77. Lo IKY, deMatt GHR, Valk JW. Intraarticular morphology of human anterior cruciate ligament disruptions: Evidence of a healing response. Paper presented at the annual meeting of the Canadian Orthopaedic Association, Hamilton, 1997.
78. Losse GM, Howard ME, Cawley PW. The effect of neurosensory training following ACL reconstruction. Paper presented at the American Or-

thopaedic Society for Sports Medicine Specialty Day, Atlanta, 1996.
79. Lutz GE, Palmitier RA, An KA, Chao EYS. Comparison of tibiofemoral joint forces during open kinetic chain and closed kinetic chain exercises. *JBJS* 75A: 732–39, 1993.
80. Marder RA, Raskind JR, Carroll M. Prospective evaluation of arthroscopically assisted anterior cruciate ligament reconstruction. *AJSM* 19: 478–84, 1991.
81. McNair PJ, Stanley SN, Strauss GR. Knee bracing: Effects on proprioception. *Arch Phys Med Rehabil* 77: 287–89, 1996.
82. Miller MD, Harner CD. The use of allograft: Technique and results. *Clinics Sports Med* 12(4): 757–70, 1993.
83. Miyatsu M, Atsuta Y, Watakabe. The physiology of mechanoreceptors in the anterior cruciate ligament: An experimental study in decerebrate spinalized animals. *JBJS* 75B(4): 653–57, 1993.
84. Newberg TA. Examination of joint position sense in knees having undergone anterior cruciate ligament reconstruction. Master's thesis, University of Oregon, Eugene, 1986.
85. O'Brien SJ, Warren RF, Pavlov H, Panariello R, Wickiewicz TL. Reconstruction of the chronically insufficient anterior cruciate ligament with central third of the patellar ligament. *JBJS* 73A(2): 278–86, 1991.
86. O'Connor BL, Palmoski MJD, Brandt KD. Neurogenic acceleration of degenerative joint lesions. *JBJS* 67A: 562–72, 1985.
87. O'Connor BL, Visco DM, Brandt KD, Myers SL, Kalasinski LA. Neurogenic acceleration of osteoarthrosis. *JBJS* 74A(3): 367–76, 1992.
88. O'Donoghue DH. Surgical treatment of fresh injuries to the major ligaments of the knee. *JBJS* 32: 721–38, 1950.
89. Oeffinger DJ, Shapiro R, Pienkowski D, Hyland J, Caborn DN, Johnson D. Proprioception in the normal and ACL-reconstructed knee.
90. Palmer I. Plastic surgery of ligaments of the knee joint. *Acta Cir Scand* 91: 37–48, 1944.
91. Palmer I. On the injuries to the ligaments of the knee joint: A clinical study. *Acta Chir Scand* 53(Suppl): 11–273, 1938.
92. Pappas AM, Zawacki RM, Sullivan TJ. Biomechanics of baseball pitching: A preliminary report. *AJSM* 13: 216, 1985.
93. Paulos LE, Rosenberg TD, Rewe SR, Tearse DS, Beck CL. The Gore-Tex anterior cruciate ligament prosthesis: A long-term follow-up. *AJSM* 20(3): 246–52, 1992.
94. Perlau R, Frank C, Fick G. The effect of elastic bandages on human knee proprioception in the uninjured population. *AJSM* 23(2): 251–55, 1995.
95. Petrella RJ, Lattanzio PJ, Nelson MG. The effect of age and activity on knee-joint proprioception.
96. Petrik J, Amendola, A, Rampersaud R, Hayes KC. The effect of effusion on H-reflex amplitude and viscoelastic properties of the ankle.
97. Pitman NU, Nainzadeh N, Menche D, Gasalberti R, Song EK. The intraoperative evaluation of the neurosensory function of the anterior cruciate ligament in humans using somatosensory evoked potentials. *Arthroscopy* 8(4): 442–47, 1992.
98. Pincivero DM, Henry TJ, Lephart SM. The effects of kinesthetic training on balance and proprioception in the anterior cruciate ligament-injured knee. *J Athletic Training* 31(2): 2–52, 1996.
99. Safran MR, Caldwell GL, Fu FH. Proprioception considerations in surgery. *J Sport Rehab* 3(l): 105–15, 1994.
100. Safran MR, Lephart SM, Allen AA, Giraldo J, Fu FH, Harner CD. Contribution of PCL mechanoreceptors to knee proprioception. Paper presented at the American Orthopaedic Society for Sports Medicine Specialty Day, Atlanta, 1996.
101. Schaible HG, Schmidt RF. Activation of groups III and IV sensory units in medial articular nerve by local mechanical stimulation of knee joint. *J Neurophysiol* 49: 35–44, 1983.
102. Schultz RA, Miller DC, Kerr CS, Micheli L. Mechanoreceptors in human cruciate ligaments: A histological study. *JBJS* 66A: 1072–1076, 1984.
103. Schutte MJ, Dabezies EJ, Zimny ML, Happel LT. Neural anatomy of the human anterior cruciate ligament. *JBJS* 69A: 243–47, 1987.
104. Simmons S, Lephart S, Rubash H, Borsa P, Barrack RL. Proprioception following total knee arthroplasty with and without the posterior cruciate ligament. *J Arthroplasty* 11(7): 763–68, 1996.
105. Simmons S, Lephart S, Rubash H, Pifer GW, Barrack R. Proprioception after unicondylar knee arthroplasty versus total knee arthroplasty. *Clin Orthop* 331: 179–84, 1996.
106. Simonet WT, Sim FH. Repair and reconstruction of rotatory instability of the knee. *AJSM* 12(2): 89–97, 1984.
107. Skinner HB, Barrack RL, Cook SD, Age-related decline in proprioception. *Clin Orthop* 184: 208–11, 1984.

108. Skinner HB, Barrack RL, Cook SD, Haddad RJ Jr. Joint position sense in total knee arthroplasty. *J Orthop Res* 1: 276–83, 1984.
109. Skinner HB, Wyatt NP, Hodgdon JA, Conard DW, Barrack RL. Effect of fatigue on joint position sense of the knee. *J Orthop Res* 4: 112–18, 1986.
110. Skinner HB, Whatt MP, Stone ML, Hodgdon JA, Barrack RL. Exercise-related knee joint laxity. *AJSM* 14: 30–34, 1986
111. Smith RL, Brunoli J. Shoulder kinesthesia after anterior glenohumeral joint dislocation. *Phys Ther* 69(2): 106–12, 1989.
112. Solomonow M, Baratta R, Zhou BH, Shoji H, Bose W, Beck C, D'Ambrosia R. The synergistic action of the anterior cruciate ligament and thigh muscles in maintaining joint stability. *AJSM* 15: 207–13, 1987.
113. Stauffer RN, Chao EYS, Gyory AN. Biomechanical gait analysis of the diseased knee joint. *Clin Orthop* 126: 246–55, 1977.
114. Strand T, Engesaeter LB, Molster AO, Raugstad TS, Stangeland L, Stray O, Alho A. Knee function following suture of fresh tears of the anterior cruciate ligament. *Acta Orthop Scand* 55: 181–84, 1984.
115. Steiner ME, Grana WA, Chillag K, Schelberg-Karnes E. The effect of exercise on anterior-posterior knee laxity. *AJSM* 14: 24–29, 1986.
116. Tibone JE, Antich TJ. Electromyographic analysis of the anterior cruciate ligament-deficient knee. *Clin Orthop* 288: 35–39, 1993.
117. Tropp H, Ekstrand J, Gillquist J. Stabilometry in functional instability of the ankle and its value in predicting injury. *Med Sci Sports Med* 16: 64–66, 1984.
118. Tropp H, Odenrick P. Postural control in single-limb stance. *J Orthop Res* 6: 833–39, 1988.
119. Tropp H, Odenrick P, Gillquist J. Stabilometry recordings in functional and mechanical instability of the ankle joint. *Int J Sports Med* 6: 180–82, 1985.
120. Tsujimoto K, Andrish JT, Kambic BE, Grabiner M, Wink C. An investigation of the neurohistology and biomechanics of ACL reconstruction in goats: A comparison of primary repair and augmentation versus primary reconstruction alone. *Transactions of the 39th annual meeting of the Orthopaedic Research Society,* San Francisco, CA, 26, 1993.
121. Vangsness CT, Ennis M, Taylor JG, Atkinson R. Neural anatomy of the glenohumeral ligament, labrum, and subacromial bursa. *Arthroscopy* 11(2): 180–84, 1995.
122. Walla DJ, Albright JP, McAuley E, Martin RK, Eldridge V, El-Khoury G. Hamstring control and the unstable anterior cruciate ligament-deficient knee. *AJSM* 13(1): 34–39, 1985.
123. Warner JJP, Caborn DN. Overview of shoulder instability. *Crit Rev Phys Rehab Med* 4: 145–98, 1992.
124. Warner JJ, Lephart S, Fu FH. Role of proprioception in pathoetiology of shoulder instability. *Clin Orthop* 330: 35–39, 1996.
125. Warner JJP, Micheli LJ, Arslanian LE, Kennedy J, Kennedy R. Patterns of flexibility, laxity, and strength in normal shoulders and shoulders with instability and impingement. *AJSM* 18(4): 366–75, 1990.
126. Wegner L, Kisner C, Nichols D. Static and dynamic balance responses in persons with bilateral knee osteoarthritis. *J Orthop Sport Phys Therapy* 25(1): 13–18, 1997.
127. Wilkerson GB, Nitz AJ. Dynamic ankle stability: Mechanical and neuromuscular interrelationships. *J Sport Rehab* 3(1): 43–57, 1994.
128. Williams, WJ. A systems-oriented evaluation of the role of joint receptors and other afferents in position and motion sense. *Crit Rev Biomed Eng* 7: 23–77, 1981.
129. Zätterström R, Fridén T, Lindstrand A, Moritz U. The effect of physiotherapy on standing balance in chronic anterior cruciate ligament insufficiency. *AJSM* 22(4): 531–36, 1994.
130. Zoltan DJ, Reinecke C, Indelicato PA. Synthetic and allograft anterior cruciate ligament reconstruction. *Clin Sports Med* 7(4): 773–84, 1988.

CHAPTER 29

The Role of Proprioception in Patients With DJD and Following Total Knee Arthroplasty

C. Buz Swanik, PhD, ATC
Harry E. Rubash, MD
Robert L. Barrack, MD
Scott M. Lephart, ATC

Introduction

In recent years an extensive body of literature has evolved, which has elucidated the complex relationship between capsuloligamentous structures, proprioception, and joint function. In addition to their mechanical role, research has shown that capsuloligamentous structures possess neurosensory properties that mediate neuromuscular control for dynamic restraint and motor coordination (Borsa et al. 1997).

Neurological feedback from the joint capsule and surrounding ligaments is utilized by the neuromuscular control apparatus to regulate muscle activity for coordinated movements and dynamic joint stability. Kålund and coworkers (1990) suggest that general motor control and coordination may be impaired if normal joint proprioception is compromised. Research on anterior cruciate ligament- (ACL-) and posterior cruciate ligament- (PCL-) deficient knees has demonstrated that proprioception is diminished and that strong correlation exists between diminished proprioception and functional tests of the knee (Barrett 1991; Lephart 1992; Safran et al. 1996).

In a normal population, proprioceptive acuity also declines with chronological age and to a greater extent in the arthritic joint (Barrack et al. 1983a; Barrett, Skinner et al. 1984b; Kleinbart et al; 1992, Kokmen et al. 1978; Warren et al. 1993). Joint laxity, inflammation, and pain are closely associated with joint pathology and have been adopted as experimental models to assess the effects of degenerative joint disease (DJD) on proprioception. Decreased joint space height and inflammation alters tension on the capsuloligamentous tissue and may cause proprioceptive deficits in the arthritic joint (Attfield et al. 1996). Joint inflammation also contributes to arthritic pain, which may impede afferent information concerning joint motion and position sense (Schaible & Schmidt 1985). Proprioceptive deficits resulting from joint pathology may have a deleterious effect on the dynamic restraint capabilities of muscles surrounding joints. These deficits are related to functional disability and limit an individual's capacity to perform activities of daily living (ADL) (Andriacchi et al. 1982; Barrack et al. 1983a; Skinner et al. 1984a; Dorr et al. 1988; Lephart et al. 1992a; Lephart et al. 1992b; Borsa et al. 1997).

Total knee arthroplasty (TKA) combined with rehabilitation may restore proprioception, neuromuscular control, and functional performance by retensioning the capsuloligamentous structures, reducing pain, and interrupting chronic inflammation. However, researchers and clinicians remain divided over the importance of retaining the cruciate ligaments for additional afferent feedback after TKA. It is argued that preservation of the cruciate ligaments restores proprioception and neuromuscular control, ultimately improving prosthesis longevity and the functional outcome of TKA.

Clinical research comparing proprioception after TKA with several prosthetic designs has been inconclusive. Subjective evaluations after bilateral TKA do not demonstrate significant differences. However, kinematic and functional scores during stair climbing slightly favor cruciate retaining designs. Ongoing research continues to examine the influence of prosthetic design for restoring joint proprioception, stability, and function.

The following discussion defines the role of sensory receptors and neuromuscular control mechanisms that contribute to joint proprioception and function in the pathological knee. The theoretical framework and clinical research concerning diminished joint sensation in patients with DJD is examined, followed by a review of literature demonstrating the impact of TKA and prosthetic design on proprioception, neuromuscular control, and functional stability.

Proprioception and Neuromuscular Control

The role of articular and tenomuscular mechanoreceptors in providing afferent feedback to the central nervous system (CNS) is well established (Freeman & Wyke1966; Finsterbush & Friedman1975; Kennedy et al. 1982; Alexiades et al. 1989). Peripheral mechanoreceptors within articular and tenomuscular structures mediate neuromuscular control by conveying joint motion and position sense to the individual. This information is used for preparatory and reactive muscle activation necessary for dynamic restraint and motor coordination. Mechanoreceptors function by transducing mechanical deformation of tissue into frequency-modulated neural signals (Grigg 1994). These signals provide sensory information concerning internal and external forces acting on the joint.

Mechanoreceptors can be classified according to their responses to mechanical stimuli as slow adapting (SA) and quick adapting (QA) (Guyton 1981, Grigg 1994). The QA mechanoreceptors decrease their discharge rate to extinction within milliseconds of the onset of a continuous stimulus, while SA mechanoreceptors continue to discharge. The QA mechanoreceptors are very sensitive to changes in stimulation and are thought to mediate the sensation of joint motion. The SA mechanoreceptors are maximally stimulated at specific joint angles and thus are thought to mediate the sensation of joint position (Freeman & Wyke 1966b; Grigg 1994).

Three morphological types of articular mechanoreceptors have been identified in the knee: Pacinian corpuscles, Meissner corpuscles, and free nerve endings (Freeman & Wyke 1966; Grigg 1994; Kennedy et al. 1982; Schultz et al. 1984). Pacinian corpuscles, found in the joint capsule, are classified as QA (Freeman & Wyke 1966; Grigg 1994). Meissner corpuscles and free nerve endings are located in ligaments, menisci, and capsular tissue and are both grouped as SA (Alexiades et al. 1989; Schultz et al. 1984). Free nerve endings are inactive during normal joint loads but become active when articular tissues are subjected to damaging mechanical deformation. Free nerve endings are also chemosensitive, especially to various inflammatory mediators present in the arthritic joint.

Debate exists over the relative contribution of articular afferents for joint sensation because mechanoreceptors in articular structures appear to be stimulated only when under considerable loads (Solomonow et al. 1987). However, Johansson and coworkers 1986) contend that articular receptors may provide continuous feedback during submaximal loading by eliciting frequent and potent effects on the gamma motor nerves that regulate muscle spindles. Muscle spindles then regulate muscle activity through modulation of the stretch reflex. Changes in joint position are accompanied by simultaneous alterations in muscle length and tension. Muscle spindles, imbedded within skeletal muscle, detect length and rate of length changes, transmitting these signals to the CNS by way of afferent nerves (Barker 1974; Clark et al. 1985; Guyton 1981). Golgi tendon organs (GTO) are also capable of regulating muscle activity and are responsible for monitoring muscle tension (Hutton & Atwater 1992). Located within the tendon and tenomuscular junction, GTOs serve to protect the tenomuscular unit by reflexively inhibiting muscle activation when excessive tension may cause structural damage. Conscious awareness of joint motion and position is essential for proper joint function in activities of daily living, while unconscious proprioception modulates muscle function and initiates reflex stabilization.

The efferent (motor) response to sensory information is termed neuromuscular control (Jonsson et al. 1989; Kandell et al. 1996). Two motor control mechanisms are involved with interpreting afferent information and coordinating efferent responses (Dunn et al. 1986; Kandell et al. 1996). Preparatory (feedforward) and reflexive (feedback) neuromuscular control mechanisms are both required for motor coordination and dynamic joint stabilization (Kandell et al. 1996; Lephart et al. 1994). Conscious awareness of joint motion and position in the knee is essential for placement of the lower extremity during ambulation, while preparatory and reflexive muscle activation provide necessary dynamic stabilization for joint protection. Balance is influenced by the same sensory information that mediates joint proprioception and is partially dependent upon the inherent ability to integrate joint position sense with neuromuscular control. Balance, therefore, is frequently used to assess functional joint stability, and deficits may result from diminished proprioception in the lower extremity. Strong correlation exists between proprioception and function in the knee (Borsa et al. 1997; Barrett 1991; Lephart et al. 1992; Safran et al. 1996).

Damage to capsuloligamentous structures creates a mechanical disturbance (instability) or uncontrolled translation of the joint surfaces relative to one another (Corrigan et al. 1992). Because these structures contain extensive neural networks, neurological feedback to the central nervous system is also disrupted (Freeman et al. 1966; Johansson et al. 1991; Katonis et al. 1991). A latency period in reflexive muscle activation has been demonstrated when capsuloligamentous structures are damaged, presumably a result of joint deafferentation (Beard et al. 1993; Wojtys & Huston 1994). Furthermore, the sequence and pattern of muscle activation is altered during functional activities (Kålund et al. 1990; Ciccotti et al. 1994; Lephart 1997). These proprioceptive and neuromuscular characteristics coupled with mechanical instability leads to functional instability or episodes of "giving way." Repeated episodes of "giving way" cause further damage to the articular cartilage and capsuloligamentous structures (see figure 29.1).

Degenerative Joint Disease

Degenerative joint disease is the most common systemic disorder in synovial joints such as the knees and hips (Kosser 1996). Patients suffering from DJD complain of joint pain, instability, and decreased function. Prolonged weight bearing and ambulation usually aggravate these symptoms. Although synovial joints are well adapted to sustain and distribute mechanical stress, joint function is dependent on the hyaline cartilage that covers the adjacent articular surfaces. Excessive joint forces can damage the articular cartilage, decreasing its capacity to endure stress and initiating the chronic cycle of disrepair. Although joint inflammation, pain, and deformity occur as a result of DJD, the mechanism for dynamic restraint is also disrupted. Disturbances in the afferent or efferent pathways impair joint proprioception and neuromuscular control. Ultimately, the

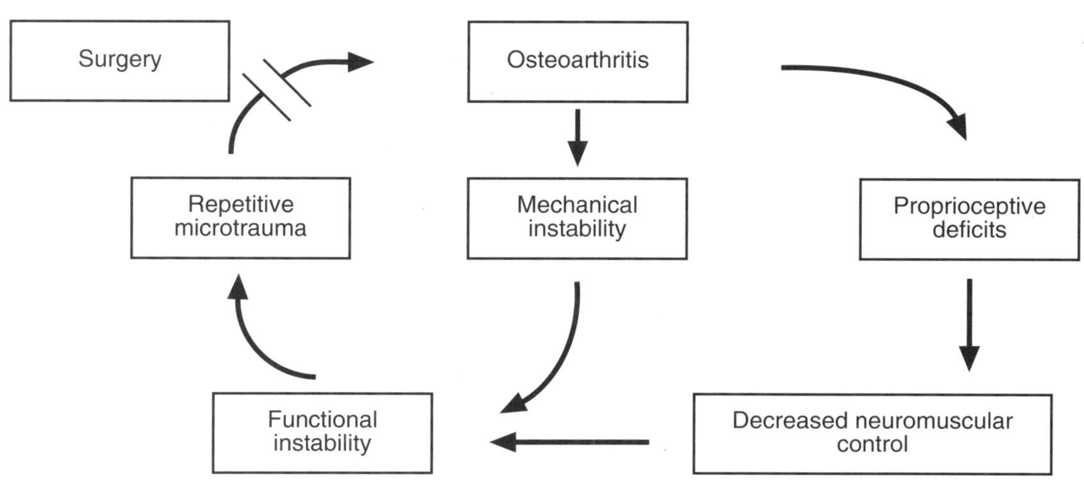

Figure 29.1 Functional stability paradigm depicting the influence of osteoarthritis on mechanical instability and proprioception, diminishing neuromuscular control and functional stability, which predisposes the knee to repetitive microtrauma. (Reproduced by kind permission of Human Kinetics, from: Lephart, SM, Henry, TJ The physiological basis for open and closed kinetic chain rehabilitation for the upper extremity. *J Sport Rehabil*, 5: 71-87, 1996.)

capability of tenomuscular structures to absorb joint forces diminishes the dynamic restraint mechanism. Consequently, excessive joint loads transmitted to the static restraints and subchondral bone accelerate the disease process. The result is an inflamed, deformed, and painful joint with diminished static and dynamic restraint capabilities.

Etiology and Pathophysiology of Degenerative Joint Disease

Articular cartilage functions to reduce peak stress and shearing forces between joint surfaces. A highly specialized tissue, it is both strong and elastic with a very low coefficient of friction (Kosser 1996). Chondrocytes maintain articular cartilage homeostasis but the intraarticular environment is avascular, and the synovial fluid must provide nutrients to these important cells. Therefore, damage to the articular surface significantly alters cartilage metabolism. Because articular cartilage exhibits poor healing qualities, it may initiate or potentiate DJD.

Chronological age is the strongest determinant of the onset and progression of DJD (Kosser 1996). In addition, a history of obesity, joint injury, participation in power sports (i.e., American football), and excessive repetitive behavior may predispose individuals to DJD. These conditions create abnormal mechanical stress, abrading the articular cartilage that is responsible for distributing joint loads to subchondral bone. Chemical mediators are released from damaged cells, initiating the acute inflammatory response. Increased arterial vasodilation and synovial membrane permeability permit degrading enzymes and growth factors to infiltrate the synovial fluid. Repair of minor articular defects may be possible; however, excessive damage to the cartilage diminishes its capacity to distribute stress. Therefore, joint loads are transmitted to subchondral bone, stimulating bone resorption and remodeling. New subchondral bone formation alters the joint surface and causes malalignment.

The chronic presence of degrading enzymes coupled with malalignment changes the length/tension relationship of capsuloligamentous structures and compromises joint stability (Schultz et al. 1984). The ACL is often lax due to pathological changes and completely absent in approximately 50% of TKA patients (Cloutier 1991; Li & Ritter 1995). The PCL remains intact in as high as 99% of TKA patients, but its mechanical properties can be compromised (Sharma & Yi-Chung 1997). Severe varus or valgus malalignment also causes capsular stretching and asymmetrical forces across the collateral ligament. These changes perpetuate the inflammatory cycle by creating abnormal mechanical stress on the articular cartilage.

Proprioception

Deficits in proprioception also occur with the normal aging process and may impair the dynamic mechanism for knee stability. Cross-sectional studies correlating age with proprioception reveal a continuous decline in the sensation of joint motion and position with increasing age (see figure 29.2) (Kokmen et al. 1978; Barrack et al. 1983a; Skinner et al. 1984a; Kaplan et al. 1985; Barrett 1991). Diminished proprioception is also identified as a contributing factor to the loss of balance and is a predictive measure for falls in the elderly (Petrella et al. 1997; Lord et al. 1991). Regular physical activity appears to attenuate the decline in proprioception with age, suggesting disuse atrophy as a possible causative factor (see figure 29.3). However, patients with DJD demonstrate greater decrements in joint sensibility when compared to age-matched controls (see figure 29.4) (Skinner et al. 1984, Skinner & Barrack 1991; Barrack et al. 1983a; Kaplan et al. 1985; Barrett et al. 1991). Contemporary research suggests that diminished proprioception may initiate or accelerate the process of DJD. Because the loss of proprioceptive acuity appears to occur early in the diseased joint, the mechanism for dynamic joint stabilization is also compromised (Barrett 1991 Simmons et al. 1996a).

Histological studies on human cruciate ligaments have discovered low populations of mechanoreceptors and neurological degeneration in arthritic joints (Schultz et al. 1984; Alexiades et al. 1989). Finsterbush and Friedman (1975) confirmed that sensory denervation of the knee precedes the pathological changes occurring throughout the joint. Barrack and coworkers (1983a) contend that disruption of proprioception and the dynamic restraint mechanism may precipitate DJD by changing one's weight-bearing patterns. Functional outcome research substantiates this theory, since Berman and coworkers (1987) documented abnormal gait patterns preceding radiographic evidence of joint pathology. The loss of joint afferents disrupts normal neuromuscular coactivation, reducing the shock absorbing capacity of dynamic structures and distributing excessive joint forces to the soft tissue restraints, articular surface, and subchondral bone (Andriacchi & Galante 1988; Warren et al. 1993). This data suggests that proprioception from capsuloligamentous tissue is lost early in the degenerative

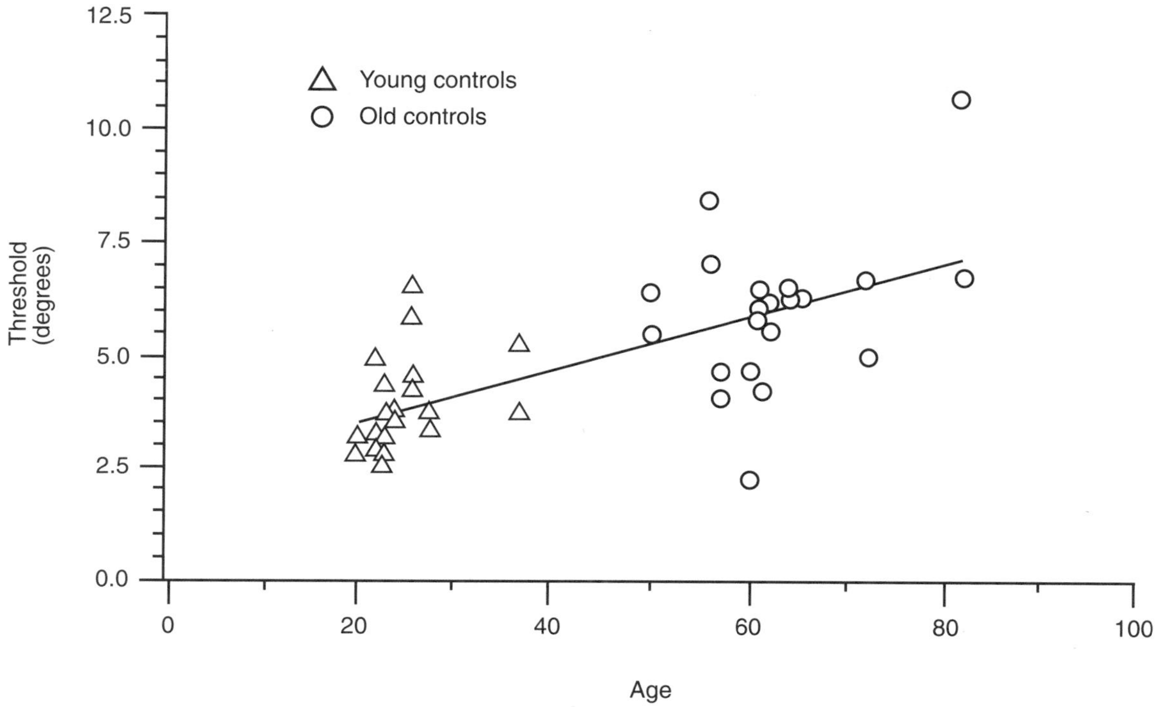

Figure 29.2 Inaccuracy in knee joint position sense increases with chronological age. (Reproduced by kind permission of Elsevier Science Ltd., from: Skinner HB, Barrack RL. Joint position sense in the normal and pathologic knee joint. *J Electromyogr Kinesiol*. 1(3): 180-190, 1991.)

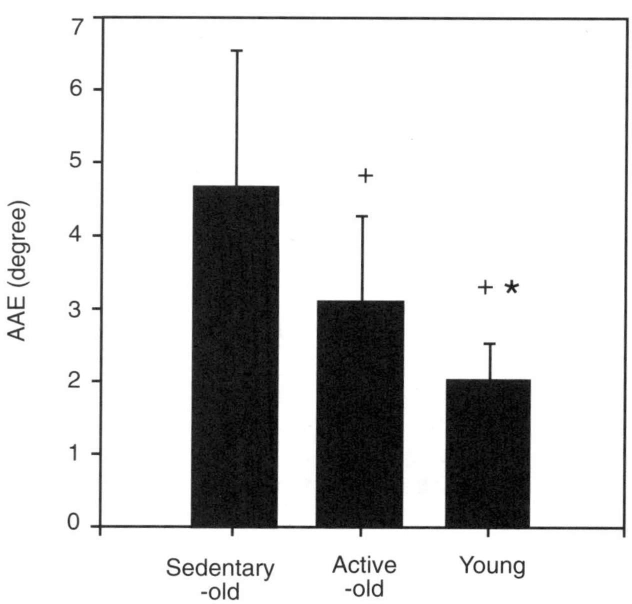

Figure 29.3 Less error in active reproduction of joint position among active young and elderly subjects when compared to sedentary elderly subjects. + = Significant difference from sedentary-old ($p < .03$). * = Significant difference from active-old ($p < .001$). (Reproduced by kind permission of Williams & Wilkins, From: Petrella RJ, Lattanzio PJ, Nelson MG. Effect of age and activity on knee joint proprioception. *Am J Phys Med and Rehabil*. 76(3):235-241, 1997.)

process, and a neurological deficit initiates or at least accelerates degenerative changes in the pathological joint (Barrett et al. 1991; Barrack et al. 1983a; Kleinbart et al. 1992; Warren et al. 1993).

Joint Laxity and Proprioception

Unequal redistribution of joint loads causes the articular surface to deteriorate, diminishing the joint space height and altering the balance of tension on the surrounding soft tissue (see figure 29.5). Inadequate tension on capsuloligamentous structures may be responsible for the deficits in proprioception demonstrated by patients with hypermobility syndrome (HMS). Hall and coworkers (1995) observed significant deficits in women with HMS when compared to age-matched controls, by measuring proprioception with ability to detect joint motion. Barrack and coworkers (1983) concluded that decreased joint position sense in professional dancers might result from joint hypermobility and consequently predispose dancers to acute and chronic injuries. In patients with DJD, capsuloligamentous laxity is created by the decrease in joint space height. Without sufficient tension, mechanoreceptors located within these structures are not stimulated and proprioceptive information is diminished (Nicholas 1970; Barrack

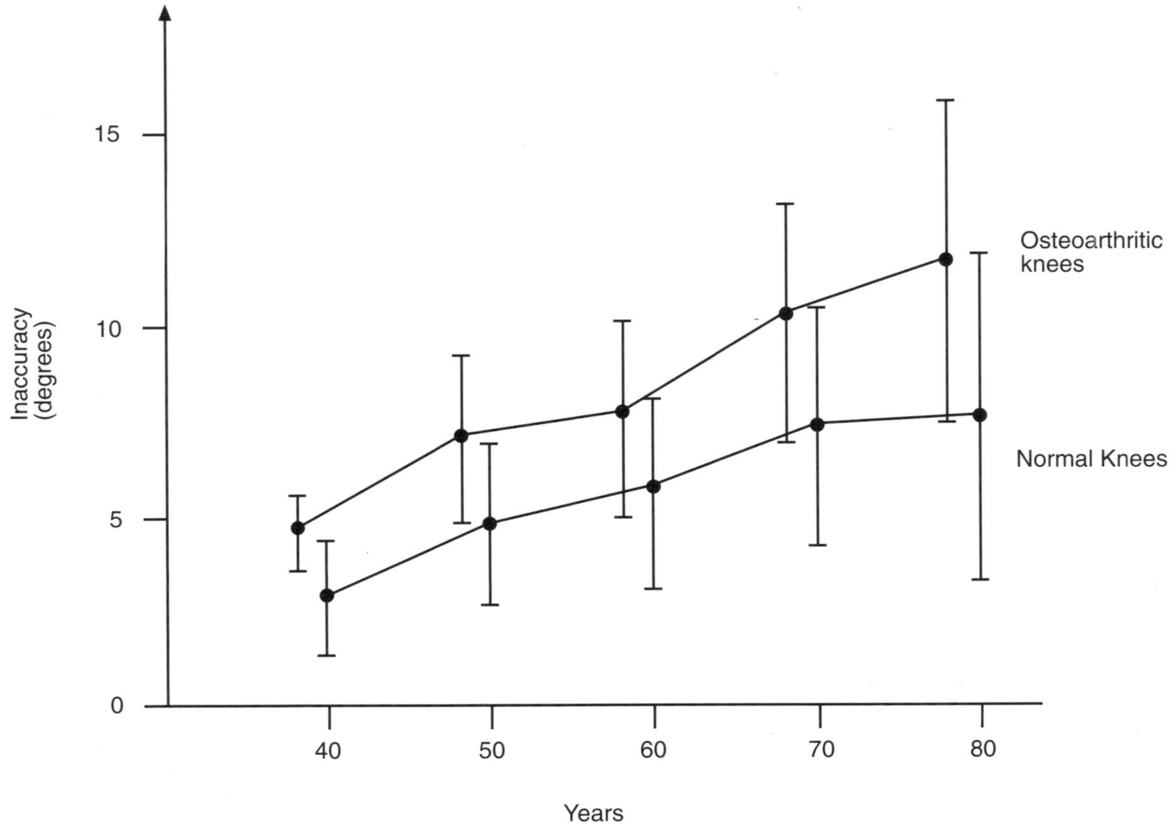

Figure 29.4 Inaccuracy detecting joint position increased to a greater extent in patients with osteoarthritis than age-matched controls. (Reproduced by kind permission of British Editorial Society of Bone and Joint Surgery, from: Barrett DS, Cobb AG, and Bentley G. Joint proprioception in normal, osteoarthritic, and replaced knees. *J Bone Joint Surg.* 73-B:55, 1991.).

et al. 1983b; Barrack et al. 1991; Barrett 1991b; Hall et al. 1995).

Inflammation and Proprioception

In the past, studies on age-related changes in the knee have focused on structural deformities of bone geometry. However, abnormal stress causes additional microtrauma to the surrounding soft tissue, exacerbating chronic swelling. Joint inflammation results in greater intraarticular pressure and increased temperature. When combined with noxious chemical substances and local ischemia, the chronic inflammatory condition can cause significant pain. Both pain and joint inflammation have the ability to disrupt joint sensibility. However, the mechanisms are unclear since most research on joint pain involves reproducing joint inflammation (Barrack et al. 1983b; Kennedy et al. 1982; Marshall et al. 1993; Sluka 1996; Guyton 1981). Joint effusion in the knee appears to decrease mechanoreceptor afference, ultimately inhibiting or significantly altering muscular activation (Barrack et al. 1983b; Kennedy et al. 1982; Marshall et al. 1993). With 60 cc of experimentally induced joint effusion, 30 to 50% reflex-evoked quadriceps inhibition has been demonstrated (Kennedy et al. 1982). Conflicting results with noninflammatory fluids suggest that joint effusion alone is not responsible for deficits in proprioception and may enhance joint sensibility if capsular tension is increased (McNair et al. 1995; Ferrell et al. 1992). An alternate mechanism that includes pain may explain deficits in proprioception.

Pain and Proprioception

Joint inflammation also produces noxious stimuli that can inhibit information concerning joint motion and position. The gate theory of pain management implies that the CNS constantly balances somatosensory and nociceptive information, each with the capability to inhibit the other (Guyton 1981; Melzack & Wall 1965). Pain also initiates primitive reflex motor reactions, "withdrawal reflexes," which

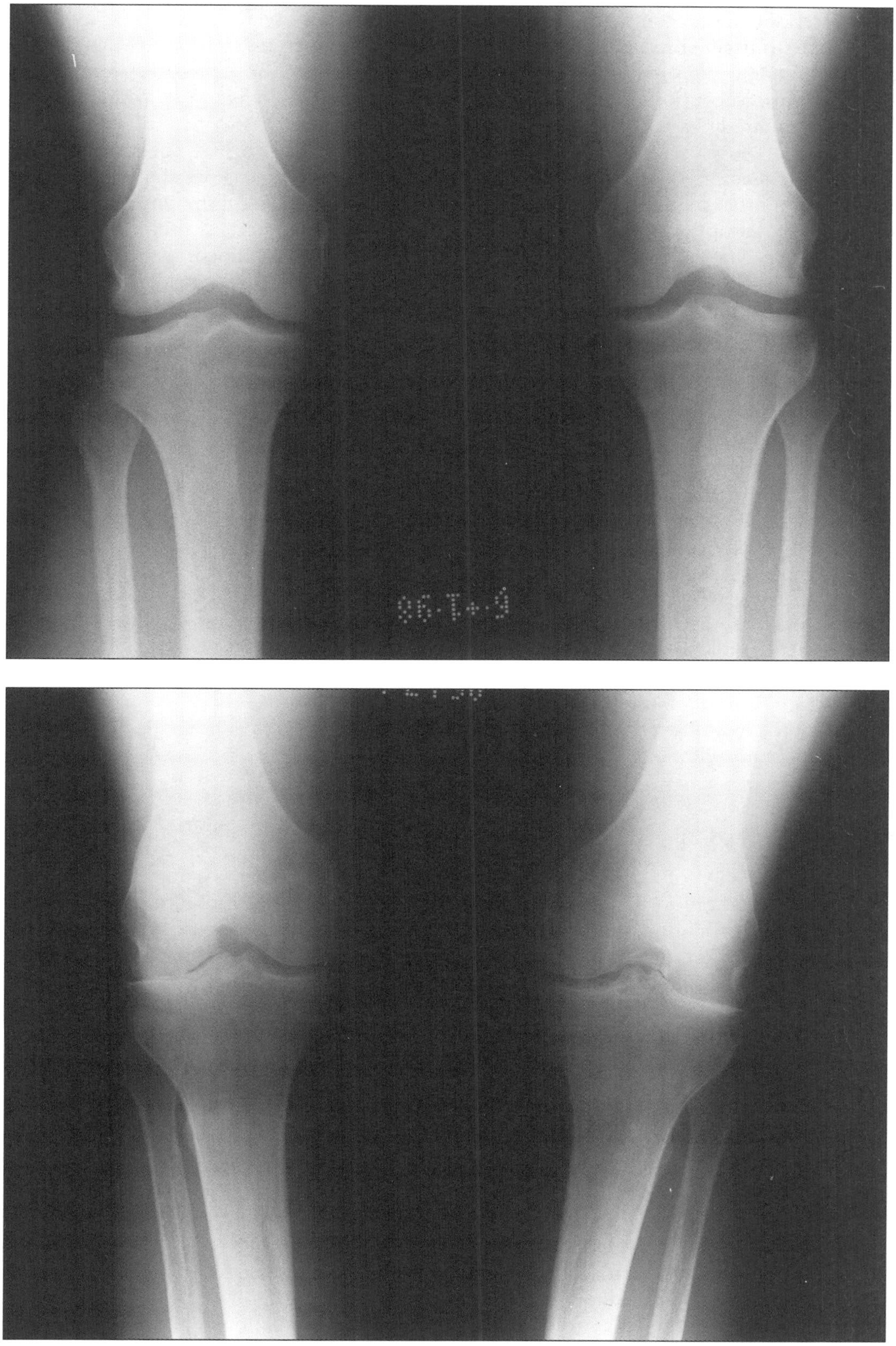

a

b

Figure 29.5 (*a*) X ray of normal knee joint alignment, (*b*) X ray of deformed joint resulting from subchondral bone remodeling.

may disrupt descending motor commands or reflex pathways from the muscle spindle system. Joint laxity, inflammation, and pain may all contribute to the deficits in proprioception among patients with DJD when compared to age-matched healthy subjects.

The process of degenerative joint disease, with the associated pain, inflammation, and decreased joint space, results in disruption of the normal neuromuscular control mechanism necessary for joint stabilization. Abnormal afferent information in the arthritic joint is believed to be responsible for the phenomenon of arthrogenous muscle inhibition (AMI), which is the inability to achieve full voluntary muscle activation (Hurley & Newham 1993; Sharma & Yi-Chung 1997). Although AMI has not been directly linked to proprioceptive deficits, the presence of AMI in arthritic patients illustrates a disruption in the neuromuscular control mechanism. Aberrations in the muscle activity necessary for dynamic restraint may contribute to excessive forces on the capsule, ligaments, and articular surfaces. Gait abnormalities demonstrated by patients with DJD may represent motor coordination deficits or attempts to augment proprioceptive information (Stauffer et al. 1977). Encouraging results assessing proprioception after intervention with TKA revealed that the loss of joint sensibility is reversible in some patients with DJD.

Total Knee Arthroplasty

Severe degenerative changes in the osteoarthritic knee are painful and debilitating, often requiring knee replacement surgery. The goals of TKA include alleviating pain, improving stability, and restoring function (Insall et al. 1989). Although mechanical stability is critical to the success of TKA, reestablishing proprioception and dynamic restraint aids in the recovery of joint function and should maximize prosthesis longevity. Clinicians continue to discuss the effect of TKA and the influence of several prosthetic designs on proprioception in patients electing primary TKA. When the cruciate ligaments are intact, PCL-retaining prostheses appear to offer certain biomechanical advantages that may result in more physiological motion. Specifically, preservation of the PCL is responsible for initiating femoral rollback during knee flexion. This serves to increase knee flexion range of motion and extensor mechanism function (Kelman et al. 1989, Mahoney et al. 1994).

In addition, retaining the cruciate for its neurosensory properties contributes to a more normal gait and "feel" of the knee after joint replacement (Galante 1973; Jefferson & Whittle 1990; Marmor 1993; Cloutier 1991; Pritchett 1996). Although PCL-retaining (CR) and PCL-substituting (PS) designs appear equal in patient satisfaction, restoration of function, and long-term clinical results, efforts to establish differences in proprioception remain inconclusive. Proprioceptive feedback from the cruciates would theoretically enhance neuromuscular control, ultimately improving dynamic restraint, functional outcome, and prosthesis longevity.

Resurfacing the articulating segments of the femur, tibia, and patella accomplishes the goals of joint replacement surgery. Reestablishing the joint line and retensioning lax capsuloligamentous structures is necessary for mechanical stability, provided the tension between collateral structures is balanced (Attfield et al. 1996). When joint forces are not balanced, excessive motion can result in prosthetic loosening, accelerated wear, and episodes of instability. Recent literature suggests that retensioning soft tissue may be important for restoring proprioception and therefore the mechanism for dynamic stability.

Proprioception

The effects of TKA on proprioception demonstrate that knee joint replacement, although traumatic, does not significantly decrease joint position or motion sense (Barrack et al. 1983; Skinner et al. 1984). Moreover, research by Barrett, Cobb, and Bentley (1991) and Warren and associates (1993) suggests that TKA may improve joint position sense when comparisons are made with the contralateral limb and an osteoarthritic control group. When a prospective study assessed proprioception by measuring the subject's ability to represent the position of the leg using a model, significant improvements were demonstrated 6 mo postoperatively (Attfield et al. 1996). It is reasonable to speculate that by alleviating pain, reestablishing the joint space, and retensioning the soft tissue, proprioception can be improved after TKA. Disuse atrophy associated with DJD may also be a contributing factor to deficits in proprioception. Several studies have demonstrated a relationship between proprioception and the level of physical activity (Petrella et al. 1997; Barrack et al. 1983b; Lephart et al. 1996). Following TKA, the response characteristics of mechanoreceptors in both capsuloligamentous and tenomuscular structures may be modified, enhancing the perception of joint motion and position.

Function

Functional assessments before and after TKA demonstrate improvements in range of motion, gait parameters, and stair climbing (Simon et al. 1983; Dorr et al. 1988; Kroll et al. 1989; Jevsevar et al. 1993). Patterns of knee movement after TKA resemble healthy knees (Jevsevar et al. 1993). Thus, the motor control mechanisms governing motion usually remain intact. Furthermore, Skinner and coworkers (1984b) found that gait parameters correlated with combined clinical and proprioception scores. These studies build a relationship between proprioception and function after TKA, suggesting that the maintenance of proprioceptive qualities is a potential mechanism for improving functional outcome after surgery (Andriacchi et al. 1982; Dorr et al. 1988; Insall 1993; Li & Ritter 1995; Simmons et al. 1996b). However, persistent abnormalities in gait parameters exist and can be construed as evidence for deficits in proprioception after TKA (Skinner et al. 1984; Stauffer et al. 1977). The presence of pain, swelling, and possibly unbalanced soft tissue tension after TKA may cause aberrations in the sensory feedback necessary for motor control. Skinner and coworkers (1984) suggest that the loss of proprioceptive function may also be responsible for discrepancies between clinical and functional outcomes following TKA. However, after TKA it is difficult to isolate gait abnormalities caused by biomechanical considerations or compensatory muscle activation strategies mediated by proprioception.

Prosthetic Design

Debate still exists regarding the criteria for selecting a prosthetic design for TKA. Three prosthetic designs appear to offer excellent outcomes for TKA. Unicondylar designs retain both the cruciate ligaments, PCL-retaining designs (CR) sacrifice only the ACL, and posterior stabilized designs (PS) sacrifice both of the cruciates. A cam mechanism substitutes for the PCL (see figure 29.6) in posterior stabilized designs. Past arguments for selecting a CR or PS knee replacement were based solely on biomechanical issues and the theoretical advantages of saving the PCL. Contemporary research suggests that the neurosensory contribution of the cruciates may be critical when selecting a type of implant design (Barrett et al. 1991; Simmons et al. 1996a; Pritchett et al. 1996; Li & Ritter 1995; Moilanen & Freeman 1995).

Currently, three general considerations exist when selecting a prosthetic design: consistency, durability, and function (Insall et al. 1989). The consistency of the result depends in part on the surgical procedure. For implantation of unicondylar designs, an island is created out of the tibial eminence. This may predispose the cruciates to potential rupture if exact restoration of the joint line is not achieved (Pritchett 1996). The PS designs are more frequently utilized for correcting large deformities. Implantation is technically less complicated for PS designs but involves excising small amount of extra bone from the intracondylar notch (Faris et al. 1988; Freeman & Railton 1988; Insall 1993). The durability of all three prostheses is design specific and is generally comparable at 8 and 10 yr follow-ups. All three designs attain survival rates of approximately 90%, although long-term data remains incomplete (Scott et al. 1988; Ritter et al. 1989; Cloutier 1991; Li & Ritter 1995). Functional outcome measures comparing CR and PS designs have established some advantages to retaining the cruciate ligaments.

During gait analysis and stair climbing, patients with the least constrained CR designs exhibit more normal range of motion, while sacrificing the cruciates results in less efficient motion and quadriceps activity (Andriacchi & Galante 1988; Dorr et al. 1988; Kelman et al. 1989; Warren et al. 1993). These differences are influenced by individual prosthetic designs imposing various strains on the surrounding soft tissue (Andriacchi et al. 1982). Both joint kinematics and proprioception would be affected, and it is their interaction that may be responsible for gait abnormalities. However, subjective data shows no significant difference in patient satisfaction or preferences for the CR or PS design (Dorr et al. 1988; Becker et al. 1991; Cameron & Jung 1988).

Proprioception

Although CR and PS models appear equal in providing satisfactory relief from pain, instability, and dysfunction, proponents of CR designs suggest that neurosensory loss from resecting the cruciates may result in additional proprioceptive, motor, and reflexive disturbances. Theoretically, the direct automatic neuromotor link between ligaments and muscles is left intact with a CR prosthesis and may

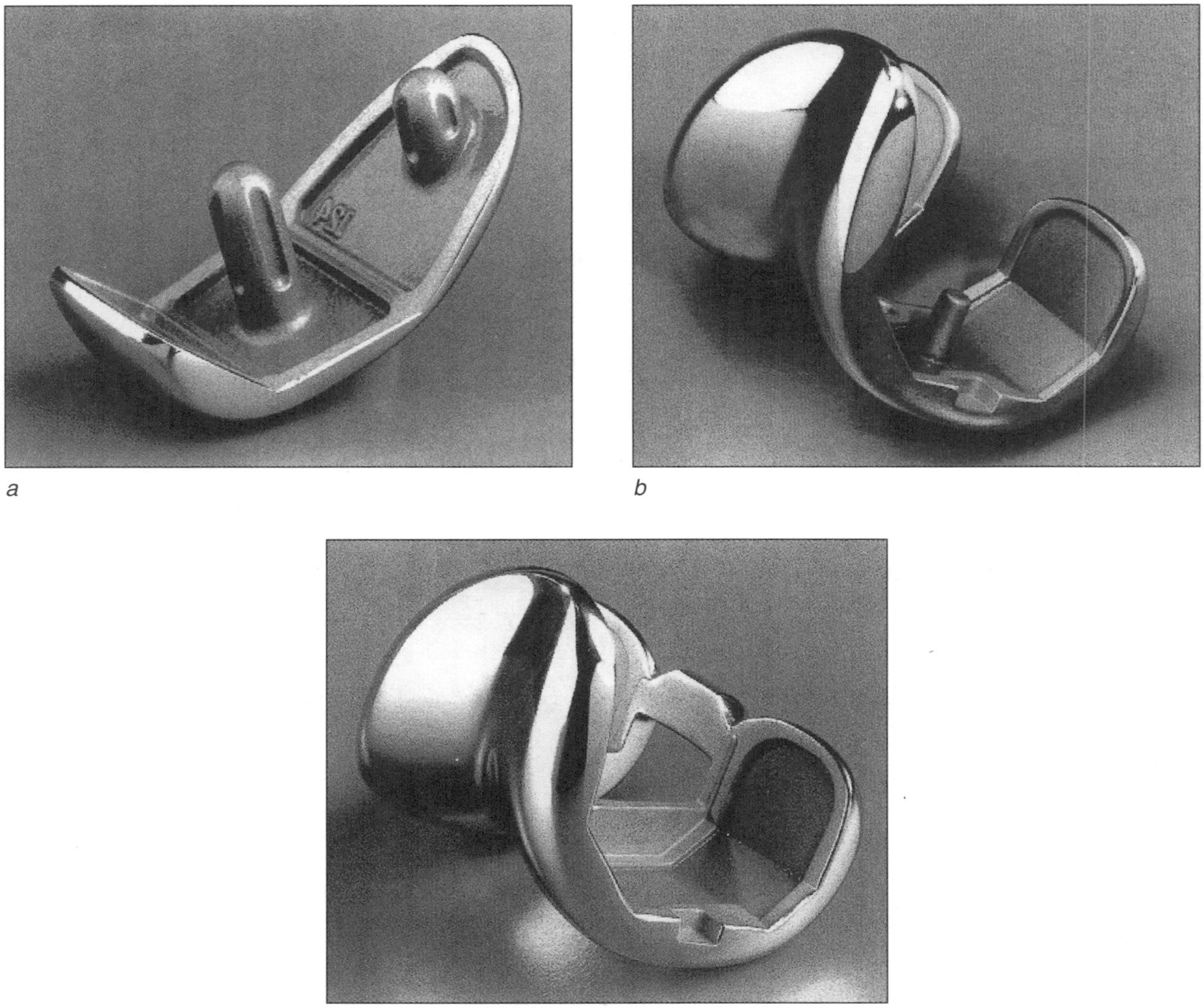

a b c

Figure 29.6 (*a*) Unicondylar prosthesis, (*b*) PCL-retaining prosthesis, (*c*) PCL-substituting prosthesis. (Photographs courtesy of Zimmer Reed Assoc.)

maximize the recovery of proprioceptive acuity with TKA. Additional sensory feedback would be utilized for cortical and reflexive muscle activation strategies, increasing motor coordination and dynamic restraint. More efficient muscular contractions would help dissipate shear forces on the joint and bone-prosthesis interface, increasing the durability of the implant and functional performance on ADLs. However, research linking proprioceptive benefits with prosthetic design has been contradictory.

Unicondylar Versus Total Knee Arthroplasty

Isolated tears of the ACL have been linked to knee proprioception deficits in otherwise-healthy adults (Barrack et al. 1989). This suggests that resecting an intact ACL with TKA may have deleterious effects on joint motion and position sense after surgery. A study that compared joint position sense in hinged (Noiles), total condylar, and CR (Polycentric) designs found no significant difference (Barrack et al. 1983a). Simmons and coworkers (1996) assessed kinesthetic sensations in the knee by measuring patients' ability to detect slow passive joint motion (TTDPM). No significant differences were found between the Miller-Galante unicondylar prosthesis and two total knee prostheses that included the Insall-Burstein II PS design and the Miller-Galante II CR design (see figure 29.7). This data suggests that capsuloligamentous destruction

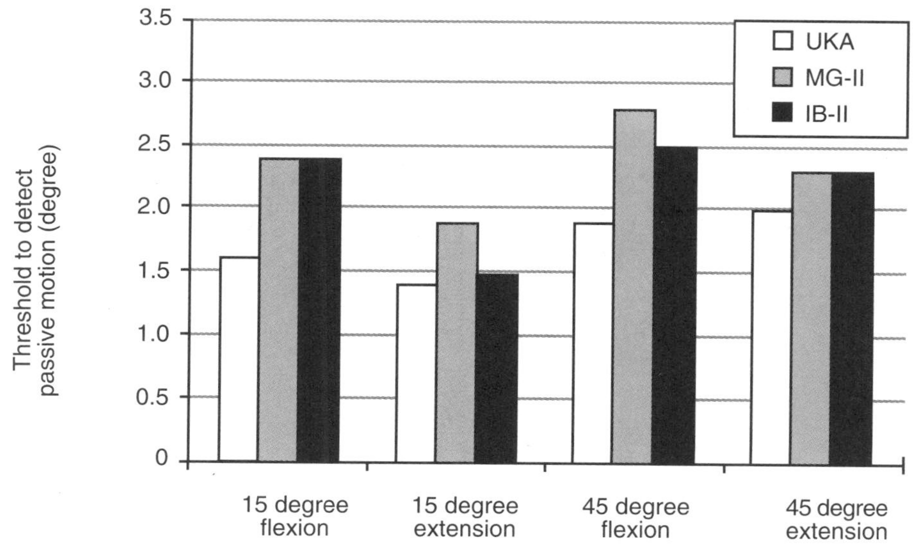

Figure 29.7 No significant differences in threshold to detect motion after unicondylar (UKA) vs. total knee arthroplasty with (M-G II) and without (I-B II) the posterior cruciate ligament. (Adapted from: Simmons S et al. *J Arthroplasty* 11(7):763-768, 1996.)

does not influence joint motion or position sense after joint replacement (Barrack et al. 1983a). However, Laurencin and associates (1991) conducted postoperative interviews and report that patients have a more normal-feeling knee with unicondylar knee arthroplasty when compared to TKA (Simmons et al. 1996). Skinner and coworkers (1984b) assessed proprioception by measuring both TTDPM and joint position sense among patients with CR Polycentric, total condylar, or Noiles prosthetic designs. Patients with the Polycentric design performed significantly better on TTDPM measurements; however, no significant differences between prostheses were found in joint position sense (see figure 29.7). Continued research applying a prospective randomized design may provide more conclusive data regarding the effect of ACL preservation on proprioception.

CR Versus PS

Like the ACL, a healthy PCL also contains an extensive neural network. It follows that a ruptured PCL creates not only a mechanical disturbance, but also interrupts neurological feedback to the central nervous system (Katonis et al. 1991). Safran and coworkers (1996) assessed proprioception in PCL-deficient patients and found significant deficits in the perception of joint motion. Retrospective studies have attempted to establish differences in proprioception after CR and PS TKA (Faris et al. 1988; Barrett et al. 1991; Warren et al. 1993; Ishii et al. 1997). Faris and associates (1988) and Simmons and coworkers (1996) compared CR vs. PS prostheses and found no significant differences in proprioception. However, Barrett, Cobb, and Bentley (1991) and Warren and associates (1993) observed significant increases in proprioception when CR designs were utilized, suggesting that it may be beneficial to save the PCL when feasible. These experiments were not randomized or prospective, which may explain the conflicting results. In addition, variables such as the degree of preoperative arthritis or soft tissue balance were not always controlled and can influence postsurgical proprioception values. Simmons and coworkers (1996) further stratified patients into groups with moderate (grade 2) and severe (grade 3) preoperative arthritis. The patients with severe DJD who received PS prostheses performed significantly better on threshold to detect passive motion (TTDPM) measurements than patients with the CR prostheses (see figure 29.8). Attfield and coworkers (1996) conducted a prospective study to determine the influence of prosthetic design but emphasized soft tissue imbalance using the Derby balancer (Attfield et al. 1994). Proprioception was assessed by measuring the subject's ability to represent knee position utilizing a large model of the leg. No significant differences were found between CR and PS. However, knees that achieved satisfactory balance ($< \pm 2^\circ$) in flexion and extension, rather than just extension, improved significantly on joint position measures (Attfield et al. 1996). This data suggests that soft tissue balance is an important factor medi-

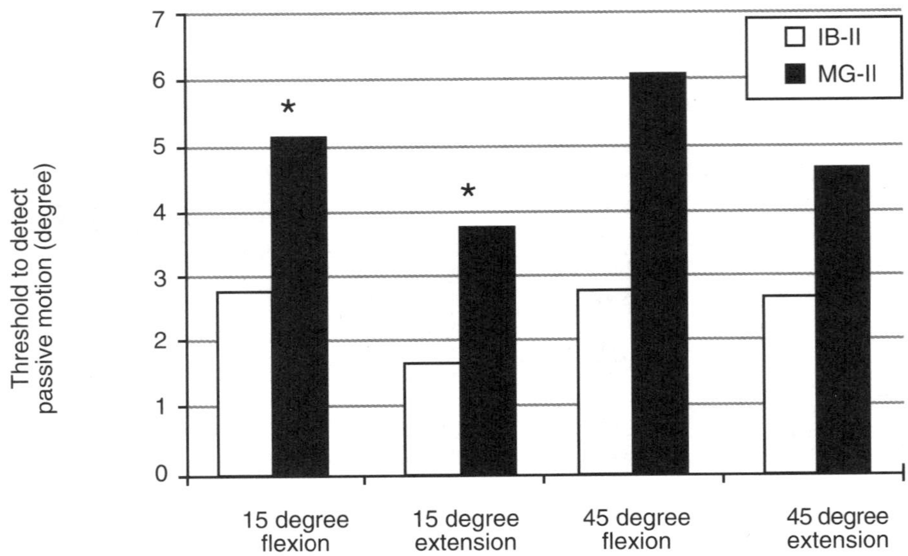

Figure 29.8 Significantly improved threshold to detect motion among patients with severe preoperative arthritis receiving the IB-II PCL-substituting design when compared to patients with MG-II PCL-retaining prosthesis. $*p < .05$. (Adapted from: Simmons S et al. *Clin Orthop,* 331:179-184, 1996.)

ating postoperative proprioception and should be controlled before comparing prosthetic design. The sample size and nonrandomized selection of prosthetic design may have compromised the results comparing PCL retension and resection in this study. Additional proprioception tests have investigated the influence of variables such as patellar replacement and the use of cement but have not shown significant differences (Ishii et al. 1997).

If proprioceptive feedback from the PCL is expected to benefit knee function, the existence of both reflexive and cortical pathways needs to be established linking the PCL and quadriceps muscle group. Raunest and coworkers (1996) demonstrated the reflexive neuromotor link in an animal model whereby loads of 200–500 N on the PCL elicited significant excitation of the quadriceps. Electromyographic (EMG) studies among patients with posterior laxity offer convincing evidence supporting cortical adaptations to quadriceps activity during gait. Cain and Schwab (1981) and Tibone and coworkers (1988) found that PCL-deficient subjects compensated for posterior laxity by unconsciously contracting their quadriceps early and for a prolonged period during gait analysis. Similarly, patients with PS prosthetics also appear to have inefficient (excessive) quadriceps activation (Dorr et al. 1988). Presumably, this aberration in muscle activity is a consequence of deafferentated mechanoreceptors from the PCL and concomitant loss of mechanical stability. If neurological degeneration of the mechanoreceptors in the PCL has not occurred and retensioning of the soft tissue is standardized, then improved proprioceptive values with CR TKA can be explained by the neurosensory properties in the PCL. In theory, restoring the cortical and reflex pathways necessary for motor coordination and dynamic stabilization will maintain intrinsic knee mechanics, avoid stress on the implant-bone interface, and increase prosthesis longevity (Andriacchi & Galante 1988, Dorr et al. 1988, Barrett 1991). To address these questions, the authors have initiated a prospective, randomized study that expects to provide objective data for surgical management decisions concerning TKA and prosthetic design. With the ability to measure proprioception, degenerative arthritis, and neuromuscular function preoperatively and compare these to postoperative measurements, a more powerful, well-controlled study may reveal results that are more conclusive. Research on proprioception must continue and is necessary to identify the effectiveness of medical treatments where joint function, cost containment, and patient satisfaction need to be considered (Ritter et al. 1995).

Summary

Mechanoreceptors in ligamentous and capsular tissue mediate joint motion and position sense. The conscious proprioceptive awareness is necessary for coordinated neuromuscular control, while unconscious awareness directs reflex muscle activity. Patients with DJD experience joint inflammation, pain, and deformity that diminish proprioception and may predispose them to episodes of joint instability and re-injury, leading to loss of function. Total knee arthroplasty may restore some proprioceptive acuity that has been lost with DJD and is associated with improved functional outcome. The neurosensory contribution of the ACL and PCL after TKA is at the center of debate concerning the selection of CR and PS prosthetic designs. Both have excellent outcome, yet research on knee proprioception has yielded inconclusive results when comparing the effects of unicondylar, CR, and PS designs. A prospective randomized design that controls for the degree of preoperative arthritis, deformity, and soft tissue balance would provide more meaningful information with respect to prosthetic design selection and proprioception.

References

1. Alexiades M, Scuderi G, Vigorita V, Scott WN. 1989. A histological study of the posterior cruciate ligament in the arthritic knee. *Am. J. Knee Surg.*, 2(4): 153–59.
2. Andriacchi TP, Galante JO, Fermier RW. 1982. The influence of total knee-replacement design on walking and stair climbing. *J. Bone Joint Surg.*, 64A: 1328.
3. Andriacchi TP, Galante JO. 1988. Retension of the posterior cruciate in total knee arthroplasty. *J. Arthroplasty*, (suppl): S13–19.
4. Attfield SF, Warren-Forward M, Wilton T, Sambatakakis A. 1994. Measurement of soft tissue imbalance in total knee arthroplasty using electronic instrumentation. *Med. Eng. Phys.*, 16: 501–505.
5. Attfield SF, Wilton TJ, Pratt DJ, Sambatakakis A. 1996. Soft tissue balance and recovery of proprioception after knee replacement. *J. Bone Joint Surg.*, 78B(4): 540–45.
6. Barker D. 1974. The morphology of muscle receptors. In *Handbook of sensory physiology*, Hunt CC, ed. Berlin: Springer-Verlag, 191–234.
7. Barrack RL, Skinner HB, Cook SD, Haddad JR. 1983a. Effect of articular disease and total arthroplasty on knee joint position sense. *J. Neurophysiol.*, 50: 684–87.
8. Barrack RL, Skinner HB, Brunet ME, Cook SD. 1983b. Joint laxity and proprioception in the knee. *Phys. Sports Med.*, 11: 130–35.
9. Barrack RL, Skinner HB, Brunet ME, Buckley SL. 1989. Proprioception in the anterior cruciate ligament deficient knee. *Am. J. Sports Med.*, 17: 1–6.
10. Barrett DS, Cobb AG, and Bentley G. 1991. Joint proprioception in normal, osteoarthritic, and replaced knees. *J. Bone Joint Surg.*, 73B: 53–56.
11. Barrett DS. 1991. Proprioception and function after anterior cruciate reconstruction. *J. Bone Joint Surg.*, 73B: 83–87.
12. Baxendale RH, Ferrell WR. 1987. Disturbances of proprioception at the human knee resulting from acute joint distension. *J. Physiol.*, 392: 60.
13. Beard DJ, Kyberd PJ, Fergusson CM, Dodd CAF. 1993. Proprioception after rupture of the anterior cruciate ligament. *J. Bone Joint Surg.*, 75B: 311–15.
14. Becker MW, Insall JN, Faris PM. 1991. Bilateral total knee arthroplasty: One cruciate retaining and one cruciate substituting. *Clin. Orthop.*, 271: 122.
15. Berman AT, Zarrto VJ, Bosacco M, Israelite C. 1987. Quantitative gait analysis after unilateral and bilateral total knee replacement. *J. Bone Joint Surg.*, 69A: 1340–345.
16. Borsa PA, Lephart SM, Irrgang JJ, Safran MR, Fu FH. 1997. The effects of joint position and direction of joint motion on proprioceptive sensibility in anterior cruciate ligament-deficient athletes. *Am. J. Sports Med.*, 25(3): 336–40.
17. Cain TE, Schwab GH. 1981. Performance of an athlete with straight posterior knee instability. *Am. J. Sports Med.*, 9: 203–208.
18. Cameron HU, Jung YB. 1988. A comparison of unicondylar knee replacement with total knee arthroplasty. *Orthop. Review*, 17: 983–88.
19. Ciccotti M, Kerlain R, Perry J, Pink, M. 1994. An electromyographic analysis of the knee during functional activities. II: The anterior cruciate ligament-deficient knee and reconstructed profiles. *Am. J. Sports Med.*, 22(5): 651–58.
20. Clark FJ, Burgess R, Chapin JW, Lipscomb WT. 1985. Role of intramuscular receptors in the awareness of limb position. *J. Neurophysiol.*, 54(6): 1529–540.
21. Cloutier JM. 1991. Long-term results after nonconstrained total knee arthroplasty. *Clin. Orthop.*, 236: 61.
22. Dorr LD, Ochsner JL, Gronley J, Perry J. 1988. Functional comparisons of posterior cruciate-retained versus cruciate-sacrificed total knee arthroplasty. *Clin. Orthop.*, 236: 36–43.
23. Dunn TG, Gillig SE, Ponser SE, Weil N. 1986. The learning process in biofeedback: Is it

feedforward or feedback. *Biofeedback Self Reg.*, 11(2): 143–55.
24. Ewald FC. 1989. The knee society total knee arthroplasty roentgenographic evaluation and scoring system. *Clin. Orthop.*, 248: 9–12.
25. Faris PM, Jiang CC, Otis JC, Manouel M. 1988. Proprioceptive input of the posterior cruciate ligament in knee prosthesis. *Trans. Orthop. Res. Soc.*, 13: 358.
26. Ferrell W, Crighton A, Sturrock R. 1992. Position sense at the interphalangeal joint is distorted in patients with rheumatoid arthritis of finger joints. *Exp. Physiol.*, 77: 675–80.
27. Finsterbush A, Friedman B. 1975. The effects of sensory denervation on rabbits' knee joints. *J. Bone Joint Surg.*, 57A: 949–56.
28. Freeman MAR, Railton GT. 1988. Should the posterior cruciate ligament be retained or resected in condylar nonmeniscal knee arthroplasty? *J Arthroplasty*, 3(suppl): S13.
29. Freeman MAR, Wyke B. 1966. Articular contributions to limb reflexes. *Brit. J. Surg.*, 53: 61–69.
30. Galante JO. 1983. Selection of prosthesis in total knee arthroplasty. *Clin. Orthop.*, 177: 307.
31. Grigg P. 1994. Peripheral neural mechanisms in proprioception. *J. Sport Rehab.*, 3: 1–17.
32. Guyton AC. 1981. *Textbook of medical physiology*, 6th ed. Philadelphia: Saunders, 534–36, 562–64, 588–95, 616.
33. Hall MG, Ferrell WR, Sturrock RD, Hamblen DL, Baxendale RH. 1995. The effect of hypermobility syndrome on knee joint proprioception. *Brit. J. Rheumatol.*, 34: 121–25.
34. Hurley MV, Newham DJ. 1993. The influence of arthrogenous muscle inhibition on quadriceps rehabilitation of patients with early, unilateral osteoarthritic knees. *Br. J. Rheumatol.*, 32:127–31.
35. Hutton RS, Atwater SW. 1992. Acute and chronic adaptations of muscle proprioceptors in response to increased use. *Sports Med.*, 14(6): 406–21.
36. Insall JN, Lawrence DD, Scott RD, Scott WN. 1989. Rationale of the knee society clinical rating system. *Clin. Orthop.*, 248: 13–14.
37. Insall JN. 1993. *Surgery of the knee*, 2d ed. New York: Churchill Livingstone, 719–38.
38. Ishii Y, Terajima K, Terashima S, Bechtold J, Laskin RS. 1997. Comparison of joint position sense after total knee arthroplasty. *J. Arthroplasty*, 12(5): 541–45.
39. Jefferson RJ, Whittle MW. 1990. Functional biomechanical results of unicompartmental knee arthroplasty compared with total condylar arthroplasty and tibial osteotomy. *J. Bone Joint Surg.*, 72B: 161–62.
40. Jevsevar DS, O'Riley PO, Hodge WA, Krebs DE. 1993. Knee kinematics and kinetics during locomotion activities of daily living in subjects with arthroplasty and in healthy control subjects. *Phys. Ther.*, 73(4): 229–39.
41. Johansson H, Sjolander P, Sojka P. 1991. A sensory role for the cruciate ligaments. *Clin. Orthop.*, 268: 161–78.
42. Jonsson H, Kärrholm J, Elmqvist LG. 1989. Kinematics of active knee extension after a tear of the anterior cruciate ligament. *Am. J. Sports Med.*, 17: 796–802.
43. Kålund S, Sinkjær T, Arendt-Nielsen A., et al. 1990. Altered timing of hamstring muscle action in anterior cruciate ligament-deficient patients. *Am. J. Sports Med.*, 18(3): 245–48.
44. Kandell ER, Schwartz JH, Jessell TM. 1996. *Principles of neural science*, 3d ed. Norwalk, CT: Appleton & Lange, 535–37, 619.
45. Kaplan FS, Nixon JE, Reitz L, Tucker J. 1985. Age-related changes in proprioception and sensation of joint position. *Acta Orthop. Scand.*, 56: 72.
46. Katonis PG, Assimakopoulos AP, Agapitos MV, Exarchou EI. 1991. Mechanoreceptors in the posterior cruciate ligament. *Acta Orthop. Scand.*, 62(3): 276–78.
47. Kelman GJ, Biden EN, Phil D, Wyatt MP, Ritter MA, Colwell CW. 1989. Gait laboratory analysis of a posterior cruciate-sparing total knee arthroplasty in stair ascent and descent. *Clin. Orthop.*, 248: 21–26.
48. Kennedy JC, Alexander IJ, Hayes KC. 1982. Nerve supply of the human knee and its functional importance. *Am. J. Sports. Med.*, 103: 329–35.
49. Kleinbart FA, Bryk E, Evangelista J, Scott WN, Vigorita VJ. 1992. A histological comparison of posterior cruciate ligaments harvested from arthritic and age-controlled knee specimens. *Orthop. Trans.*, Summer: 583.
50. Kokmen E, Bossemyer RW, Williams WJ. 1978. Quantitative evaluation of joint motion perception in an aging population. *J. Gerontol.*, 33: 62–67.
51. Kosser JR. 1996. *Orthopaedic knowledge update 5*. American Academy of Orthopaedic Surgeons, Rosemont, IL, 193–166.
52. Kroll MA, Otis JC, Sculco TP, Lee AC, Paget SA, Buckenstein R, Jensen DA. 1989. The relationship of stride characteristics to pain before and after total knee arthroplasty. *Clin. Orthop.*, 239: 191–95.

53. Laurencin CT, Zelicof SB, Scott RD, Ewald FC. 1991. Unicompartmental versus total knee replacement in the same patient. *Clin. Orthop.*, 273: 151–56.
54. Leksell L. 1945. The action potential and excitatory effects of the small ventral root fibers to skeletal muscle. *Acta Physiol. Scand.*, 10(suppl 31): 1–84.
55. Lephart, SM. 1997. EMG profile of the functional ACL-deficient patient during dynamic activities. Paper presented at the annual meeting of the American Orthopaedic Society for Sports Medicine, San Francisco.
56. Lephart SM, Fu FH, Borsa PA. 1994. *Proprioception in sports medicine: Advances in operative orthopaedics,* vol 2. St. Louis: Mosby Year Book.
57. Lephart SM, Giraldo JL, Borsa PA, Fu FH. 1996. Knee joint proprioception: A comparison between female intercollegiate gymnasts and controls. *Knee Surg Sports Traumatol Arthroscopy,* 4: 121–24.
58. Lephart SM, Kocher MS, Fu FH, Borsa PA, Harner CD. 1992a. Proprioception following ACL reconstruction. *J. Sports Rehabil.*, 1: 188–96.
59. Lephart SM, Perrin DH, Fu FH, Gieck JH, McCue FC, Irrgang JJ. 1992b. Relationship between selected physical characteristics and functional capacity in the anterior cruciate-insufficient athlete. *JOSPT,* 16: 174–80.
60. Li E, Ritter MA. 1995. The case for retension of the posterior cruciate ligament. *J. Arthroplasty,* 10: 560–63.
61. Lord SR, Clark RD, Webster IW. 1991. Physiological factors associated with falls in an elderly population. *J. Am. Geriatr. Soc.*, 39: 1194–1200.
62. Mahoney OM, Noble CN, Rhoads DD, Alexander JW, Tullos HS. 1994. Posterior cruciate function following total knee arthroplasty: A biomechanical study. *J. Arthroplasty,* 9(6): 569–78.
63. Marmor L. 1993. Unicompartmental knee replacement. In *Total knee arthroplasty,* Rand JA, ed. New York: Raven Press, 245–80.
64. Marshall RN, McNair PJ, Maguire K. 1993. Effects of knee effusion on muscle activity and kinematics of walking. *Proc. Int. Soc. Biomech.*, 826–27.
65. McNair PJ, Marshall RN, Maguire K, Brown C. 1995. Knee joint effusion and proprioception. *Arch. Phys. Med. Rehabil.*, 76: 566–68.
66. Melzack R, Wall PD. 1965. Pain mechanisms: A new theory. *Science,* 15: 971.
67. Moilanen T, Freeman MAR. 1995. The case for retension of the posterior cruciate ligament. *J. Arthroplasty*, 10: 564–67.
68. Nicholas JA. 1970. Injuries to knee ligaments: Relationship to looseness and tightness in football players. *JAMA*, 212: 2236–239.
69. Palmer I. 1958. Pathophysiology of the medial ligament of the knee joint. *Acta Chir. Scand.,* 115: 312–18.
70. Petrella RJ, Lattanzio PJ, Nelson MG. 1997. Effect of age and activity on knee joint proprioception. *Am. J. Phys. Med. Rehabil.*, 76(3): 235–41.
71. Pritchett JW. 1996. Anterior cruciate-retaining total knee arthroplasty. *J. Arthroplasty.*, 11: 194–97.
72. Raunest J, Sager M, Burgener E. 1996. Proprioceptive mechanisms in the cruciate ligaments: An electromyographic study on reflex activity in the thigh muscles. *J. Trauma Inj. Inf. Crit. Care,* 41(3): 48–493.
73. Resnick D, Niwoyama G. 1981. *Diagnosis of bone and joint disorders*. Philadelphia: Saunders, 1276.
74. Ritter MA, Campbell, Faris PM, Keating EM. 1989. Long-term survival analysis of the posterior cruciate condylar total knee arthroplasty. *J. Arthroplasty*, 4: 293–96.
75. Safran MR, Lephart SM, Fu FH, Harner CD. 1996. Proprioception in the posterior cruciate deficient knee. Paper presented at the annual meeting of the American Academy of Orthopaedic Surgeons on, Atlanta, GA.
76. Schaible HG, Schmidt RF. 1985. Effects of an experimental arthritis on the sensory properties of fine articular afferent units. *J. Neurophysiol.*, 54(5): 1109–122.
77. Schultz RA, Miller DC, Kerr CS, Micheli L. 1984. Mechanoreceptors in human cruciate ligaments. *J. Bone Joint Surg.*, 66A: 1072–1076.
78. Scott NW, Rubinstein M, Scuderi G. 1988. Results after knee replacement with posterior cruciate-substituting prosthesis. *J. Bone Joint Surg.*, 70A: 1163–173.
79. Sharma L, Yi-Chung P. 1997. Impaired proprioception and osteoarthritis. *Current Op. Rheumatol.*, 9: 253–58.
80. Sherrington CS. 1911. *The integrative action of the nervous system*. New Haven, CT: Yale University Press.
81. Simmons S, Lephart S, Rubash H, Borsa P, Barrack R. 1996a. Proprioception following total knee arthroplasty with and without the posterior cruciate ligament. *J. Arthroplasty,* 11(7): 763–68.
82. Simmons S, Lephart S, Rubash H, Pifer GW, Barrack R. 1996b. Proprioception following unicondylar knee arthroplasty versus total knee arthroplasty. *Clin. Orthop.*, 331: 179–84.

83. Simon SR, Triesmann HW, Burdett RG, Ewald FC, Sledge CB. 1983. Quantitative gait analysis after total knee arthroplasty for monarticular degenerative arthritis. *J. Bone Joint Surg.*, 65A: 605–13.
84. Skinner HB, Barrack RL. 1991. Joint position sense in the normal and pathological knee joint. *J. Electromyogr. Kinesiol.*, 1(3): 180–90.
85. Skinner HB, Barrack RL, Cook SD. 1984a. Age-related decline in proprioception. *Clin. Orthop.*, 184: 208–11.
86. Skinner HB, Barrack RL, Cook SD, et al. 1984b. Joint position sense in total knee arthroplasty. *J. Orthop. Res.*, 1: 276–83.
87. Sluka KA. 1996. Pain mechanisms involved in musculoskeletal disorders. *JOSPT*, 24(4): 240–54.
88. Solomonow M, Baratta R, Zhou BH, Shoji H, Bose W, Beck C, D'Ambrosia R. 1987. The synergistic action of the anterior cruciate ligament and thigh muscles in maintaining joint stability. *Am. J. Sports Med.*, 15(3): 207–13.
89. Stauffer RN, Chao EYS, Gyory AN. 1977. Biomechanical gait analysis of the diseased knee joint. *Clin. Orthop.*, 126: 246–55.
90. Tibone JE, Antich TJ, Perry J, Moynes D. 1988. Functional analysis of untreated and reconstructed posterior cruciate ligament injuries. *Am. J. Sports Med.*, 16: 217–23.
91. Walla DJ, Albright JP, McAuley E, et al. 1985. Hamstring control and the unstable anterior cruciate ligament-deficient knee. *Am. J. Sports Med.*, 13: 34–39.
92. Warren PJ, Olanokun TK, Cobb AG, Bentley G. 1993. Proprioception after knee arthroplasty: The influence of prosthetic design. *Clin. Orthop.*, 297: 182–87.
93. Wojtys E, Huston L. 1994. Neuromuscular performance in normal and anterior cruciate ligament-deficient lower extremities. *Am. J. Sports Med.*, 22: 89–104.

CHAPTER 30

Overview of the Neuromuscular Control of the Shoulder, Its Status in Patients With Degenerative Joint Disease and After Shoulder Arthroplasty

Jorge L. Giraldo, MD
Christian Fink, MD
Ivan Vassilev, MD
Jon J.P. Warner, MD
Scott M. Lephart, PhD, ATC

Introduction

Peripheral sensations originating from mechanoreceptors are integrated in the central nervous system, where they are processed to generate a coordinated motor response. This muscle activity serves as a protective mechanism to maintain dynamic stabilization of the joints, thereby protecting them from injury. This mechanism of neuromuscular control of the joints also includes proprioception, which is especially important in the shoulder where bony constraint is minimal, so muscles surrounding the shoulder joint play an important role as dynamic stabilizers.

In order to describe the complex neurological process involved in the motor control of the shoulder, the following topics are discussed in this chapter:

- The histological evidence of shoulder structures participating in neuromuscular control
- The three levels of motor control in the central nervous system (spinal cord, brain stem, and cortex levels), with special emphasis on the shoulder
- The effect of degenerative joint disease on shoulder motor control
- The status of motor control in patients after prosthetic shoulder arthroplasty

Histological Evidence of Shoulder Contribution to Proprioception

The role of proprioception in the shoulder has been examined by histological studies demonstrating the presence of mechanoreceptors in shoulder tissues. The first histological report of shoulder mechanoreceptors was made by Jerosch and associates (23). They demonstrated not only axons located in the subsynovial layer of the ligaments, but also type II (Pacinian) mechanoreceptors positioned directly beneath the synovial membrane and close to the humeral insertion of the glenohumeral ligaments. Two years later Vangsness and coworkers (39) described shoulder mechanoreceptors in more detail.

By evaluating the glenohumeral (superior, middle, inferior, and posterior), coracoclavicular, and coracoacromial ligaments, glenoid labrum, and subacromial bursa, these authors observed three types of mechanoreceptors and free nerve endings. The first type they described was the classical Ruffini receptor, the second type was the Ruffini end organ, and the third type was the fast adapting Pacinian corpuscle. In their study, the Pacinian corpuscle was the most abundant mechanoreceptor in the glenohumeral ligaments, while free nerve endings were noted primarily in the subdeltoid bursa. More recently, Jerosch and associates (21) reported the presence of axons with no relation to the vessels and type II mechanoreceptors (Pacinian corpuscles) in the capsule and the glenohumeral ligaments. Solomonow and coworkers (37) studied a feline model and found Golgi tendon organs, Ruffini endings and Pacinian corpuscles.

In summary, identification of shoulder mechanoreceptors has progressed from the initial description of type II sensory receptors, to the most recent publication, which reports type I, II, and III mechanoreceptors in animal models. Conversely, in human shoulders Golgi organ tendons have not been well identified.

Neuromuscular Control of the Shoulder

As stated previously, current understanding of neuromuscular control of the joints expresses the concept that joints are controlled by complex neural mechanisms, which ultimately provide dynamic stabilization as a protective mechanism. In order to develop this protective mechanism, neuromuscular control is carried out at three different levels of the central nervous system: at the spinal level, where activities that encourage reflex joint stabilization take place; at the brain stem, where the balance and postural activities are developed; and at the cerebral cortex, where the conscious sensations of motion and position occur (13, 29, 31).

Spinal Level

At the lowest level of neuromuscular control, the spinal cord contains neuronal circuits that mediate automatic and stereotyped reflexes. Moreover, these reflexes can function even when the cord is disconnected from the rest of the brain. It has been widely demonstrated that almost all reflexes integrate activation and inhibition of activity in different muscle groups in order to develop specific motor functions. In other words, to execute forward flexion of the shoulder, the antagonist muscles must be relaxed. Even simple descending commands can produce complex effects through these interneurons. It is now known that the same networks of neurons that organize reflex behavior also are involved in voluntary movements. Ultimately, however, all interneuronal controls converge on the motor control that innervates the skeletal muscles (13).

To evaluate the first level of motor control, electrophysiological studies have been conducted to elucidate the reflex activity of the muscles surrounding the shoulder. Muscle activity plays an important role in shoulder function. Contraction of some of the muscles creates joint compression and increases the concavity compression fit of the humeral head into the glenoid (41), while contraction of other shoulder muscles produces humeral motion. Consequently, shoulder muscles are classified in two different groups: stabilizers and effectors.

Basmajian and Bazant (5) demonstrated the synergism between supraspinatus and posterior fibers of the deltoid with the glenoid and capsule, which prevents the shoulder from downward dislocation. The role of the muscles surrounding the joint during other movements was described by Kronberg and coworkers (28). They evaluated the muscle activity during abduction in the coronal plane, external and internal rotation in neutral position, and at 45° and 90° of abduction, flexion, and extension. They suggested that muscle coordination plays an important role in developing stabilization of the joint. As a result, in abduction the muscles of motion are the supraspinatus and anterior and middle deltoid, and the stabilizers are the infraspinatus, subscapularis, and latissimus dorsi. In external rotation the movers are the infraspinatus and supraspinatus, and the stabilizer is the subscapularis. In internal rotation the movers are the subscapularis, latissimus dorsi, and pectoralis major, and no stabilizer was identified. This delicate synergism between the two groups of muscles seems to be altered under pathological conditions, which leads the shoulder to develop muscular imbalance.

Glousman and coworkers (14) evaluated 15 throwing shoulders with chronic glenohumeral instability. They assessed the EMG activity of 8 muscles surrounding the shoulder while pitching a baseball and reported that subjects with shoulder instability had imbalance in the shoulder muscles. Ballantyne and coworkers (3) have demonstrated that, in addition to the instability, the painful shoulders present muscular imbalance. Muscular balance plays an important role, because it allows the shoulder to develop sports activities. Jobe and associates (27), in 1983, described not only the phases of pitching, but also the muscle patterns of the deltoid, supraspinatus, subscapularis, and infraspinatus/teres minor during these phases. In a later study, the Jobe group (26) included more muscles and reported the major muscles that control the shoulder during pitching and described their altered EMG patterns as a result of impingement, instability, and poor technique (15). In addition to the analysis of muscular balance of the shoulder during pitching, muscle balance has been described for other sport activities such as golfing (25) and swimming. Furthermore, the EMG evaluation of this level of motor control has led to the description of therapeutic exercises that have been incorporated into modern rehabilitation programs.

Moseley and coworkers (33) described the four shoulder exercises that do not neglect the activation of scapular muscles. Those exercises are scaption, rowing, push-up with plus, and press-up. Similarly, exercises promoting humeral motion have also been described. The most challenging exercises for humeral motion are elevation in the scapular plane with thumbs down, flexion, horizontal abduction with arms externally rotated, and the press-up (38). In addition, the two-handed overhead medicine ball throw is an ideal technique for dynamic muscular reeducation in a protected manner while closely simulating portions of the throwing motion (9).

An additional role of the shoulder muscles includes dynamic stabilization of the joint. This function can be developed, thanks to the spinal level of motor control. Evaluating this level, Guanche and associates (16), in a feline model, demonstrated the reflex arc that exists between capsule and biceps, subscapularis, supraspinatus, and infraspinatus. Similarly, in a clinical trial, Jerosch and coworkers (22) compared the humeral anteroposterior and inferior translation in shoulders, with intraarticular anesthesia and without anesthesia. They found significantly more translation in shoulders under local anesthesia. This study also demonstrated the reflex arc between intraarticular mechanoreceptors and muscles of the shoulder, which means that passive restrains are ligaments and active restraints are the muscles. These findings confirm the idea that joint stability is not an exclusive function of the ligaments.

In summary, the assessment of the reflex activity of the muscles surrounding the shoulder has been useful in understanding the muscle firing patterns under normal and pathological conditions. Moreover, this knowledge is invaluable in designing more effective rehabilitation programs, which must be focused on developing strength, the endurance of specific muscles (10, 42), and regaining muscular balance (2).

Brain Stem Level

The second level of neuromuscular control is the brain stem. It contains three neuronal systems (medial, lateral, and aminergic) whose axons project and regulate the segmental network of the spinal cord. Since the brain stem system integrates visual and vestibular information with somatosensory input, it plays an important role in modulating spinal motor circuits. Moreover, the reticular formation of the brain stem participates in the regulation of skeletal muscle tone, reflexes, and body posture. In addition, eyes and head movements are controlled at this level. Consequently, the input from the reticular formation, the vestibulospinal projections, and other motor system components are integrated in the brain stem to provide a continuously adapting background of muscle tone and body posture, which facilitates voluntary motor actions (13).

This level of motor control has been widely studied for the lower extremity by using unstable platforms, because it is important for equilibrium and balance. In the upper extremity this level of motor control has been used in the therapeutic area, in order to promote adequate balance between compression and shear forces of the shoulder girdle (7). Strengthening of the joint in a closed kinetic fashion meets these requirements. Due to the properties of closed kinetic chain exercises, it results in less stress to the capsuloligament complex and facilitates the co-contraction of the dynamic stabilizers (7). Therefore, the use of unstable platforms for the upper extremity in a closed chain exercise seems to facilitate dynamic and static control of the scapula and the glenohumeral joint. These types of exercises are most commonly used in modern rehabilitation programs, because they produce adequate strengthening of the stabilizers of the scapula (11). Under conditions in which an external load is applied, but the extremity is fixed on the floor (e.g., a push-up), these advantages have been described: co-contraction of the scapular and humeral force couples, promotion of dynamic stabilization, joint compression, facilitation of proprioceptors, minimal shear forces, and some functional specificity (30).

Brain Cortex Level

The highest level of motor control consists of three areas of the cerebral cortex: the primary motor cortex, the lateral premotor area (premotor cortex), and the supplementary motor area. Each area projects directly to the spinal cord through the corticospinal tract as well as indirectly through the brain stem motor systems. The premotor and supplementary motor areas are important for coordinating and planning sequences of movement. Both areas receive information from the posterior parietal and prefrontal association cortices (13).

This level of motor control is generally known as proprioception, which is considered the sense of position and movement of the extremities. Consequently, there are two modalities of limb proprioception: the sense of stationary position of the limbs (limb position sense) and the sense of limb movement (kinesthesia). These sensations are important for maintaining balance, controlling limb movements, and evaluating the shape of grasped objects. Proprioceptive sensations of the limbs generally occur as a consequence of voluntary (or reflexive) movement. For this reason it was long thought that limb proprioception depended, not on signals from peripheral receptors, but rather on signals from brain regions controlling limb movements. Thus, limb proprioception was thought to differ from other somatosensory modalities, which are mediated by peripheral receptors. Three main types of peripheral receptors signal the stationary position of the limb, as well as the speed and direction of limb movement:

- Mechanoreceptors located in joint structures
- Mechanoreceptors in muscle that are specialized to transduce stretch of the muscle, the muscle spindle receptors
- Cutaneous mechanoreceptors

Consequently, while the contribution of muscle spindle receptors to limb proprioception is clearly important, full proprioceptive sensitivity depends on combined actions of the muscle receptors, joint receptors, and cutaneous mechanoreceptors. Although the pathways for proprioceptive information from the arms and legs to the medulla are somewhat different, they all synapse on neurons in the thalamus. The thalamus plays a key role in transforming sensory information that will eventually reach the cerebral cortex. In the primary somatic sensory cortex the axons from the thalamus terminate on pyramidal cells and excite them strongly. They also terminate on interneurons whose axons are oriented perpendicular to the surface and parallel to the apical dendrites of the pyramidal cells (13).

Therefore, as Guyton (17) states, "proprioceptive sensations are those having to do with the physical state of the body, including position sensations, tendon and muscle sensations, pressure sensations from the bottom of the feet and even the sensation of equilibrium, which generally is considered to be a special sensation rather than somatic sensation." These sensations arise through activity in sensory neurons located in the skin, muscles, and joint tissues.

Several studies have been conducted under clinical and pathological conditions, looking at shoulder sensation of motion and position (kinesthesia and joint position sense). In 1983, Hall and McCloskey (18) assessed the shoulder, the elbow, and the distal joint of the middle finger for detection of passive motion. Their conclusions suggest that the muscular mechanoreceptors are important determinants in proprioceptive performance. Jerosch and coworkers (24) evaluated the proprioceptive ability of 27 volunteers in different shoulder positions. They found better proprioception when the shoulders were tested above the shoulder level. They explain their findings as a result of stretching the glenohumeral capsule and the inferior ligaments, which may lead to an increase in mechanoreceptor response. On the other hand, Blasier and associates (6) reported that detection of passive motion in external rotation is significantly more sensitive than detection in internal rotation. They propose capsular tightening as a mechanism for this finding.

Proprioceptive patterns can also be influenced as a result of aging. Hearn and coworkers (19) reported that younger subjects are able to more accurately detect position of the dominant upper extremity compared to older subjects. Under pathological conditions, it has been suggested that loosening of the capsule can cause a diminished mechanical deformation of mechanoreceptors, which leads to a proprioceptive deficit. Allegrucci and coworkers (1) reported that overhead-sport athletes had a kinesthetic deficit when the throwing shoulder was compared to the contralateral nondominant shoulder. Also, Smith and Brunolli (36) reported a kinesthetic deficit after glenohumeral dislocation, which may result in abnormal neuromuscular coordination and subsequent re-injury. Forwell and Carnahan (12) suggest that patients with shoulder instability have a proprioceptive deficit. Muscular fatigue has been advocated to have negative influence on joint proprioception. Although Voight and associates (40) reported no significant difference between dominant and nondominant shoulders, they found a significant decrease in active and passive reproduction of position after muscle fatigue. Moreover, surgical correction of shoulder instability has a positive influence on shoulder proprioception. Lephart and coworkers (32) compared shoulder proprioceptive patterns in normal subjects, in patients with unilateral instability, and after surgical repair of the instability. They found that the surgical procedure restores shoulder proprioception to near normal levels.

In summary, the ability of the joint to detect motion and position can be affected by multiple factors such as instability, fatigue, training, and surgical correction of instability. However, another pathological condition that needs to be studied is the effect of degenerative shoulder disease on shoulder motor control.

Effect of Degenerative Joint Disease on Shoulder Motor Control

Although osteoarthritis is the most common disorder of synovial joints, primary degenerative arthritis is definitely less common in the shoulder girdle than in the hip or the knee (20). Osteoarthritis probably represents the final common pathology of a variety of mechanisms, which lead the joint to a failure. The essential macroscopic features of the disease include cartilage injury with the development of loss of cartilage and subsequent exposure of subchondral bone, formation of subchondral cysts surrounded by areas of sclerotic bone (these cysts often are connected to the joint cavity by narrow channels), and the development of bony growths at the margins of the joint. All of these changes, and the wear of the exposed subchondral bone, distort the shape of the articular surface (35). Concomitant histological and biochemical changes occur, which explain the pathological features. On the other hand, those main pathological features match the radiological changes. Although the knees and the small joint of the hands are the most commonly involved, this condition can be seen in any of the articulations of the shoulder.

With osteoarthritis of the sternoclavicular joint patients often complain of swelling and pain, which affect only some overhead activities. Consequently, they are able to develop activities of daily living. Radiological studies may reveal a high incidence of osteoarthritic changes; but not all of them have clinical significance.

Osteoarthritis of the acromioclavicular joint is very frequent. Pain is the most common clinical finding. Its main characteristic is that it increases with abduction of the arm and with axial load of the joint (abduction of the arm across the chest). As the disease progresses the patient develops impingement of the subacromial space. This impingement results not only from formation of osteophytes at the distal end of the clavicle and the acromion, but also from traction spurs developed from the coracoacromial ligament.

Osteoarthritis of the glenohumeral joint is not rare. Extensive cartilage changes are more commonly located in the glenoid than in the humeral head. Patients often complain of pain in the shoulder and, particularly, of loss of internal rotation. Abduction may be limited, as the inferior recess is stretched across osteophytes (34).

Although the effect of shoulder osteoarthritis on proprioception and motor control has not been as widely studied as in the knee and the hip, it seems that the degenerative changes of the shoulder have a negative influence of shoulder proprioception. Cuomo and coworkers presented a paper at the annual meeting of the American Academy of Orthopaedic Surgeons in 1996 on a prospective comparative study reporting a decline in proprioception in osteoarthritic shoulders. This reported proprioceptive deficit might be due to the pathological changes (loss of cartilage, bone cysts, and osteophytes) developed in osteoarthritic shoulders. Under this condition, damage to the shoulder mechanoreceptors may occur. This damage to the articular mechanoreceptors may lead to the same proprioceptive deficit as seen in hips or knees. Research done on those joints suggests that diminished proprioception initiates or accelerates the process seen in osteoarthritis (4), by compromising the dynamic stabilization of the joint. Another source of proprioceptive deficit could result from soft tissue contractures, which prevent the mechanoreceptors from deforming, leading to a diminished afferent signal to the nervous central system. In addition, older people develop neurological changes as a consequence of diminished perfusion to the neurological tissues. Under the aforementioned condition damage to the three levels of motor control can occur.

Effect of Total Shoulder Arthroplasty on Shoulder Motor Control

Although the neurological effects of shoulder arthroplasty have not been well studied, it seems that the procedure has a positive effect on shoulder proprioception and neuromuscular control. Cuomo and coworkers, in the study that was mentioned previously, reported a significant improvement of kinesthesia and shoulder position sense 6 mo after the arthroplasty. There are two probable explanations for restoring proprioception after the arthroplasty:

- Correction of capsular and ligament contractures and restoring motion permits the joint to deform the mechanoreceptors, with subsequent decreasing of the afferent threshold.
- *Pain relief*: The afferent input from joints, tendons, and muscles, as well as descending impulses from the brain, can influence the excitability of motoneurons and hence muscle stiffness determined by motoneuronal control (43). Since the arthroplasty produces pain relief, it is able to break the cycle and therefore reduces the muscle stiffness.

References

1. Allegrucci M, Whitney SL, Lephart SM, Irrgang J, Fu FH. Shoulder kinesthesia in healthy unilateral athletes participating in upper extremity sports. *J Orthop Sports Phys Ther* 21(4): 220–26, 1995.
2. Baker L, Parker K. Neuromuscular electrical stimulation of the muscles surrounding the shoulder. *Phys Ther* 66(12): 1930–937, 1986.
3. Ballantyne BT, O'Hare SJ, Paschall JL, Pavia-Smith MM, Pitz AM, Gillon JF, et al. Electromyographic activity of selected shoulder muscles in commonly used therapeutic exercises. *Phys Ther* 73(10): 668–77, 1993.
4. Barret DS, Cobb AG, Bentley G. Joint proprioception in normal, osteoarthritic, and replaced knees. *J Bone Joint Surg* 73B: 53–56, 1991.
5. Basmajian JV, Bazant FJ. Factors preventing downward dislocation of the adducted shoulder joint: An electromyographic and morphological study. *J Bone Joint Surg* 41A(7): 1182–186, 1959.
6. Blasier RB, Carpenter JE, Huston LJ. Shoulder proprioception: Effect of joint laxity, joint position, and direction of motion. *Orthop Rev* 23(1): 45–50, 1994.
7. Borsa PA, Lephart SM, Kocher MS, Lephart SP. Functional assessment and rehabilitation of shoulder proprioception for glenohumeral instability. *J Sports Rehab* 3: 84–104, 1994.
8. Conn M. *Neuroscience in medicine.* Philadelphia: Lippincott, 1995.
9. Cordasco FA, Wolfe IN, Wooten ME, Bigliani LU. An electromyographic analysis of the shoulder during medicine ball rehabilitation program. *Am J Sports Med* 24(3): 386–92, 1996.
10. Davies GJ, Dickoff-Hoffman S. Neuromuscular testing and rehabilitation of the shoulder complex. *J Sports Phys Ther* 18(2): 449–58, 1993.
11. Diaz MP, Sosa H, Yanez R, Dines DM, Levinson M. The conservative management of the unstable shoulder including rehabilitation. [Review] *Clin Sports Med* 14(4): 797–816, 1995.
12. Forwell LA, Carnahan H. Proprioception during manual aiming in individuals with shoulder instability and controls. *J Orthop Sports Rehab* 23(2): 111–19, 1996.
13. Ghez C: The control of movement. In *Principles of neural science,* Kandel ER, Schwartz JH, Jessell TM (eds). East Norwalk, CT: Appleton & Lange, 533–47, 1991.
14. Glousman R, Jobe FW, Tibone J, Moynes D, Antonelli D, et al. Dynamic electromyographic analysis of the throwing shoulder with glenohumeral instability. *J Bone Joint Surg* 70A(2): 220–26, 1988.
15. Gowan ID, Jobe FW, Tibone JE, Perry J, Moynes D. A comparative electromyographic analysis of the shoulder during pitching: Professional versus amateur pitchers. *Am J Sports Med* 15(6): 586–90, 1987.
16. Guanche C, Knatt T, Solomonow M, Lu Y, Baratta R. The synergistic action of the capsule and the shoulder muscles. *Am J Sports Med* 23(3): 301–306, 1995.
17. Guyton A. *Textbook of medical physiology,* 9th ed. Philadelphia: Saunders, 595, 1996.
18. Hall LA, McCloskey DI. Detection of movements imposed on finger, elbow, and shoulder joints. *J Physiol* 335: 519–33, 1983.
19. Hearn M, Crowe A, Keessen W. Influence of age on proprioceptive accuracy in two dimensions. *Percep Motor Skills* 69(3, part 1): 811–18, 1989.
20. Jaffe H. *Metabolic, degenerative, and inflammatory diseases of the bones and joints.* Philadelphia: Lea & Febiger, 1972.
21. Jerosch J, Castro WHM, Grosse-Hackman A, Clahsen H. [Function of the glenohumeral ligaments in active protection of shoulder stability]. *Zeitschrift für Orthopadie und Ihre Grenzgebiete* 133(1): 67–71, 1995.
22. Jerosch J, Castro WHM, Halm H, Drescher H. Does the glenohumeral joint capsule have proprioceptive capability? *Knee Surg Sports Traumatol Arthroscopy* 1(2): 80–84, 1993.

23. Jerosch J, Steinbeck J, Clahsen H, Schmitz-Nahrath M, Grosse-Hackmann A. Function of the glenohumeral ligaments in active stabilization of the shoulder joint. *Knee Surg Sports Traumatol Arthroscopy* 1(3–4): 152–58, 1993.
24. Jerosch J, Thorwesten L, Steinbeck J, Reer R. Proprioceptive function of the shoulder girdle in healthy volunteers. *Knee Surg Sports Traumatol Arthroscopy* 3(4): 219–25, 1996.
25. Jobe FW, Perry J, Pink M. Electromyographic shoulder activity in men and women professional golfers. *Am J Sports Med* 17(6): 782–87, 1989.
26. Jobe FW, Radovich M, Tibone J, Perry J. An EMG analysis of the shoulder in pitching: A second report. *Am J Sports Med* 12(3): 218–20, 1984.
27. Jobe FW, Tibone JE, Perry J, Moynes D. An EMG analysis of the shoulder in throwing and pitching: A preliminary report. *Am J Sports Med* 11(1): 3–5, 1983.
28. Kronberg M, Gunnar N, Broström L. Muscle activity and coordination in the normal shoulder: An electromyographic study. *Clin Orthop* 257: 76–85, 1990.
29. Lephart SM, Fu FH. The role of proprioception in the treatment of sports injuries. *Sports Exer Inj* 1: 96–102, 1995.
30. Lephart SM, Henry T. The physiological basis for open and closed kinetic chain rehabilitation for the upper extremity. *J Sports Rehab* 5(1): 71–87, 1996.
31. Lephart SM, Pincivero D, Giraldop JL, Fu FH. The role of proprioception in the management and rehabilitation of athletic injuries. *Am J Sports Med* 25(1): 130–37, 1997.
32. Lephart SM, Warner JJP, Borsa PA, Fu FH. Proprioception of the shoulder joint in healthy, unstable, and surgically repaired shoulders. *J Shoulder Elbow Surg* 3(6): 371–80, 1994.
33. Moseley BJ, Jobe FW, Pink M, Perry J, Tibone J. EMG analysis of the scapular muscles. *Am J Sports Med* 20(2): 128–34, 1992.
34. Moskowitz RW. *Osteoarthritis, diagnosis and medical/surgical management,* 2d ed. Philadelphia: Saunders, 567–78, 1994.
35. Salisbury JR, Woods C, Byers PD. *Diseases of bones and joints,* 1st ed. London: Chapman & Hall, 1994.
36. Smith RL, Brunolli J. Shoulder kinesthesia after anterior glenohumeral joint dislocation. *Phys Ther* 69(2): 106–12, 1989.
37. Solomonow M, Guanche C, Wink C, Knatt T, Baratta RV, et al. Mechanoreceptors and reflex arc in the feline shoulder. *J Shoulder Elbow Surg* 5(2, part 1): 139–46, 1996.
38. Townsend H, Jobe FW, Pink M, Perry J. Electromyographic analysis of the glenohumeral muscles during a baseball rehabilitation program. *Am J Sports Med* 19(3): 264–72, 1991.
39. Vangsness CT Jr, Ennis M, Taylor JG, Atkinson R. Neural anatomy of the glenohumeral ligaments, labrum, and subacromial bursa. *Arthroscopy* 11(2): 180–84, 1995.
40. Voight ML, Hardin JA, Blackburn TA, Tippett S, Canner GC. The effects of muscle fatigue on and the relationship of arm dominance to shoulder proprioception. *J Orthop Sports Phys Ther* 23(6): 348–52, 1996.
41. Warner JJP, Lephart S, Fu FH. Role of proprioception in pathoetiology of shoulder instability. *Clin Orthop* (330): 35–39, 1996.
42. Wilk KE, Arrigo C. Current concepts in the rehabilitation of the athletic shoulder. [Review] *J Orthop Sports Phys Ther* 18(1): 365–78, 1993.
43. Zimmermann M. Basic mechanisms of pain and pain therapy related to osteoarthritis and other disorders of the musculoskeletal system. In *Osteoarthritis,* Schumacher RH Jr (ed). New York: Springer-Verlag, 1988.

SECTION 4

Role of Rehabilitation in Reestablishing Proprioception and Neuromuscular Control

Section Leaders: David H. Perrin, PhD, ATC,
and James J. Irrgang, PhD, PT, ATC

Section Participants: Louis Osternig, PhD, ATC, Lynn Snyder-Mackler, ScD, PT,
Scott M. Lephart, PhD, ATC, Timothy J. Henry, PhD, ATC,
Kevin E. Wilk, PT, Pongsak Yuktanandana, MD

This section provides a clinical perspective of the mechanisms and therapeutic means by which neuromuscular control can be restored to provide dynamic restraint to ligament-deficient joints. The authors also discuss the effects of surgical intervention on the sensorimotor system and the specific rehabilitation considerations that are needed. Models of clinical research are also presented to investigate the sensorimotor system's adaptive characteristics following injury and rehabilitation.

Perrin and Shultz discuss various clinical research models that are available for the investigation of injury and rehabilitation following joint injury. Irrgang and Neri provide a basis for the integration of closed and open kinematic chain exercises for the purpose of restoring sensorimotor characteristics and functional joint stability. Rozzi and associates next provide a theoretical paradigm for the influence of fatigue on the sensorimotor system along with the potential risk factor associated with joint injury.

The role of coactivation and eccentric activity in the ACL-injured knee is addressed by Osternig, followed by a discussion of the role of the dynamic restraint in the ACL-deficient knee and models for restoration of neuromuscular control by Snyder-Mackler's group. Lephart and Henry continue with an overview of sensorimotor mechanisms responsible for shoulder stability and a basis for the restoration of functional stability. In conclusion, Wilk presents a specific protocol designed for the restoration and testing of shoulder function in the overhead-sport athlete.

This group engaged in extensive discussion about the need for clinical research models to assess the efficacy of rehabilitation intervention. Many of the topics of future direction focus on enhancing the reliability and validity of our current research instruments and the need for improved specificity of measurement as it relates to the function of the patient. The following recommendations are set forth for future directions of research in the area of measurement and rehabilitation.

Directions for Future Research

1. Develop a common language that is consistent with the model developed during the workshop and presented in this text, which classifies tests of sensorimotor impairment based on physiological functions.
2. Develop innovative methods for assessing sensory motor impairment that take into consideration weight-bearing vs. nonweight-bearing modes of assessment, alternate methods of perturbation, and the like.
3. Methods of assessment should include laboratory measures that can be used as criterion measures against which clinically applicable measures can be validated.
4. Establish reliability and validity of measures of sensorimotor impairment. Validity should demonstrate the relationship of the test score to functional instability, functional outcome (i.e., functional limitations, disability), and tissue homoestasis and should also provide evidence for discrimination, prediction, and evaluation over time. Further evidence should be provided for responsiveness, accuracy, and precision. Designs to validate measures of sensorimotor impairment should be prospective in nature for a variety of pathologies as well as regions of the body and levels of activity.
5. Provide normative data for comparison and interpretation of tests to assess sensory motor impairment. This should include comparison to contralateral limb and noninjured healthy subjects, as well as to those who demonstrate effective strategies of functional stability.
6. Research methodologies should assess long-term implications of sensory motor impairment.
7. Validation of tests should demonstrate clinical relevance.
8. Establish the effectiveness of interventions to enhance sensorimotor function.
9. Develop taxonomy for the classification of activities to enhance sensorimotor function that are consistent with the model developed at the workshop and presented in this text.
10. Establish criteria for selecting intervention strategies to enhance sensorimotor function.
11. Test the effectiveness of interventions to improve sensorimotor impairment (i.e., improvement in measures of sensory motor impairment), functional outcomes (i.e., functional limitations and disability), and tissue homeostasis and their cost effectiveness.

CHAPTER 31

Models for Clinical Research Involving Proprioception and Neuromuscular Control

David H. Perrin, PhD, ATC
Sandra J. Shultz, PhD, ATC

Introduction

The previous chapters in this book have discussed neurosensory and neuromuscular contributions to joint stability and the effects of ligament injury on proprioception and neuromuscular control. Special issues related to proprioception at the ankle, knee, and shoulder and the effects of orthoses and arthroplasty on neuromuscular control have also been addressed. This and the following chapters will focus on several issues related to assessment and rehabilitation of proprioception and neuromuscular control.

The accurate assessment of proprioception and neuromuscular control is necessary to determine the efficacy of therapeutic interventions following musculoskeletal injury. This chapter presents several techniques useful for assessing proprioception and neuromuscular control. Research studies conducted at the University of Virginia's Sports Medicine/Athletic Training Research Laboratory are offered as examples of clinical research involving proprioception.

Instrumentation

Joint proprioception has traditionally been assessed by determining perception of joint movement (kinesthesia) or joint position sense. Kinesthesia is measured by determining the threshold to detection of passive motion. Joint position sense is assessed by documenting an individual's ability to reproduce a predetermined angle in the joint's range of motion. This can best be accomplished through the use of sophisticated instrumentation designed specifically for this purpose. The joint proprioception-testing device developed at the University of Pittsburgh is one good example of such a device (see figure 31.1). Assessment of proprioception and neuromuscular control in the absence of instrumentation designed for this purpose presents a challenge for most clinicians and many researchers. Examples of innovative ways to assess proprioception include the use of isokinetic dynamometers, electrogoniometers, flexometers, balance devices, and postural stability systems.

Isokinetic Dynamometers

Isokinetic dynamometers are designed primarily for the rapid and reliable quantification of human muscle performance (20), which is accomplished by the dynamometer's force-sensing apparatus and internal goniometer. The internal goniometer has also been used for passive and active assessment of joint reposition sense of the ankle (see figure 31.2)

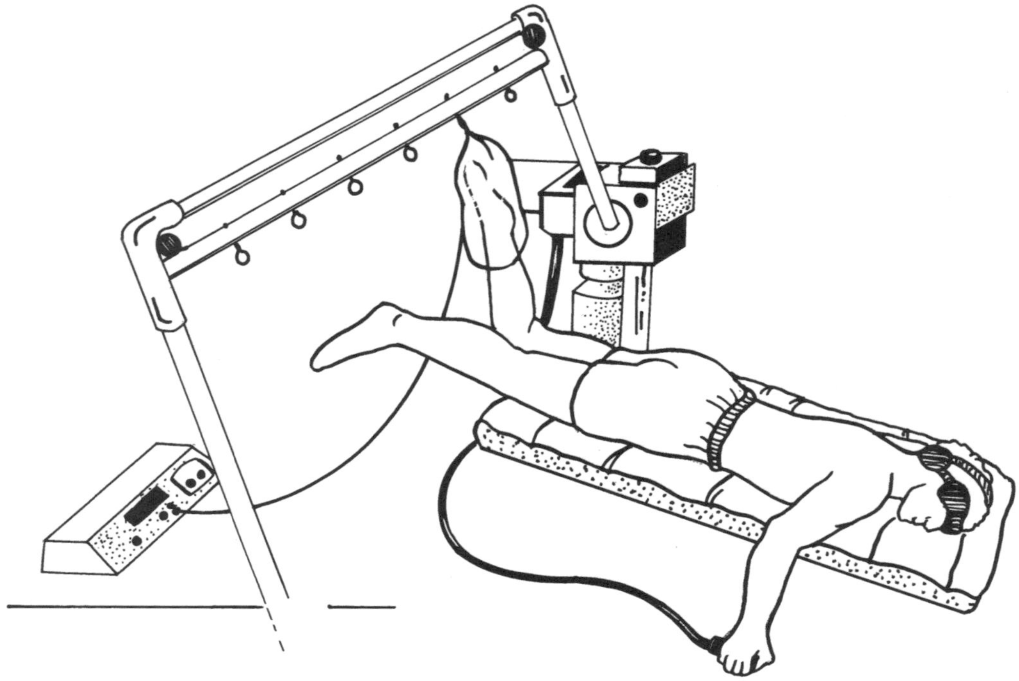

Figure 31.1 University of Pittsburgh joint proprioception testing device (with permission).

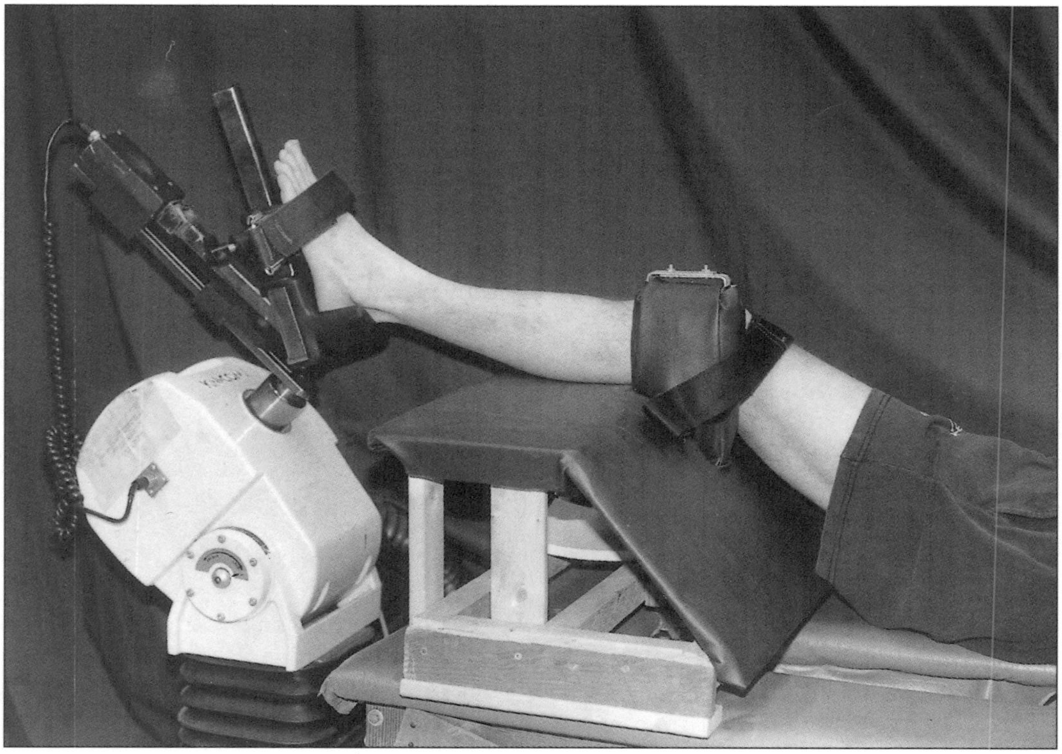

Figure 31.2 Internal goniometer of an isokinetic dynamometer used for ankle joint position sense testing.

(1, 11, 23), knee (see figure 31.3) (13, 24), and shoulder (see figure 31.4) (6).

Szczerba and coworkers (23) used a Kinetic Communicator (Kin Com, Chattanooga Group, Hixson, TN) to establish intertester reliability of active and passive joint position sense testing of the ankle. Twenty healthy subjects, free from history of ankle sprain, were positioned supine for examination of inversion and eversion joint position sense testing (see figure 31.2). Testing occurred at 10° eversion, 0° subtalar neutral, 15° inversion, and 5° from maximum inversion. An investigator initially moved the ankle through its entire range of motion, and the joint was then passively positioned in one of the four test positions for 15 s. The joint was then returned to the starting position, followed by passive movement back in the direction of the test position. When the subject felt the ankle had moved to the test position, he or she performed a quick contraction in the direction opposite the passive motion. This effort produced a spike on the Kin Com's force-velocity curve that enabled the recording of degrees of error from the test position. Active joint position sense testing followed a similar protocol except that the subject actively replicated the test position. Error scores were averaged from two test trials for each condition. The study found that the average ankle joint position sense error scores were significantly smaller for passive than active reposition testing (see table 31.1). A wide range of intraclass correlation reliability estimates for active (.03–.51) and passive (.08–.87) reposition test conditions was found, which suggests that further research is needed to refine this technique.

Hertel and associates (11) examined the effect of induced anesthesia of the lateral ankle joint on passive joint position sense as well as center of balance and postural sway, using a balance device under both static and dynamic conditions. The rationale for this study was that joint deafferentation is believed to occur with injury to the lateral ligaments of the ankle. Passive joint position sense testing followed a protocol similar to that described by Szczerba and coworkers (23) except that the test angles were 10° eversion, 20° and 30° inversion, and the error scores were the average of three trials for each condition. Eight ml of 1% lidocaine were injected into the anterior talofibular ligament and lateral joint capsule of the ankle in each of 16 subjects free from previous injury to the lower extremity. Subjects were tested for joint position sense and balance before and 5 min following injection. The study found no alteration in passive joint position sense or postural sway following lateral ankle joint anesthesia. The subjects did, however, assume a

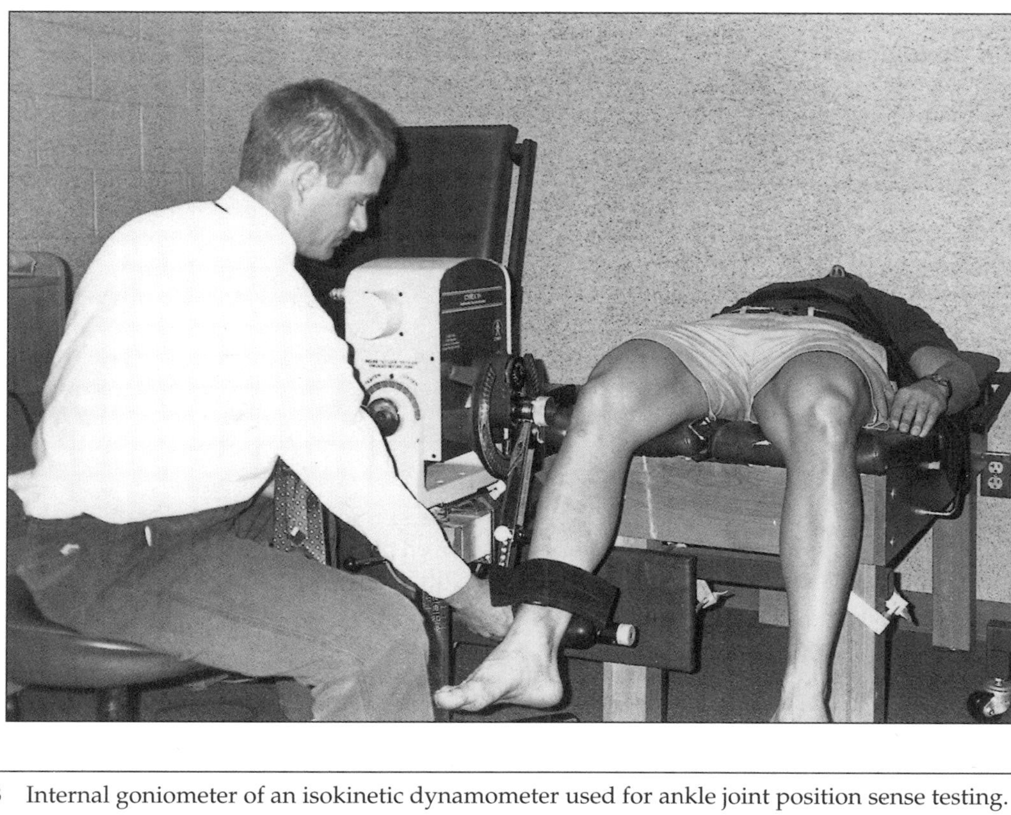

Figure 31.3 Internal goniometer of an isokinetic dynamometer used for ankle joint position sense testing.

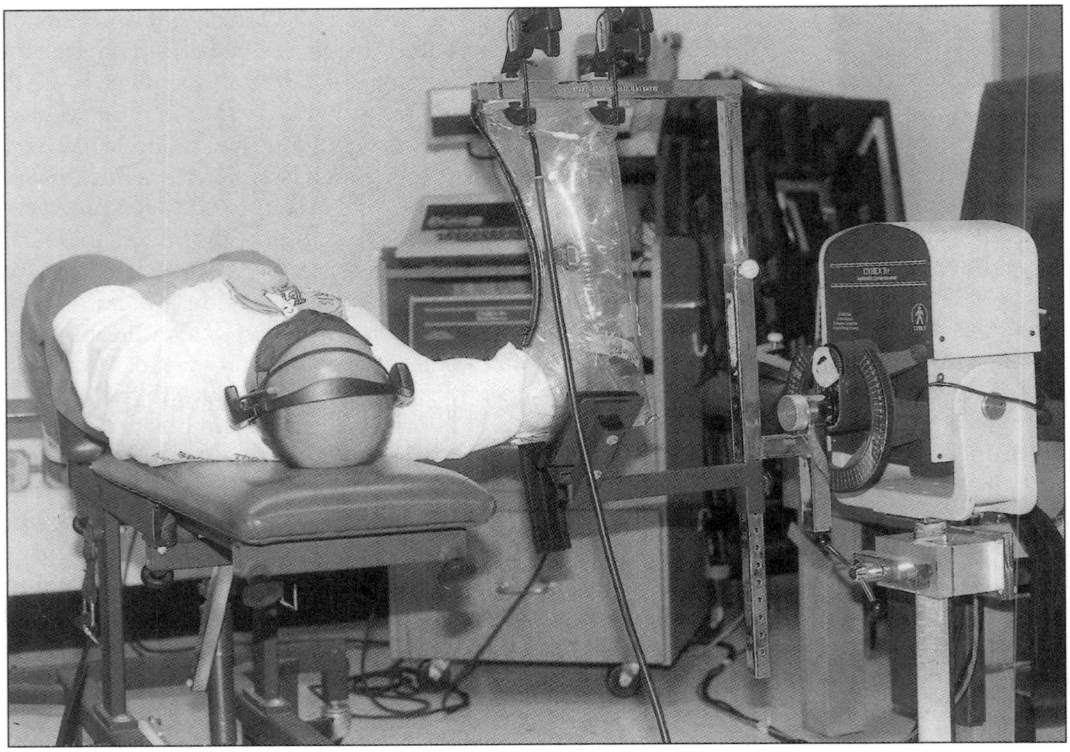

Figure 31.4 Internal goniometer of an isokinetic dynamometer used for shoulder joint position sense testing.

Table 31.1 Means and Standard Deviations for Ankle Joint Position Sense Measurements in Degrees of Error for Two Testers From Szczerba (23)

		Tester 1		Tester 2	
Position	Mode	M	*SD*	M	*SD*
5° from max inversion	Passive	4.50	5.41	4.55	3.00
	Active	8.55	6.71	7.58	4.27
15° inversion	Passive	6.60	5.02	5.63	4.04
	Active	6.95	5.09	5.65	4.25
0° neutral	Passive	5.20	3.46	6.68	5.86
	Active	5.50	4.73	6.55	4.20
10° eversion	Passive	8.00	6.23	6.60	5.91
	Active	6.80	4.23	6.62	4.86

different center of balance following anesthesia. This finding would seem to support the need for assessment of multiple parameters of proprioception.

Bernier and Perrin (1) examined the effects of a 6 wk coordination training program on active and passive joint position sense in 45 subjects with functional instability of the ankle. Postural stability in the form of sway index and a modified equilibrium score were also assessed before and after the training program. Functional instability was defined as at least one significant inversion ankle sprain followed by repeated injury or episodes of giving way within 12 mo prior to testing. Subjects were assigned to either a control group, a sham electrical stimulation treatment group, or a balance and coordination training group. Active and passive joint position sense testing followed a protocol similar to Szczerba and associates (23). Active and passive joint repositioning were assessed with a Kinetic Communicator at 15° inversion, 0° neutral, and 10°

eversion at 0° and 25° of plantar flexion. Maximum inversion was also assessed with the ankle in 25° of plantar flexion. Error scores were the average of two trials for each test condition and can be seen in table 31.2. This study found that 6 weeks of coordination and balance training did not affect joint position sense or sway index but did improve the subject's modified equilibrium balance scores. As with the Hertel group study (11), this study suggests that assessment of joint position sense alone may be insufficient for detection of changes in proprioception.

Kaminski and Perrin (13) determined the effect of a prophylactic knee guard on balance and joint position sense of the knee in 36 healthy male subjects. The authors hypothesized that the knee guard would enhance knee proprioception based on previous work that found improvement in proprioception with the use of a neoprene sleeve (14) and elastic bandage (19). In this repeated measures design study, subjects were tested under both braced and unbraced conditions for active and passive joint position sense and for balance (see figures 31.3 and 31.5). The internal goniometer of a Cybex II isokinetic dynamometer (Cybex, Division of Lumex, Inc., Ronkonkoma, NY) was used to assess joint position sense. The starting position for each subject was 90° of knee flexion. The leg was then passively extended at 12.5°/s, which corresponded to the weigh-limb velocity on the dynamometer's digital speed control box. The target angles were 15°, 25°, 35°, and 75° in the range of motion. Each target angle was maintained for 5 s, and the subject's limb was then returned to the starting position. The subject's limb was then passively moved, or he was asked to actively return to the target angle and to verbally indicate when he felt he had attained the previous angle. The zero velocity button on the speed control box was depressed at this point, and the joint angle was recorded from the dynamometer's computer. The error score was recorded as the difference between the target and repositioned angles. Balance testing (see figure 31.5) consisted of measurement of sway index and center of balance under single-leg and double-leg stance conditions with stable and dynamic platform conditions. Subjects were tested with bare feet to enhance somatosensory feedback from foot contact with the support surface. The findings indicated that bracing had no effect on active or passive joint repositioning (see figure 31.6). Knee bracing improved center of balance under one dynamic condition (double-leg stance), but no differences were found for any of the other balance conditions.

Tamburello (24) determined the effect of a knee joint effusion on isokinetic concentric torque and active and passive joint position sense. The author hypothesized that a reflex inhibition would occur from the induced knee effusion. Muscle performance and joint position sense were assessed on a Cybex II isokinetic dynamometer before and following injection of 30 ml of saline into the knee joint of each of 8 healthy females. Assessment of passive and active joint position sense

Table 31.2 Means and Standard Deviations for Ankle Joint Position Sense Measurements in Degrees of Error From Bernier et al. (1)

		Control				Sham				Treatment			
		Active		Passive		Active		Passive		Active		Passive	
Position		*X*	*SD*	*X*	*SD*	*X*	*SD*	*X*	*SD*	*X*	*SD*	*X*	*SD*
Pre	0°, inv	7.21	(5.33)	5.03	(4.16)	8.04	(4.56)	6.71	(4.56)	5.38	(3.11)	5.85	(3.60)
Post	0°, inv	7.28	(6.26)	4.46	(3.12)	6.21	(4.76)	5.79	(3.17)	5.26	(3.70)	5.85	(4.35)
Pre	0°, neu	4.17	(3.12)	4.17	(3.12)	5.39	(3.67)	5.39	(3.67)	5.41	(3.53)	5.41	(3.53)
Post	0°, neu	4.00	(3.32)	4.89	(2.80)	5.57	(2.45)	4.39	(2.35)	5.76	(3.94)	3.62	(2.13)
Pre	0°, ev	7.25	(4.38)	5.07	(3.47)	7.82	(4.54)	5.86	(1.90)	7.09	(4.24)	5.88	(4.01)
Post	0°, ev	5.85	(3.46)	5.50	(3.96)	4.14	(2.81)	4.25	(2.68)	5.56	(3.58)	3.79	(3.04)
Pre	25°, inv	8.75	(6.00)	6.46	(3.57)	8.71	(6.08)	6.71	(4.20)	6.38	(4.45)	4.47	(2.98)
Post	25°, inv	7.61	(3.96)	4.29	(3.51)	7.54	(4.63)	6.39	(3.63)	5.24	(4.61)	4.44	(4.35)
Pre	25°, neu	6.54	(4.24)	5.46	(4.18)	6.82	(4.99)	3.64	(4.31)	5.26	(2.97)	6.71	(4.85)
Post	25°, neu	5.14	(2.82)	5.32	(4.40)	6.71	(4.67)	8.07	(6.28)	4.76	(2.81)	5.74	(3.95)
Pre	25°, ev	6.43	(4.70)	4.89	(3.23)	6.93	(3.68)	4.79	(2.99)	7.97	(4.87)	7.00	(4.76)
Post	25°, ev	5.61	(3.69)	5.11	(2.87)	7.71	(5.80)	5.25	(3.62)	6.18	(3.70)	4.74	(2.87)
Pre	25°, max inv	9.36	(6.82)	3.57	(2.81)	7.82	(4.95)	5.29	(4.07)	8.47	(7.71)	4.71	(2.87)
Post	25°, max inv	7.54	(5.78)	4.64	(3.81)	6.68	(3.19)	4.71	(2.57)	7.24	(5.95)	4.29	(2.76)

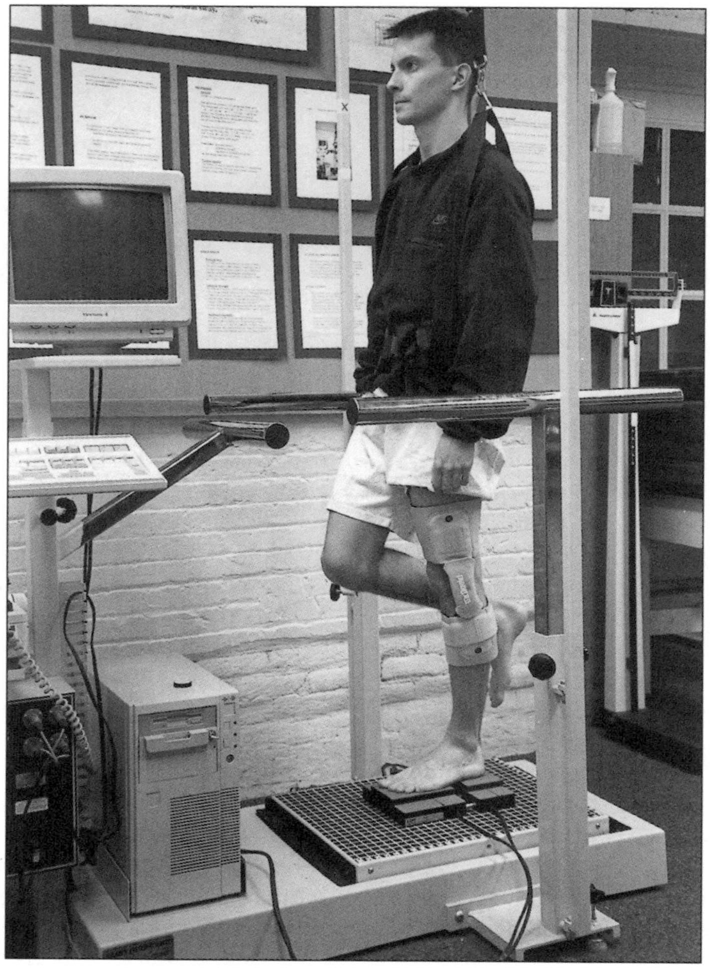

Figure 31.5 Single-limb postural stability testing on a Chattecx Balance System.

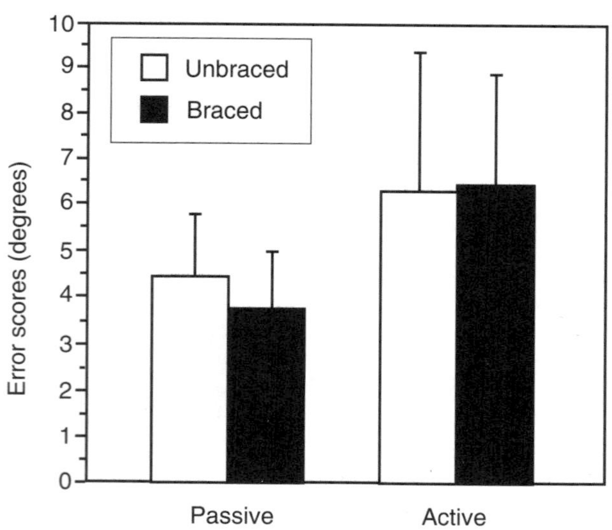

Figure 31.6 Knee joint position error scores during passive and active modes of repositioning from Kaminski and Perrin (13).

began with the knee in full extension. The limb was actively or passively moved through a full range of motion at a speed of approximately 10°/s and then positioned at 15° of knee flexion for 15 s. The limb was again moved through a full range of motion and the subject was asked to indicate when she felt she had reproduced the 15° angle. Error scores averaged over 3 trials were used for analysis. Muscle performance testing occurred at 60°/s and consisted of 3 submaximal and 1 maximal warm-up contractions, followed by a 1 min rest, and then 4 maximal reciprocal concentric knee extension and flexion contractions. Measures of peak torque and total work were recorded for analysis. The study found no decrement in strength or active joint position sense following inducement of the effusion. However, the subjects did have a significant reduction in passive joint position sensitivity with the knee effusion.

Giunta and coworkers (6) compared joint position sense in the shoulders of overarm-trained athletes with a group of untrained control subjects. The rationale for this study was to determine if training of the upper extremity had a positive impact on joint proprioception. Active and passive joint position sense were assessed at angles of 25–30° of internal rotation, 25–30° of external rotation, and 5–10° from maximal external rotation using the Cybex II internal goniometer. The subjects were positioned supine with each test beginning in neutral rotation. The limb was then passively or actively moved to the test angle, held in that position for 5 s and then returned to the neutral position. Immediately following, the limb was again passively or actively moved toward the target angle, and the subject indicated verbally when he or she believed the desired angle had been achieved. The error scores were the average of 2 trials for each test condition. The study found overarm-trained athletes were able to reproduce the targeted joint angles with significantly less error than control subjects were. The significant main effect for the group found mean angular reproduction error scores of 3.35 ±2.33° for the trained group and 4.29 ±2.43° for the untrained group. No difference was found in error scores between active and passive joint repositioning.

The aforementioned studies demonstrate assessment of joint proprioception at the ankle, knee, and shoulder using isokinetic dynamometry. For the most part, healthy subjects were studied. However, Hertel and coworkers (11) attempted to induce a deafferentation of the lateral ankle ligaments with injections of lidocaine, and Tamburello (24) created a knee joint effusion with injections of saline. The validity of these models in replicating the injury state for joint proprioception research requires additional study. The findings of Szczerba and coworkers (23) also suggest that additional research is needed to optimize the reliability of measurements using this technology. Isokinetic dynamometry for assessment of joint proprioception would seem to be a reasonable option in the absence of more sophisticated instrumentation designed specifically for this purpose.

Electrogoniometers and Flexometers

Electrogoniometers and flexometers have also been used to assess joint position sense of the knee (see figures 31.7 & 31.8) (5, 12) and shoulder (see figure 31.9) (21). These devices are advantageous, especially for the lower extremity joints, as they permit assessment of joint position sense in either open or closed kinetic chain positions.

Higgins and Perrin (12) used a Leighton flexometer (Leighton, Spokane, WA) and Cybex II to compare active knee joint position sense in weight-bearing and nonweight-bearing conditions. The protocol for assessment of nonweight-bearing position sense was similar to the procedure used by Kaminski and Perrin (13), with a target angle of 30° in the range of motion. The limb was passively placed at the target angle for 15 s followed by placement at full extension for 15 s. The subject was then asked to reposition the limb at the target angle. Error scores over 3 trials were obtained. For the weight-bearing test, a Leighton flexometer was attached to the distal thigh of the dominant extremity approximately 1 in. above the knee joint line (see figure 31.8). Each subject stood on a 6 in. box with the back against a wall and was blindfolded to eliminate visual cues. Using the angular display on the flexometer, the subjects squatted to 30° of knee flexion, held this position for 15 s, and returned to the starting position of 0° knee extension. Following a 15 s rest period the subjects then attempted to reposition themselves at the predetermined angle. The degree of error from the 30° knee flexion target angle was recorded, and the average of 3 trials was used for data analysis. The reliability of the measurements was also computed from the 3 trials. The intraclass coefficients were $R = .97$ and $R = .93$ for the weight-bearing and nonweight-bearing tests, respectively. The study found that joint position sense assessed from the weight-bearing position was more sensitive than from the nonweight-bearing position (WB error = 1.7° vs. NWB error = 4.05°). The authors postulated that this was due to multiple contributions from the muscular, capsular, and cutaneous cues during joint movement and approximation at the ankle, knee, and hip during squatting. This would seem to be a disadvantage in the isolated assessment of joint position sense yet would appear to be a more "functional" position for assessment of proprioception.

Fisher and coworkers (5) studied the effect of slide board (Don Courson Enterprises, Inc.) exercise on open and closed chain knee joint proprioception in 16 female (8 experimental, 8 control) subjects free from injury to the lower extremity. Closed chain knee joint position sense was assessed during a squat movement with an electrogoniometer (Penny & Giles, Inc., Santa Monica, CA) attached to the lateral aspect of the knee. Open chain joint position sense was assessed with a Cybex II isokinetic dynamometer using a protocol similar to Kaminski and Perrin (13) and Tamburello (24). The target angles for joint position sense testing were 30° and 70° of knee flexion. The exercise protocol consisted of an interval type program 3 days per wk for 4 wks. Intensity of training was progressively increased based on exercise duration, slide rate, and

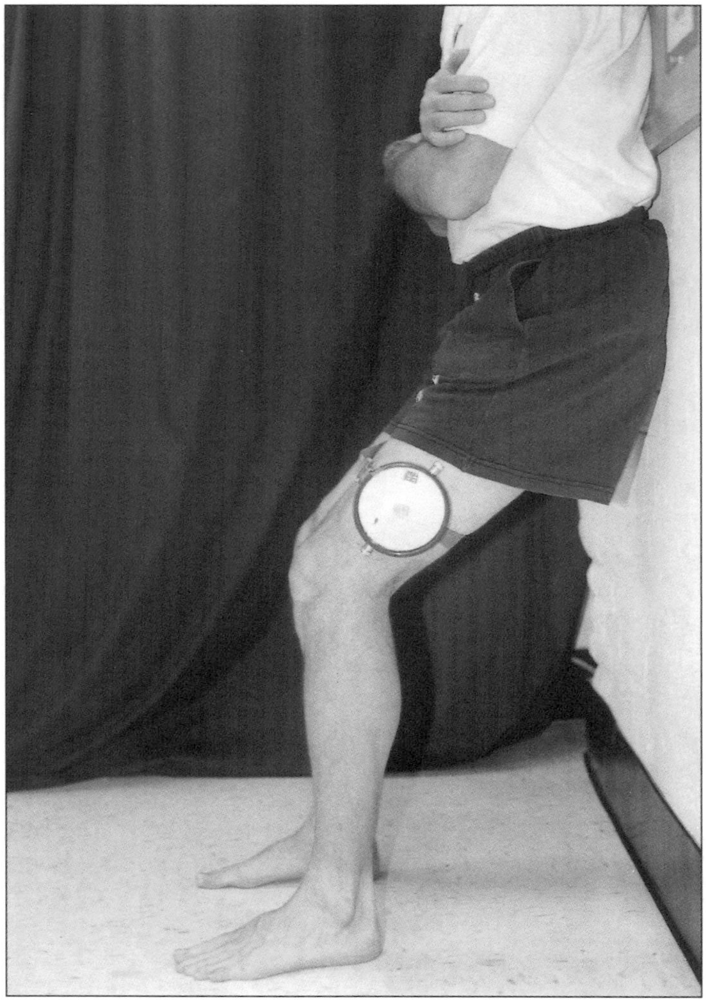

Figure 31.7 A Leighton flexometer used for weight-bearing knee joint position sense testing.

board length. The results indicated that open and closed chain joint position sense significantly improved at both the 30° and 70° target angles for the experimental subjects in comparison to the control group. The authors concluded that slide board training was effective in improving knee joint proprioception in healthy university females.

Open and closed chain exercises have historically been of primary interest as they relate to the lower extremity. More recently, the relevance of these exercises to the shoulder joint complex has interested clinicians and researchers. Rogol and coworkers (21) compared the effects of open versus closed chain exercise on shoulder joint proprioception in 39 injury-free male cadets at a military academy. The subjects were randomly assigned to an open chain exercise group, a closed chain exercise group, or a comparison group. A Cybex II dynamometer and a flexometer were used to assess shoulder joint active and passive position sense at 30° internal rotation, 30° external rotation, and 10° from full external rotation (see figure 31.9). The subjects assigned to the closed chain exercise group performed 3 sets of 15 repetitions of standard push-ups. The open chain exercise group performed the same number of supine dumbbell press repetitions. All subjects trained 3 days per wk for a 6 wk period. The findings of the study were that both the open and closed chain groups improved joint position sensibility in comparison to the control group. The authors concluded that both open and closed chain exercises were effective in improving open chain shoulder joint proprioception in a group of healthy males.

The vast majority of proprioception research has assessed joint position sense from a nonweight-bearing, or open kinetic chain position. This would seem to be the preferred method for isolation of the proprioceptive mechanism at a specific joint. However, the func-

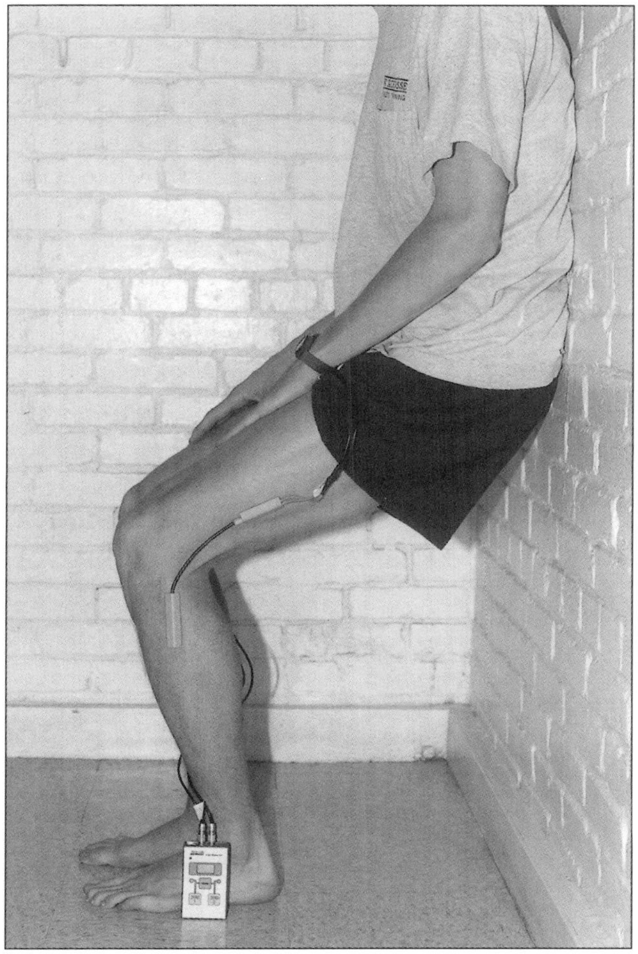

Figure 31.8 An electrogoniometer used for knee joint position sense testing.

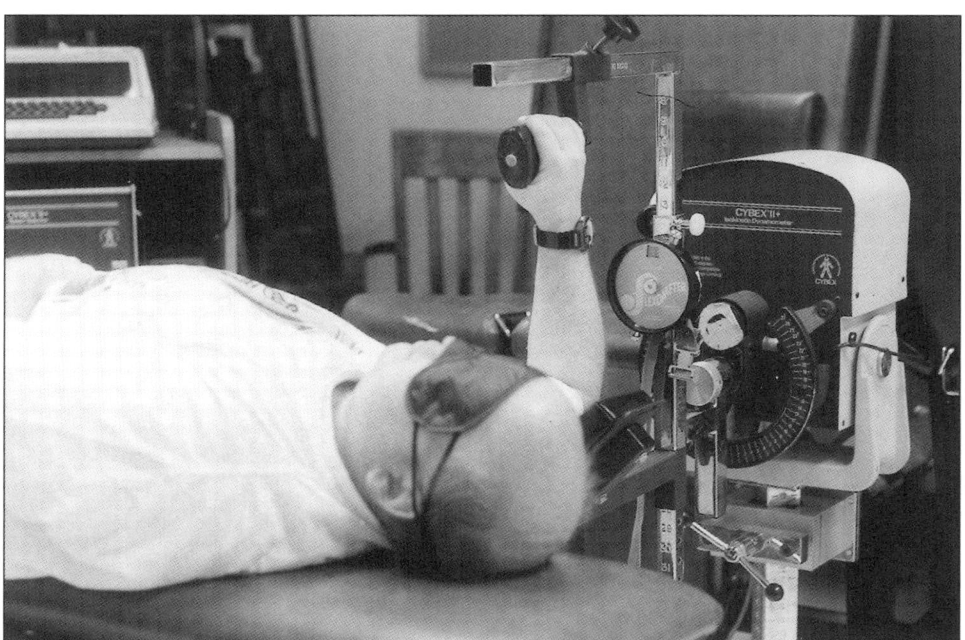

Figure 31.9 A Leighton flexometer attached to a Cybex isokinetic dynamometer for shoulder joint position sense testing.

tional application of this technique may be questionable. The aforementioned studies provide examples of the potential application of weight-bearing, or closed kinetic chain, assessment of joint proprioception. Additional research is needed to refine the technique and validity of closed chain assessment of joint proprioception for both the upper and lower extremities.

Balance and Postural Stability Systems

Feedback from the vestibular, visual, and proprioceptive (somatosensory) systems is necessary for the maintenance of postural stability. Musculoskeletal injury to the lower extremity involving disruption of the joint proprioceptors at the hip, knee, or ankle has the potential to cause partial deafferentation, which can alter one's postural sway (9). Several studies have used posturography to assess the effects of injury (2, 16), exercise (1), ligament anesthesia (11), orthotic intervention (8), fatigue (18), and bracing (13) on postural stability. Postural sway can be assessed in single- or double-leg stances under static and dynamic conditions with eyes open or closed. Mattacola and associates (17) found good reliability under some of these conditions while a wide range exists under other conditions.

Mattacola and coworkers (16) compared the effects of anterior cruciate ligament reconstruction (ACLR) on postural stability, a single-leg hop test, and muscle strength in 20 subjects with 20 matched controls possessing otherwise similar physical characteristics. Postural stability was measured as a stability index with a Biodex Stability System (Biodex Medical Systems, Shirley, NY) (see figure 31.10). The mean time from surgery for the ACLR subjects was 18 mo. No significant differences were found between the ACLR subjects and the matched controls for stability index and knee flexion strength scores. However, the ACLR subjects hopped for less distance and produced less torque when compared to the matched control group limb. The authors felt that these findings support the notion that functional exercise is an essential component of both rehabilitation and assessment of ACL-injured patients.

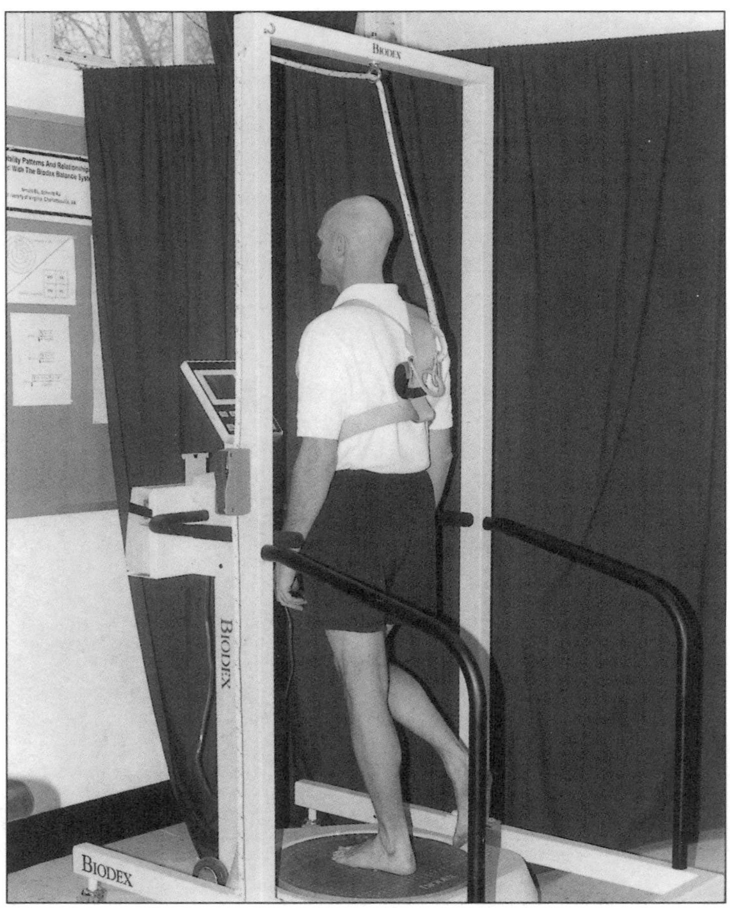

Figure 31.10 Postural stability assessed with a Biodex Stability System.

Bernier and coworkers (2) determined if subjects with a unilateral functional instability of the ankle had decreased postural sway and decreased concentric and eccentric strength of the ankle invertors and evertors when compared to an uninjured population. Functional instability was defined as a history of significant ankle inversion sprain followed by repeated episodes of "giving way." Nine subjects meeting this criterion were compared with 9 subjects with no history of lower extremity injury. Sway index was assessed in dual- and single-limb stances under static and dynamic conditions with a Chattecx Balance System (Chattanooga Group Inc., Hixson, TN) (see figure 31.11). No significant differences in single-limb postural sway and muscle strength were found between the functional instability subjects and the uninjured controls. The authors postulated that a more sensitive means of assessing proprioception may be needed to detect deficits in subjects with functional instability of the ankle.

In the study by Bernier and associates (1) previously discussed in this chapter, subjects with ankle functional instability participated in a 6 wk coordination and balance training program (see table 31.3). In addition to joint position sense testing, subjects were assessed for postural sway on a Chattecx Balance System under the following conditions: stable platform with eyes open and eyes closed and an inversion/eversion tilting platform with eyes open and eyes closed. The dependent measures for postural sway were sway index and modified equilibrium score. The sway index is defined as a numerical value of the standard deviation of the distance the subject spends away from the center of balance. The modified equilibrium score is a unitless measure of the actual anterior-posterior or medial-lateral sway in relation to the theoretical limits of sta-

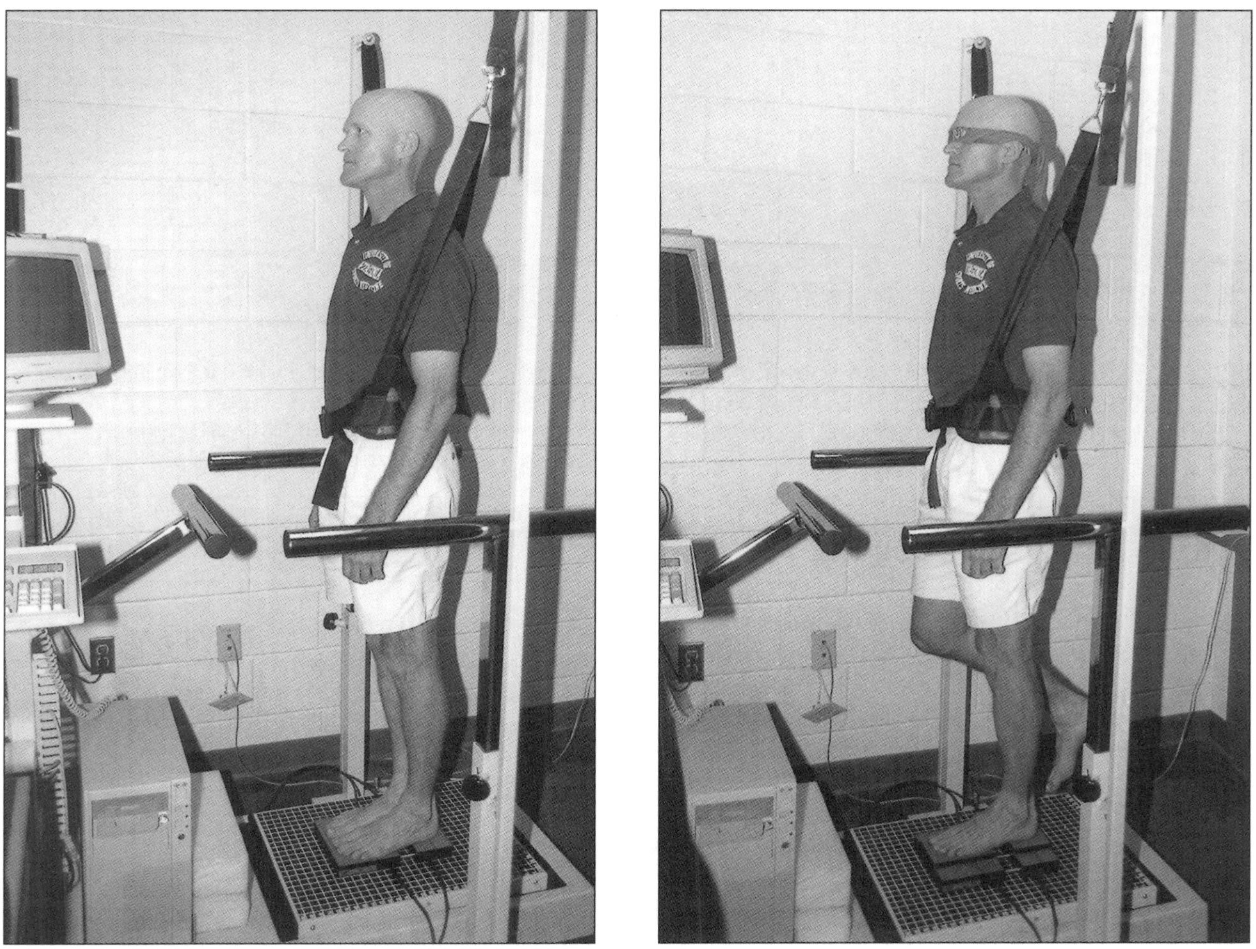

a b

Figure 31.11 Postural stability assessed with a Chattecx Balance System under (*a*) double-leg, eyes-open, and (*b*) single-leg, eyes-closed conditions.

Table 31.3 Coordination and Balance Training Protocol From Bernier et al. (1)

Week 1 15 s each, 45 s rest between exercises	Week 2 20 s each 40 s rest between exercises	Week 3 25 s each 35 s rest between exercises	Week 4 30 s each 30 s rest between exercises	Week 5 30 s each 30 s rest between exercises	Week 6 30 s each 30 s rest between exercises
1. Fixed surface, eyes open (FEO)	Same as week 1	FEO FEC	FEC FPO	FEC FPO	FEC FPO
2. Fixed surface, eyes closed (FEC)		FPO TEO2	TEO2 × 2 TEC2 × 2	TEO2 TEC2	TEO2 TEC2
3. Fixed surface, picking up objects (FPO)	Add wobble board	TEC2 TEO3	WEO × 2 WEC × 2	WEO × 2 WEC × 2	WEO WEC
4. Tilt board, dorsi/plantar, eyes open (TEO1)	10. Wobble, eyes open (WEO) × 2	TEC3 WEO × 2 11. Wobble, eyes closed (WEC)		12. Functional hop, eyes open (FHO) × 2	FHO × 2 13. FHC × 2 (eyes closed only *after* landing)
5. Tilt board, dorsi/plantar, eyes closed (TEC1)					
6. Tilt board, inv/ev, eyes open (TEO2)					
7. Tilt board, inv/ev, eyes closed (TEC2)					
8. Tilt board, diag placement, eyes open (TEO3)					
9. Tilt board, diag placement, eyes closed (TEC3)					

inv = inversion, ev = eversion, diag = diagonal

bility. The study found that the 6 wk training program significantly improved the modified equilibrium scores of balance in both the anterior-posterior and medial-lateral directions but had no effect on sway index or joint position sense of the ankle.

Guskiewicz and Perrin (8) determined if orthotics would reduce postural sway in 13 subjects with acute ankle sprains when compared with 12 uninjured controls. Acute ankle injury was defined as an injury that had occurred within 21 days of participation in the study. Additional criteria included a pain-free range of motion and the ability to fully bear weight at the time of data collection. Postural sway during single-limb stance was assessed with the Chattecx Balance System with and without orthotics that were custom produced by Foot Management, Inc. (Pittsville, MD). Subjects were assessed with a stable platform, and under inversion/eversion, plantar/dorsiflexion, and medial/lateral platform movement conditions. The mean postural sway values are presented in table 31.4. The study found that the intervention of orthotics significantly reduced postural

Table 31.4 Mean Postural Sway Measurements for Ankle-Injured and Uninjured Subjects Presented as Sway Index in CM (±*SD*) From Guskiewicz and Perrin (8)

	No orthotics		With orthotics	
Stable				
Injured	.80	(.22)	.82	(.32)
Uninjured	.63	(.18)	.87	(.32)
Inversion/eversion				
Injured	1.07	(.31)	.86	(.19)*
Uninjured	.89	(.19)	.87	(.21)
Plantar/dorsiflex				
Injured	1.39	(.49)	1.33	(.48)
Uninjured	1.14	(.27)	1.13	(.33)
Medial/lateral				
Injured	1.63	(.27)	1.26	(.21)*
Uninjured	1.39	(.35)	1.34	(.32)

*Significantly different ($p < .05$).

sway in ankle-injured subjects as compared to uninjured subjects under the inversion/eversion and medial/lateral movement conditions.

McGuire and coworkers (18) examined the effect of hip and knee extensor muscle fatigue on postural sway in 16 healthy male athletes. A Kinetic Communicator isokinetic dynamometer was used to induce concentric muscle fatigue to 50% of an initial maximal voluntary contraction in a "closed chain" manner (see figure 31.12). A Chattecx Balance System was used to assess postural sway in a single-limb stance under static, medial/lateral, inversion/eversion, anterior/posterior, and plantar/dorsiflexion movement conditions. The study found that the fatigue protocol for the hip and knee musculature did not influence postural sway. The authors speculated that the ankle musculature might provide a more prominent role in controlling postural sway.

The assessment of postural stability is a highly complex process involving multiple neurological and musculoskeletal systems. Feedback from the proprioceptive (somatosensory) system plays a crucial role in the maintenance of postural stability. As such, assessment of this component of somatosensory input seems justified when studying musculoskeletal injury and proprioception. The aforementioned studies provide examples of research involving assessment of postural stability and proprioceptive feedback from the ankle and knee.

Summary

This chapter provides examples of several techniques that can be used for assessing proprioception and neuromuscular control in a clinical or research setting. The studies presented in this chapter should generate many questions for the clinician and researcher. For example, which test protocols are practical and accessible while at the same time have good reproducibility (reliability) of measurement? When are statistically significant findings clinically relevant when dealing with measurements of joint position sense in degrees and postural sway in centimeters? How many subjects are necessary for adequate statistical power when using these units of measurement? What is the generalizability of findings to a broader population, especially when healthy or injured subjects are studied? Finally, when considering future research methodology, can a clinical model of injury be utilized for studies involving joint proprioception and neuromuscular control? For example, a model of experimentally induced delayed onset muscle soreness (DOMS) has been used to study the effects of various therapeutic interventions on pain, strength, and range of motion associated with DOMS (3, 4, 7, 10, 15, 22). Would DOMS be a useful model for studying joint proprioception and neuromuscular control in subjects who have many of the same features seen with an actual injury such as tis-

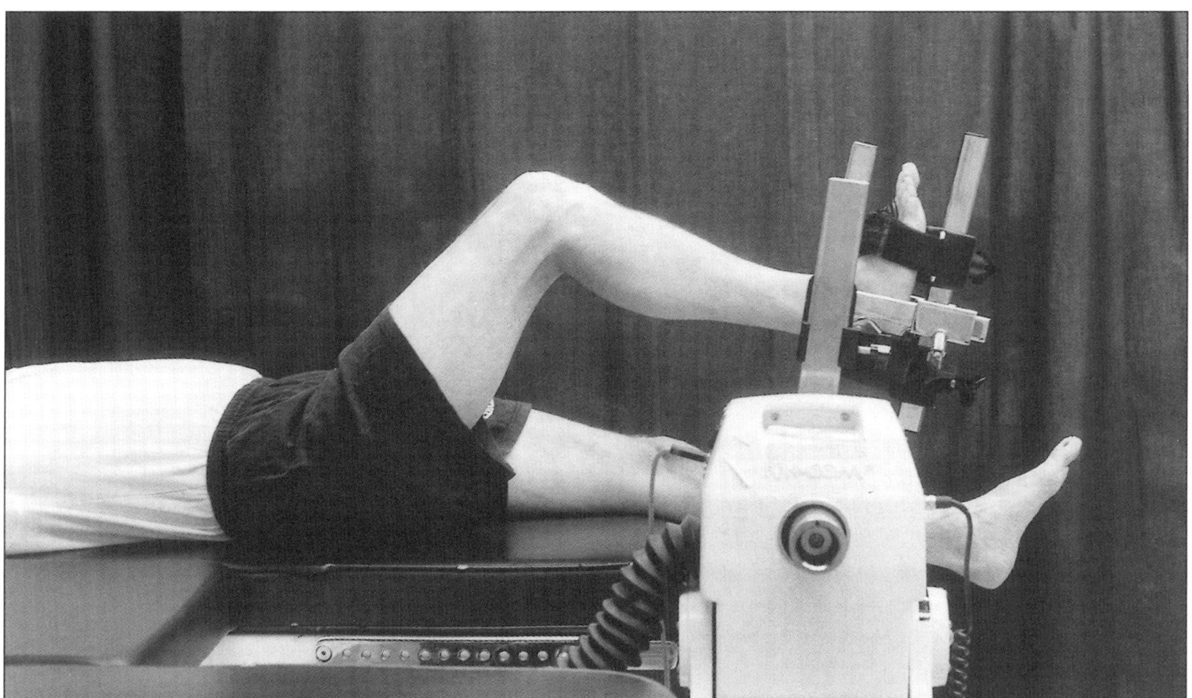

Figure 31.12 Isokinetic dynamometer used to induce closed chain fatigue of the hip and knee extensor muscle groups.

sue microtrauma, pain, swelling, and loss of motion? Hopefully, these questions and the clinical research presented in this chapter will stimulate others to contribute to the limited body of knowledge related to joint proprioception and neuromuscular control.

References

1. Bernier, J.N., & Perrin, D.H. Effect of coordination training on proprioception of the functionally unstable ankle. Manuscript submitted for publication.
2. Bernier, J.N., Perrin, D.H., & Rijke, A. 1997. Effect of unilateral functional instability of the ankle on inversion and eversion strength and postural sway. *Journal of Athletic Training* 32: 226–32.
3. Denegar, C.R., & Perrin, D.H. 1992. Effect of transcutaneous electrical nerve stimulation, cold, and a combination treatment on pain, decreased range of motion, and strength loss associated with delayed onset muscle soreness. *Journal of Athletic Training* 27: 200–206.
4. Denegar, C.R., Perrin, D.H., Rogol, A D., & Rutt, R.R. 1989. Influence of transcutaneous electrical nerve stimulation on pain, range of motion, and serum cortisol concentration in females experiencing delayed onset muscle soreness. *Journal of Orthopaedic and Sports Physical Therapy* 11: 100-103.
5. Fisher, D.C., Moore, J.H., & Perrin, D.H. Effect of slide board exercise on proprioception of the knee. Manuscript submitted for publication.
6. Giunta, S.L., Bernier, J.N., & Perrin, D.H. Joint position sense in the trained and untrained shoulder. Manuscript submitted for publication.
7. Grossman, J.M., Arnold, B.L., Perrin, D.H., & Kahler, D.M. 1995. Effect of ibuprofen use on delayed onset muscle soreness of the elbow flexors. *Journal of Sport Rehabilitation* 4: 253–63.
8. Guskiewicz, K.M., & Perrin, D.H. 1996. Effect of orthotics on postural sway following inversion ankle sprain. *Journal of Orthopedic and Sports Physical Therapy* 23: 326–31.
9. Guskiewicz, K.M., & Perrin, D.H. 1996. Research and clinical applications of assessing balance. *Journal of Sport Rehabilitation* 5: 45–63.
10. Haynes, S.C., & Perrin, D.H. 1992. Effect of a counterirritant on pain and restricted range of motion associated with delayed onset muscle soreness. *Journal of Sport Rehabilitation* 1: 13–18.
11. Hertel, J.N., Guskiewicz, K.M., Kahler, D.M., & Perrin, D.H. 1996. Effect of lateral ankle joint anesthesia on center of balance, postural sway, and joint position sense. *Journal of Sport Rehabilitation* 5: 111–19.
12. Higgins, M.J., & Perrin, D.H. 1997. Comparison of weight-bearing and nonweight-bearing conditions on knee joint reposition sense. *Journal of Sport Rehabilitation* 6: 327–34.
13. Kaminski, T.W., & Perrin, D.H. 1996. Effect of prophylactic knee bracing on balance and joint position sense. *Journal of Athletic Training* 31: 131–36.
14. Lephart, S.M., Kocher, M.S., Fu, F.H., & Harner, C.D. 1992. Proprioception following anterior cruciate ligament reconstruction. *Journal of Sport Rehabilitation* 1: 188–96.
15. Mattacola, C.G., Perrin, D.H., Gansneder, B.M., Allen, J.D., & Mickey, C.A. 1997. A comparison of visual analog and graphic rating scales for assessing pain following delayed onset muscle soreness. *Journal of Sport Rehabilitation* 6: 38–46.
16. Mattacola, C.G., Perrin, D.H., Gansneder, B.M., Gieck, J.H., Saliba, E.N., & McCue, F.C. 1997. Dynamic postural stability following anterior cruciate ligament reconstruction. *Journal of Athletic Training* 32: S9.
17. Mattacola, C.G., Lebsack, D.A., & Perrin, D.H. 1995. Intertester reliability of assessing postural sway using the Chattecx Balance System. *Journal of Athletic Training* 30: 237–42.
18. McGuire, B.A., Mattacola, C.G., Perrin, D.H. Effects of closed chain induced fatigue of the hip and knee extensors on postural sway. Manuscript submitted for publication.
19. Perlau, R., Frank, C., & Fick, G. 1995. The effect of elastic bandages on human knee proprioception in the uninjured population. *American Journal of Sports Medicine* 23: 251–55.
20. Perrin, D.H. 1993. *Isokinetic exercise and assessment*. Champaign, IL: Human Kinetics.
21. Rogol, I.M., Ernst, G.P, & Perrin, D.H. Effect of open versus closed kinetic chain shoulder exercise on proprioception. Manuscript submitted for publication.
22. Schmitz, R.J., Martin, D.M., Perrin, D.H., Iranmanesh, A., & Rogol, A.D. 1997. Effect of interferential current on perceived pain and serum cortisol associated with delayed onset muscle soreness. *Journal of Sport Rehabilitation* 6: 30–37.
23. Szczerba, J.E., Bernier, J.N., Perrin, D.H., & Gansneder, B.M. 1995. Intertester reliability of active and passive ankle joint position sense testing. *Journal of Sport Rehabilitation* 4: 282–91.
24. Tamburello, M. 1992. The effect of a small knee effusion on concentric isokinetic muscle performance and joint reposition sense. Doctoral dissertation, University of Virginia, Charlottesville.

CHAPTER 32

The Rationale for Open and Closed Kinetic Chain Activities for Restoration of Proprioception and Neuromuscular Control Following Injury

James J. Irrgang, PhD, PT, ATC
Randy Neri, PT, ATC

Introduction

Proprioception is a specialized sense of touch that is mediated by mechanoreceptors located in the skin, muscles, tendons, ligaments, and joint capsules. Movement results in mechanical deformation of these structures, which in turn results in generation of action potentials that travel to the central nervous system (CNS). Once in the CNS, the afferent information is processed to result in conscious awareness of movement and position. Proprioceptive information also serves to mediate voluntary and involuntary motor responses to permit smooth coordinated movement. It has been hypothesized that injury to capsuloligamentous structures results in partial deafferentation of the joint, which leads to proprioceptive deficits and loss of neuromuscular control. Loss of neuromuscular control, in turn, may result in functional instability and repeated ligamentous injury. Recognition of the effects of joint injury on loss of neuromuscular control has led to an emphasis in rehabilitation on restoring proprioception to enhance dynamic joint stability.

Over the last 10 years there has been a greater emphasis on the use of closed kinetic chain (CKC) exercises for rehabilitation of lower and upper extremity injuries. The rationale for use of CKC exercises is based upon the premise that CKC exercises are more functional in terms of the loads placed upon the joint and the types of muscle contraction that result. This paper discusses the use of open and closed kinetic chain exercises to enhance proprioception and restore dynamic joint stability in the rehabilitation of capsuloligamentous injuries. We provide a brief overview of current concepts related to proprioception and a comparison of open versus closed kinetic chain exercises. Finally, we provide recommendations for incorporation of open and closed chain exercises in the rehabilitation process, to enhance proprioception and dynamic joint stability.

Overview of Proprioception

Proprioception is the cumulative neural input to the CNS from mechanoreceptors located in the joint capsules, ligaments, muscles, tendons, and the skin (53). Other terms that are often used synonymously with proprioception include kinesthesia and balance. Kinesthesia is the conscious awareness of joint position and movement resulting from proprioceptive input to the CNS (17). Balance refers to the ability to maintain the center of gravity over the base of support without falling (36). The ability to maintain balance requires the integration of proprioceptive input from the periphery with afferent information from the eyes and the vestibular apparatus in the inner ear. Appropriate use of this terminology is important among clinicians to enhance communication and understanding in this area.

Mechanoreceptors are specialized neuroepithelial structures, embedded in connective tissue, that transduce mechanical deformation into an encoded neural signal that is transmitted to the CNS. Mechanoreceptors are located in the joint capsules, ligaments, muscles, tendons, and skin.

Mechanoreceptors located within the joint capsule include Ruffini and Paciniform endings as well as free nerve endings. Ruffini endings are located within the joint capsule, predominantly on that side of the joint that is under tension when the joint is extended (48). Ruffini endings are slow adapting mechanoreceptors, which implies that they fire continuously at a specified frequency that is dependent on the stress placed upon them. They are therefore thought to be responsible primarily for providing information concerning joint position. Ruffini endings respond to stress (i.e., load) rather than strain (i.e., displacement) (21). The posterior aspect of a joint is slack in most positions of the joint and becomes stressed only when the joint is moved near the limit of extension. Capsular stress is dependent upon the degree of extension (i.e., the extension moment) and the response of the Ruffini endings is proportional to stress applied to the tissue. For example, in the knee, Ruffini endings are excited only during extreme extension. As a result, they primarily serve as limit detectors (21). Microstimulation of nerve fibers arising from Ruffini endings has been associated with the sensation of joint movement (23, 34).

Paciniform endings are widely distributed throughout the joint capsule and periarticular connective tissue (48). They respond primarily to compression of the tissues in which they lie (21). Paciniform endings are rapidly adapting mechanoreceptors that respond to changes in movement with a burst of activity that quickly declines. They are thought primarily to provide information concerning acceleration and deceleration of joint movement. Microstimulation of nerve fibers originating from Paciniform endings has been associated with the sensation of compression (23, 34).

Free nerve endings are associated with small nerve fibers and respond primarily to noxious stimuli; thus they are nociceptors rather than proprioceptors (21). Free nerve endings may respond at the extremes of joint rotation (41). Also supporting the notion that the free nerve endings are nociceptors is the fact that they are sensitized when the joint is inflamed (21).

Mechanoreceptors in the musculotendinous unit include the muscle spindle and Golgi tendon organ. The muscle spindle is composed of intrafusal muscle fibers that are innervated by gamma sensory and motor neurons. Response of the muscle spindle afferents is a function of the length of the muscle, and as such, the muscle spindle provides information concerning joint motion (21). Vibration of a muscle stimulates the primary sensory afferent nerve fibers from the muscle spindle and produces the sensation of joint movement in the direction that would stretch the muscle being vibrated (20). When sensory nerves from the joint and cutaneous tissues are anesthetized, sensation of joint movement may be diminished but not lost as a result of sensory input from the muscle spindle (11, 15). Tensing muscles around the joint increases the muscle spindle's sensitivity to stretch and can dramatically enhance proprioception at the joint (16, 21).

The Golgi tendon organ is a mechanoreceptor that is located in tendons and serves to protect the muscle from overloading. The Golgi tendon organ responds to loading of the tendon, which occurs through contraction of the muscle or by passive lengthening of the muscle. Stimulation of the Golgi tendon organ results in inhibition of the motor neurons supplying the muscle in which the Golgi tendon organ lies and excitation of the motor neurons supplying the antagonistic muscles (32).

Afferent information from mechanoreceptors is conducted to the CNS by different nerve fiber types that are specific for each modality of sensation. Information concerning joint position and movement from mechanoreceptors located in the joint capsule and ligaments is conducted along large diameter nerve fibers, A(cc) fibers (3). Proprioceptive information from the muscle spindle is conducted to the CNS by the A(y) nerve fibers. Afferent stimulation from the free nerve endings is conducted to the CNS by the smaller diameter pain fibers, A(6) fibers. Proprioceptive input is conducted to the CNS via the dorsal root ganglion, where it is integrated segmentally or conducted via the posterior columns to the cerebral cortex in the postcentral gyrus (3).

Once in the CNS, proprioceptive input provides for conscious awareness of joint position and motion and also promotes voluntary and involuntary movement. There is a high degree of spatial orientation of information reaching the cerebral cortex, which facilitates conscious awareness of position sense and motion (3). Animal research has supported the notion that proprioceptive information from the joint capsule and ligaments may result in reflex muscle contraction, most likely mediated through a spinal reflex. In 1987 Solomonow and coworkers (45) demonstrated a ligament-muscle reflex arc involving the anterior cruciate ligament (ACL) and the hamstring and quadriceps muscles in an anesthetized cat. Loading of the ACL resulted in reflex contraction of the hamstrings and electrical silence in the quadriceps. This response was evident only when high loads were produced on the ACL. Low to moderate loading of the ACL failed to result in any alteration of muscle activity. The reflex arc between the ACL and hamstrings leads one to speculate that the hamstrings function as a load regulator during extension of the knee. As such, hamstring activity is increased on demand when the ligament is overloaded. The fact that the ACL-hamstring reflex arc is elicited when high loads are applied is consistent with the anatomical fact that most of the mechanoreceptors in the ACL are located near the insertions of the ligament, which corresponds to the region of the ligament that becomes stressed only with high loading of the ACL (42, 45). A similar reflex arc between the articular branches of the axillary nerve and the biceps, supraspinatus, infraspinatus, subscapularis, and deltoid has been demonstrated in the cat model (22).

Solomonow and coworkers (45) also demonstrated inhibition of quadriceps torque and electrical activity and increased hamstring electrical activity during a maximal isokinetic contraction of the quadriceps in individuals with a midsubstance tear of the ACL. This alteration in muscle activity corresponded to the point in the range of knee extension at which the quadriceps caused anterior subluxation of the tibia (i.e., at approximately 45° of knee flexion). These findings indicate that there are mechanoreceptors other than those in the ACL that are capable of producing changes in muscle activity. The mechanoreceptors responsible for these changes may be located in the joint capsule or musculotendinous structures. However proprioceptive input from these secondary sources is less than optimal in stabilizing the joint, since the alterations in muscle activity were unable to prevent the joint from subluxing.

The exact mechanism by which these reflex muscle changes are initiated is unknown. Some have hypothesized that input from mechanoreceptors results in direct stimulation of the alpha motor neuron, which in turn alters muscle activity (3). Others have hypothesized that input from mechanoreceptors primarily stimulates gamma motor neurons, which enhances sensitivity of the muscle spindle. Enhanced muscle spindle activity in turn influences activity of the muscle in which the muscle spindle lies. Johansson and coworkers (26–28) concluded that input from mechanoreceptors in the knee increased the level of responsiveness of the muscle spindle, which was primarily responsible for appropriate patterns of muscle firing to stabilize the joint and protect it from injury under moderate loading conditions.

Proprioceptive input also projects to higher centers in the CNS, including the brain stem and cerebral cortex. In the brain stem proprioceptive input from mechanoreceptors located in the skin, ligaments, joint capsule, and musculotendinous units combines with vestibular and visual input to maintain balance and posture. Proprioceptive input reaching the cerebral cortex results in conscious awareness of body position and movement and may be involved in initiating voluntary movements.

To enhance dynamic joint stability following ligament injury with subsequent loss of proprioceptive feedback from the involved ligament, rehabilitation should be designed to maximize use of proprioceptive input from these secondary sources. To accomplish this, the rehabilitation program must be developed to simulate the conditions under which the individual must function, which in turn necessitates the need for appropriate use of open and closed kinetic chain exercises.

Overview of Open and Closed Chain Exercises

Over the last 5 to 10 years there has been increased interest in the use of closed chain exercises for rehabilitation of injuries involving the upper and lower extremities. Proponents of closed chain exercises have advocated their use in rehabilitation to better simulate the functional demands placed on the limb during a variety of activities. Closed chain exercises result in simultaneous motion of all joints in the extremity, which requires coordinated muscle activity to control all segments in the limb. This is accomplished through concentric and eccentric co-contraction of muscles throughout the extremity in a manner similar to that found during weight-bearing activities. Closed chain exercises also result in compression of joint surfaces, which facilitates muscular coactivation that in turn enhances joint stability. These theoretical benefits of closed chain exercises have led some to rely solely on the use of closed chain exercises to rehabilitate injuries. While closed chain exercises may appear to be more functional, they may not result in maximal activation of muscles to allow for optimal strength development (38). Additionally, some functional activities occur as a result of isolated joint movements (i.e., knee extension during swing phase of gait) and are not simulated by closed chain exercises. Therefore it is important to consider both open and closed chain exercises to ensure full rehabilitation and return to function.

Often there is confusion concerning the definition of open and closed chain exercises. Traditionally, open chain exercises have been defined as those exercises in which the distal segment is free to move, and closed chain exercises have been defined as those activities in which the distal segment is fixed or those activities in which the distal segment meets considerable resistance (46). These definitions, however, may be misleading. For example, when pedaling a bike or stationary ergometer, the foot is not considered to be fixed, but the resulting motion is considered to be closed chain in nature since motion is occurring at multiple segments and involves co-contraction of muscles throughout the lower extremity.

Lephart and Henry (30) have developed a classification system for upper extremity exercises, which defines the position of the extremity, the load, and direction of the force. The system is divided into four categories based on a fixed or moveable boundary and the load and direction of the force. The classification system includes (1) fixed boundary with an external axial load, such as when performing a push-up on an unstable platform, (2) moveable boundary with an external axial load, such as rhythmic stabilization or a traditional bench press, (3) moveable boundary with an external rotary load, such as with resistive tubing exercises in a functional diagonal pattern, and (4) moveable boundary with no load, such as exercise that involves active and passive positioning. This classification system can also be easily applied to the lower extremity (30).

In order to minimize confusion in this paper, open chain exercise will be defined as that exercise in which the distal segment is free to move, resulting in isolated motion of a given joint. Open chain movement occurs as a result of contraction of the agonist. For example, open chain knee extension occurs as a result of isolated contraction of the quadriceps, and open chain knee flexion occurs as a result of isolated contraction of the hamstrings. Baratta and coworkers (2) and Draganich and associates (12) have demonstrated low levels of hamstring EMG activity during the terminal range of open chain knee extension and hypothesized that the hamstrings were functioning eccentrically to decelerate knee extension, thus protecting the ACL. Similar hamstring activity occurs with open chain knee extension during the swing phase of gait, in which the hamstrings function eccentrically to decelerate knee extension prior to heel strike.

Closed chain exercises are defined as those exercises that result in simultaneous motion of all joints in the limb. For example, the descending phase of squat occurs as a result of simultaneous dorsiflexion of the ankle and flexion of the knee and hip joints. Closed chain motion results in co-contraction of muscles throughout the limb. For example, when squatting there is co-contraction of the quadriceps and hamstrings. The quadriceps contract to counter the flexion moment arm at the knee, and the hamstrings contract to counter the flexion moment arm at the hip. As a result, a two-joint muscle may contract concentrically across one joint and eccentrically across another joint. For example, during the ascending phase of a squat, the hamstrings shorten across the hip and lengthen across the knee. Palmitier and coworkers (39) coined the term "pseudoisometric contraction" to describe the condition in which a muscle contracts concentrically and eccentrically at opposite ends. This "pseudoisometric" contraction can only be simulated with closed chain exercises; thus the statement by some that closed chain exercises are more functional. Wilkerson and Nitz (53) use the term "econcentric" to describe a similar situation, in which muscles function eccentrically at one joint and concentrically at another joint within a closed kinetic chain.

Much has been written in the rehabilitation literature of the advantage of closed chain over open chain exercises for rehabilitation of the lower extremity. Most of the evidence to support use of the closed chain exercises has been related to the effects of open versus closed chain exercises on the patellofemoral and tibiofemoral joints.

Hungerford and Barry (24) developed a mathematical model that compared the effects of open chain exercise (knee extension against a 9 kg weight boot) to closed chain exercise (squatting under body weight). The results revealed that patellofemoral contact stress (load per unit area) was less during the closed chain condition in the range from 0° to 53° of knee flexion, while patellofemoral contact stress was less during the open chain condition in the range from 53° to 90° of flexion. Steinkamp and coworkers (47) demonstrated similar findings in a biomechanical study comparing the effects of a leg press to a leg extension exercise in 20 normal subjects.

During open chain knee extension from 90° of flexion to full extension, the flexion moment arm increases, requiring greater quadriceps and patellar tendon force to extend the knee, which results in increasing patellofemoral joint reaction forces. Reilly and Martens (40) calculated peak patellofemoral joint reaction force during open chain knee extension against a 9 kg weight boot to be 120 kg at 36° of knee flexion. At this angle of knee flexion, the patellofemoral joint reaction forces are concentrated on a relatively small patellofemoral contact area, thus creating relatively large patellofemoral contact stresses.

During closed chain exercises, the flexion moment arm increases as the angle of knee flexion increases. Greater quadriceps and patellar tendon forces are required as the angle of knee flexion increases. The increasing quadriceps and patellar tendon forces result in increasing patellofemoral joint reaction forces as the knee flexes; however, these increasing forces are distributed over a larger patellofemoral contact area, which minimizes the increase in contact stress.

Closed chain exercises are also thought to be superior to open chain exercises in terms of reduced tibial translation and reduced stress and strain on the ACL. Closed chain exercises are thought to reduce tibial translation as a result of joint compression and co-contraction of the hamstring and quadriceps (see figure 32.1) (39). Compressive loading of the joint enhances joint stability due to approximation of the joint surfaces, thus reducing tibial translation. The resulting hamstring contraction during closed chain exercise is thought to counteract the anterior translation produced by the quadriceps, thus reducing tibial translation during closed chain exercises. During open chain exercises, the angle of force application is perpendicular to the lower leg, while during closed chain exercises the force is more axially aligned with the lower leg. Resolving the resultant force on the knee into its shear and compressive components reveals decreased posterior shear force of the femur (i.e., decreased anterior shear of the tibia) during closed chain exercises when compared to open chain exercises (39). Voight and coworkers (52) demonstrated decreased tibial translation during a maximal isometric leg press at 30° of flexion compared to maximal isometric leg extension at 30° of knee flexion in normal and ACL-reconstructed subjects. Several investigators have studied the effects of open chain exercises on the ACL in vitro (1) and in vivo (7, 8). In these studies, ACL strain was found to be significantly greater during active and resisted open chain knee extension in the range from 45° to 0° of knee extension over the strain produced in the ACL during passive motion. The magnitude of the strain produced on the ACL during open chain knee extension was on the order of 3 TO 4% more strain when compared to ACL strain when the knee was in full passive extension.

Thus, it appears that closed chain exercises are preferable to open chain exercises in terms of tibial

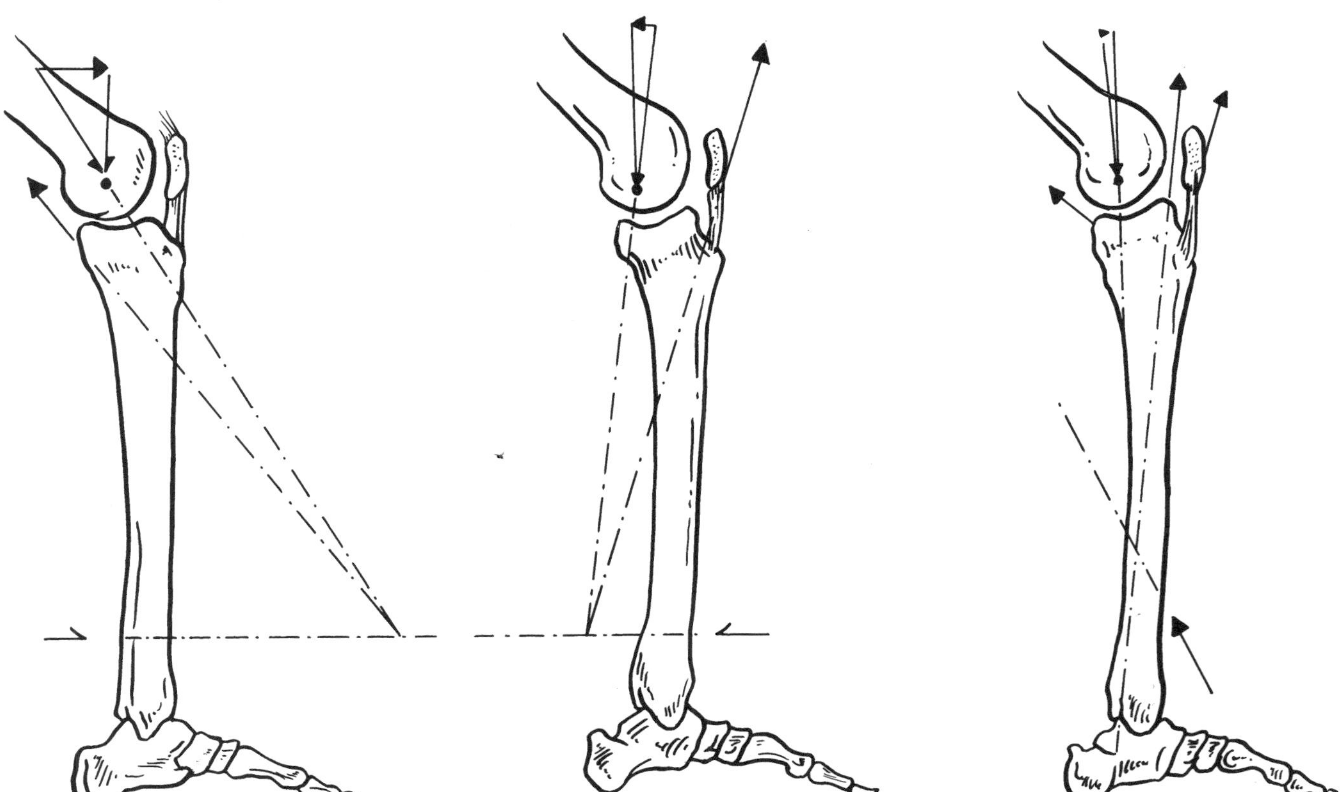

Figure 32.1 Closed chain exercises are thought to reduce tibial translation as a result of joint compression, hamstrings and quadriceps co-contraction and the angle at which forces are applied.

translation and ACL strain. However, recent evidence from Beynnon and coworkers (9) demonstrates significant strain on the ACL during closed chain exercises with and without resistance. The magnitude of strain on the ACL during closed chain exercises was found to be on the order of 4 to 6% more strain on the ACL than when the knee is in full passive extension. Meglan and coworkers (35) utilized EMG, motion analysis, and force plates to calculate the net load on the capsular and ligamentous structures about the knee during a variety of closed chain exercises commonly used in weightlifting. When a quadriceps only model was used, the results revealed an anteriorly directed shear load on the capsule and ligamentous structures about the knee between 20° to 40° of flexion. However, when the model was expanded to include quadriceps and hamstring co-contraction, the anterior shear force increased between the range of 20° to 60° of knee flexion. Meglan and associates (35) hypothesized that during closed chain exercises the hamstrings contract to offset the flexion moment arm at the hip and simultaneously increase the quadriceps force necessary to extend the knee. Therefore, contraction of the hamstrings is insufficient to negate the anteriorly directed shear force produced by the quadriceps. Thus, it is unknown if closed chain exercises are safer than open chain exercises for rehabilitation following ACL reconstruction. Furthermore, it is unknown if the stresses produced on the ACL graft during open and closed chain exercises are harmful or helpful, since some level of loading is necessary to induce remodeling of the graft.

Another issue related to the use of closed chain exercises for rehabilitation of lower extremity injuries is the magnitude of muscle activity that is produced. Ninos and coworkers (38) demonstrated that the magnitude of quadriceps EMG activity is on the order of 25 to 30% of maximum voluntary isometric contraction of the quadriceps, when performing an Olympic squat with 25% body weight added to the shoulders in normal individuals without a history of lower extremity pathology. It is doubtful that this level of loading would be sufficient to improve the ability of the quadriceps to generate muscle force. Therefore, relatively high levels of loading may be required during closed chain exercises to produce a training effect for the quadriceps. Further evidence concerning the ineffectiveness of closed chain exercise to improve quadriceps function was provided by Snyder-Mackler and associates (44). These investigators demonstrated electrically induced open chain quadriceps exercises to be superior to closed chain exercises in restoring quadriceps function following ACL reconstruction. Thus it appears that complete rehabilitation for the lower extremity requires judicious use of both open and closed chain exercises.

Use of Open and Closed Chain Exercises to Restore Proprioception

Injury to ligamentous and capsular structures has been demonstrated to reduce proprioceptive response from the involved structures. It has been hypothesized that this reduced proprioceptive response occurs as a result of direct injury to the mechanoreceptors or as a result of residual ligamentous and capsular laxity that reduces sensitivity of the mechanoreceptors to stretch. Freeman (13) used the term "articular deafferentation" to describe the reduced proprioceptive response that occurs as a result of ligamentous and capsular injury. Furthermore, Freeman (13) hypothesized that this articular deafferentation reduced neuromuscular control of the joint, resulting in functional instability.

Numerous researchers have demonstrated decreased proprioception following ligamentous injury, using a variety of approaches. Loss of conscious awareness of joint position and movement has been demonstrated as deficits in the threshold to detection of passive motion and reproduction of passive positioning (4, 5, 31, 33, 43). This research has demonstrated loss of proprioception by isolating movement of the injured joint, using open chain movements to test the ability of an individual to detect motion or reproduce joint position.

Deficits in balance have also been used to demonstrate loss of proprioception following joint injury. In these studies, loss of balance, expressed as increased postural sway, has been demonstrated during single-limb support on a stationary or moving force-sensing platform. The ability to demonstrate loss of proprioception with balance testing is confounded by the fact that visual and vestibular input also contributes to maintenance of balance. Despite this fact, several researchers have demonstrated decreased balance following ankle sprains (19, 49–51) and following ACL injury (14, 18).

Loss of neuromuscular control following joint injury has been operationalized as increased latency of muscle firing when the joint is subjected to a sudden unexpected perturbation. This research paradigm generally involves unexpected perturbation of the joint while the subject is weight bearing in unilateral stance. Latency of muscle firing is defined as the period of time from perturbation of the joint until the onset of muscle activity to stabilize the joint. Use of this paradigm is the most direct approach to assess the effects of loss of proprioceptive input on loss of neuromuscular control and, thus, functional instability. Konradsen and Ravn (29), Lephart and coworkers (32), and Nawoczenski and coworkers (37) demonstrated increased latency of firing of the peroneal muscles following sudden inversion in individuals who have suffered an ankle sprain. Similarly, Beard and associates (6) and Wojtys & Huston (54) demonstrated increased latency of firing of the hamstrings in response to a sudden anteriorly directed force applied to the proximal tibia in individuals with an anterior cruciate-deficient knee.

Proprioceptive training is generally thought to be limited to single-leg balance exercises that are performed on a multiaxial balance board for the purpose of enhancing neural mechanisms that will compensate for lost proprioceptive input following injury (13). This definition of proprioceptive training is quite limited, since all forms of exercise that result in deformation of mechanoreceptors will result in sensory input, which may enhance development of neural mechanisms to compensate for lost proprioceptive input following injury. Exercise that will result in deformation of mechanoreceptors includes all forms of passive, active-assisted, active and resisted open and closed chain exercises. The key to successful rehabilitation is to chose the correct form of exercise to progressively simulate the demands required during functional activities in which the individual participates. It is likely that this will include a combination of open and closed chain exercises since most activities, including gait, combine open and closed chain movements.

Lephart and coworkers (32) described a taxonomy for classification of proprioceptive exercises that includes activities designed to enhance conscious awareness of joint position and movement, activities to enhance balance, and activities to enhance neuromuscular control of movement. All forms of exercise will enhance conscious awareness of position and movement, and in our clinical experience it is rare to prescribe exercises solely for this purpose.

Balance activities include those activities that are performed in a closed chain fashion for the purpose of improving one's ability to maintain one's center of gravity within the base of support. Balance exercises include those activities in which the individual attempts to maintain his or her center of gravity within the base of support while standing in double- or single-limb support on a stationary or moving surface with or without visual input. Initially these activities should be performed while the individual concentrates on his or her sense of body position, muscle control, and joint position and movement. Over time as the individual's balance improves, activities to distract the individual from concentrating on balance, such as catching and throwing a ball, may be incorporated into the balance training activities (25). Exercises designed to enhance balance may improve one's awareness of the location of the center of gravity, increase strength in a functional "econcentric" mode, and increase the responsiveness and sensitivity of mechanoreceptors, thereby increasing proprioceptive input to the CNS (53).

Neuromuscular control of joint motion requires development of muscle strength and endurance, as well as development of appropriate recruitment patterns to regulate the timing and force of contraction to produce efficient movement and provide dynamic joint stabilization. As discussed previously, it is believed that proprioceptive input acting at the spinal, brain stem, and cortical levels provides information that influences voluntary and involuntary motor responses. Development of neuromuscular control of joint motion requires simulation of the conditions under which the individual must function. This necessitates use of both open and closed chain activities to simulate the type of muscle activity that is required by the functional activities in which the individual participates (i.e., principle of specificity of exercise). Additionally, the stresses imposed by these activities must be progressed gradually in order to give the individual time to adapt to the stresses that are being imposed (i.e., SAID principle).

General guidelines for progression of activities to enhance neuromuscular control require that activities be progressed from slow speed to fast speed, from low force to high force, and from controlled to uncontrolled activities. It is expected that introduction of more complex activities will require conscious effort on part of the individual to develop the appropriate movement pattern; however, over time, with repetition, it is expected that the individual will be able to perform the movement without conscious effort.

Initially, activities to enhance neuromuscular control should be performed within the safe ranges of joint motion (i. e., those positions in which the joint is not susceptible to episodes of instability). As the individual develops control of movement with the joint in the position of stability, activities can be progressed to positions in which the joint is more vulnerable to episodes of instability. Control of motion in positions vulnerable to instability requires gradual introduction of activities that perturb the joint to initiate proprioceptively mediated reflexes that dynamically stabilize the joint. To illustrate this concept, consider an individual with functional instability of the glenohumeral joint in the position of abduction and external rotation (i.e., anterior instability). Research has indicated that the posterior rotator cuff (infraspinatus and teres minor) serves as a dynamic restraint to anterior translation of the humeral head with the arm in abduction and external rotation (10). To enhance the ability of the rotator cuff to stabilize the glenohumeral joint, one might begin with rhythmic stabilization performed with the joint in a position of stability (i.e., elevation in the scapular plane to 80–100°) (see figure 32.2). In this position, the rhythmic stabilization activities should initially be performed in a slow, controlled manner with application of low levels of force. Over time, the level and speed of the applied forces can be increased. As the individual develops the ability to dynamically stabilize the joint in this position, the rhythmic stabilization activities can be progressed toward the vulnerable range of motion (i.e., toward abduction and external rotation) (see figure 32.3). As one moves toward the range of vulnerability, the rhythmic stabilization activities are again gradually progressed in terms of the level and speed of the applied forces. Application of forces to suddenly displace the joint toward the position of vulnerability (i.e., in the direction of abduction and external rotation) requires reflex contraction of the rotator cuff to dynamically stabilize the joint.

The activities used to develop neuromuscular control are dependent on the type of activities that the individual will engage in and may include a variety of open and closed chain activities. To illustrate this, consider the individual who has an ACL-deficient knee with anteriolateral laxity and complaints of instability during activities that require cutting and pivoting. Closed chain activities that mimic demands of the stance phase of gait may be used to enhance neuromuscular control of abnormal joint motion. These closed chain activities may include a variety of running and cutting activities such as running straight ahead and backward, stopping and starting, running circles and figure eights, and activities that require a change in direction and rotation of the body over the foot (i.e., the carioca). Open chain activities may be incorporated to mimic the swing phase of gait. For example, the function of the hamstrings to decelerate knee extension prior to heel strike may be enhanced through the use of open chain eccentric hamstring exercises using the Inertial Impulse Machine (Totem Inc, by EMA, Newman, Georgia) (see figure 32.4) or Thera-Band (Hygenic Corporation, Akron, Ohio) (see figure 32.5).

Progression of activities to enhance neuromuscular control requires careful monitoring of the individual. Factors to consider when progressing the program include symptoms (i.e., pain, swelling, and

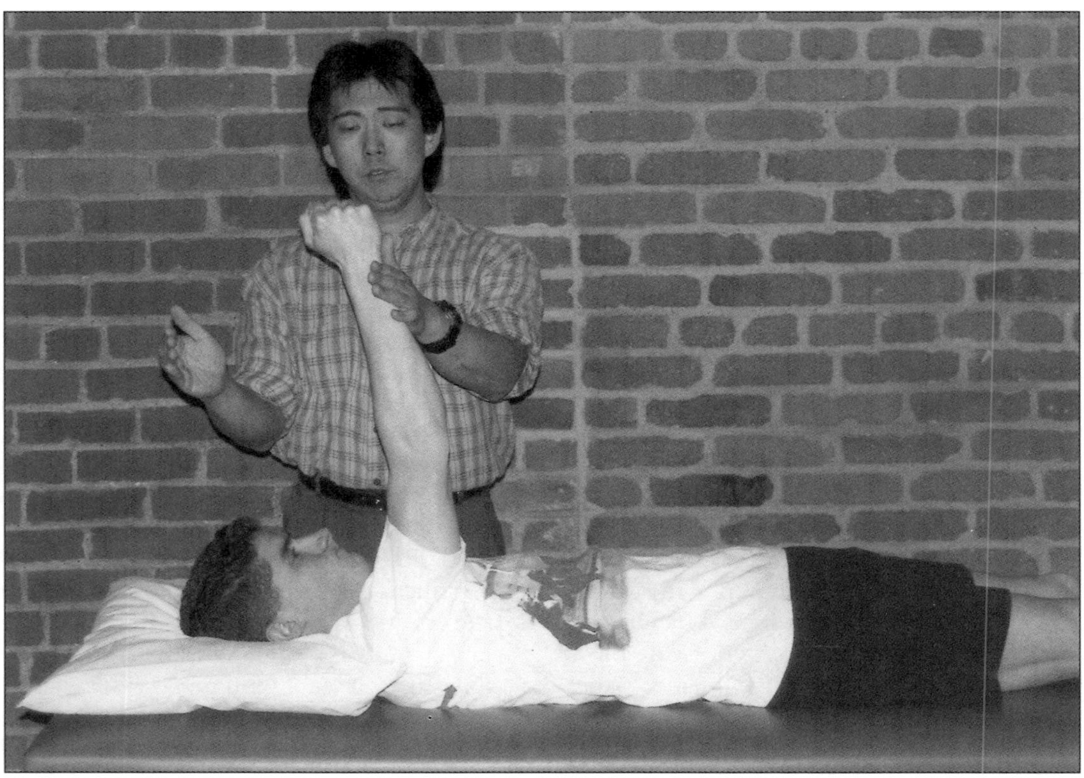

Figure 32.2 Rhythmic stabilization with the arm elevated at 90°.

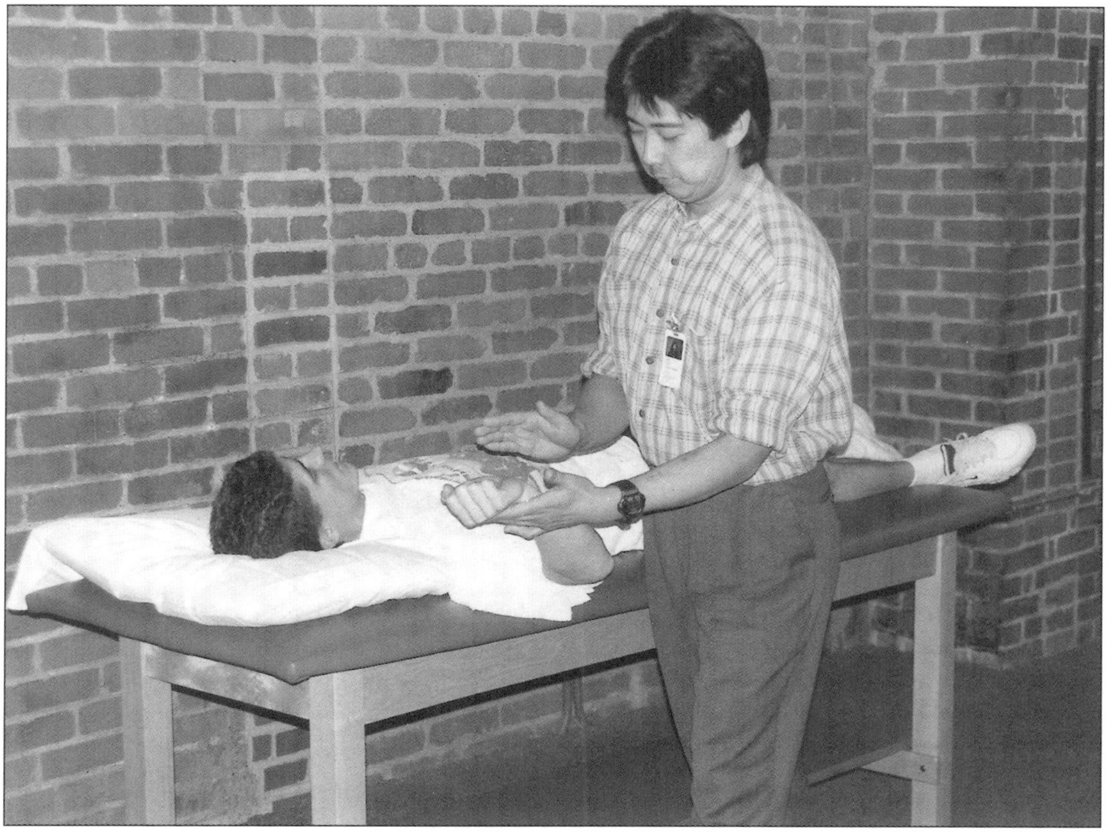

Figure 32.3 Rhythmic stabilization with arm positioned at 90° abduction and external rotation.

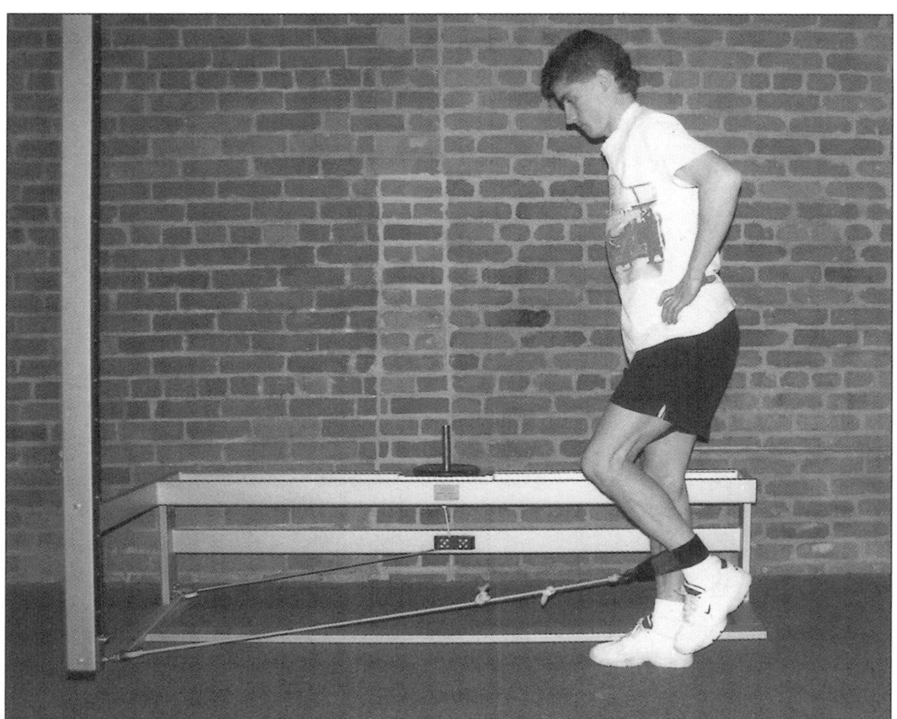

Figure 32.4 Open chain eccentric hamstring exercise using Inertial Impulse Machine.

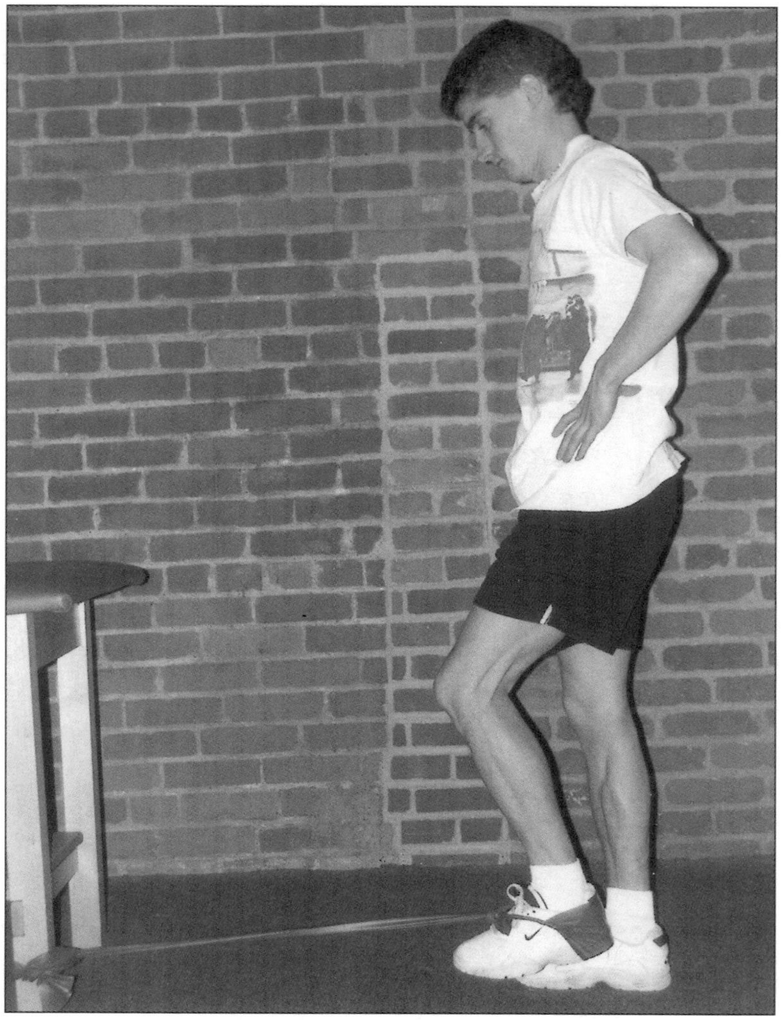

Figure 32.5 Open chain hamstring exercise using theraband.

instability), as well as the quality of the movement pattern. Development of symptoms or use of abnormal movement patterns is a sign that the individual does not have the necessary neuromuscular control to perform the activities safely, and the program should be modified accordingly.

Summary and Conclusions

In summary, we have provided an overview of proprioception and open and closed chain exercises. The evidence suggests that injury may lead to proprioceptive deficits, which, in turn, may adversely affect neuromuscular control of joint motion and lead to functional instability. Furthermore, the evidence for open and closed chain exercises indicates that rehabilitation should include a combination of open and closed chain exercises to restore optimal levels of muscle function. The effectiveness of open and closed chain exercises to enhance proprioception and restore neuromuscular control requires further investigation. This research should determine the effects of open and closed exercises on individuals who have identified proprioceptive deficits with complaints of functional instability. In addition, this research must use appropriate measures of outcome, including changes in the proprioceptive characteristics of the subjects as well as changes in their level of function.

References

1. Arms, S.W., M.H. Pope, R.J. Johnson, R.A. Fischer, I. Arvidsson, and E. Eriksson. The bio-

mechanics of anterior cruciate ligament rehabilitation and reconstruction. *AJSM* 12(1): 8–18, 1984.

2. Baratta, R., M. Solomonow, B.H. Zhou, D. Letson, R. Chuinard, and R. D'Ambrosia. Muscular coactivation: The role of the antagonist musculature in maintaining knee stability. *AJSM* 16(2): 113–22, 1988.
3. Barrack, R.L., P.J. Lund, and H.B. Skinner. Knee joint proprioception revisited. *J Sport Rehab* 3: 18–42, 1994.
4. Barrack, R.L., H.B. Skinner, and S.L. Buckley. Proprioception in the anterior cruciate-deficient knee. *AJSM* 17(1): 1–6, 1989.
5. Beard, D.J., P.J. Kyberd, C.M. Fergusson, and C.A.F. Dodd. Proprioception after rupture of the anterior cruciate ligament: An objective indication of the need for surgery? *J Bone Joint Surg* 75(2): 311–15, 1993.
6. Beard, D.J., P.J. Kyberd, J.J. O'Conner, C.M. Fergusson, and C.A.E. Dodd. Reflex hamstring contraction latency in anterior cruciate ligament deficiency. *J Orthop Res* 12(2): 219–28, 1994.
7. Beynnon, B., J.G. Howe, M.H. Pope, R.J. Johnson, and B.C. Fleming. The measurement of anterior cruciate ligament strain in vivo. *Int Orthop (SICOT)* 16(16): 1–12, 1992.
8. Beynnon, B.D., B.C. Fleming, R.J. Johnson, C.E. Nichols, P.A. Renstrom, and M.H. Pope. Anterior cruciate ligament strain behavior during rehabilitation exercises in vivo. *AJSM* 23(1): 24–34, 1995.
9. Beynnon, B.D., R.J. Johnson, B.C. Fleming, C.J. Sankewich, P.A. Renström, and C.E. Nichols. The strain behavior of the anterior cruciate ligament during squatting and active flexion-extension: A comparison of an open and a closed kinetic chain exercise. *AJSM* 25: 823–29, 1997.
10. Cain, P.R., T.A. Mutschler, F.H. Fu, and S.K. Lee. Anterior stability of the glenohumeral joint: A dynamic model. *AJSM* 15(2): 144–48, 1998.
11. Clark, F.J., K.W. Horch, S.M. Bach, and G.F. Larson. Contributions of cutaneous and joint receptors to static knee-position sense in man. *J Neurophys* 42(3): 877–88, 1979.
12. Draganich, L.F., R.J. Jaeger, and A.R. Kralj. Coactivation of the hamstrings and quadriceps during extension of the knee. *J Bone Joint Surg* 71A(7): 1075–1081, 1989.
13. Freeman, M.A.R. Instability of the foot after injuries to the lateral ligament of the ankle. *J Bone Joint Surg* 47B: 669–77, 1965.
14. Fridén, T., R. Zätterström, A. Lindstrand, and U. Moritz. Disability in anterior cruciate ligament insufficiency: An analysis of 19 untreated patients. *Acta Orthop Scand* 61(2): 131–35, 1990.
15. Gandevia, S.C., and D. I. McCloskey. Joint sense, muscle sense, and their combination as position sense, measured at the distal interphalangeal joint of the middle finger. *J Physiol* 260: 387–407, 1976.
16. Gandevia, S.C., D.I. McCloskey, and D. Burke. Kinesthetic signals and muscle contraction. *Trends Neurosci* 15(2): 62–65, 1992.
17. Garn, S.N., and R. A. Newton. Kinesthetic awareness in subjects with multiple ankle sprains. *Phys Ther* 68(11): 1667–671, 1988.
18. Gauffin, H., and H. Tropp. Altered movement and muscular-activation patterns during the one-legged jump in patients with an old anterior cruciate ligament rupture. *AJSM* 20(2): 182–92, 1992.
19. Gauffin, H., H. Tropp, and P. Odenrick. Effect of ankle disk training on postural control in patients with functional instability of the ankle joint. *Int J Sports Med* 9: 141–44, 1988.
20. Goodwin, G.M., D.I. McCloskey, and P.B.C. Matthews. The contribution of muscle afferents to kinesthesia shown by vibration induced illusions of movement and by the effects of paralyzing joint efferents. *Brain* 95: 705–48, 1972.
21. Grigg, P. Peripheral neural mechanisms in proprioception. *J Sport Rehab* 3: 2–17, 1994.
22. Guanche, C., T. Knatt, M. Solomonow, Y. Lu, and R. Baratta. The synergistic action of the capsule and the shoulder muscles. *AJSM* 23(3): 301–306, 1995.
23. Hullinger, M., E. Nordh, A. Thelin, and A.B. Vallbo. The responses of afferent fibers from the glabrous skin of the hand during voluntary finger movements in man. *J Physiol* 291: 233–49, 1979.
24. Hungerford, D. S., and M. Barry. Biomechanics of the patellofemoral joint. *Clin Orthop* 144: 9–15, 1979.
25. Irrgang, J.J., S.L. Whitney, and E. Cox. Balance and training for the lower extremity. *J Sports Rehab* 3: 68–83, 1994.
26. Johansson, H. Role of knee ligaments in proprioception and regulation of muscle stiffness. *J Electromyog Kinesiol* 1(3): 158–79, 1991.
27. Johansson, H., P. Sjolander, and P. Sojka. Receptors in the knee joint ligaments and their role in the biomechanics of the joint. *Biomed Eng* 18(5): 341–67, 1991.
28. Johansson, H., P. Sjolander, and P. Sojka. A sensory role for the cruciate ligaments. *Clin Orthop* 268: 161–78, 1991.

29. Konradsen, L., and J.B. Ravn. Ankle instability caused by prolonged peroneal reaction time. *Acta Orthop Scand* 61(5): 388–90, 1990.
30. Lephart, S.M., and T.J. Henry. The physiological basis for open and closed kinetic chain rehabilitation for the upper extremity. *J Sport Rehab* 5: 71–87, 1996.
31. Lephart, S.M., M.S. Kocher, F.H. Fu, P.A. Borsa, and C.D. Harner. Proprioception following anterior cruciate ligament reconstruction. *J Sport Rehab* 1: 188–96, 1992.
32. Lephart, S.M., D.M. Pincivero, J.L. Giraldo, and F.H. Fu. The role of proprioception in the management and rehabilitation of athletic injuries. *AJSM* 25(1): 130–37, 1997.
33. Lephart, S.M., J.J.P. Warner, P.A. Borsa, and F.H. Fu. Proprioception of the shoulder joint in health, unstable, and surgically repaired shoulders. *J Shoulder Elbow Surg* 3: 371–80, 1994.
34. Macefield, G., S.C. Gandevia, and D. Burke. Perceptual responses to microstimulation of single afferents innvervating joints, muscles, and skin of the human hand. *J Physiol* 429: 113–29, 1990.
35. Meglan, D., G. Lutz, and M. Stuart. Effects of closed kinetic chain exercises for ACL rehabilitation upon the load in the capsular and ligamentous structures of the knee. *Orthopaedic Transactions of the J Bone Joint Surg* VIII(3): 719–20, 1993.
36. Nashner, L.M., and G. McCollum. The organization of human postural movements: A formal basis and experimental synthesis. *Behav Brain Sci* 8: 135–72, 1985.
37. Nawoczenski, D.A., M.G. Owne, ML. Ecker, B. Altman, and M. Epler. Objective evaluation of peroneal response to sudden inversion stress. *JOSPT* 7(3): 107–109, 1985.
38. Ninos, J.C., J.J. Irrgang, R. Burdett, and J.R. Weiss. Electromyographic analysis of the squat performed in self-selected lower extremity neutral rotation and 30° of lower extremity turnout from the self-selected neutral position. *JOSPT* 25(5): 307–315, 1997.
39. Palmitier, R.A., K. An, S.G. Scott and E.Y.S. Chao. Kinetic chain exercise in knee rehabilitation. *Phys Sportsmed* 11(6): 402–13, 1991.
40. Reilly, D.T., and M. Martens. Experimental analysis of the quadriceps muscle force and patellofemoral joint reaction force for various activities. *Acta Orthop Scand* 43: 126–37, 1972.
41. Schaible, H., and R.F. Schmidt. Responses of fine medial articular nerve afferents to passive movements of knee joint. *J Neurophysiol* 49(5): 1118–126, 1983.
42. Schultz, R. A., D.C. Miller, C. S. Kerr, and L. Micheli. Mechanoreceptors in human cruciate ligaments: A histological study. *J Bone Joint Surg* 66A: 1072–1076, 1984.
43. Smith, R.L., and J. Brunolli. Shoulder kinesthesia after anterior glenohumeral joint dislocation. *Phys Ther* 69(2): 106–112, 1989.
44. Snyder-Mackler, L., A. Delitto, S.L. Bailey, and S.W. Stralka. Strength of the quadriceps femoris muscle and functional recovery after reconstruction of the anterior cruciate ligament. *J Bone Joint Surg* 77A(8): 1166–173, 1995.
45. Solomonow, M., R. Baratta, B.H. Zhou, H. Shoji, W. Bose, C. Beck, and R. D'Ambrosia. The synergistic action of the anterior cruciate ligament and thigh muscles in maintaining joint stability. *AJSM* 15(3): 207–13, 1987.
46. Steindler, A. *Kinesiology of the human body: Under normal and pathological conditions,* 3d ed. Springfield, IL: Charles C Thomas, 1955.
47. Steinkamp, L.A., M.F. Dillingham, M.D. Markel, J.A. Hill, and K.R. Kaufman. Biomechanical considerations in patellofemoral joint rehabilitation. *AJSM* 21(3): 438–44, 1993.
48. Strassmann, T., and Z. Halata. Applications for 3-D image processing in functional anatomy: Reconstruction of the cubital joint region and spatial distribution of mechanoreceptors surrounding this joint in *Monodelphis domestica*, a laboratory marsupial. *Eur J Cell Biol* 25: 107–10, 1988.
49. Tropp, H., J. Ekstrand, and J. Gillquist. Stabilometry in functional instability of the ankle and its value in predicting injury. *Med Sci Sports Exer* 16(1): 64–66, 1984.
50. Tropp, H., and P. Odenrick. Postural control in single-limb stance. *J Orthop Res* 6(6): 833–39, 1988.
51. Tropp, H., P. Odenrick, and J. Gillquist. Stabilometry recordings in functional and mechanical instability of the ankle joint. *Int J Sports Med* 6: 180–82, 1985.
52. Voight, M., S. Bell, and D. Rhoades. Instrumented testing of anterior tibial translation in open versus closed chain activity. *Phys Ther* 71: S98, 1991.
53. Wilkerson, G.B., and A.J. Nitz. Dynamic ankle stability: Mechanical and neuromuscular interrelationships. *J Sport Rehab* 3: 43–57, 1994.
54. Wojtys, E.M., and L.J. Huston. Neuromuscular performance in normal and anterior cruciate ligament-deficient lower extremities. *AJSM* 22(1): 89–104, 1994.

CHAPTER 33

Role of Fatigue on Proprioception and Neuromuscular Control

Susan Rozzi, PhD, ATC
Pongsak Yuktanandana, MD
Danny Pincivero, PhD
Scott M. Lephart, PhD, ATC

Introduction

Fatigue is defined simply as an inability to maintain a power output or force during repeated muscle contraction, which may be attributed to either metabolic or nonmetabolic peripheral factors (3, 25). Muscle fatigue has been shown to adversely alter joint proprioception and neuromuscular control in both the upper and lower extremities (8, 33, 46, 48, 55, 60, 63, 76). This chapter describes fatigue in conjunction with its effect on joint proprioception and neuromuscular control.

Muscle Fatigue

Numerous investigators have discussed the concept of muscle fatigue in an attempt to provide a concise definition for this term. Bills (14) first proposed that fatigue be divided into three categories: (1) subjective fatigue, defined by mental concentration and other psychological factors, (2) objective fatigue, characterized by a decline in work output, and (3) physiological fatigue, which represents changes in physiological processes. Merton (51) later suggested that the onset of fatigue may have its source peripherally (in the muscle) or centrally (in the central nervous system). Chaffin (18) identified localized muscular fatigue as being isolated to a group of muscles performing a contraction that manifests external signs such as an inability to maintain a desired force output, muscular tremor, and localized pain.

Although the concise definition of muscle fatigue as a failure to maintain a required or expected force output has been adopted by some (21), it may be it may be more appropriately represented as a failure point in work performance (19). Since it has been demonstrated that fatigue is time dependant and involves the impairment of many different processes at various rates, external signs such as work output decrements may not be indicative of physiological alterations during sustained muscular contractions (19). The existence of an appropriate definition is critical to the understanding of muscle fatigue; however, such a definition may not seem plausible. Winter (75) has recently referred to muscle fatigue as occurring when the muscle tissue cannot support metabolism at the contractile element, because of either ischemia (insufficient oxygen) or local depletion of any of the metabolic substrates.

Enoka (22) has generally denoted muscle fatigue as a class of acute effects that impair performance, which includes both an increase in the perceived effort necessary to exert a desired force and an eventual inability to produce this force. The muscle fatigue concepts outlined by Winter (75) and Enoka (22) appear to be more appropriate than the traditional definition of Edwards (21),which does not appear to be an accurate description of the numerous physiological processes involved.

Peripheral Nonmetabolic Fatigue

Physiological processes that ultimately drive operation of the contractile machinery of the cell are often referred to as the nonmetabolic factors that contribute to muscle fatigue. Such factors include impairments in neuromuscular and sarcolemma excitation and propagation, and excitation-contraction coupling. These nonmetabolic factors appear to be partially the underlying cause of alterations in EMG and force output during fatiguing conditions.

Examination of the electromyogram under fatiguing contractions has yielded consistent results since the early part of the century (19). During sustained contractions, a shift in the EMG power spectrum towards lower frequencies has been demonstrated repeatedly. Komi and Tesch (37) observed this phenomenon in the vastus lateralis muscle in subjects performing 100 repeated isokinetic knee extensions at an angular velocity of 180°/s. A significantly greater reduction in torque and mean frequency was observed in a group of subjects displaying a predominance of fast twitch (FT) muscle fibers. Since FT motor units demonstrate fast-fatiguing characteristics, it appears that a greater reduction in their firing frequency may explain this observed shift (37). This finding has also been observed recently by Gerdle and Elert (24) in subjects performing 3 bouts of 70 maximal isokinetic knee extensions at an angular velocity of 180°/s. An early shift in the EMG power spectrum towards lower frequencies was observed that corresponded to significant reductions in peak torque. Lindström and coworkers (46) further justified these findings as they observed significant early reductions in peak torque and mean EMG frequency during 100 repeated knee extensions at 180°/s.

It has been suggested that a reduction in the conduction velocity of the muscle fiber membrane is the major cause behind this shift in the mean EMG frequency (24). It has also been proposed that an increase in integrated EMG area under fatiguing conditions at constant tension levels, as well as an increase in motor unit recruitment (75), is a result of this decrease in conduction velocity. This increase in recruitment of new motor units to compensate for a decreased firing rate of the already recruited units in order to maintain constant tension appears to be a likely explanation of the changes that occur within the first 20 s of exercise (24, 46, 71, 75). However, a reduction in the conduction velocity corresponds to a widening of the action potential pulse width, therefore increasing the area under the IEMG curve (75). Conduction velocity decreases have been attributed to an increased potassium ion concentration $[K^+]$ in the extracellular compartment, a decrease in $[K^+]$ inside the muscle cell, as well as an increase in extracellular sodium ion concentration $[Na^+]$ (16, 45). This effect has been demonstrated to reduce the number and rate of opening of Na^+ channels as well as prolonging the repolarization phase of muscle contraction (31, 57). McComas and coworkers (50) noted such an effect after sustained isometric contractions following blood flow occlusion via compression. The decrease in torque output appeared to correspond with a reduction in M-wave amplitude, which was restored following the return of blood flow. It was concluded that the rapid increase in M-wave amplitude was due to a "washing out" of accumulated extracellular K^+ (50).

Excitation-contraction coupling refers to a series of processes that are involved in the conversion of muscle fiber membrane excitation to a muscle fiber force (22). It appears that impairments in this process contribute to a greater degree to a decline in muscle force generation during prolonged periods of recovery. Baker and coworkers (4) demonstrated that after 15 to 20 min of intermittent maximal contractions of the ankle dorsiflexors, tetanic force remained depressed after 15 min of recovery. Since their results did not demonstrate significant changes in EMG activity, intracellular pH, or accumulation of inorganic phosphate molecules following this period of recovery, it was concluded that impaired excitation-contraction coupling beyond the cell membrane is a major factor contributing to force decrements (4). Similar conclusions were derived by Moussavi and associates (53), who found persistent reductions in tetanic twitch force of the tibialis anterior muscle in the absence of significant metabolic and EMG changes.

Researchers have proposed that an altered excitation-contraction process is manifested as a reduction in neuromuscular efficiency (NME). NME, defined as the force per unit of rectified integrated EMG at 50% of maximal force, has been shown to be depressed after 60 min of recovery following a 4 min period of maximal contractions for the adductor pollicis longus muscle (52). Miller and coworkers (52) suggested that a prolonged recovery of NME with a complete restoration of the maximum voluntary contraction, pH, phosphocreatine (PCr), and EMG is related to altered excitation-contraction coupling. Much evidence has recently suggested an impairment in calcium ion (Ca^{++}) release and reuptake by the SR under fatiguing conditions (1, 2, 73). Plausible explanations for this mechanism include depolarization alterations in the T-tubule system. Changes in the normal, resting function of these nonmetabolic processes as a result of prolonged muscular contractions are not exclusive events. Instead, they appear to be a major contributor to performance decrements in conjunction with various metabolic factors.

Peripheral Metabolic Fatigue

As indicated earlier, ATP resynthesis is a necessary process in order for muscles to perform mechanical work. However, a reduced ability to contract muscles does not appear to be a result of decreases in intracellular ATP levels. In fact, it has been demonstrated that it is impossible to deplete ATP stores more than 20–25% in voluntary exercise (27, 28). With respect to changes in ATP, it has been suggested that it is the total free energy available from this molecule rather than its total concentration that contributes to fatigue (50). A reduction in this free energy availability has been attributed to the accumulation of ADP and inorganic phosphate (P_i) (50). The recovery, or resynthesis, of ATP during maximal contractions is a key element for the continuation of muscular work. Since PCr is the immediate and only substrate for ATP resynthesis during the early stages (< 10 s) of intense exercise, rapid degradation of this compound has been shown to affect exercise performance (65). Hultman and coworkers (34) demonstrated a rapid decrease in intracellular PCr levels within the first 2 min of continuous exercise, which was followed by a complete restoration of this compound within a few minutes during rest. Following 30 min of an intense heavy resistance exercise program that consisted of squats, leg presses, and leg extensions, Tesch (67) found significant reductions in PCr in the vastus lateralis muscles of 9 strength-trained athletes. Miller and coworkers (52) found similar results in the adductor pollicis muscle during 4 min of sustained maximal exercise. Significant reduction in the concentration of PCr was found in the first minute of exercise, and it further declined to 10% of the control value by the end of 4 min (52). A rapid increase in PCr concentration occurred within the first 2 min of recovery, whereas intramuscular pH remained depressed up to 3 min postexercise. Jansson and coworkers (35) demonstrated significant decreases in intramuscular PCr of the vastus lateralis following 30 isokinetic knee extension repetitions performed at 180°/s. These results also demonstrated that the recovery of PCr was highly correlated with the aerobic oxidative potential of the muscle (35). Bendahan and coworkers (12) observed that submaximal isometric contractions at 60% of the maximum voluntary contraction (MVC) resulted in a linear reduction in the PCr concentration of the forearm flexor muscles. Significant linear relationships were also found between the decrease in PCr concentration and energy in the low frequency band of the EMG power spectrum (12). Takahashi and associates (66) have recently demonstrated that exhausting exercise of the vastus lateralis muscle resulted in a significant reduction in muscle PCr. This reduction was followed by a time constant of PCr resynthesis of 46.4 ±3.8 s and 69.2 ±4.9 s in trained runners and matched nontrained subjects, respectively (66).

High-intensity exercise activities that exceed a duration of 10 s appear to develop a more progressive reliance on the anaerobic glycolytic pathway for ATP resynthesis (49, 56). This notion is based on measures of blood lactate and intramuscular H^+ accumulation observed following high-intensity exercise bouts. Tesch (67) found an 8-fold increase in muscle lactate following 50 isokinetic knee extension repetitions, which was also positively correlated with a decline in force output. High positive correlation ($r = .82 - .94$) between muscle fatigue and LDH and M-LDH activity in the vastus lateralis muscle was also reported. Since the M-LDH isozyme facilitates the conversion of pyruvate to lactate, elevated concentrations of this chemical compound, as typically found in FT muscle fibers, have been shown to be positively correlated to the onset of muscle fatigue (32, 64, 67). The increase in H^+ concentration during prolonged high-intensity activities has also been shown to directly interfere with the contractile machinery of muscle by competing for the Ca^{++} binding sites on troponin C (23, 27, 58). Boska and coworkers (15) found a linear relationship between the decline in MVC of the tibialis anterior muscle during a sustained 4 min isometric contraction and H^+

accumulation. These results were confirmed by Douris (20), who demonstrated a significant increase in blood lactate during a 1 min isokinetic protocol for knee extension and flexion as a function of contraction velocity. Furthermore, a positive correlation ($r = .82$) was also found between muscle fatigue and the accumulation of blood lactate (20).

The role of the diprotonated form of inorganic phosphate ($H_2PO_4^-$) has proved to be significant in the reduction of force output. It appears that the accumulation of this molecule occurs as a result of the following buffering reaction, which occurs at a lower physiological pH: $HPO_4^{-2} + H^+ = H_2PO_4^-$ (15, 52, 53, 74). The excessive production of this metabolite has been postulated to be a direct inhibitor of the actomyosin ATPase system in which the removal of inorganic phosphate (P_i) from the myosin globular head is reduced (30, 74). The manifestation of this hypothesis was observed by Boska and associates (15), who noted that decreases in MVC and $H_2PO_4^-$ accumulation during the onset of muscle fatigue were highly correlated, as was their rapid restoration during recovery. A loss in force production with a change in protonated phosphate was also found to have a temporal correspondence, by Miller and coworkers (52).

It is apparent that the onset of muscle fatigue is a progressive process that manifests nonmetabolic and metabolic changes. Although these factors appear to be the underlying cause for muscle contractile failure during maximal sustained contractions, they have also been found to occur during submaximal contractions in the absence of force decrements. Therefore, decreases in force production alone may not provide an objective and accurate indication for the onset of muscle fatigue as represented by physiological changes in the muscle.

Proprioception and Neuromuscular Control

The central nervous system (CNS) is the primary mediator for the perception and execution of musculoskeletal control and movement. Perception and sensation of joint movement are monitored by three main subsystems: (1) the somatosensory system, (2) the vestibular system, and (3) the visual system. The somatosensory system, often referred to as proprioception, receives input from peripheral articular and musculotendinous receptors concerning changes in muscle length and tension, in addition to information regarding joint position and motion. The vestibular system receives information from the vestibules and semicircular canals of the ear, which aid in keeping the body in balance, while the visual system provides the body with visual cues, contributing to balance by providing reference points for orientation (68).

Information gathered by the somatosensory system, in addition to that from vestibular and visual systems, is processed at three distinct levels of motor control: the spinal level, the brain stem, and the higher centers such as the motor cortex, basal ganglia, and cerebellum (38, 41, 42, 68). The spinal level provides dynamic muscular stabilization and synchronized muscle activation patterns based on spinal reflexes and activity received from higher levels of the CNS. The brain stem, where input originates from the visual, vestibular, and somatosensory systems via the cerebellum nuclei, mediates CNS activity for the maintenance of posture and balance. The higher brain centers are responsible for motor movements that are voluntary but are performed without continual reference to consciousness. This level of motor control is often referred to as cognitive programming. The culmination of information gathered and processed from articular and musculotendinous neural receptors results in unconscious joint stabilization through protective spinal-mediated reflexes, in addition to conscious appreciation of joint position sense, and the maintenance of posture and balance (38, 41, 42, 68).

Proprioception and neuromuscular control may be assessed clinically through evaluation of the afferent and efferent neuromuscular pathways. The afferent pathway is qualified through the examination of joint kinesthesia and joint position sensibility, which provide the researcher with a measurement of conscious appreciation of joint motion and position sensibility. Joint kinesthesia is determined clinically by establishing the threshold to detection of passive motion (TTDPM), an assessment of the ability to detect relatively slow passive joint motion (6–8, 38–44, 61, 62). Testing joint position sense, another method of assessing the afferent pathway, determines the ability of the subject to comprehend a presented joint angle and then once removed, actively or passively reproduce the joint angle. Assessment of the efferent pathway is conducted through measurements of balance and muscle activity, which provide a direct determination of the efferent response to afferent stimulation (9, 10, 36). Balance may be qualified utilizing a variety of clinical assessment tools or with the use of commercially available testing devices, while muscle activity is best studied with the use of electromyography. EMG, which can be defined as the electrical signals associated with the contraction of a muscle, can be used to study the quality, sequence, and timing of muscular activity.

Effect of Fatigue on Joint Proprioception

Muscular fatigue has been suggested to alter joint proprioception by increasing the threshold for muscle spindle discharge and through changes in alpha-gamma coactivation (5, 47, 72). Changes in the neural drive to the muscle, which may involve altered descending supraspinal drive and changes resulting from the influence of segmental spinal reflexes, can potentially exacerbate the fatigue state. Alpha motoneurons receive monosynaptic and polysynaptic input from sensorimotor cortex projections, brain stem nuclei, and type Ia, II, III, and IV sensory afferents (59). Alterations in the afferent input to alpha motoneurons may potentially alter muscle function, resulting in a joint unable to produce protective reactive muscular activation. The ability of the joint to sense forces imparted on the surrounding articular structures and to mediate appropriate muscular responses believed to provide dynamic joint stabilization is essential for functional joint stability.

Research suggests that in both upper and lower extremity joints, muscular fatigue worsens or impairs joint position sensibility while having no apparent effect on joint motion sensibility, which is often referred to as joint kinesthesia (46, 60, 63). Marks and Quinney (48) investigated the effects of isokinetically induced quadriceps muscular fatigue on knee joint position sensibility. They concluded that, while fatigue did not impair absolute knee joint position sensibility in the experimental subjects, it did undermine the relative proficiency attainable by learning, as was demonstrated by the control group. However, utilizing a comprehensive lower-extremity fatigue protocol, Skinner and coworkers (63) demonstrated that fatigue significantly worsened joint position sensibility while joint motion sensibility was unaffected. In this investigation both threshold to detection of passive motion (TTDPM) and reproduction of passive positioning (RPP) of the knee joint were measured in 11 healthy males in response to a high-load fatigue-inducing protocol, which included running and isokinetic exercise.

Sharpe and Miles (60) utilized the elbow joint to investigate the effect of fatigue on joint position sense in the upper extremity. In this investigation of 13 subjects the ability of the test arm to match the elbow angle of the contralateral arm was determined prior to and subsequent to a fatigue protocol, which induced fatigue with a series of maximal voluntary contractions of the elbow flexors. Since the results of this investigation revealed inconsistent findings, the authors attributed the observed changes in the fatigued state to proprioceptive alterations as well as central fatigue processes. Diminished joint position sense as a result of muscular fatigue has also been demonstrated in studies of the shoulder. Voight and coworkers (69) investigated the effect of isokinetically induced muscle fatigue on shoulder joint position sensibility and concluded that shoulder joint proprioception, as determined through the assessment of joint position sense, was significantly diminished in the presence of muscular fatigue.

Effect of Fatigue on Neuromuscular Control

In addition to deleteriously affecting joint proprioception, muscular fatigue has been suggested to affect adversely the neuromuscular control of the joint. Electromyographical studies of fatigued muscles have demonstrated an extended latency of muscle firing (55) and less efficient muscular processes (29), when compared to unfatigued muscle. Measurements of lower extremity balance, another means of quantifying the efferent neuromuscular pathway, also appear to be altered by muscular fatigue (33).

When an athlete encounters a dangerous situation, the speed with which the muscles can generate force so that the athlete can move away from that situation is very important; and when an abnormal movement occurs, one that is nearly beyond the limit of anatomical restraint, a fast reaction time for muscle contractions to prevent anatomical disruption of the capsuloligamentous structure will prevent severe injuries. Researchers have reported that the response time is related to the rate of force development. Muscle force generation is dependent on central and peripheral factors (11). Central factors include the proportion of the available total motor unit pool that is recruited during contraction, motor neuron excitability, and the type of motor unit recruited during contraction. Peripheral factors include the cross-sectional area of the contracting muscle and the biochemical and the electrical events associated with the joining-sliding-relaxation of the contractile proteins. The response time delay consists of the time interval between stimulus and change in electrical activity in skeletal muscle and the time delay between the change in electrical activity and actual force generation by the muscle.

Electromechanical delay (EMD) is defined as the delay between onset of EMG activity and the onset of mechanical response (11, 17, 26, 54). In studies of human movement, electromyography is being used widely to assess muscle firing patterns and recruitment of motor units during various activities. Norman and Komi (54) proposed that the length of the EMD primarily is affected by the time necessary to stretch the series of elastic components of a muscle to a point where muscle force can be detected, and factors such as initial muscle length, type of contraction, and velocity of contraction influence this phase lag. However, the EMD values are still in a wide range even when reported for the same muscle, same muscle length, and same type of contraction. A weak point in this analysis is that one should define the level of both EMG onset and threshold level of mechanical response. Most of the studies were predominantly focused on the rising limb of force production. Then it is important to verify signal between muscle activation and deactivation phase. In the EMG studies, EMD would be collected by shifting of the phase between EMG signal and torque signal. Vos and coworkers (70) found longer relaxation delay in fatiguing knee extension protocol in vastus medialis, rectus femoris, and vastus lateralis muscles. Zhou and coworkers (78) also found significant prolonged EMD of knee extensors in isometric contraction after fatiguing exercise. They stated that the mechanisms of EMD lengthening during fatigue could have been due to the deterioration in muscle conductive, contractile, or elastic properties and require further study.

Wojtys and coworkers (76) investigated the effect of quadriceps and hamstring muscle fatigue on anterior tibial translation and muscle reaction time in 10 healthy subjects. They defined muscle reaction time as the time between onset of passive anterior tibial translation and onset of muscle firing. During fatigue they found an average increase of 32.5% in anterior tibial translation and the response times in the gastrocnemius, hamstring, and the quadriceps originating at the spinal cord and cortical level were slower. However, the recruitment order of the lower extremity muscles in response to anterior tibial translation did not change with muscle fatigue. They proposed that the lengthening of muscle reaction time was in agreement with both Woods and coworkers (77) and Bigland-Ritchie and coworkers (13), who reported a decrease in motoneuron firing rates during muscle fatigue in the upper extremities. The reason for this outcome was thought to be that, as motoneuron firing rate decreases, muscle reaction time should lengthen. They believed that muscle fatigue affects the dynamic stability of the knee, alters the neuromuscular response to anterior tibial translation, and may play an important role in the pathomechanics of knee injuries in physically demanding sports.

Nyland and coworkers (55) investigated the effect of muscular fatigue on the muscle firing patterns of female athletes who performed a run and rapid stop maneuver. It was demonstrated that a longer time to the onset of muscle activation occurred following the fatigue test trials than during the nonfatigue trials. The authors suggest a delayed rate of firing may create a moment when the knee joint is unable to stabilize against joint forces resulting in ligamentous injury. Additionally, decreased neuromuscular control, as determined through the assessment of balance, has been demonstrated in healthy individuals subsequent to the induction of knee joint muscular fatigue (33).

References

1. Allen DG, Westerblad H, Lee JA, Lannergren J. Role of excitation-contraction coupling in muscle fatigue. *Sports Med* 13(2): 116–26, 1992.
2. Allen DG, Lannergren J, Westerblad H. Muscle cell function during prolonged activity: Cellular mechanisms of fatigue. *Exp Physiol* 80: 497–527, 1995.
3. Assmusen E. Muscle fatigue. *Med Sci Sport* 11: 313–21, 1979.
4. Baker AJ, Kustov KG, Miller RG, Weiner MW. Slow force recovery after long-duration exercise: Metabolism and activation factors in muscle fatigue. *J Appl Physiol* 74(5): 2294–2300, 1993.
5. Balestra C, Duchateau J, Hainaut K. Effects of fatigue in the stretch reflex in a human muscle. *EMG and Clin Res* 85: 46–52, 1992.
6. Barrack RL, Lund PJ, Skinner HB. Knee joint proprioception revisited. *J Sport Rehab* 3(1): 18–42, 1994.
7. Barrack RL, Skinner HB, Brunet ME, Cook SD. Joint kinesthesia in the highly trained knee. *J Sports Med* 24: 18–20, 1984.
8. Barrack RL, Skinner HB, Cook SD. Proprioception of the knee joint: Paradoxical effect of training. *Am J Phys Med* 63(4): 175–81, 1984.
9. Beard DJ, Kyberd PJ, Fergusson CM, Dodd CA. Proprioception after rupture of the anterior cru-

ciate ligament: An objective indication of the need for surgery? *J Bone Joint Surg* 76B: 654–59, 1994.
10. Beard DJ, Kyberd PJ, O'Connor JJ, Fergusson CM, Dodd CA. Reflex hamstring contraction latency in anterior cruciate ligament deficiency. *J Bone Joint Surg* 12: 219–28, 1994.
11. Bell DG, Jacobs IRS. Electromechanical response times and rate of force development in males and females. *Med Sci Sports* 18(1): 31–36, 1986.
12. Bendahan D, James Y, Salvan AM, Badier M, Confort-Gouny S, Guillot C, Cozzone PJ. Combined electromyography and ^{31}P magnetic resonance spectroscopy study of human muscle fatigue during static contraction. *Muscle Nerve* 19: 715–21, 1996.
13. Bigland-Ritchie B, Jones DA, Johansson R, Lippold OCJ. Reflex origin for the slowing of motoneuron firing rates in fatigue of human voluntary contractions. *J Physiol* (London) 379: 451–59, 1986.
14. Bills, AG. *The psychology of efficiency.* New York: Harper & Row, 1943.
15. Boska MD, Moussavi RS, Carson PJ, Weiner MW, Miller RG. The metabolic basis of recovery after fatiguing exercise of human muscle. *Neurol* 40: 240–44. 1990.
16. Cairns SP, Dulhunty AF. High-frequency fatigue in rat skeletal muscle: Role of extracellular ion concentrations. *Muscle Nerve* 18: 890–98. 1995.
17. Cavanagh PR, Komi PV. Electromechanical delay in human skeletal muscle under concentric and eccentric contraction. *Eur J Appl Physiol* 45: 159–63, 1979.
18. Chaffin DB. Localized muscle fatigue: Definition and measurement. *J Occup Med* 15: 346, 1973.
19. DeLuca CJ. Myoelectrical manifestations of localized muscular fatigue in humans. *CRC Crit Rev Biomed Eng* 11(4): 251–79, 1984.
20. Douris PC. The effects of isokinetic exercise on the relationship between blood lactate and muscle fatigue. *J Orthop Sports Phys Ther* 17(1): 31–35, 1993.
21. Edwards RHT. Human muscle function and fatigue. In *Human muscle fatigue: Physiological mechanisms,* Porter R, Whelan J (eds). London: Pitman Medical, 1–18, 1981.
22. Enoka RM. *Neuromechanical basis of kinesiology,* 2d ed. Champaign, IL: Human Kinetics, 151–73, 1994.
23. Fabiato A, Fabiato F. Effects of pH on the myofilaments and the sarcoplasmic reticulum of skinned cells from cardiac and skeletal muscle. *J Physiol* (London) 276: 233–55, 1978.
24. Gerdle B, Elert J. The temporal occurrence of the mean power frequency shift of the electromyogram during maximum prolonged dynamic and static working cycles. *Int J Sport Med* 15(1): S32–S37. 1994.
25. Gibson H, Edwarts RHT. Muscle exercise and fatigue. *Sports Med* 2: 120–32, 1985.
26. Graniber MD. Bioelectrical characteristics of the electrical delay preceding concentric contraction. *Med Sci Sports Exerc* 18: 37–43, 1986.
27. Green HJ. Metabolic determinants of activity induced muscular fatigue. In *Exercise metabolism,* Hargreaves M. (ed). Champaign, IL: Human Kinetics, 211–56.
28. Hackney DD, Clark PF. Steady state kinetics of high enzyme concentrations: The myosin Mg ATPase. *J Biol Chem* 260: 5505–510, 1985.
29. Hagbarth KE, Bongiovanni LG, Nordin M. Reduced servocontrol of fatigued human finger extensor and flexor muscles. *J Physiol* 485(3): 865–72, 1995.
30. Hibberd MG, Dantzig JA, Trentham DR, Goldman YE. Phosphate release and force generation in skeletal muscle fibers. *Science* 228: 1317–319, 1985.
31. Hodgkin AL, Horowicz P. Movements of Na^+ and K^+ in single muscle fibers. *J Physiol* (London) 145: 405–32, 1995.
32. Houston ME. *Biochemistry primer for exercise science.* Champaign, IL: Human Kinetics, 13–20, 1995.
33. Howard, Crawlsy, Losse. Effect of lower extremity muscular fatigue on motor control performance in a group of normal subjects. *AAOS Program,* 196, 1996.
34. Hultman E, Sjöholm H. Energy metabolism and contraction force of human skeletal muscle in situ during electrical stimulation. *J Physiol* (London) 345: 525–32, 1983.
35. Jansson E, Dudley GA, Norman B, Tesch PA. Relationship of recovery from intense exercise to the oxidative potential of skeletal muscle. *Acta Physiol Scand* 139: 147–52, 1990.
36. Jenning AG, Seedhom BB. Proprioception in the knee and reflex hamstring contraction latency. *J Bone Joint Surg* [Br] 76B: 491–94, 1994.
37. Komi PV, Tesch P. EMG frequency spectrum, muscle structure, and fatigue during dynamic contractions in man. *Eur J Appl Physiol* 42: 41–50, 1979.
38. Lephart SM, Fu FH. The role of proprioception in the treatment of sports injuries. *Sports Exerc Inj* 1: 96–102, 1995.
39. Lephart SM, Fu FH, Borsa PA. Proprioception in sports medicine. In *Advances in operative orthopaedics.* 2, 1994.

40. Lephart SM, Fu FH, Irrgang JJ, Borsa PA. Proprioception characteristics of trained and untrained college females. [Abstract] *Med Sci Sport Exerc* 23(4): S113, 1991.
41. Lephart SM, Henry TJ. Functional rehabilitation for the upper and lower extremity. *Orthop Clin N Amer* 26(3): 579–92, 1995.
42. Lephart SM, Henry TJ. The physiological basis for open and closed kinetic chain rehabilitation for the upper extremity. *J Sport Rehab* 1: 188–96, 1992.
43. Lephart SM, Kocher MS, Fu FH, Borsa PA, Harner CD. Proprioception following anterior cruciate ligament reconstruction. *J Sport Rehab* 1: 188–96, 1992.
44. Lephart SM, Warner JP, Borsa PA, Fu FH. Proprioception of the shoulder joint in healthy, unstable, and surgically repaired shoulders. *J Shoulder Elbow Surg* 3(6): 371–80, 1994.
45. Lindinger MI, McKelvie RS, Heigenhauser GJF. K^+ and lactate distribution in humans during and after high-intensity exercise: Role in muscle fatigue attenuation? *J Appl Physiol* 78(3): 765–77, 1995.
46. Lindström B, Karlsson S, Gerdle B. Knee extensor performance of dominant and nondominant limb throughout repeated isokinetic contractions, with special reference to peak torque and mean frequency of the EMG. *Clin Physiol* 15: 275–86, 1995.
47. Macefield G, Gandevia SC, Burke D. Perceptual response to microstimulation of single afferents innervating joint, muscle, and skin of the human hand. *J Physiol* 429: 113–29, 1990.
48. Marks R, Quinney HA. Effect of fatiguing maximal isokinetic quadriceps contractions on ability to estimate knee position. *Perc Motor Skills* 77: 1195–1202, 1993.
49. McArdle WD, Katch FI, Katch VL. *Exercise physiology: Energy, nutrition, and human performance,* 3d ed. Philadelphia: Lea & Febiger, 348–66, 1991.
50. McComas AJ, Galea V, Einhorn RW, Hicks AL, Kuiack S. The role of the NA^+, K^+ pump in delaying muscle fatigue. In *Neuromuscular fatigue,* Sargeant AJ, Kernell D, (eds). Amsterdam: North-Holland, 35–43, 1993.
51. Merton PA. Voluntary strength and fatigue. *J Physiol* 123: 553–64, 1954.
52. Miller RG, Boska MD, Moussavi RS, Carson PJ, Weiner M. ^{31}P nuclear magnetic resonance studies of the high energy phosphates and pH in human muscle fatigue: Comparison of aerobic and anaerobic exercise. *J Clin Invest* 81(4): 1190–196, 1988.
53. Moussavi RS, Carson PJ, Boska MD, Weiner MW, Miller RG. Nonmetabolic fatigue in exercising human muscle. *Neurol* 39: 1222–226, 1989.
54. Norman RW, Komi PV. Electromechanical delay in skeletal muscle under normal movement conditions. *Acta Physiol Scan* 106: 248, 1979
55. Nyland JA, Shapiro R, Stine RL, Horn TS, Ireland ML. Relationship of fatigued run and rapid stop to ground reaction forces, lower extremity kinematics, and muscle activation. *J Orthop Sports Phys Ther* 20(3): 132–37, 1994.
56. Powers SK, Howley ET. *Exercise physiology: Theory and application to fitness and performance.* Dubuque, IA: Brown, 149–72, 1990.
57. Renaud JM, Light P. The effects of K^+ on the twitch and tetanic contractions in the sartorius muscle of the frog, *Rana pipiens*: The implication for fatigue in vivo. *Can J Physiol Pharmacol* 70: 1236–246, 1992.
58. Sahlin K. Metabolic aspects of fatigue in human skeletal muscle. In *Muscle fatigue mechanisms in exercise and training,* vol 34, Marconnet P, Komi PV, Saltin B, Sejersted O (eds). Basel: Karger, 54–68, 1992.
59. Schomburg ED. Spinal sensorimotor system and their supraspinal control. *Neurosci Res* 7: 265–340, 1990.
60. Sharpe MH, Miles TS. Position sense at the elbow after fatiguing contractions. *Exp Brain Res* 94: 179–82, 1993.
61. Skinner HB, Barrack RL, Cook SD, Haddad RJ. Joint position sense in total knee arthroplasty. *J Orthop Res* 1: 276–83, 1984.
62. Skinner HB, Barrack RL, Cook SD. Age-related decline in proprioception. *Clin Orthop* 184: 208, 1984.
63. Skinner HB, Wyatt MP, Hodgdon JA, Conard DW, Barrack RL. Effect of fatigue on joint position sense of the knee. *J Orthop Res* 4: 112–18, 1986.
64. Skinner JS, McLellan TH. The transition from aerobic to anaerobic metabolism. *Res Quart* 51(1): 234–48, 1980.
65. Spriet LL. Anaerobic metabolism during high-intensity exercise. In *Exercise metabolism,* Hargreaves M (ed). Champaign, IL: Human Kinetics, 1–40, 1995.
66. Takahashi H, Mitsuharu I, Fujimoto K, Katsuta S, Anno I, Niitsu M, Itai Y. Control of the rate of phosphocreatine resynthesis after exercise in trained and untrained human quadriceps muscles. *Eur J Appl Physiol* 71: 396–404, 1995.
67. Tesch PA. Muscle fatigue in man with special reference to lactate accumulation during short-

term intense exercise. *Acta Physiol Scand* 480(Suppl): 1–40, 1980.

68. Tyldesley B, Grieves JI. *Muscle, nerves and movement: Kinesiology in daily living.* Cambridge, MA: Blackwell Scientific, 1989.
69. Voight ML, Harden JA, Blackburn TA, Tippet S, Canner GC. The effect of muscle fatigue on the relationship of arm dominance to shoulder proprioception. *J Orthop Sports Phys Ther* 23(6): 348–52, 1996.
70. Vos EJ, Harlaar J, Van Ingen Schenau GJ. Electromechanical delay during knee extensor contractions. *Med Sci Sports Exerc* 23(10): 1187–193, 1991.
71. Vredenbregt J, Rau G. Surface electromyography in relation to force, muscle length, and endurance. In *New developments in electromyography and clinical neurophysiology,* vol 1, Desmedt JE (ed). Basel: Karger, 607–22, 1973.
72. Watson JD, Colebatch JG, McCloskey DI. Effects of externally imposed elastic loads on the ability to estimate position and force. *Behav Brain Res* 13: 267–71, 1984.
73. Williams JH, Klug GA. Calcium exchange hypothesis of skeletal muscle fatigue: A brief review. *Muscle Nerve* 18: 421–34, 1995.
74. Wilson JR, McCully KK, Mancini DM, Boden B, Chance B. Relationship of muscular fatigue to pH and diprotonated P_i in humans: A ^{31}P NMR study. *J Appl Physiol* 64(6): 2333–339, 1988.
75. Winter DA. *Biomechanics and motor control of human movement,* 2d ed. New York: Wiley, 191–212, 1990.
76. Wojtys EW, Wylie BB, Huston LJ. The effects of muscys fatigue on neuromuscular function and anterior tibial translation in healthy knees. *Am J Sports Med* 24(5): 615–21, 1996.
77. Woods JJ, Furbish F, Bigland-Ritchie B. Evidence for a fatigue-induced reflex inhibition of motoneuron firing rates. *J Neuro Physiol* 58(1): 125–37, 1987.
78. Zhou S, McKenna MJ, Lawson DL, Morrison WE, Fairweather I. Effect of fatigue and sprint training on electromchanical delay of knee extensor muscles. *Eur J Appl Physiol Occup Physiol* 72(5–6): 410–16, 1996.

CHAPTER 34

The Role of Coactivation and Eccentric Activity in the ACL-Injured Knee

Louis Osternig, PhD, ATC

Introduction

The knee is a complex, multiaxial joint that must absorb and transmit large forces while simultaneously permitting intricate rotations that allow locomotion and pivoting. The seemingly diametric functions of stability and mobility apparently occur due to interactions of joint ligamentous and muscular structures controlled by the nervous system (21). Noncoordination of these operations may lead to articular and soft tissue damage (7, 27, 35). Because the knee is critical to lower extremity function and because of its vulnerability to injury, there has been renewed interest about the mechanisms that control knee actions (32).

The anterior cruciate ligament (ACL) is critical to normal knee function, and its disruption often leads to early-onset osteoarthritis (13, 14, 33, 40). Despite these associated problems, there is considerable variability in functional outcome among the ACL-deficient population (9,41,42). Young, physically active ACL-deficient patients may be considered candidates for ACL reconstructive surgery due to the relatively low percentage of satisfactory outcomes from conservative treatment and the relatively high percentage of good surgical results in this population (4).

Previous studies have shown evidence of an antagonistic effect by the hamstring musculature to anterior tibial load generated by quadriceps contractions in knee extension or external loads (7, 18, 27, 39, 46,58, 60, 61). These studies suggest that the hamstrings work synergistically with knee ligaments to assist in joint stability and reduce the magnitude of net anterior shear. Although the mechanisms for hamstring coactivation during knee extension appear to be complex and have not been fully elucidated, it has been postulated that afferent discharge from ligamentous mechanoreceptors may be stimulated by motion-induced tension in the anterior cruciate ligament and other knee ligaments (20, 30, 31, 51, 53, 56, 57). Such tension may exert reflex effects on neuronal circuits, possibly via the gamma system, which controls muscles around the knee joint (29, 36, 61).

Histological research by Krauspe and coworkers (36) suggested that stretching the anterior or posterior cruciate ligament produces a change in the activity of gamma motor neurons of the leg and thigh, indicating that the innervation of the cruciate ligaments may be important for sensory control of movement and for protecting ligamentous tissue. Other research, conducted in vivo (58), shows that direct stress to the anterior cruciate ligament produces quadriceps inhibition and hamstring facilitation. These studies have clinical significance in that knee ligament disruption and postinjury surgical reconstruction of the knee may disrupt ligamentous mechanoreceptors and consequently influence extremity function (8, 25, 35–37).

Adaptations to Anterior Cruciate Ligament Deficiency

Neuromuscular adaptations to anterior cruciate ligament deficiency have been recognized for several years (42), although little is known about the nature of these adaptations (12). It has been postulated that the adaptations of lower extremity function exhibited by ACL-deficient and ACL-postsurgical patients represent early accommodations to the loss of ACL function after injury and subsequent reprogramming of the locomotor process, so that excessive anterior displacement of the tibia is prevented (12).

Noyes and coworkers (42) found substantial discrepancy among 84 ACL-deficient patients in ability to compensate to the injury during a nonsurgical rehabilitation regimen. They found that approximately one-third of the group improved and compensated well to the injury, another one-third became worse and failed the program, and one-third partially compensated but needed to discontinue some activities. Berchuck and coworkers (12) assessed 16 patients with unilateral ACL deficiency and observed substantial differences from normal controls in several variables associated with walking, jogging, and ascending and descending stairs. They reported that 75% of the ACL-deficient patients exhibited a quadriceps avoidance gait during level walking. It was suggested that these patients altered their gait to avoid the anterior displacement of the proximal end of the tibia, which is normally produced when the quadriceps contracts while the knee is in nearly full extension. This finding was indirectly supported in an electromyographic study by Sinkjaer and Arendt-Nielsen (52) who reported that, prior to heel contact in walking, ACL-injured subjects demonstrated earlier and longer onset times for knee flexor muscles compared to controls. They speculated that the earlier recruitment and longer burst duration may be compensatory mechanisms, perhaps stabilizing the knee in preparation for foot contact with the ground.

Berchuck and coworkers (12) also found significantly greater maximum flexor moments about the hip in the ACL-deficient group compared to controls. Andriacchi and coworkers (4) had previously found greater than normal flexion of the hip and knee in ACL-insufficient subjects during a side step cutting maneuver. It was suggested that the when the knee is flexed the hamstrings become better positioned to stabilize the tibia and reduce anterior translation. The apparent compensatory maneuver increases moments at the hip and knee, necessitating greater activity of the quadriceps to maintain stability. Snyder-Mackler and coworkers (54) reported an extended knee flexion period during the stance phase of walking in patients who had recently undergone ACL surgical reconstruction. This finding was strongly correlated to quadriceps weakness, which has been shown to persist for several months after surgery (19). More recently, Snyder-Mackler and coworkers (55) also reported that ACL-postsurgical patients exhibit a flexed knee gait during the stance phase of walking, with less flexion excursion and a failure to return to a normal knee extended position. They found similarly that the gait variations were significantly correlated to the strength of the quadriceps femoris muscle.

Muscle Control of Anterior Tibial Displacement and ACL Strain

In recent years, particular interest has been focused on the role of the knee flexor musculature in the control of anterior tibial displacement elicited by quadriceps activity and passive shear forces. It has been postulated that knee flexor coactivation provides a mode of dynamic joint stiffness necessary to protect internal joint structures during knee extension (50, 58, 62). Hirokawa and associates (27) used cadaver specimens to show that hamstring coactivation progressively reduced anterior tibial displacement induced by the quadriceps musculature between 15° and about 80° of knee flexion. Within this range, a progressive reduction in anterior tibial displacement was noted as hamstring coactivating force increased. However, no such attenuation was noted at positions of 0° to 15° of knee flexion, suggesting that quadriceps-induced anterior tibial displacement is less restricted by the hamstrings as the knee approaches full extension.

The effect of coactivation on reducing anterior tibial displacement also suggests that knee flexor muscle activity may reduce the load on the ACL during knee extension (7, 25, 39, 43, 56). Renstrom and colleagues (50) measured ACL strain during simulated quadriceps and hamstring activity (see figure 34.1). They found that ACL strain increased significantly between 0° and 45° of knee flexion under the quadriceps-activity-alone condition compared to passive knee extension. With simulated quadriceps and hamstring coactivation, ACL strain was reduced significantly between 30° and 90° of knee flexion but not between 0° and 30° when compared to the quadriceps-activity-alone condition, suggesting that any potential ACL protection effect from flexor coactivation may only be present at knee mid ranges of motion. This finding is supported by the data from Hirokawa and associates (27), who found that hamstring coactivation was less effective in reducing quadriceps-induced anterior tibial displacement near full knee extension.

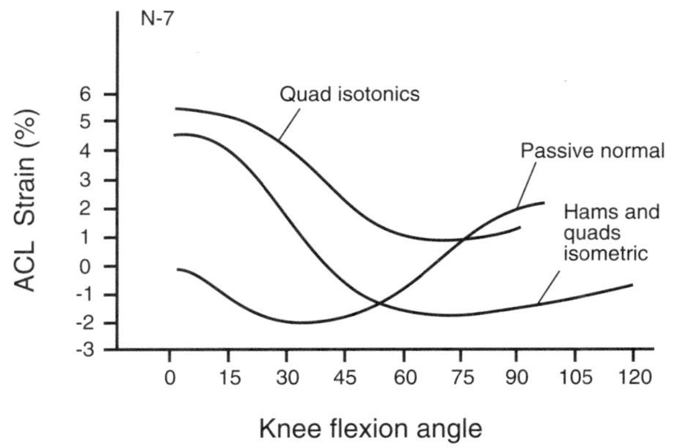

Figure 34.1 Mean passive, normal, simulated quadriceps isotonic and simulated simultaneous quadriceps and hamstring isometric strain patterns. (Reproduced from Renström P, Arms SW, Stanwyck TS, et al. Strain within the anterior cruciate ligament during hamstring and quadriceps activity. *Am J Sports Med* 14:83-87, 1986.)

O'Connor (43) and Collins (15) produced models indicating that both flexors (hamstrings and gastrocnemius) can restrain extensor torque and possibly unload the cruciate ligaments throughout the range of knee motion, except at near full extension (43). Their calculations assumed isometric (43) or closed chain activity (15), and direct application of the quantitative results requires further study.

While knee flexor muscles are considered to be important in the control of anterior tibial displacement elicited by knee extensors, the magnitude of quadriceps-induced ACL strain may not be significant. Beynnon and associates (11) found a significant increase in ACL strain resulting from maximal quadriceps force administered at 20° of knee flexion in vivo. However, the peak strain of 2.8% was well below tissue failure values. Howell (28) measured the effect of maximum isometric quadriceps contractions on anterior tibial translation in healthy subjects and reported that the tension in the ACL was no greater than the tension produced during instrumented laxity testing. Using human cadaveric knee models flexed to 30°, Aune and colleagues (6) found that a quadriceps muscle contraction of 889 N resulted in an anterior tibial translation force of only 69 N, which was less than that produced by a Lachman test. This finding was consistent with a prior animal study conducted in vivo by Aune and coworkers (5) in which tetanic quadriceps muscle contraction did not affect anterior shear force to ACL failure. It was reported in this same study, however, that when the hamstring muscles were tetanically stimulated, the anterior tibial shear load to ACL failure was 1.5 times greater than when the hamstrings were relaxed. These studies suggest that external rather than internal force mechanisms are the predominant cause of ACL failure and that knee flexor activation can resist anterior shear force and thus potentially protect the ACL.

It has been postulated that this knee flexor coactivation function may be compromised by a loss of afferent neural activity from traumatic or surgical denervation of the anterior cruciate ligament (25, 35–37, 47). Beard and associates (10) found a significantly increased reflex latency in the hamstrings of ACL-deficient subjects compared to the uninjured contralateral extremity. They also reported that functional instability of the knee was directly related to the increase in reflex latency (9). DiFabio and colleagues (17) recorded the automatic postural response from the tibialis anterior, quadriceps, and hamstrings muscles in a group of subjects with ACL deficiency. They found that an externally induced backward body sway induced selective activation of the hamstrings in the ACL-deficient limb as an apparent addition to the synergistic structure of the lower extremity. It was postulated that a capsular hamstring reflex might be integrated into the existing structure of a preprogrammed postural synergy, in ACL-deficient limbs, to compensate for ligamentous laxity.

Eccentric Muscle Actions and Joint Stability

Coactivation of antagonist knee flexors during active knee extension is thought to aid in maintaining joint stability by exerting an opposing torque to anterior tibial displacement induced by the quadriceps (7). This opposing torque is believed to be generated by eccentric muscle actions that stiffen the knee during voluntary extension, thereby attenuating strain to joint ligaments (7, 25, 39, 58). Eccentric muscle actions (lengthening contractions) exhibit force-velocity relationships that are distinct from those occurring during concentric actions (shortening contractions), and this may affect the capacity of knee flexors to counter tibial anterior shear and rotation, which may strain the ACL (see figure 34.2).

While concentric muscle actions function primarily to move bodily parts, eccentric actions function to decelerate and control skeletal motion. Since tension generated in the musculotendinous unit is greatest during eccentric compared to concentric or isometric actions (see figure 34.2), muscles undergoing lengthening contractions are well suited to resist opposing forces. Muscles under active ten-

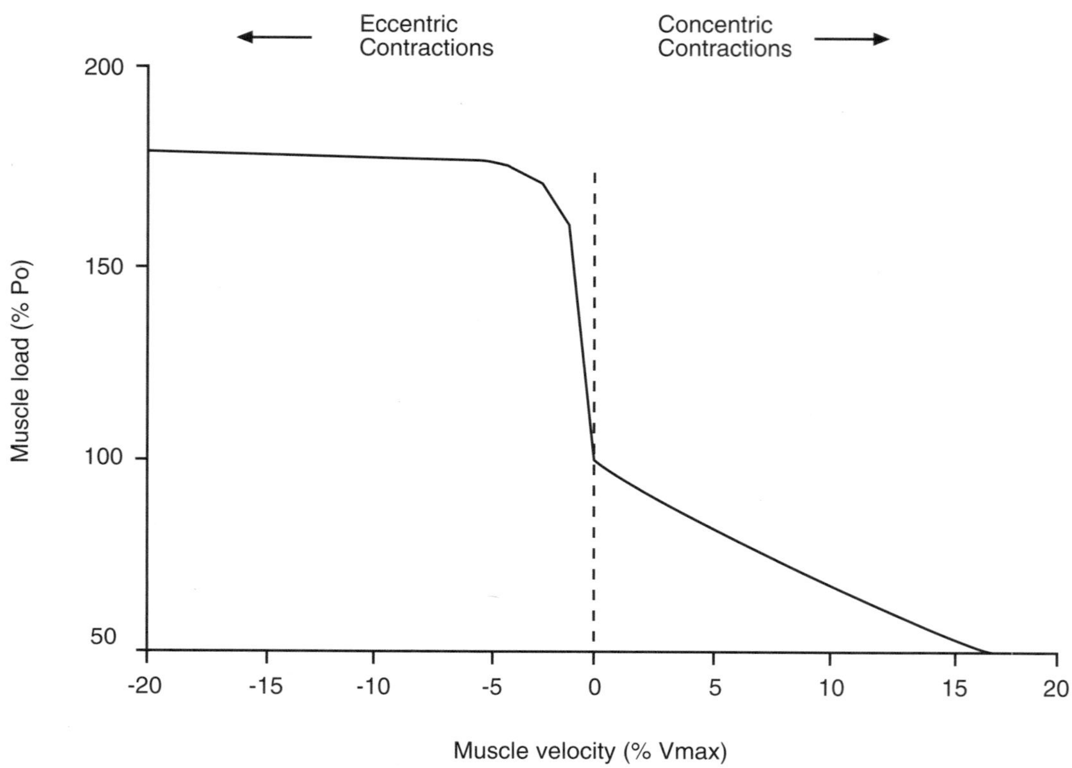

Figure 34.2 Force-velocity relationships for concentric and eccentric contractions. Note that for shortening velocities (velocities greater than zero) force drops relatively slowly as velocity increases. However, for lengthening velocities (velocities less than zero) force increases rapidly. (Reproduced from Fridén J, and Lieber RL. Structural and mechanical basis of exercise-induced muscle injury. *Med Sci Sports Exerc* 24:521-530, 1992.)

sion are highly resistive to forced lengthening. It has been estimated that a muscle lengthening at 1% Vmax can increase tension by 50% over its maximum isometric contractile tension (23). In this case, tension rises about 10 times faster for lengthening than for an equivalent velocity of shortening.

In a study on ankle muscle proprioception, Condon and Hutton (16) speculated that rapid movement speeds might facilitate the active contractile components in muscles that resist stretch. Hagood and colleagues (26) reported that as knee extension velocity increased to 240°/s there was a substantial EMG rise in the antagonist musculature, suggesting an increase in joint stiffness and reduction in laxity. Lestienne (38) found that triceps brachii activity during fast ballistic elbow flexion was proportional to the velocity of movement above a certain speed. Freund and Budingen (22) found that antagonist coactivation is typical with the onset of most rapid and vigorous isometric forces.

It has been shown previously in normal subjects that eccentric electromyographic activity of the hamstrings during rapid knee extension averaged 15 to 33% of the hamstring activity generated during maximal concentric knee flexion (45, 46). A similar study of eccentric hamstring EMG activity in subjects with unilateral ACL dysfunction revealed that coactivation of the injured limb hamstrings averaged less than half of the normal contralateral limb hamstrings during maximal knee extension (47) (see figure 34.3). It is possible that the injured limb subjects may have suffered denervation of ligamentous tissue from trauma or operative repair, thus reducing afferent activity that triggers neuronal circuitry relevant for joint stability. It has been suggested that loss of ACL innervation due to traumatic or operative denervation may be followed by a loss of afferent activity and neuronal control (35, 36). Such asymmetry in eccentric knee flexor coactivation may indicate an attenuation of the restraining role that these muscle play in ACL dysfunctional limbs.

Deficits in kinesthesia have been reported for subjects with ACL-deficient knees and for those who have undergone ACL reconstructive surgery. Barrack and associates (8) found deficits of more than 25%

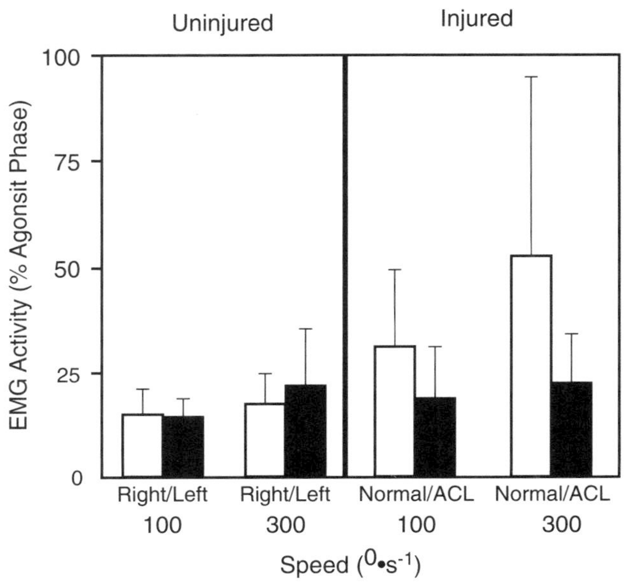

Figure 34.3 Mean hamstring coactivation (EMG activity) during maximal knee joint extension for uninjured group right and left limbs and for injured group normal and ACL-postsurgical limbs at 100°/s and 300°/s. (Adapted from Osternig LR, Caster BL, and James CR. Contralateral hamstring (biceps femoris) coactivation patterns and anterior cruciate ligament dysfunction. *Med Sci Sports Exerc* 28:805-808, 1995.)

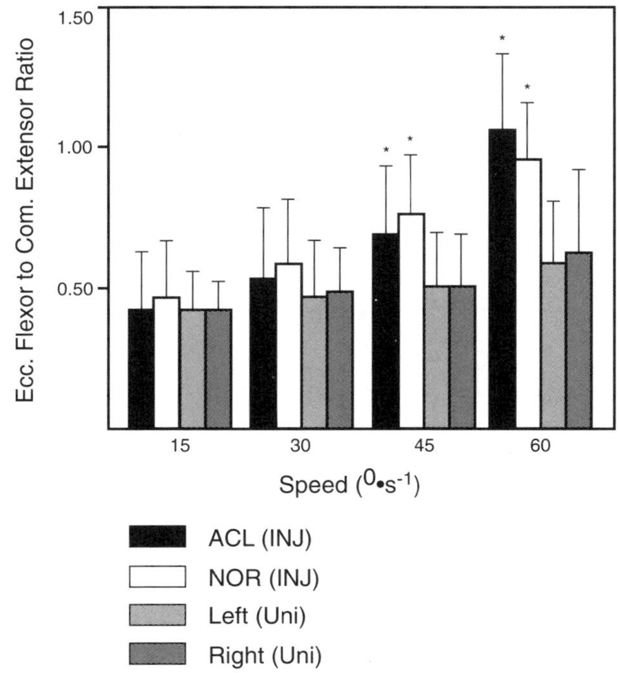

Figure 34.4 Means and standard deviations for ratio of eccentric (Ecc) flexor torque to concentric (Con) extensor torque for injured (INJ) group contralateral ACL-postsurgical and normal (NOR) limbs, and uninjured (UNI) group left and right limbs. Asterisks indicate values are significantly greater than corresponding uninjured left and right limbs ($p < .05$). (Reproduced from Osternig LR, James CR, and Bercades DT: Eccentric knee flexor torque following anterior cruciate ligament surgery. *Med Sci Sports Exerc* 28: 1229-1234, 1996.)

between contralateral normal and ACL-deficient knees on a test of proprioception. Lephart and colleagues (37) reported decreased kinesthetic awareness among 12 patients who were 11 to 26 months ACL-postreconstructive surgery. If adequate coactivation of knee flexors and extensors is necessary for knee stability and control, attenuation of this role, due to injury and surgery, may be a factor in the rate and degree of recovery following ACL injury and surgery.

Concentric hamstring/quadriceps torque ratios have been studied extensively (49) with reported averages ranging from about 0.5 to 0.75. However, although the knee flexors are activated eccentrically against the concentrically activated extensors, little has been reported on the eccentric knee flexor torque relative to concentric knee extensor torque.

Aagaard and associates (1) found that the eccentric hamstring/concentric quadriceps ratio was close to 1.0 at fast speeds (240°/s) and dropped to 0.27 at 30°/s. Osternig and coworkers (48) reported that the ratio of eccentric flexor torque to concentric extensor torque in ACL-postsurgical subjects increased with speed of movement and approached 1.0 at 60°/s, nearly twice that of normal controls (see figure 34.4). These studies suggest that as speed of motion increases, the potential restraining action of the eccentrically contracting flexors may have an increasing capacity to counter the tibial anterior shear moment created by forcefully contracting knee extensors or external loads.

Muscle Function and Joint Position

As the length of knee musculature changes with changes in joint position, the agonist/antagonist forces may differ from one knee joint position to another. The knee flexor and extensor muscles exert maximum force at particular muscle lengths according to the length-tension relationship (24) that corresponds to a particular joint position, about 30° of knee flexion for flexors and about 60° of knee flexion for extensors when measured concentrically from the seated position (34, 44, 59). Consequently, the capacity of the knee flexors to counter knee extensor activity may vary throughout the joint range. Furthermore, since the knee flexors are activated eccentrically in this function, their exerted force may be greater at a given joint position than when activated concentrically. Since the interactions of knee antagonist musculature occur at various points throughout the joint range, it is important to understand better the relationships between concentric and eccentric actions of the knee flexors and extensors at specific joint intervals.

Summary

In summary, it is apparent that the knee flexor and extensor muscles act synergistically to play important roles in controlling tibiofemoral articulations and guard ligamentous structures. The processes of flexor-extensor coactivation and eccentric flexor torque, which protectively stiffen the knee and help regulate knee motions, are controlled by the nervous system. Afferent responses induced by ligament strain appear to influence the quality of knee muscle synergy through reflex or spinal-mediated pathways. Stretching cruciate ligaments produces a change in gamma motor neuron activity of the lower extremity, and direct stress to the ACL has been shown to inhibit the quadriceps and facilitate the hamstrings. Although the neurological mechanisms for knee muscle control have not been fully explained, it is plausible that knee function is compromised by a loss of afferent neural activity from traumatic or surgical denervation of the anterior cruciate ligament.

References

1. Aagaard, P., E.B. Simonsen, M. Trolle, J. Bangsbo, and K. Klausen. Isokinetic hamstring/quadriceps strength ratio: Influence from joint angular velocity, gravity correction and contraction mode. *Acta Physiol. Scand.* 154: 421–27, 1995.
2. Abbott, B., B. Bigland, and J. Ritchie. The physiological cost of negative work. *J. Physiol.* 117: 380–90, 1952.
3. Asmussen, E. Positive and negative muscular work. *Acta Physiol. Scand.* 28: 364–82, 1953.
4. Andriacchi, T., P. Sabiston, and K. DeHaven. Ligament: Injury and repair. In *Injury and repair of the musculoskeletal soft tissues,* S.L. Woo and J.A. Buckwalter (Eds). Park Ridge, IL: American Academy of Orthopaedic Surgeons, 1987, 103–28.
5. Aune, A.K., A. Ekeland, and L. Nordsletten. Effect of quadriceps or hamstring contraction on the anterior shear force to anterior cruciate ligament failure: An in vivo study in the rat. *Acta Orthop. Scand.* 66: 261–65, 1995.
6. Aune, A.K., R.W. Cawley, and A. Ekeland. Quadriceps muscle contraction protects the anterior cruciate ligament during anterior tibial translation. *Am. J. Sports Med.* 25: 187–90, 1997.
7. Baratta, R.M., B.H. Solomonow, E.D. Zhou, R. Letson, R. Chuinard, and R. D'Ambrosia. Muscular coactivation: The role of the antagonist musculature in maintaining knee stability. *Am. J. Sports Med.* 16: 113–22, 1988.
8. Barrack, R.L., H.B. Skinner, and S.L. Buckley. Proprioception in the anterior cruciate ligament deficient knee. *Am. J. Sports Med.* 17: 1–6, 1989.
9. Beard, D., R. Kyberd, C. Fergusson, and C. Dodd. Proprioception after rupture of the anterior cruciate ligament. *J. Bone Joint Surg.* 75B: 311–15, 1993.
10. Beard, D., R. Kyberd, J. O'Connor, C. Fergusson, and C. Dodd. Reflex hamstring contraction latency in anterior cruciate ligament deficiency. *J. Orthop. Res.* 12: 219–28, 1994.
11. Beynnon, B., J.G. Howe, M.H. Pope, R.J. Johnson, and B.C. Fleming. The measurement of anterior cruciate ligament strain in vivo. *Int. Orthop.* 16: 1–12, 1992.
12. Berchuck, M., T. Andriacchi, B. Bach, and B. Reider. Gait adaptations by patients who have a deficient anterior cruciate ligament. *J. Bone and Joint Surg.* 72A: 871–77, 1990.
13. Brandt, K. Transection of the anterior cruciate ligament in the dog: A model of osteoarthritis. *Sem. Arthritis Rheum.* 21(3 Suppl. 2): 22–32, 1991.
14. Brandt, K., S. Myers, D. Burr, and M. Albrecht. Osteoarthritic changes in canine articular cartilage, subchondral bone, and synovium fifty-four months after transection of the anterior cruciate ligament. *Arthritis Rheum.* 34: 1406–415, 1991.
15. Collins, J.J. Antagonistic-synergistic muscle action at the knee during competitive weightlifting. *Med. Biol. Eng. Comput.* 32: 168–74, 1994.
16. Condon, S.A., and R. S. Hutton. Soleus muscle electromyographic activity and ankle dorsiflexion range of motion during four stretching procedures. *Phys. Ther.* 67: 24–30, 1987.
17. DiFabio, R.P., B. Graf, M.B. Badke, A. Breunig, and K. Jensen. Effect of knee joint laxity on long-loop postural reflexes: Evidence for a human capsular-hamstring reflex. *Exp. Brain Res.* 90: 189–200, 1992.

18. Draganich, L.F., R.J. Jaeger, and A.R. Kralj. Coactivation of the hamstrings and quadriceps during extension of the knee. *J. Bone Joint Surg.* 71A: 1075–1081, 1989.
19. Elmqvist, L., R. Lorentzon, C. Johansson, M. Langstrom, M. Fagerlund, and A. Fugl-Meyer. Knee extensor muscle function before and after reconstruction of anterior cruciate ligament tear. *Scand. J. Rehabil. Med.* 21: 131–39, 1989.
20. Elmqvist, L., R. Lorentzon, C. Johansson, and A. Fugl-Meyer. Does a torn anterior cruciate ligament lead to change in the central nervous drive of the knee extensors? *Eur. J. App. Physiol.* 58: 203–207, 1988.
21. Frank, C., S. Woo, and T. Andriacchi. Normal ligament: Structure, function, and composition. In *Injury and repair of the musculoskeletal soft tissues,* S.L. Woo and J.A. Buckwalter (Eds). Park Ridge, IL: American Academy of Orthopaedic Surgeons, 1987, 45–101.
22. Freund, H.J., and H.J. Bundingen. The relationship between speed and amplitude of the fastest voluntary contractions of human arm muscles. *Exp. Brain Res.* 31: 1–12, 1978.
23. Friden, J., and R.L. Lieber. Structural and mechanical basis of exercise-induced muscle injury. *Med. Sci. Sports Exerc.* 24: 521–30, 1992.
24. Gordon, A.M., A.F. Huxley, and F.J. Julian. The variation in isometric tension with sarcomere length in vertebrate muscle fibers. *J. Physiol.* 184: 17–192, 1966.
25. Harter, R.A., L.R. Osternig, and K.M. Singer. Knee joint proprioception following anterior cruciate ligament reconstruction. *J. Sports Rehabil.* 1: 103–10, 1992.
26. Hagood, S., M. Solomonow, R. Baratta, B.J. Zhou, and R. D'Ambrosia. The effect of joint velocity on the contribution of the antagonist musculature to knee stiffness and laxity. *Am. J. Sports Med.* 18: 182–87, 1990.
27. Hirokawa, S., M. Solomonow, Z. Luo, Y. Lu, and R. D'Ambrosia. Muscular co-contraction and control of knee stability. *J. Electromyog. Kinesiol.* 1: 199–208, 1991.
28. Howell, S.M. Anterior tibial translation during a maximum quadriceps contraction: Is it clinically significant? *Am. J. Sports Med.* 18: 573–78, 1990
29. Johansson, H., P. Sjolander, and P. Sojka. Activity in receptor afferents from the anterior cruciate ligament evokes reflex effects on sensorimotor neurons. *Neurosci. Res.* 8: 54–59, 1990.
30. Johansson, H., P. Sjolander, and P. Sojka. A sensory role for the cruciate ligaments. *Clin. Orthop.* 268: 161–78, 1991.
31. Johansson, H., P. Sjolander, and P. Sojka. Receptors in the knee joint ligaments and their role in the biomechanics of the joint. *Crit. Rev. Biomed. Eng.* 18: 341–68, 1991.
32. Johansson, H. Role of knee ligaments in proprioception and regulation of muscle stiffness. *J. Electromyog. Kinesiol.* 1: 158–79, 1991.
33. Johnson, R., B. Beynnon, C. Nichols, and P. Renstrom. The treatment of injuries of the anterior cruciate ligament. *J. Bone Joint Surg.* 74A: 140–51, 1992.
34. Kannus, P., M. Jarvinen, and R. Johnson. Function of the quadriceps and hamstrings muscles in knees with chronic partial deficiency of the anterior cruciate ligament. *Am. J. Sports Med.* 20: 162–68, 1992.
35. Kennedy, J.C., I.J. Alexander, and K.C. Hayes. Nerve supply of the human knee and its functional importance. *Am. J. Sports Med.* 10: 329–35, 1982.
36. Krauspe, R., M. Schmidt, and H. Schaible. Sensory innervation of the anterior cruciate ligament. *J. Bone Joint Surg.* 74A: 390–97, 1992.
37. Lephart, S.M., M.S. Kocher, F.H. Fu, P. Borsa, and C.D. Harner. Proprioception following anterior cruciate ligament reconstruction. *J. Sports Rehabil.* 1: 188–96, 1992.
38. Lestienne, F. Effects of inertial load and velocity on the braking process of voluntary limb movements. *Exp. Brain Res.* 35: 407–18, 1979.
39. More, R.C., B.T. Karras, R. Neiman, D. Fritschy, S. Woo, and D.M. Daniel. Hamstrings: An anterior cruciate ligament protagonist. *Am. J. Sports Med.* 21: 231–37, 1993.
40. Myers, S., K. Brandt, B. O'Connor, D. Visco, and M. Albrecht. Synovitis and osteoarthritic changes in canine articular cartilage after anterior cruciate ligament transection. *Arthritis Rheum.* 33: 1406–415, 1990.
41. Noyes, F., P. Mooar, D. Matthews, and D. Butler. The symptomatic anterior cruciate-deficient knee. Part I: The long-term functional disability in athletically active individuals. *J. Bone Joint Surg.* 65A: 154–62, 1983.
42. Noyes, F., D. Matthews, P. Mooar, and E. Grood. The symptomatic anterior cruciate-deficient knee. Part II: The results of rehabilitation, activity modification, and counseling on functional disability *J. Bone Joint Surg.* 65A: 163–74, 1983.
43. O'Connor, J. Can muscle co-contraction protect knee ligaments after injury or repair? *J. Bone Joint Surg.* 75B: 41–48, 1993.
44. Osternig, L.R., J.A. Sawhill, B.T. Bates, and J. Hamill. Function of limb speed on torque: Pat-

terns of antagonistic muscles. *Biomechanics* VIIIA, Champaign, IL: Human Kinetics, 1983, 251–57.
45. Osternig, L., J. Hamill, D. Corcos, and J. Lander. Electromyographic patterns accompanying isokinetic exercise under varying speed and sequencing conditions. *Am. J Phys. Med.* 63: 289–97, 1984.
46. Osternig, L.R., J. Hamill, J.E. Lander, and R. Robertson. Coactivation of sprinter and distance runner muscles in isokinetic exercise. *Med. Sci. Sports Exerc.* 18: 431–35, 1986.
47. Osternig, L., B. Caster, and C. James. Contralateral hamstring (biceps femoris) coactivation patterns and anterior cruciate ligament dysfunction. *Med. Sci. Sports Exerc.* 27: 805–808, 1995.
48. Osternig, L., C. James, D. Bercades. Eccentric knee flexor torque following anterior cruciate ligament surgery. *Med. Sci. Sports Exerc.* 28: 1229–234, 1996.
49. Perrin, D. *Isokinetic exercise and assessment.* Champaign, IL: Human Kinetics, 1993, 153–58.
50. Renstrom, P., S.W. Arms, T.S. Stanwyck, R.J. Johnson, and M.H. Pope. Strain within the anterior cruciate ligament during hamstring and quadriceps activity. *Am. J. Sports Med.* 14: 83–87, 1986.
51. Schultz, R.A., D. Miller, C.S. Kerr, and L. Micheli. Mechanoreceptors in human cruciate ligaments: A histological study. *J. Bone Joint Surg.* 66A: 1072–1076, 1984.
52. Sinkjaer, T., and L. Arendt-Nielsen. Knee stability and muscle coordination in patients with anterior cruciate ligament injuries: An electromyographic approach. *J. Electromyogr. Kinesiol.* 1: 209–17, 1991.
53. Sjolander, P., H. Johansson, P. Sojka, and A. Rehnholm. Sensory nerve endings in the cat cruciate ligaments: A morphological investigation. *Neurosci. Lett.* 102: 33–38, 1989.
54. Snyder-Mackler, L., A. Delitto, S. Bailey, and S. Stralka. Strength of the quadriceps femoris muscle and functional recovery after reconstruction of the anterior cruciate ligament. *J. Bone Joint Surg.* 77A: 1166–173, 1995.
55. Snyder-Mackler, LZ Ladin, A. Schepsis, and J. Young. Electrical stimulation of the thigh muscles after reconstruction of the anterior cruciate ligament. *J. Bone Joint Surg.* 73A: 1025–1036, 1991.
56. Sojka, R., P. Sjolander, H. Johansson, and M. Djupsjobacka. Influence from stretch-sensitive receptors in the collateral ligaments of the knee joint on the gamma muscle spindle systems of flexor and extensor muscles. *Neurosci. Res.* 11: 55–62, 1991.
57. Sojka, P., H. Johansson, P. Sjolander, R. Lorentzon, R, and M. Djupsjobacka. Fusimotor neurons can be reflexly influenced by activity in receptor afferents from the posterior cruciate ligament. *Brain Res.* 483: 177–83, 1989.
58. Solomonow, M., R. Baratta, and B.H. Zghou. The synergistic action of the anterior cruciate ligament and thigh muscles in maintaining joint stability. *Am. J. Sports Med.* 15: 207–13, 1987.
59. Westing, S. H., and J.Y. Seger. Eccentric and concentric torque-velocity characteristics, torque output comparisons, and gravity effect torque corrections for the quadriceps and hamstring muscles in females. *Int. J. Sports Med.* 10: 175–80, 1989.
60. Yasuda, K., and T. Sasaki. Exercise after anterior cruciate ligament reconstruction: The force exerted on the tibia by the separate contractions of the quadriceps or the hamstrings. *Clin. Orthop.* 220: 275–83, 1987.
61. Yasuda, K., and T. Sasaki. Muscle exercise after anterior cruciate ligament reconstruction: Biomechanics of the simultaneous isometric contraction method of the quadriceps and the hamstrings. *Clin. Orthop.* 220: 266–74, 1987.
62. Zimny, M., M. Schutte, and E. Dabezies. Mechanoreceptors in the human anterior cruciate ligament. *Anat. Rec.* 214: 204–209, 1986.

CHAPTER 35

Restoration of Dynamic Stability in the ACL-Deficient Knee

Katherine S. Rudolph, MS, PT
Kelley Fitzgerald, MS, PT, OCSS
Lynn Snyder-Mackler, ScD, PT

Introduction

The most predictable impairment resulting from anterior cruciate ligament (ACL) rupture is anterior tibiofemoral laxity. The assumptions have been that joint laxity (the clinical sign) leads inexorably to instability (the symptom), and instability leads to disability and progressive arthritic changes. Many patients require reconstructive surgery to control the symptoms of instability. Some elect to be treated nonoperatively. For some of these patients, instability continues to be a problem that is controlled only by adapting their physical activities to the disability: curtailing activities that provoke instability. Factors that influence successful nonoperative management include intercurrent injury, age, and activity level (5, 6, 9). We have recently identified a select subgroup of ACL-deficient patients (10% of the population) who are able to return to all pre-injury activities at the same level, including high-level sport activities, without surgery. These patients, whom we term copers, differ from those described by others (5, 6, 9) in that they did not adapt to the injury, but rather were able to return to all activity without restriction and without surgery. Study of the strategies by which copers are able to stabilize their knees across a wide range of demanding activities can provide better templates for rehabilitation for the 40% of those with ACL injuries who elect nonoperative management.

Most of the studies of gait in persons with ACL deficiency fail to distinguish copers from noncopers. Studies of gait patterns in individuals with ACL deficiency are most notable for the inconsistency in their results. When published results are reconsidered with respect to differing functional abilities, more consistent movement patterns begin to emerge. In general, the more stressful the activity, the more clearly the patterns appear. Two basic strategies emerge from the literature. The first strategy is one where the subjects stiffen their knee joints, which we hypothesize is accomplished as the activity of all muscles crossing the knee joint increases (co-contraction) to quasistatically stabilize the knee. This is a mechanically inefficient strategy that has a very limited capacity to respond to unexpected perturbations. The second strategy, which we term coordinated activation, involves coordination of muscles around the knee, hip, and ankle. This strategy involves muscle activity patterns, possibly idiosyncratic, which cause selective, short duration joint stabilization (without stiffening), to allow more normal joint motion during functional activities.

In noncopers, the joint stiffens, as manifested by an attenuation of the knee joint excursions during loading. This pattern has been described in the literature and is underscored in our recent study of copers and noncopers. In our study, 16 ACL-deficient subjects were studied; 8 were copers (who had returned to all cutting and pivoting sports) and 8 were noncopers (scheduled for ACL reconstruction) (26). There was no difference in the passive anterior knee joint laxity or strength of the involved quadriceps femoris muscles of the two groups.

The most striking differences in the movement patterns between copers and noncopers appeared during weight acceptance. We found that both groups mitigated their vertical ground reaction forces (GRF) in walking, but only the noncopers reduced the range of motion on the involved side, landing with less knee flexion at initial contact and flexing the knee less during weight acceptance. Both groups had lower internal knee extensor moments and lower power absorption on the involved side. Ankle power absorption, however, was negligible in the coper group on both sides while the noncopers had slightly greater ankle power absorption on the involved side.

The less dynamic pattern was more pronounced when the subjects were jogging, with the noncopers continuing to show reduced vertical GRF (see figure 35.1), less knee flexion at initial contact and during weight acceptance (see figure 35.2), and they maintained less knee flexion throughout the entire stance phase.

Berchuck, Andriacchi, and Bach (2) introduced the notion of the "quadriceps avoidance" gait pattern, similar to the gait pattern seen in our noncoper subjects. We feel, however, that the lower knee moment seen in our subjects does not represent reduced quadriceps activity but rather an increased knee flexor activity. Since joint moments are net moments, that is, the sum of the moments generated by opposing muscle groups, we feel that the reduced knee extensor moment seen in *some* ACL-deficient individuals more likely reflects a greater relative contribution of the knee flexors, including hamstrings and gastrocnemius muscles, as they contract concurrently.

As the heel contacts the floor the ground reaction force tends to displace the tibia anteriorly (7, 19), and a strong eccentric quadriceps muscle contraction follows in order to control the normal knee flexion. The potential for knee instability at this point in the gait cycle is substantial when the anterior cruciate ligament is ruptured, since the quadriceps activity may lead to anterior tibial translation. In the noncopers, the concurrent activation of knee flexors and extensors results in the attenuation of joint motion: a strategy of stiffening co-contraction.

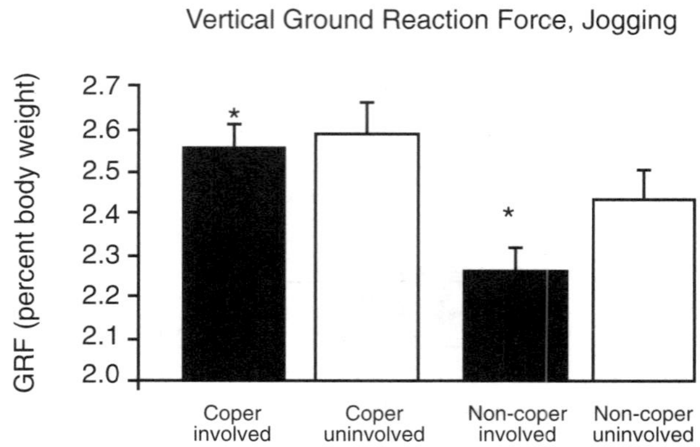

Figure 35.1 Vertical ground reaction force normalized to body weight. Both groups have lower vertical GRF on the involved side. (*F = 7.696, $p = .015$.)

These individuals attempt to stabilize the anterior cruciate ligament-deficient limb by co-contracting all muscles surrounding that joint to stiffen the knee, which is similar to the strategy we all adopt when we walk on slippery surfaces.

Other investigators have described the pattern of co-contraction that we assume to be responsible for the decreased knee flexion in the noncopers (6, 8, 21). Ciccotti and coworkers (6) found that anterior cruciate ligament-deficient subjects had less vastus lateralis, rectus femoris, and gastrocnemius muscle activity, along with greater biceps femoris activity during knee loading. Simultaneous activation of the knee flexors and knee extensors may result in joint stiffening and increased joint compression forces (32). In our noncoper sample the stiffening co-contraction was generally a more crude compensation tactic, which was incapable of stabilizing the knee under all conditions. The incidences of giving way experienced by the noncopers would lead to greater shear forces in the knee. These two forces, compression and shear, contribute significantly to the biochemical and metabolic changes that characterize degeneration of articular cartilage. Recent work by Setton and colleagues (26) demonstrates that even small shear forces lead to changes in the viscoelastic behavior of articular cartilage after anterior cruciate ligament transection in a canine model. The noncopers not only have knee joint instability with the associated excessive shear forces, they also use the stiffening co-contraction strategy with increased joint compression, which together may lay the unfavorable ground work for further articular damage.

The copers, on the other hand, appear to use a more precisely tuned strategy to stabilize the ACL-

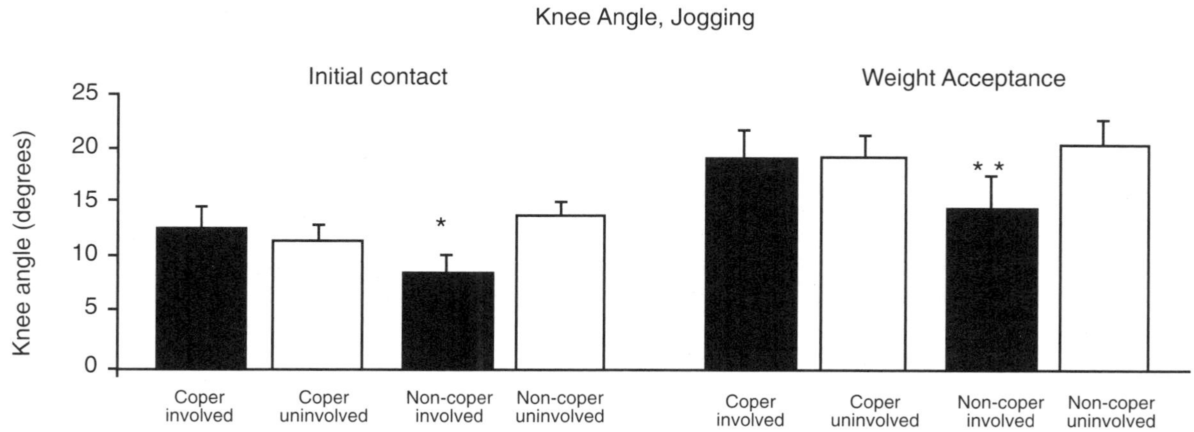

Figure 35.2 Knee flexion at initial contact and during weight acceptance. Noncopers landed in less knee flexion and achieved less flexion during weight acceptance. (*$F = 4.452$, $p = .053$, **$F = 4.659$, $p = .049$.)

deficient knee, one that reduces the knee extensor moment while maintaining joint motions similar to those reported for young healthy subjects (22). This reduction in knee moment is probably achieved by a strategy of coordinated activation of the anterior cruciate ligament agonists (hamstrings), which act strategically to stabilize the knee without stiffening the joint. The copers showed a much more pronounced attenuation of knee extensor power absorption than that seen in the noncopers; the involved limb's value was less than half of that in the uninvolved limb. The ankle power absorption seen at peak knee flexion was the least in the copers. The kinetic differences seen in the copers and noncopers indicate that differences in the synchronization of muscles at the knee and ankle may be in effect. Further kinematic, kinetic, and EMG study involving the hip musculature may further elucidate this stabilization strategy.

One successful stabilization strategy involving ankle musculature has been suggested in the literature. Ciccotti and coworkers (6) studied a group of anterior cruciate ligament-deficient individuals who had successfully returned to all previous activities without re-injury after participating in a 6 mo rehabilitation program. The subjects in Ciccotti's group appear to be more similar to our coper group than those reported in other studies, and they showed increased tibialis anterior activity during both terminal swing and terminal stance. Perhaps this well-rehabilitated group, like our copers, used the increased tibialis anterior activity to "set the ankle" in a posture to allow the gastrocnemius to work more precisely to protect the knee from pivoting during loading. Sinkjaer and Arendt-Nielsen (28) found that subjects who had reported "good/excellent" knee stability recruited the medial head of the gastrocnemius and lateral hamstrings earlier than did those with poor stability. The combined activity of the tibialis anterior and medial gastrocnemius could act as a force couple whereby the tibialis anterior rotates the tibia externally and the medial gastrocnemius rotates the femur internally to help keep the knee from pivoting. Our data suggest that the reduced ankle power absorption seen in the copers reflects the contribution of the dorsiflexors in acting synchronously with the plantarflexors to allow the well-coordinated stabilization of the knee without compromising knee motion.

The normal joint motion seen in our coper subjects occurs despite side-to-side knee laxity measurements that were no different than those of the noncopers (22). The coper's ability to maintain normal joint motion through a well-coordinated activation strategy should minimize the compression and shear forces. Daniel and coworkers (9) suggested that the development of arthritic changes after anterior cruciate ligament injury is *not* inevitable and that there are individuals who are stable and free of arthritic changes despite their anterior cruciate deficiency. The ability of the copers to mitigate contact forces without compromising joint motion may bode well for favorable knee function in the long term.

The results of our study clearly indicate that, in a small number of individuals, anterior cruciate ligament deficiency does not necessarily lead to functional deficits that require surgical stabilization. The copers are able to induce the appropriate compensatory pattern to achieve dynamic functional stability. Further investigation of joint kinematics and kinetics with simultaneous electromyography is necessary to more fully elucidate these differences.

Muscle Activity and Motor Control

There are conflicting reports regarding reflex activation of the muscle stabilizers in the ACL-deficient knee. Increased joint laxity or afferent input from the ACL may activate α motor neurons in the muscles that cross the knee joint in order to stabilize the knee (1, 29, 30). Disruption of afferent input from the ACL, however, may be insufficient to interfere with the protective mechanisms of the knee joint during stressful activity (15). Reflexive activity, however, involves more than just the α motor neurons of the musculoskeletal system. The afferent activity likely involves the γ system to a greater degree, which shows its effects on muscle stiffness. Johansson and coworkers (17) postulated that the γ system plays a large part in regulating stiffness of the muscles around the knee joint, which in turn serves to regulate joint stability, particularly in response to sudden perturbations. They also suggested that the γ system is responsible for the integration of different muscle activity, which is well suited for synchronized recruitment of specific muscles in response to greater joint laxity. Nichols and Steeves (23) studied decerebrate cats and found that the stiffness of a muscle at a given length and contractile force may vary. The change in muscle stiffness may reflect a higher state of readiness, allowing an individual to better compensate for increased joint laxity. In previous work done in our laboratory, we found a change in the physiological characteristics of the quadriceps muscles in noncopers. Evidence suggests that the muscle of the involved limb undergoes a physiological slowing, paradoxically, without morphological changes. The presence of fast, high-force muscle contractions in the quadriceps muscles of copers may also contribute to the readiness of the muscle to compensate for ACL deficiency. Motor control mechanisms that employ selective stiffening and coordinated activation of muscles with adequate contraction times and force generating capabilities could produce a sophisticated stabilization strategy at the knee to allow more dynamic joint excursions rather than static co-contraction.

The work of Lawrence, Nichols, and English (19), English and Letbetter (12), and English (13) on muscle compartmentalization in cats showed that, within one muscle, different compartments may be selectively activated during particular activities. Botterman and associates (4) found a functional compartmentalization in the cat biceps femoris muscle where the caudal compartments were strong knee flexors and the rostral compartments were almost exclusively hip extensors. English and Letbetter (12) found differing EMG activity at proximal and distal ends of biarticular forearm muscles, which may represent the selective activation of neuromuscular compartments within a muscle. It may be necessary to record EMG from different parts of biarticular muscles to fully elucidate the strategies adopted by those who compensate well for ACL injury.

Training and Rehabilitation

Traditionally, rehabilitation for those who elect nonsurgical treatment of the ACL injury includes initial treatment of the inflammation, followed by treatments directed at impairments (quadriceps strengthening, ROM) and those directed at reinforcing the missing ligament (hamstring strengthening, functional bracing.) Gait training largely consists of teaching patients to walk like healthy subjects with a "normal gait pattern." The literature and our pilot work suggest that the "abnormal" walking patterns seen in some ACL-deficient people may be related to the ability to stabilize the knee during stressful activities. Training a more "normal" pattern may actually be the wrong tactic and may lead to dynamic instability in individuals with no ACL (6, 28, 29). Those who compensate well for this injury appear to adopt a unique strategy, likely involving changes in muscle activity patterns. Training paradigms, which are directed at teaching adaptations that would mimic the coper's stabilization strategies, provide the best hope for successful return to high level functional activities.

One mechanism for training is directly mimicking the muscle activities and ground reaction force patterns of the good compensators using EMG and limb-load biofeedback (33). Researchers have used EMG biofeedback training on a very small scale to train patients with ACL deficiency to alter lower extremity EMG patterns and improve function. Sinkjaer and associates (28) used a biofeedback training protocol to teach two patients with poor stability to activate their medial gastrocnemius muscles earlier and for greater duration during the stance phase of gait. This was accomplished by having patients observe their medial gastrocnemius EMG signal on a monitor during treadmill ambulation and instructing them to activate the medial gastrocnemius at heel strike by using a slight medially rotation of the involved limb's foot. These two patients exhibited increased medial gastrocnemius activity during the stance phase of gait and improved their Lysholm scores to good stability after 15 wks of training. Although a study based on two subjects is not conclusive, it does suggest that it is possible to alter muscle activity patterns in a manner that induces functional compensation in patients with ACL deficiency.

Although Sinkjaer and coworkers (28) reported success using EMG biofeedback training in their two subjects, there are factors to consider that limit the success of this type of training on a broad scale. Ciccotti and associates (6) suggest that an adequate compensatory muscle activation pattern that improves dynamic stability will involve selective, coordinated activation of several muscle groups and not a simple co-contraction strategy. Moreover, Ciccotti and associates found that specific compensatory patterns were dependent on both the type of functional activity and the phase of the activity. The implication of these findings is that an EMG biofeedback training approach, in many cases, may be impractical for inducing appropriate alterations in muscle activity patterns to improve knee stability. The patient would have to learn how to alter the activity of several muscle groups, each of which may have to be activated at different times and at different magnitudes. The effectiveness of EMG biofeedback training becomes drastically reduced when the patient has to try and control more than one variable at a time (3).

A second problem with EMG biofeedback training is that there does not seem to be a typical or "correct" pattern for improving dynamic knee stability. Shiavi and associates (27) have reported that there may be several different strategies in lower extremity muscle activity patterns that enhance functional compensation for a given activity in ACL-deficient patients. The same alterations in muscle recruitment are not employed across individuals to enhance dynamic knee stability. Even if patients could learn to alter several muscle groups simultaneously with EMG biofeedback training, there is no standard muscle recruitment pattern on which to base the development of the training programs. Given the inherent limitations in implementing a successful EMG biofeedback training program, other treatment approaches need to be explored that would enhance patient ability to develop appropriate compensatory muscle activation patterns.

The coordination of interjoint muscle activity to maintain joint stability during weight-bearing tasks of the lower extremity may be mediated by a "force-feedback" mechanism (23). Muscle activation patterns in the lower extremity are influenced by the magnitude and direction of force or torque being applied to the joints and their associated structures during a functional task (e.g., walking, running, jumping). With experience, the nervous system develops stereotypical activation patterns for each activity based on the force or torque that is typically encountered during that activity. Rupturing the ACL changes the patterns of force or torque transmission through the knee during functional activity and the activation patterns of muscles affecting these joints would, therefore, have to change if joint stability were to be maintained.

The force-feedback theory of muscle recruitment has important clinical implications for rehabilitation of patients with joint instability. Altering the magnitude and direction of force applied to the lower extremity could induce alterations in the lower extremity muscle activation patterns in a manner that improves dynamic stability of the joint. Patients would be encouraged to develop individualized compensatory patterns rather than be forced to adopt a standard pattern that may not be successful for them.

Treatment techniques that involve perturbing support surfaces allow altered forces and torques to be applied to the lower extremity in multiple directions and in a controlled manner. These techniques can induce compensatory muscle activation patterns in ACL-deficient patients. DiFabio and associates (11) have reported altered hamstring activity in the ACL-deficient limbs of patients during anterior and posterior translational perturbations of a platform. When the support surface was translated anteriorly, a posterior postural sway was induced in the subjects. Subjects in a control group activated the quadriceps femoris muscles and the anterior tibialis muscle to correct this posterior sway. In subjects with ACL-deficient limbs the hamstring muscles also were activated, probably to control anterior shear forces that would be created by the quadriceps femoris and anterior tibialis muscle groups and would normally be countered by an intact ACL. Potential compensatory muscle activation patterns may, therefore, be induced by subjecting patients to support surface perturbations.

Ihara and Nakayama (15) and Beard and associates (1) have used perturbations of tilt boards and roller boards to improve the reaction time of the hamstring muscles in the injured limbs of patients with ACL deficiency. Only Beard and coworkers (1) have attempted to determine whether treatment programs that include perturbation training are more effective than more traditional treatment programs for patients with ACL deficiency. Subjects with ACL deficiency were randomly assigned to either a group that received a standard rehabilitation program or a group that received a standard program plus the perturbation training. Reflex hamstring contraction latencies (RHCL) and scores on the Lysholm rating scales were used as outcome measures. The Beard team reported that improvement in RHCL and Lysholm ratings occurred in both groups; however, improvement was significantly greater in the group receiving the perturbation training.

Use of the Lysholm rating scale by the Beard team as a functional outcome measure reflects the success of the perturbation training in restoring knee stability in activities of daily living. This perturbation training program focused on improving hamstring reaction time response to forces that might challenge anterior knee stability. Although the program appeared to improve performance in activities of daily living, treatment success may be limited in restoring higher levels of function. During more challenging activities, coordinated activation patterns of several muscle groups seem to be more effective in enhancing dynamic knee stability than simple co-contraction patterns (6, 28). Perturbation training techniques might be more successful in restoring high level function if they were modified to encourage the selected activation of several lower extremity muscle groups to perturbing forces that challenge knee stability in multiple directions and magnitudes, rather than the activation of a single muscle group (i.e., hamstrings).

Vereijken and associates (32) reported that in the early stages of motor skill acquisition, individuals may simplify problems with motor coordination by rigidly fixing joint angles, or even the whole extremity, via massive co-contraction of muscles during performance of the task ("freezing" degrees of freedom). As the skill level of the individual improves this rigid fixation is released, allowing for greater variety of movement options and more selective responses to forces encountered during the activity. Vereijken and associates demonstrated this phenomenon in subjects learning to perform slalom ski movements on a ski apparatus. Co-contraction was the predominant control strategy during beginning levels of skill acquisition. As skill level improved the co-contraction patterns were replaced with more selective motor responses.

We developed a training program that we believed would enhance performance at higher skill levels by encouraging selective muscle activation patterns ("unfreezing" degrees of freedom) in response to varying forces applied to the lower extremity. The techniques used are similar to those reported by Ihara and Nakayama (16) and Beard and coworkers (1), who used roller boards and tilt boards as the support surfaces. The training programs described by Ihara and Nakayama (16) and Beard and associates (1) were modified by applying perturbation forces in multiple directions and at a variety of magnitudes to evoke responses from other muscle groups (such as the gastrocnemius and tibialis anterior muscles) in addition to the hamstring muscles. We believed that with the proper patient instruction, and with the appropriate magnitude and direction of perturbing forces, muscle activity patterns that dynamically stabilize the knee could be induced and functional outcome would be improved. Before proceeding with a treatment outcome study we felt it was necessary to determine if these techniques really would yield varying responses in muscle activation patterns in the target muscles between coper and noncoper populations.

We performed a preliminary study in which EMG activity was recorded from selected muscles of the lower extremity during the perturbation training techniques. Electromyographic activity of the quadriceps femoris, hamstring, anterior tibialis, and gastrocnemius muscle groups were recorded from the right lower extremity in one subject who was not injured and from the injured lower extremity in three subjects with ACL deficiency, during application of the perturbation training techniques. One subject was a true coper who had been participating in level I and II activities for 15 yrs after complete, unilateral ACL rupture. One subject was a noncoper who had had episodes of giving way with activities of daily living and was scheduled for surgery. The third subject was a starting Division IAA middle linebacker who had sustained a complete, unilateral rupture of his ACL in the beginning of the season. He was identified as a patient with rehabilitation potential based on a screening exam that we use to distinguish between surgical candidates and patients with rehabilitation potential. He underwent 10 sessions of perturbation training in addition to standard ACL rehabilitation and then completed the remainder of the football season (7 games) without an episode of giving way. We hypothesized that the healthy subject, the coper, and the patient who had received training would respond to perturbations with selected activation of muscles that were consistent with those necessary to resist the applied forces. We hypothesized that the noncoper would use a co-contraction strategy to resist the perturbing forces, a strategy that would provide knee stability but would not allow for the performance of higher level function.

An 8-channel telemetric EMG instrument (B and L Engineering, San Diego, CA) was used for EMG recordings. Active surface electrodes were placed over the muscle bellies of the lateral hamstring, vastus lateralis, tibialis anterior, and medial gastrocnemius muscles. Exact electrode placement site for each muscle was determined, based on the method described by Delagi and coworkers (10). EMG signals were full wave rectified and filtered at a frequency of 50 Hz. Signal processing was performed using a custom written Labview (National Instruments, Austin, TX) software program. An electronic switch was used by the examiner during the perturbations to indicate the start and completion of the perturbations, which could be displayed on the EMG data graphic printout.

The EMG data for the anterior-posterior perturbations with the injured leg on the roller board is presented to illustrate typical differences between the subjects. The EMG recording from the noninjured subject during a single trial of anterior-posterior translation of the roller board is displayed in figure 35.3. During the anterior translation the hamstrings, quadriceps femoris, and tibialis anterior muscles were activated. The gastrocnemius muscle was silent. During the posterior translation the hamstrings were electrically silent, while the quadriceps femoris, gastrocnemius, and tibialis anterior muscles were activated. The change in response of the hamstrings and gastrocnemius muscles with the change in direction of perturbation force indicates a selective activation pattern in response to the perturbing forces. The co-contraction observed in the thigh muscles during anterior translation, which is not observed during the posterior translation, is hard to explain. The activity of the ankle muscles may be explained by an attempt to stabilize the ankle and promote better foot contact with the board, so that the thigh musculature can function mainly to resist the perturbation forces.

The EMG recording from the coper subject on the first trial of anterior-posterior roller board translation is displayed in figure 35.4. During this trial the subject exhibited a general co-contraction pattern for all four sampled muscles in response to perturbations in both directions. The subject indicated that he attempted to hold his test leg rigid to overcome the perturbation force applied to the roller board. The subject was then instructed to match rather than overcome the perturbation force and keep the board steady. The EMG recording from the next trial is shown in figure 35.5. When the board was perturbed anteriorly,

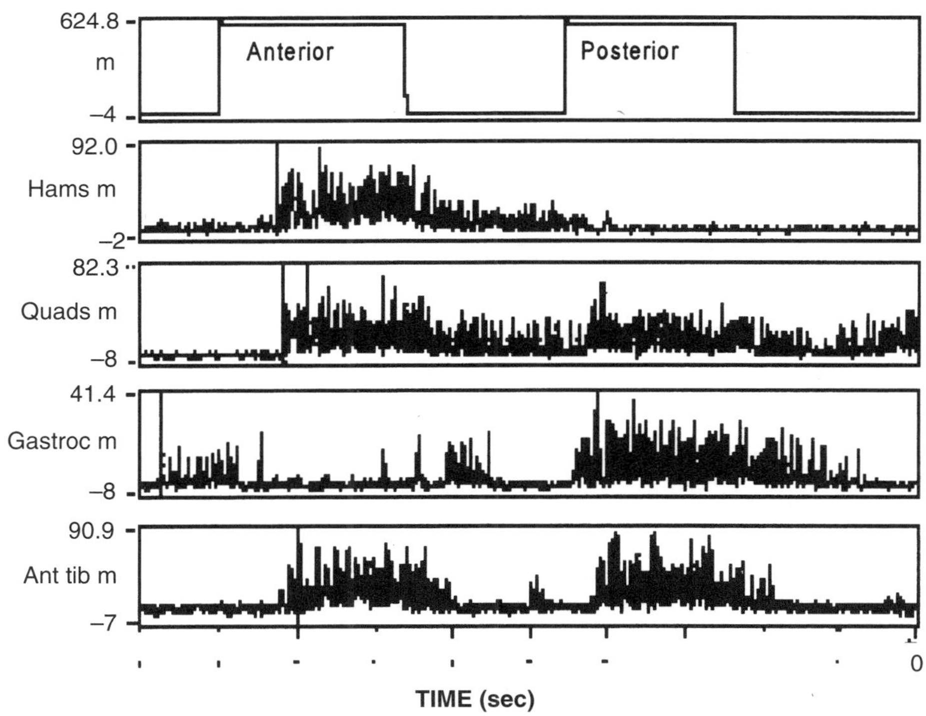

Figure 35.3 EMG response from an uninjured subject's right lower extremity during anterior and posterior perturbations of the roller board. The right lower extremity is on the roller board and the left lower extremity is on a stationary platform. The first box above the EMG signals indicates the time of the anterior perturbation and the second box indicates the time of the posterior perturbation.

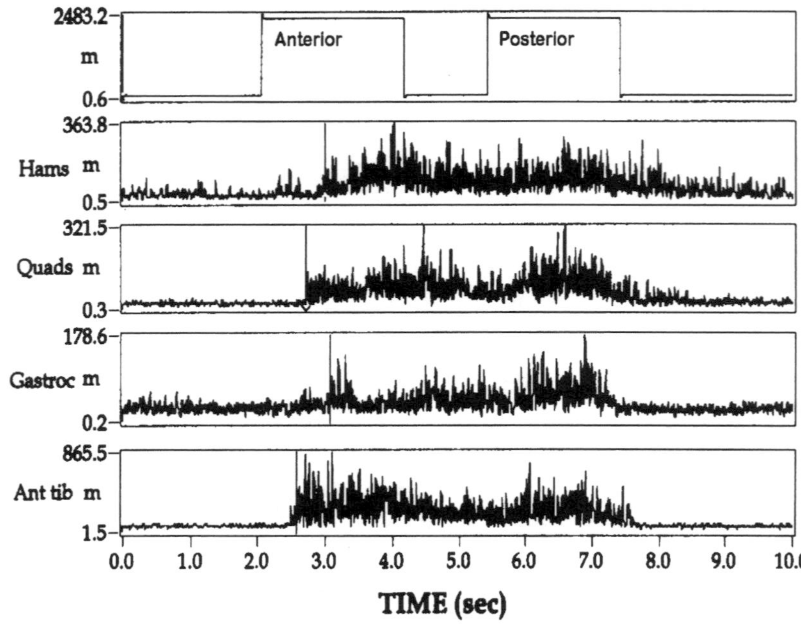

Figure 35.4 EMG response from a coper's ACL-deficient lower extremity during the first trial of anterior and posterior perturbations of the roller board. The ACL-deficient limb is on the roller board and the uninjured limb is on a stationary platform. The first box above the EMG signals indicates the time of the anterior perturbation and the second box indicates the time of the posterior perturbation.

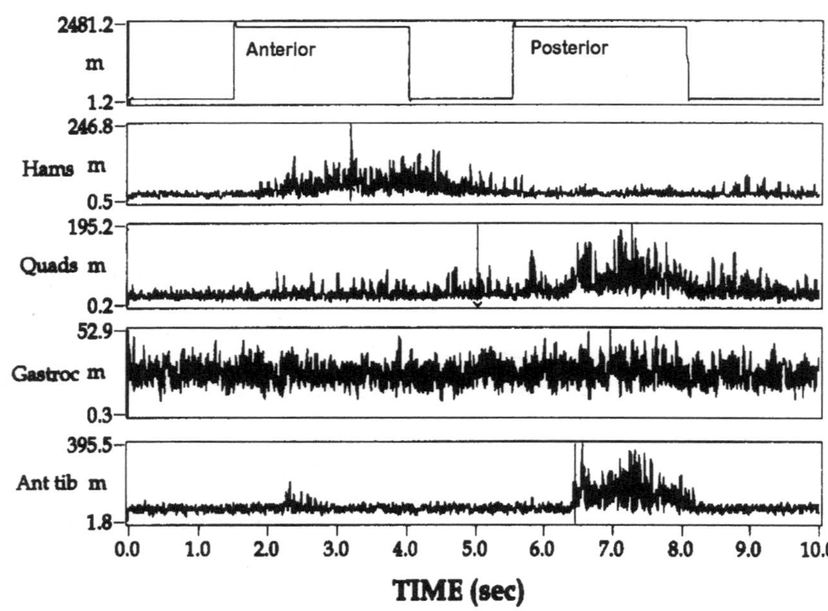

Figure 35.5 EMG response from a coper's ACL-deficient lower extremity during the second trial of anterior and posterior perturbations of the roller board. The ACL-deficient limb is on the roller board and the uninjured limb is on a stationary platform. The first box above the EMG signals indicates the time of the anterior perturbation and the second box indicates the time of the posterior perturbation.

the subject selectively activated the hamstrings, as expected, to resist the perturbation force. A low level activation of the gastrocnemius muscle was also present but did not appear to change with the perturbation. When the direction of the force was reversed, hamstring activity ceased and, as expected, there was a selective activation of the quadriceps femoris and anterior tibialis muscle groups. Low level activation of the gastrocnemius muscle remained throughout this perturbation. These figures demonstrate that the coper

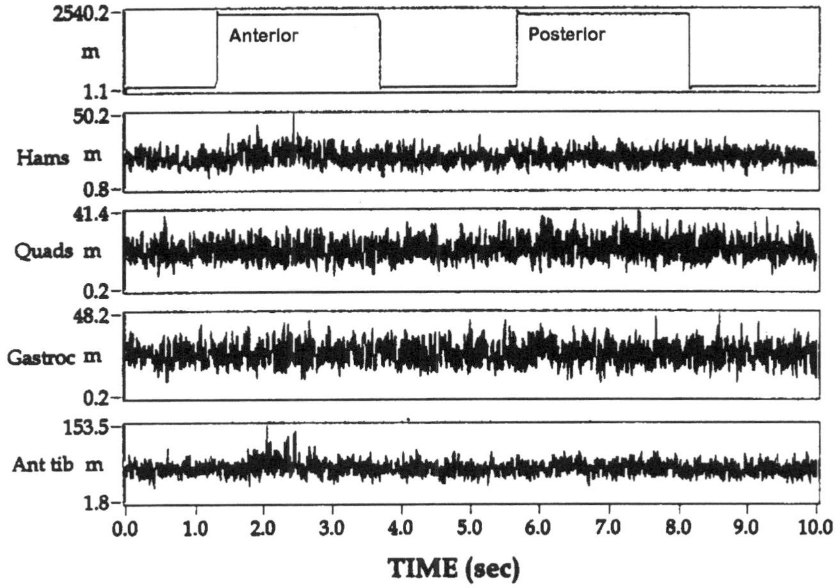

Figure 35.6 EMG response from a noncoper's injured lower extremity during anterior and posterior perturbations of the roller board. The ACL-deficient limb is on the roller board and the uninjured limb is on a stationary platform. The first box above the EMG signals indicates the time of the anterior perturbation and the second box indicates the time of the posterior perturbation.

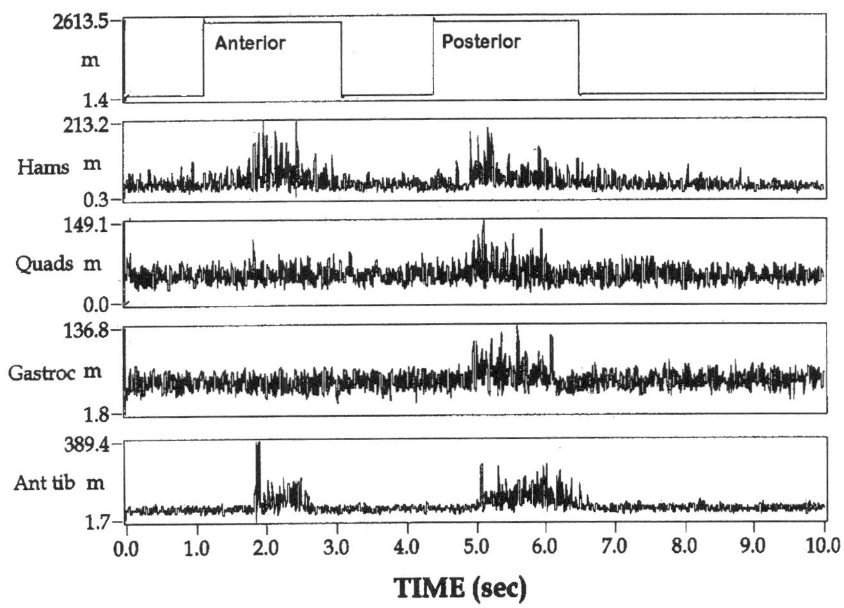

Figure 35.7 EMG response from a trained subject's ACL-deficient limb during anterior and posterior perturbations of the roller board. The ACL-deficient limb is on the roller board and the uninjured limb is on a stationary platform. The first box above the EMG signals indicates the time of the anterior perturbation and the second box indicates the time of the posterior perturbation.

had the ability to change the activation pattern from a general co-contraction to that of selective muscle activation to complete the task.

The EMG recording from the noncoper during the same perturbation technique is shown in figure 35.6. There appears to be a general co-contraction response of all four muscles during the perturbations. When the board was moved anteriorly, there appears to be a slight increase in activation of the hamstrings and anterior tibialis, but this occurs with contractions of the other muscles as well. Reversing direction of the perturbation force did not change the pattern.

The EMG recordings from the subject who underwent 10 sessions of perturbation training is shown in figure 35.7. Testing occurred approximately 1.5 mo after the training program. During the anterior translation of the board there is contraction of all muscle groups; however, the hamstrings and the anterior tibialis seem to dominate. When the board is perturbed posteriorly there is relatively less hamstring activation and relatively more quadriceps femoris activation. The gastrocnemius and anterior tibialis muscles also increased activity with the change in direction of force. This would indicate that the subject selectively changed the muscle activation patterns according to changes in the direction of perturbation force. During the patient's rehabilitation program he exhibited general lower extremity muscle co-contractions, based on visual observations and palpation, in the initial sessions. After 3–4 sessions, muscle activation responses appeared to be more selective. Based on this observation, we believe that the perturbation training assisted the patient to acquire more selected muscle activation patterns, and that he maintained this characteristic, to some degree, over time.

Observations of these three subjects provide some validation of perturbation training techniques as a mechanism to induce selective muscle activation patterns in response to forces that might alter knee stability. Patients who have potential for rehabilitation might be taught to acquire the desired activation patterns and may obtain higher levels of function at faster rates than those who do not receive this training. A randomized clinical trial is currently underway to compare treatment outcome between subjects who are treated with a standard ACL rehabilitation program and those whose standard program is augmented with the perturbation training.

Another method of applying the "force-feedback" theory to enhance the development of appropriate compensatory muscle activation patterns is the use of vertical ground reaction forces as a mode of biofeedback training. There is evidence that vertical ground reaction forces at initial contact during walking and jogging are greater on the involved limb in ACL-deficient patients who are noncopers, compared to those who are copers. The increased ground reaction force in noncopers probably reflects inadequate kinematic and muscle activity patterns to compensate for the loss of the ACL. The increased ground reaction force would also place the involved knee of the noncopers at greater risk for degenerative joint changes (16, 24). It seems that training techniques could be developed that teach subjects to alter ground reaction forces in the involved limb in a manner that results in more adequate compensatory responses in kinematics and muscle activity to improve functional knee stability. One possibility is the use of limb-load monitors that could be inserted in the patient's shoes, which would indicate when the desired load was achieved. Using vertical ground reaction forces as a mode of biofeedback training to enhance compensatory responses merits further investigation.

Summary

Movement abnormalities that occur after ACL rupture may result from an attempt to avoid positions of instability or from an inability to dynamically stabilize the knee. These abnormalities may be learned or may be the direct result of alterations in neural feedback from the injured knee. A clear picture of how those who function well differ from those who do not and how surgery changes the disability could profoundly affect rehabilitation and surgical strategies and decision making. We have attempted to describe how our work, and our reinterpretation of the work of others, can shed some light on the effects of ACL injury on movement and joint stability. There seem to be a variety of potential treatment alternatives for inducing compensatory muscle recruitment patterns in rehabilitation programs for patients with ACL deficiency. The science provides evidence for the way that treatments can be applied to yield muscle recruitment patterns that can dynamically stabilize the knee across a range of activities in the ACL-deficient patient.

Future Directions

Is successful rehabilitation just predicated on picking out those who should not try?

Can screening be successfully implemented in other joints (ankle, shoulder, spine)?

If force-feedback works, can it be used systematically as a treatment for instability? Is there a dose response relationship that can be established?

How long does the training last?

Are there markers of successful training strategies that can be measured?

References

1. Beard, D.J; Dodd, C.A.F.; Trundle, H.R.; Simpson, A.H.R.W. Proprioception enhancement for anterior cruciate ligament deficiency. *J Bone and Joint Surg* [Br] 76B: 654–59, 1994.
2. Berchuck, M.; Andriacchi, T.P.; Bach, B.R. Gait adaptations by patients who have a deficient anterior cruciate ligament. *J Bone and Joint Surg* 72A: 871–77, 1990.
3. Binder-Macleod, S.A. Electromyographic biofeedback to improve voluntary motor control. In: Robinson, A.J., and Snyder-Mackler, L. (Ed), *Clinical electrophysiology: Electrotherapy and electrophysiologic testing,* 2d Ed. Baltimore: Williams & Wilkins. 1995.
4. Botterman, B.R; Hamm, T.M.; Reinking, R.M.; Stuart, D.G. Localization of monosynaptic Ia excitatory postsynaptic potentials in the motor nucleus of the cat biceps femoris muscle. *J Physiol* [London] 338: 355–77, 1983.
5. Buss, D.D.; Min, R.; Skyhar, M.; Galinat, B.; Warren, R.F.; Wickiewicz, T.L. Nonoperative treatment of acute anterior cruciate ligament in a selected group of patients. *Am J Sports Med* 23: 160–65, 1995.
6. Ciccotti, M.G.; Kerlan, R.K.; Perry, J.; Pink, M. An electromyographic analysis of the knee during functional activities: Part II. *Am J Sports Med* 22: 651–58, 1994.
7. Ciccotti, M.G.; Lombardo, S.J.; Nonweiler, B.; Pink, M. Nonoperative treatment of ruptures of the anterior cruciate ligament in middle-aged patients. *J Bone and Joint Surg* 76A: 1315–321, 1994.
8. Czerniecki, J.M.; Lippert F.; Olerud J.E. A biomechanical evaluation of tibiofemoral rotation in anterior cruciate-deficient knees during walking and running. *Am J Sports Med* 16(4): 327–31.
9. Daniel, D.M.; Stone, M.L.; Dobson, B.E.; Fithian, D.C.; Rossman, D.J.; Kaufman, K.R. Fate of the ACL-injured patient. *Am J Sports Med* 22: 632–44, 1994.
10. Delagi, E.F.; Iazzetti, J.; Perotto, A.; Morrison, D. *Anatomic guide for the electromyographer.* Springfield, IL: Charles C Thomas, 1981.
11. DiFabio R.P., et al. Effect of knee joint laxity on long-looped postural reflexes: Evidence for a human capsular-hamstring reflex. *Exp Brain Res* 90: 189–200, 1992.
12. English, A.; Letbetter, W. A histochemical analysis of identified compartments of cat lateral gastrocnemius. *Anat Rec* 204: 123–30, 1994.
13. English, A.; An electromyographic analysis of compartments in cat lateral gastrocnemius muscle during unrestrained locomotion. *J Neurophysiol* 52(1): 114–25, 1989.
14. Grabiner, M.D.; Koh, T.J.; Miller, G.F. Further evidence against a direct automatic neuromotor link between the ACL and hamstrings. *Med Sci Sports Exer* 24: 1075-1079, 1992.
15. Ihara, H.; Nakayama, A. Dynamic joint control training for knee ligament injuries. *Am J Sports Med* 14: 309–15, 1986.
16. Jefferson, R.J.; Collins, J.J.; Whittle, M.W.; Radin, E.L.; O'Connor, J.J. The role of the quadriceps in controlling impulsive forces around heel strike. *J Eng Med* 204: 21–28, 1990.
17. Johansson, H.; Sjolander, P.; Sojka, P. A sensory role for the cruciate ligaments. *Clin Orthop Rel Res* 268: 161–77, 1991.
18. Kadaba, M.P.; Ramakrishnan, H.R.; Gainey, J.C. Gait adaptation in patients with anterior cruciate ligament deficiency. *Trans Orthop Res Soc* 39: 361, 1993.
19. Lawrence, J.H.; Nichols, T.R.; English, A.W. Cat hind limb muscles exert substantial torques outside the sagittal plane. *J Neurophys* 69(1): 282–85, 1993.
20. Limbird, T.J.; Shiavi R.; Frazer, M.; Borra, H. EMG profiles of knee joint musculature during walking: Changes induced by anterior cruciate ligament deficiency. *J Orthop Res* 6: 630–38, 1988.
21. Murray, M.P.; Drought, A.B.; Kory, R.C. Walking patterns of normal men. *J Bone Joint Surg* 46: 335–60, 1964.
22. Nichols, T.R. A biomechanical perspective on spinal mechanisms of coordinated muscular action: An architecture principle. *Acta Anatom* 151: 1–13. 1994.
23. Nichols, T.R.; Steeves, J.D. Resetting of resultant stiffness in ankle flexor and extensor muscles in the decerebrate cat. *Exp Brain Res* 62: 401–10, 1986.
24. Radin, E.; Yang, K.; Kish, V.; O'Conner, J. Relationship between lower-limb dynamics and knee joint pain. *J Orthop Res* 9: 398–405, 1991.
25. Rudolph, K.S.; Eastlack, M.E.; Axe, M.J.; Snyder-Mackler, L. Functional performance after ACL injury: A comparison of patients who compensate well for the injury and those who require operative stabilization. Manuscript submitted for publication.
26. Setton, L.A.; Mow, V.C.; Howell, D.S. Mechanical behavior of articular cartilage in shear is altered by transection of the anterior cruciate ligament. *J Orthop Res* 13: 473–82, 1995.
27. Shiavi, R.; Zhang, L.; Limbird, T.; Edmonstone, M.A. Pattern analysis of electromyographic linear envelopes exhibited by subjects with

uninjured and injured knees during free and fast speed walking. *J Orthop Res* 10: 226–36, 1992.
28. Sinkjaer T.; Arendt-Nielsen, L. Knee stability and muscle coordination in patients with anterior cruciate ligament injuries: An electromyographic approach. *J Electromyog Kinesiol* 1(3): 209–17, 1991.
29. Solomonow, M.; Baratta, R.; Zhou, B.H.; Shoji, H.; Bose, W.; Beck, C.; D'Ambrosia, R. The synergistic action of the anterior cruciate ligament and thigh muscles in maintaining joint stability. *Am J Sports Med* 15: 207–13, 1987.
30. Solomonow, M.; Baratta, R.; D'Ambrosia, R. The role of the hamstrings in the rehabilitation of the anterior cruciate ligament-deficient knee in athletes. *Sports Med* 7: 42–48, 1989.
31. Strickland, E.M.; Fares, M.; Krebs, D.E.; Riley, P.O.; Givens-Heiss, D.L.; Hodge, W.A.; Mann, R.W. In vivo acetabular contact pressures during rehabilitation. Part I: Acute phase. *Phys Ther* 72: 691–99, 1992.
32. Vereijkin, B.; van Emmerik, R.E.A.; Whiting, H.T.A.; Newell, K.M. Freezing degrees of freedom in skill acquisition. *J Motor Behav* 24: 133–42, 1992.
33. Wolf, S.L.; Binder-Macleod, S.A. Use of the Krusen limb-load monitor to quantify temporal and loading measurements of gait. *Phys Ther* 62: 976–83, 1982.

CHAPTER 36

Restoration of Proprioception and Neuromuscular Control of the Unstable Shoulder

Scott M. Lephart, PhD, ATC
Timothy J. Henry, PhD, ATC

Introduction

The kinetic complexity of the shoulder requires an intricate synergy between the static and dynamic structures in order to maintain functional stability. (8, 12, 14, 15, 20, 28–30, 32) This requires a balance of muscular strength, endurance, and flexibility, coordinated through neuromuscular control. Functional stability of the shoulder joint is the result of proper scapular stabilization, glenohumeral stabilization, and humeral control, all mediated by neuromuscular controlling mechanisms. If any of these factors are compromised, functional instability results, and injuries occur. (2, 4, 5, 7, 14, 15, 20, 27, 29, 30)

The role of the static and dynamic mechanisms have been very well documented. (5, 6, 10, 12, 15, 20, 35–37) The static mechanism consists of the joint capsule, labrum, and ligaments, each serving both a mechanical and sensory role. The dynamic mechanism is provided by the musculature and serves a stabilizing role as well as a functional role. Interruption of any of these mechanisms contributes to functional instability in the athlete. Thus, the integration of each of these restraining and functional mechanisms is imperative in order to maintain a functionally stable shoulder joint.

The static structures guide joint kinematics by providing mechanical restraint to abnormal joint motion. (5, 34) This mechanical role has been the primary concern with regard to injury to these structures. (5) In addition to this mechanical role, Baxendale and associates (3) and Kennedy and coworkers (19) observed that these articular structures provide important neurological feedback that directly mediates muscular reflex stabilization about the joint. Following injury to the articular ligaments, neuromuscular joint stabilization has been shown to be inhibited. This is due to the disruption of articular mechanoreceptors, resulting in partial deafferentation of the joint. The combination of compromised mechanical restraint and the inhibited neuromuscular stabilization capabilities renders the shoulder unstable and leads to progressive decline of the joint. (5, 21–23)

The role of the dynamic mechanism (muscle) is also twofold and includes humeral control and stabilization. Humeral control encompasses humeral acceleration and deceleration. The stabilizing role of the musculature occurs through the integration of force couples that act upon the shoulder. A force couple involves two or more muscles contracting simultaneously, producing a resultant force that promotes stability within that joint. (16) In the shoulder the dynamic force couples serve to increase joint compression, which in turn provides for maximum congruency of the articulating surfaces. The two primary glenohumeral force couples include the deltoid superiorly, opposed by the infraspinatus and teres minor inferiorly, while the subscapularis anteriorly is opposed by the infraspinatus and teres minor posteriorly. (12, 16) The serratus anterior and upper trapezius act in unison to stabilize the scapula and provide a stable base for the glenohumeral articulation.

Without the proper integration of both these dynamic and static mechanisms, aberrations in normal shoulder function and kinematics occur. The combination of mechanical instability and decreased neuromuscular control of the joint results in an insidious pattern of functional shoulder instability. (5, 21–23) Restoration of the neuromuscular mechanisms responsible for functional stability is necessary in order to properly return an athlete with shoulder instability to his or her desired activity.

Effects of Injury on Proprioception and Neuromuscular Control of the Shoulder

Functional instability that occurs following injury to the capsuloligamentous structures is in part the result of deafferentation. The excessive joint laxity associated with capsuloligamentous injury and the resulting microtrauma damage to the neural receptors within this structure leads to deafferentation. Deafferentation results in interruption of the afferent signal altering transmission to the CNS. Even partial deafferentation can result in neuromuscular deficits. These neuromuscular deficits impair reflexive muscular stabilization, predisposing the shoulder to episodes of functional instability. In the shoulder, these neuromuscular deficits have been demonstrated to result in diminished joint position sense, kinesthetic awareness, and abnormal humeral and scapular muscular firing patterns. (5, 20)

Smith and Brunoli (30) were among the first to investigate the effect of capsuloligamentous injury on proprioception in the shoulder. They reported that patients with unilateral, recurrent, traumatic anterior shoulder instability demonstrated proprioceptive sensory deficits. Lephart and coworkers[23] performed the first study comparing shoulder proprioception in groups of individuals with normal, unstable, and surgically repaired shoulders. The results revealed significant proprioceptive deficits in patients who have had chronic, traumatic anterior shoulder instability and show that surgical stabilization of such a shoulder normalizes proprioceptive sensibility. These two studies are among the few studies that have investigated the effect of injury on proprioception.

While Smith and Brunoli (32) and Lephart and coworkers (23) identified afferent proprioceptive deficits, the effect of injury on neuromuscular control has been investigated through the use of electromyography to assess resulting aberrations in muscular firing patterns. Specifically, latency in the muscle firing patterns has been identified. The latency is a measure of the motor response to sensory feedback as an unconscious muscular reflex to abnormal joint stress. Electromyographic studies have suggested that a complex, coordinated synergistic function of the shoulder musculature is required for normal function of the shoulder.

Bradley and Tibone (8) revealed that swimmers with painful shoulders demonstrate significant differences in the amplitude levels in 7 of 12 muscles examined. Glousmann and coworkers (13) performed an EMG analysis of the throwing shoulder with glenohumeral instability and revealed firing pattern abnormalities in these individuals. Glousmann and coworkers demonstrated a marked decrease in the activity of the pectoralis major, subscapularis, latissimus dorsi, and serratus anterior during the late cocking phase, during which the upper extremity is in maximum external rotation. Increased activity was described for the biceps and the supraspinatus, suggesting that these muscles may help to compensate for the laxity associated with anterior glenohumeral instability.

Each of the previous findings supports the hypothesis by Lephart and Henry (20) and others, which suggests the following injury paradigm. This paradigm (see figure 36.1) suggests that injury to the static structures ultimately affects both afferent and efferent responses to joint loads, resulting in an insidious pattern of shoulder instability.

Restoration of Functional Stability

Following injury to the shoulder, the reestablishment of functional stability is paramount. Traditional rehabilitation programs for the unstable shoulder have focused on voluntarily activated strengthening exercises for the prime movers. These types of rehabilitation programs described by Townsend and coworkers (33) and Moseley and associates (26) provide "core strengthening" exercises for both the scapular and humeral muscles. The exercises described in these studies have provided the basis for strengthening of the shoulder musculature and form the core of traditional rehabilitation programs for the unstable shoulder.

However, considering the neuromuscular mechanisms providing for dynamic stabilization and functional stability of the shoulder joint, it would appear that these traditional rehabilitation programs

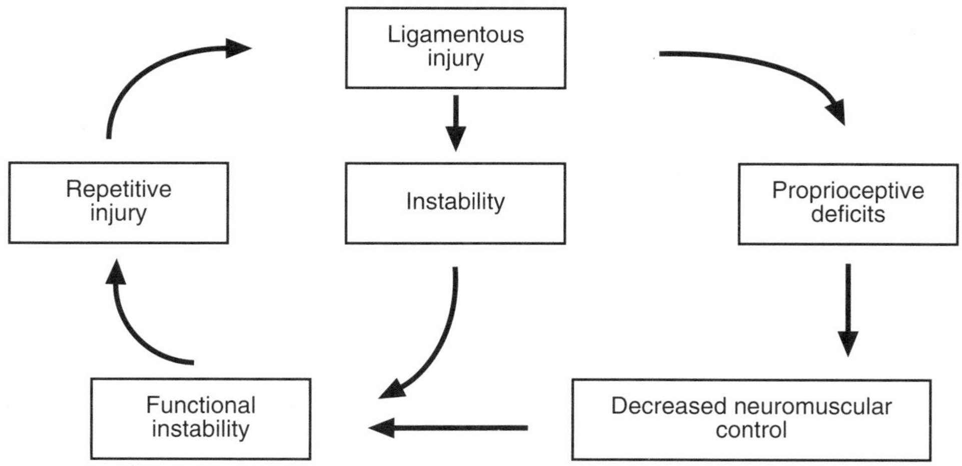

Figure 36.1 Functional instability paradigm.

do not specifically address the neuromuscular deficits contributing to shoulder instability and result in incomplete rehabilitation of the unstable shoulder. Functional stability of the shoulder is dependent upon coactivation of the musculature surrounding the joint as well as reactive neuromuscular characteristics. In order to eliminate the neurosensory deficits and restore dynamic stabilization to the unstable shoulder, exercises that stimulate the neuromuscular mechanisms are necessary.

Lephart and Henry (20) have proposed a functional classification system to serve as a guide for restoring proprioceptive deficits and reestablishing neuromuscular control. This system describes four elements that are necessary in order to restore functional stability. Each of these four elements addresses specific objectives in restoring proprioception and neuromuscular control and includes commonly described rehabilitation activities. The system is designed specifically to integrate all subsystems of movement and all levels of motor control. The subsystems that should be included are the peripheral somatosensory, the visual, and the vestibular. The three levels of motor control to be included are the spinal reflex, cognitive programming, and the brain stem.

At the spinal level, proprioception and neuromuscular control function unconsciously with reflexes subserving movement patterns that are received from the descending pathways of the higher centers. This provides for reflex stabilization of the muscles acting on the joint, thus maintaining a protected stiffness during activity. (17) This integration of input from the receptors of the joint and muscles along with the descending pathways converge at the first order neurons within the interneuronal pool. The efferent response modulates muscle function.

The second level of motor control occurs at the brain stem where joint afference converges with the second order neurons and is subsequently relayed to the motor cortex or cerebellum for processing. The afferent input at this level emanates from the joint and muscle receptors and the vestibular centers in the ears and the eyes. This information is used to maintain balance and posture of the body.

The third level of motor control includes the highest level of CNS function, the motor cortex. Here conscious awareness of joint motion and position contribute to proprioception and neuromuscular control. The higher centers (motor cortex, cerebellum, and basal ganglia) initiate and program motor commands for voluntary movements. Movement patterns that are repetitive in nature are stored as central commands and can be performed without continuous reference to consciousness. This cognitive function is a training or learning effect in response to motor programming. The higher centers are linked to the lower motor neurons via the descending pathways (corticospinal, pyramidal, and extrapyramidal) where efferent output will inhibit or facilitate motor activity. (5, 20)

Each of these levels of motor control needs to be specifically addressed during rehabilitation for the upper extremity. At the spinal level, activities that induce reflex joint stabilization should be included. These activities should include sudden alterations in joint positioning that require reflex muscular stabilization. These types of activities stimulate both articular and muscular mechanoreceptors for reflex stabilization.

Cognitive appreciation of joint position should also be addressed in the rehabilitation program. These activities are initiated at the cognitive level and include programming motor commands for voluntary movement. The repetition of movements will initiate the conversion of conscious programming to unconscious programming. This information is then stored as central commands and can be performed without conscious reference. (20)

In order to fulfill the objective of stimulating all subsystems of movement and all levels of motor control four elements have been created. Each of these elements addresses specific objectives and utilizes common rehabilitation activities. Clinicians such as Borsa and coworkers, (5) Wilk and Arrigo, (37) Litchfield and coworkers, (24) and others have described innovative rehabilitation activities in order to rehabilitate the unstable shoulder. These techniques have been categorized as addressing one or more of the four elements according to the objective they are fulfilling and the mechanism by which they function. The four elements in the Functional Classification System include dynamic stabilization, joint position sensibility, reactive neuromuscular control, and functional motor patterns.

The first element that needs to be addressed in an athlete with an unstable shoulder is dynamic stabilization. The objective of dynamic stabilization is to promote the coactivation of the force couples about the shoulder in order to center the head of the humerus on the glenoid. The glenohumeral force couples, the deltoid opposed by the infraspinatus and teres minor, and the subscapularis opposed by the infraspinatus and teres minor, serve not only to center the head of the humerus but also to compress the head of the humerus into the glenoid. Coactivation of the muscular force couples is stimulated by compression of the head of the humerus within the glenoid. The coactivation of the force couples further compresses the head of the humerus into the glenoid surface, providing for maximum congruency of the articulating joint surfaces. In addition to the glenohumeral force couples, the musculature that provides a stable scapulothoracic articulation must be addressed. Without the stable base of support provided by the scapula, glenohumeral stability is not plausible. Activities in this category need to include axial loading, resulting in joint compression, and activation of the force couples.

The dynamic stabilization is the first element that needs to be restored during shoulder rehabilitation. Due to the lack of inherent bony stability provided in the glenohumeral joint, muscular stabilization through the activation of the force couples is vital. Without dynamic stabilization, progression to more reactive and functional activities is not plausible.

The second element is joint position sensibility. The objective is to restore joint position awareness in the unstable shoulder. This element should emphasize both conscious and unconscious pathways. The activities in this category enhance the muscles' ability to provide joint stability and refine movement patterns. Joint position awareness is especially important in the upper extremity for the purpose of placing the hand in the overhead position of abduction and external rotation. Overhead throwing athletes require a great deal of precision in their movement patterns, which is mediated by proprioceptive acuity. This element, like the dynamic stabilization, needs to be addressed early in the rehabilitation program. These types of activities may begin very early without compromising the injured structures in the shoulder.

The third element that needs to be addressed to reestablish proprioception and neuromuscular control is reactive neuromuscular characteristics. The objective is to initiate reflex muscular stabilization. This reflexive muscular splinting or stabilization is induced by sudden alterations in joint position. These sudden alterations trigger the articular and muscular mechanoreceptors, which initiate the muscle splinting system. These types of reflex stabilization exercises provide a mechanism for developing dynamic joint stability. Activities in this category may be performed on some type of unstable platform or surface that will provide for sudden, unpredictable changes in the position and load upon the joint. With specific regard to the upper extremity, stretch-shortening or plyometric type activity may also be placed within this category. This type of activity involves joint loading in somewhat extreme positions. Plyometric activity also emphasizes eccentric muscle activity. Eccentric muscular activity is vital to maintaining stability and normal kinematics in the overhead throwing athlete. Eccentric activity of the shoulder musculature is necessary in order to decelerate the arm through the throwing motion and prevent injury. Eccentric loading of the rotator cuff places high stress on the musculature and may reduce injury by permitting higher levels of dynamic stability. Before commencing these reactive type activities, restoration of dynamic stabilization by the muscular force couples is necessary.

The fourth element that needs to be addressed is functional motor patterns. As with any type of rehabilitation program, functional specificity is vital. The objective of any rehabilitation program is to return the athlete to his or her desired level of sport activity. With specific regard to the overhead throwing athlete, a functional progression to the actual throwing activity is very important. Therefore, the objective of this category is to restore the functional motor patterns that the athlete will encounter during actual sport participation. The specificity of training principle is not as clearly defined in the upper extremity as it is in the lower extremity. In the lower extremity the majority of all functional activity is performed in a closed kinetic chain or weight-bearing position. This is not the case in the upper extremity. The functional positioning and resultant joint loading that occurs in upper extremity activity varies greatly and does not lend itself to traditional kinetic chain terms. The positioning and loading for a baseball pitcher is totally different from a gymnast or a football lineman. A baseball pitcher would certainly not be performing with the upper extremity in a weight-bearing position, but he does have a load on the distal extremity with the weight of the baseball. Likewise, a football lineman may not perform with the upper extremity in a weight-bearing position but he may have a considerable load on the upper extremity with the hands being fixed on another player. Therefore it is somewhat difficult and inappropriate to concentrate upper extremity functional activities on either traditional closed or open kinetic chain exercises.

The authors believe that an alternative classification system would be the most appropriate for classifying upper extremity rehabilitation activities. This classification utilizes the direction of the force, the amount of loading, the resultant muscle action, and the direction of the load. This would include activities such as a push-up, which would provide a fixed boundary, with a considerable axial load being applied to the shoulder resulting in coactivation of the force couples surrounding the joint. This type of classification appears to be more appropriate for upper extremity activity, considering the debate over traditional kinetic chain terms.

As a result of the controversy surrounding upper extremity rehabilitation, the functional phase or element should emphasize rehabilitating the shoulder in functional planes of motion. The type of activity that the athlete with the unstable shoulder will be partaking in should be considered and the functional motor patterns should be tailored to this. In addition, muscular control of the arm must be attained in the deceleration phase of throwing. Many overhead injuries occur during eccentric loading of the muscle, and this must be addressed during the functional aspect of the program. (24)

Shoulder Proprioception and Neuromuscular Control Rehabilitation Techniques

Joint position sensibility exercises focus on restoring both kinesthesia and joint position sense. This can be accomplished through joint repositioning types of exercises. These exercises may be performed on

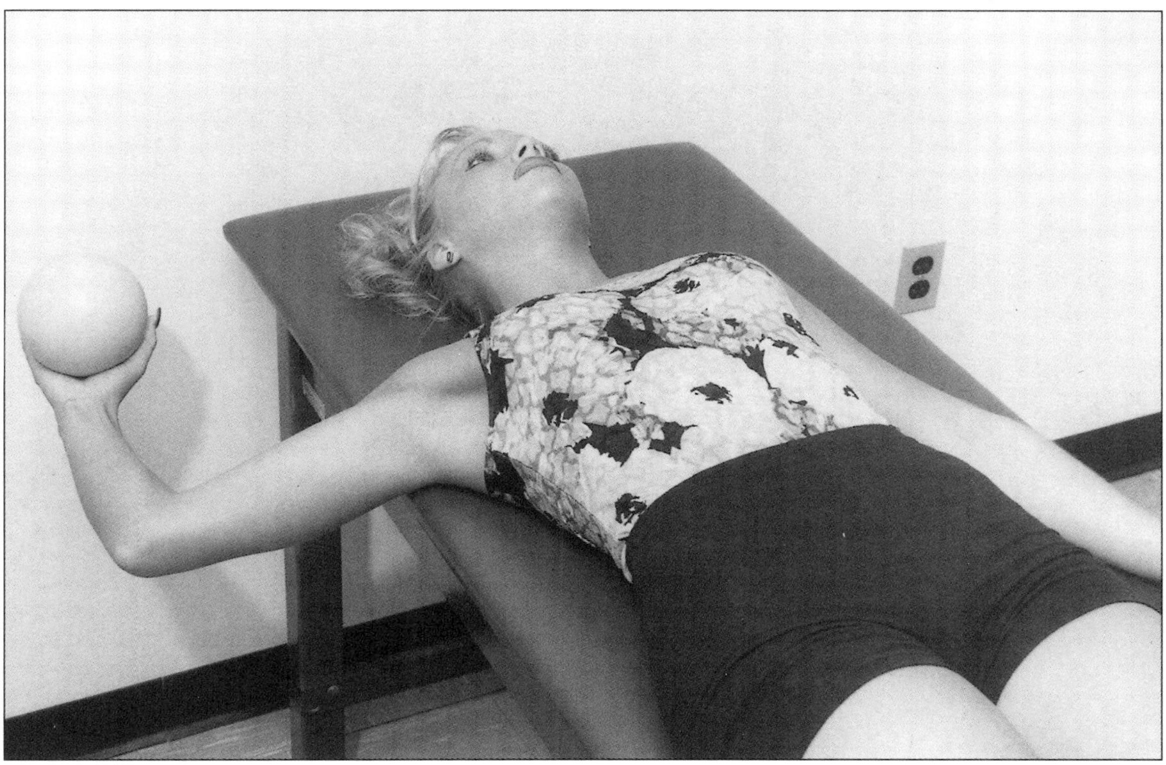

Figure 36.2 Joint position sensibility technique.

an isokinetic dynamometer or with devices such as a shoulder multiaxial machine or with a simple goniometer. Both active and passive repositioning and reproduction of angles should be included. In order to progress, the eyes should be closed in order to eliminate any visual cues during the exercise. These types of joint repositioning exercises should emphasize functional positioning and especially overhead hand placement for the throwing athlete. A light dumbbell or plyoball may be added to the hand in order to apply a load while performing the exercise (see figure 36.2). The joint position sensibility exercises can begin very early in the rehabilitation program and continue throughout the entire process.

Techniques employed for the restoration of *dynamic stabilization* are designed to promote force couple coactivation. Recent research by the authors investigating these dynamic stabilizing activities revealed that exercises that provide a significant axial load to the shoulder are necessary in order to evoke the muscular coactivation. These types of activities should include exercises that place the upper extremity in a weight-bearing position. The exercises can include activities such as push-ups and exercises on a slide board (see figure 36.3). These types of activities may begin with the athlete in the quadruped position, on hands and knees, and progress to the traditional push-up position, which significantly increases the load being placed upon the shoulder. These activities may be progressed by adding boxes or different levels for the push-ups and performing different movement activities on the slide board or similar surface. The important concept for this category is the weight-bearing position, which provides an axial load to the shoulder, initiating the force couple coactivation.

The third element required for functional stability of the shoulder is *reactive neuromuscular control.* Techniques designed to restore these characteristics attempt to stimulate reflex muscular stabilization. This is initiated by activities that provide sudden alterations in joint position and place the shoulder in vulnerable positions. These reactive types of activities should commence after dynamic stabilization has been restored. In order to induce the alteration in joint position, unstable surfaces are used. Activities that place the upper extremity in a quadruped or push-up position on an unstable platform

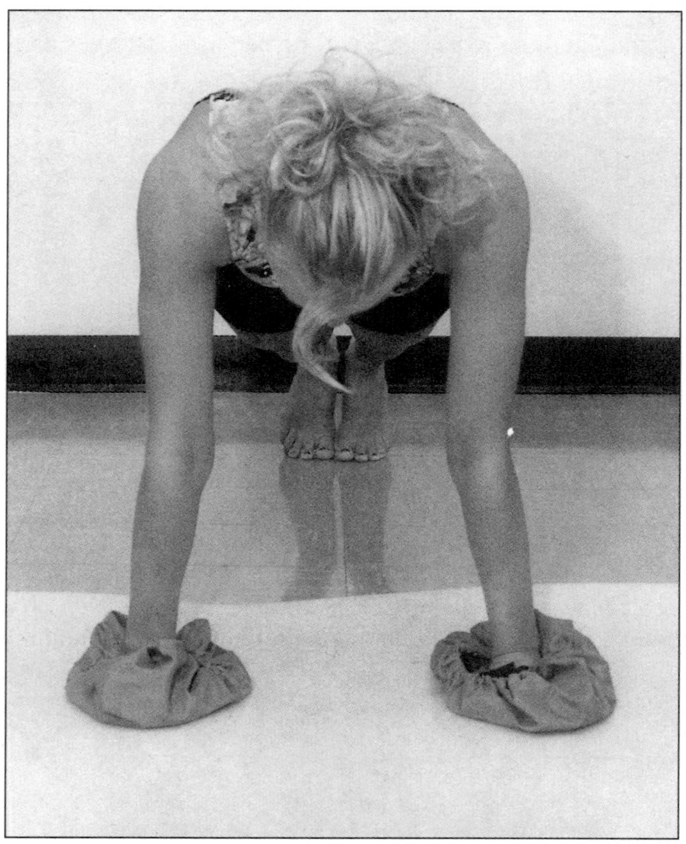

Figure 36.3 Dynamic stabilization techniques.

such as the BAPS board or instrumented stability platform are ideal for this category. An exercise such as performing a push-up on a plyoball will also necessitate the athlete reflexively responding to the alterations in shoulder position (see figure 36.4). Plyometric exercises with lightweight plyoballs should also be included. Activities that involve catching the plyoball, eccentrically decelerating, and then concentrically accelerating in order to throw should be included. This requires the athlete to stabilize and eccentrically stabilize in order to prevent injury to the shoulder. These can be performed with a pitchback or with a partner. This type of activity can begin with the athlete lying supine on the floor in order to stabilize the trunk and progress to the actual throwing position. It is important to consider that these types of reactive activities do impart a great deal of stress on the shoulder and should follow a distinct progression as well as consultation with the athlete during these activities.

The last element is *functional motor control.* The objective of techniques for restoration of functional motor control is to reaccommodate the athlete to the patterns and stresses they will encounter during actual sport participation. This category follows the specificity of training principle. The plyometric activity mentioned in the reactive category can also be progressed into this functional category as the athlete moves to more functional positioning and functional speeds (see figure 36.5). Many current isokinetic dynamometers have attachments that allow for exercise in a functional diagonal pattern. This allows the clinician to expose the athlete to a functional pattern with a variety of angular velocities, as well as providing the clinician with some objective measure of the athlete's progress. Exercises performed with rubber tubing can also be utilized in this category. The rubber tubing can be used through the throwing motion and other patterns that occur for different types of athletes. Proprioceptive neuromuscular facilitation exercise that occurs in functional patterns may also be useful. Finally, a progression to the actual overhead throwing activity is necessary for the throwing athlete. This begins with long, low-intensity tossing and progresses to short, high-intensity throws. This functional progression should be closely monitored, and close consultation with the athlete as to the response to the activities is necessary. It is also important that the athlete is sufficiently stressed during this phase of the rehabilitation program to ensure that when she returns to the actual sport participation she is confident in her ability to withstand the rigors of the activity and that she does not encounter anything more stressful than what she endured during the rehabilitation program. This fourth element provides the clinician and the athlete with the opportunity to assess the athlete's readiness to return and her response to the functional activity.

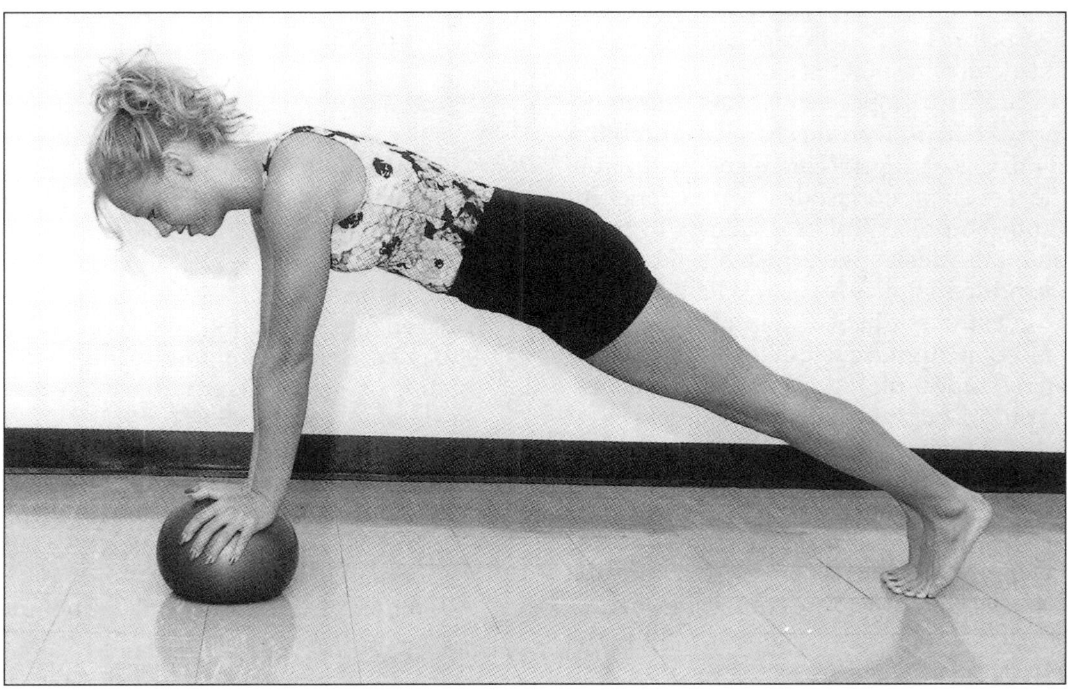

Figure 36.4 Reactive neuromuscular control techniques.

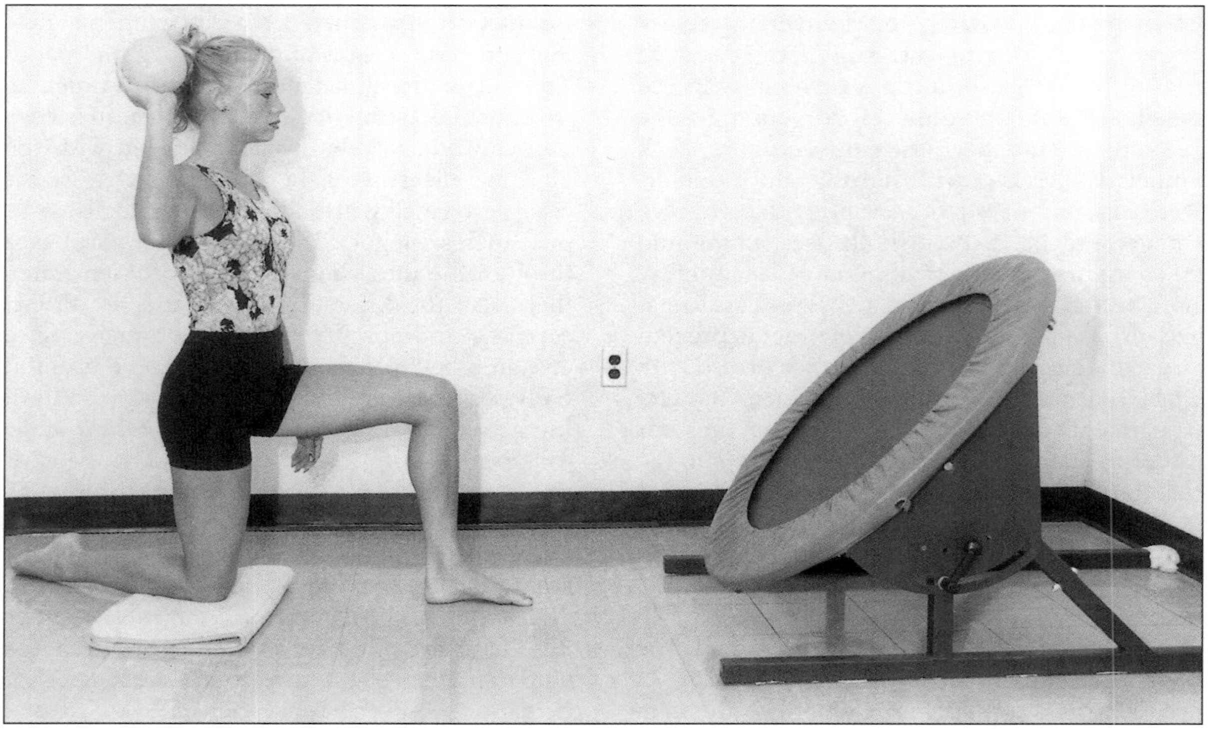

Figure 36.5 Functional motor control techniques.

Summary

Rehabilitation of the unstable shoulder must be performed with regard to the complex kinematics and the delicate integration between the static and dynamic structures of the shoulder. Injury to the articular structures results not only in mechanical instability but also in proprioception and neuromuscular control deficits. The mechanical instability coupled with these proprioceptive and neuromuscular deficits results in episodes of functional instability and the possibility of re-injury. To properly rehabilitate athletes with unstable shoulders, we need to address not only the mechanical instability and the strength deficits, but also the proprioceptive and neuromuscular deficits.

The rehabilitation plan outlined here for reestablishing proprioception and neuromuscular control provides a simple baseline for designing the rehabilitation program. The four elements described—dynamic stabilization, joint position sensibility, reactive neuromuscular characteristics, and functional motor patterns—each meet a specific objective in restoring proprioception and neuromuscular control. These four elements allow the clinician to perform specific exercises within each category in order to stimulate all subsystems of movement and all levels of motor control. Considering the objectives of each element and performing these types of activities ensures complete and successful rehabilitation for the athlete with an unstable shoulder.

References

1. Andrews JR, Gidamel RH: Shoulder arthroscopy in the throwing athlete: Perspective and prognosis. *Arthroscopy* 6: 656–61, 1987.
2. Barrack RL, Skinner HB: The sensory function of knee ligaments. In *Knee ligaments: Structure, function, and injury*, D. Daniel (ed.). New York: Raven Press, 95–114, 1990.
3. Baxendale RA, Ferrell WR, Wood L: Responses of quadriceps motor units to mechanical stimulation of knee joint receptors in the decerebrate cat. *Brain Res* 453: 150–56, 1988.
4. Beard DJ, Kyberd PJ, Fergusson CM, Dodd CA: Proprioception after rupture of the anterior cruciate ligament. *J Bone Joint Surg* 75B: 311–15, 1993.
5. Borsa PA, Lephart SM, Kocher MS, Lephart SM: Functional assessment and rehabilitation of shoulder proprioception for glenohumeral instability. *J Sport Rehab* 3: 84–104, 1994.
6. Bost FC, Inman VT: The pathological changes in recurrent dislocation of the shoulder. *J Bone Joint Surg* 24A: 595, 1942.

7. Bowen MK, Derg XH, Warner JJP, Warren RF: The effect of joint compression on stability of the glenohumeral joint. *Trans Orthop Res Soc* 17: 289, 1992.
8. Bradley JP, Tibone JE: Electromyographic analysis of muscle action about the shoulder. *Clin Sports Med* 10: 789–805, 1991.
9. Cain PR, Mutschler TA, Fu FH, et al: Anterior stability of the glenohumeral joint: A dynamic model. *Am J Sports Med* 15: 144–48, 1987.
10. Dempster WT: Mechanisms of shoulder movement. *Arch Phys Med Rehab* 46: 49–70, 1965.
11. Dickoff-Hoffman S: Functional subluxation of the glenohumeral joint in a college pitcher. *Isokin Exerc Sci* 3: 162–65, 1991.
12. Dillman CJ: Proper mechanics of pitching. *Sports Med Update* 5: 15–18, 1990.
13. Glousmann R, Jobe FW, Tibone J, et al: Dynamic electromyographic analysis of the throwing shoulder with glenohumeral instability. *J Bone Joint Surg* 70: 220–26, 1988.
14. Harryman DT, Sidles JA, Clark JM, et al: Translation of the humeral head on the glenoid with passive glenohumeral motion. *J Bone Joint Surg* 72: 1334–343, 1990.
15. Hawkins RJ, Schutte JP, Huckell GJ: The assessment of glenohumeral translation using manual and fluoroscopic techniques. *Orthop Trans* 12: 727–29, 1988.
16. Inman VT, Saunders JR, Abbott JC: Observations on the function of the shoulder joint. *J Bone Joint Surg* 26: 1–30, 1944.
17. Johansson H, Sjolander P, Sojka P: A sensory role for the cruciate ligaments. *Clin Orthop* 268: 161–78, 1991.
18. Kalund S, Sinkjaer T, Arendt-Nielsen L, Simonsen O: Altered timing of hamstring muscle action in anterior cruciate deficient patients. *Am J Sports Med* 18: 245–48, 1990.
19. Kennedy JC, Alexander IJ, Hayes KC: Nerve supply of the human knee and its functional importance. *Am J Sports Med* 10: 329–35, 1982.
20. Lephart SM, Henry TJ: The physiological basis for open and closed kinetic chain rehabilitation for the upper extremity. *J Sport Rehab* 5: 71–87, 1996.
21. Lephart SM, Kocher MS, Fu FH, Borsa PA, Harner CD: Proprioception following ACL reconstruction. *J Sport Rehab* 1: 188–96, 1992.
22. Lephart SM, Kocher MS: The role of exercise in the prevention of shoulder disorders. In *The shoulder: A balance of mobility and stability,* FA Matsen, FH Fu, RJ Hawkins (eds). Rosement, IL: American Academy of Orthopaedic Surgeons, 597–620, 1993.
23. Lephart SM, Warner JJP, Borsa PA, Fu FH: Proprioception in the shoulder of healthy, unstable, and surgically repaired shoulder. *J Shoulder Elbow Surg* 3: 371–81, 1994.
24. Litchfield R, Hawkins R, Dillman CJ, Atkins J, Hagerman G: Rehabilitation for the overhead athlete. *JOSPT* 18: 433–41, 1993.
25. McLaughlin HL: Recurrent anterior dislocation of the shoulder: Morbid anatomy. *Am J Surg* 99: 628–32, 1960.
26. Moseley JB, Jobe FW, Pink M, Perry J, Tibone J: EMG analysis of the scapular muscles during a shoulder rehabilitation program. *Am J Sports Med* 20: 128–34, 1992.
27. O'Brien SJ, Neves MC, Arnoczky SP, et al: The anatomy and histology of the inferior glenohumeral ligament complex of the shoulder. *Am J Sports Med* 18: 449–56, 1990.
28. Schwartz RE, O'Brien SJ, Warren RF: Capsular restraints to anterior-posterior motion of the abducted shoulder; a biomechanical study. *Orthop Trans* 12: 727, 1988.
29. Simonet WT, Cofield RH: Prognosis of anterior shoulder dislocation. *Am J Sports Med* 12: 19–24, 1984.
30. Smith RL, Brunolli J: Shoulder kinesthesia after anterior glenohumeral dislocation. *Phys Ther* 69: 106–12, 1989.
31. Solomonow M, Baratta R, Zhou B, et al: The synergistic action of the anterior cruciate ligament and thigh muscles in maintaining joint stability. *Am J Sports Med* 15(3): 207–13, 1987.
32. Townley CO: The capsular mechanisms in recurrent dislocation of the shoulder. *J Bone Joint Surg* 32A: 370–80, 1950.
33. Townsend H, Jobe FW, Pink M, Perry J: Electromyographic analysis of 72 glenohumeral muscles during a baseball rehabilitation program. *Am J Sports Med* 19: 264–72, 1991.
34. Turkel J, Panio JL, Marshall, Girgis FG: Stabilizing mechanisms preventing anterior dislocation of the glenohumeral joint. *J Bone Joint Surg* 63A: 1028–217, 1981.
35. Warner JJP, Deng XH, Warren RF, Torzilli PA: Static capsuloligamentous restraints to superior-inferior translation of the glenohumeral joint. *Am J Sports Med* 20: 675–85, 1992.
36. Warren RF, Kornblatt IB, Marchand R: Static factors affecting posterior shoulder instability. *Orthop Trans* 8: 1–89, 1984.
37. Wilk KE, Arrigo C: Current concepts in the rehabilitation of the athletic shoulder. *JOSPT* 18: 365–78, 1993.

CHAPTER 37

Restoration of Functional Motor Patterns and Functional Testing in the Throwing Athlete

Kevin E. Wilk, PT

Introduction

The overhead throwing motion is a highly skilled movement; however, it is also extremely stressful on the shoulder joint complex. The overhead throwing athlete places extraordinary demands on the shoulder joint complex. These excessively high stresses are applied to the shoulder joint because of the unnatural movements frequently performed by the overhead thrower. The overhead thrower's shoulder must be excessively lax; this is to allow the excessive external rotation required to throw a baseball. Thus, the thrower's shoulder must be "loose enough to throw" but still stable enough to prevent humeral head subluxation. Therefore, the thrower's shoulder is in delicate balance between mobility and functional stability.

Throwing creates repetitive microtraumatic stresses to the shoulder joint. Due to the repetitive nature of the activity, the thrower pushes the shoulder joint to its physiological limits. Frequently, alterations in mechanics, muscular fatigue, or muscular imbalances may lead to subsequent injury. Often injury occurs to the glenohumeral ligaments, glenoid labrum, or to the rotator cuff muscles. To decrease the probability of injury, the thrower should focus on a training program that balances functional stability and mobility of the shoulder and emphasizes the need for dynamic functional stabilization.

The thrower's shoulder requires the surrounding musculature to enhance dynamic functional stability. The surrounding musculature works synergistically with the glenohumeral joint capsule to provide functional stability. The overhead throwing motion places tremendous demands on the shoulder complex musculature to produce functional dynamic stability. The shoulder musculature must function and react while the arm and shoulder joint are moving at incredibly high angular velocities. Furthermore, the shoulder muscles must function effectively throughout the entire range of motion, especially at the end ranges and at tremendously fast speeds.

The Overhead Throw

Overhead throwing is a highly skilled, extremely stressful and violent activity that requires flexibility, strength, power, endurance, coordination, and timing. The throwing action requires precisely coordinated movement and a synchronized muscular firing pattern, all of which occur at an angular velocity faster than any other upper extremity sport movement. The overhead throw (pitching) can be divided into five distinct phases (see figure 37.1). During the throw, kinetic energy is generated from the legs and trunk and is transferred upward to the shoulder and arm (see figure 37.2). At ball release and follow-through, the generated energy is trans-

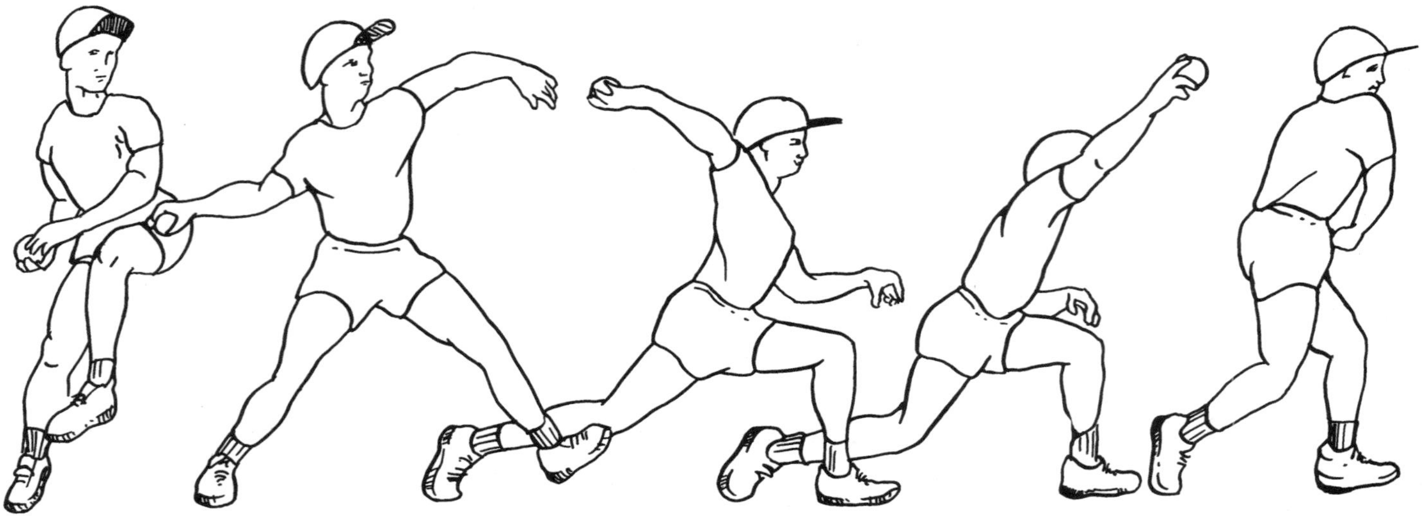

Figure 37.1 The five phases of the pitching motion.

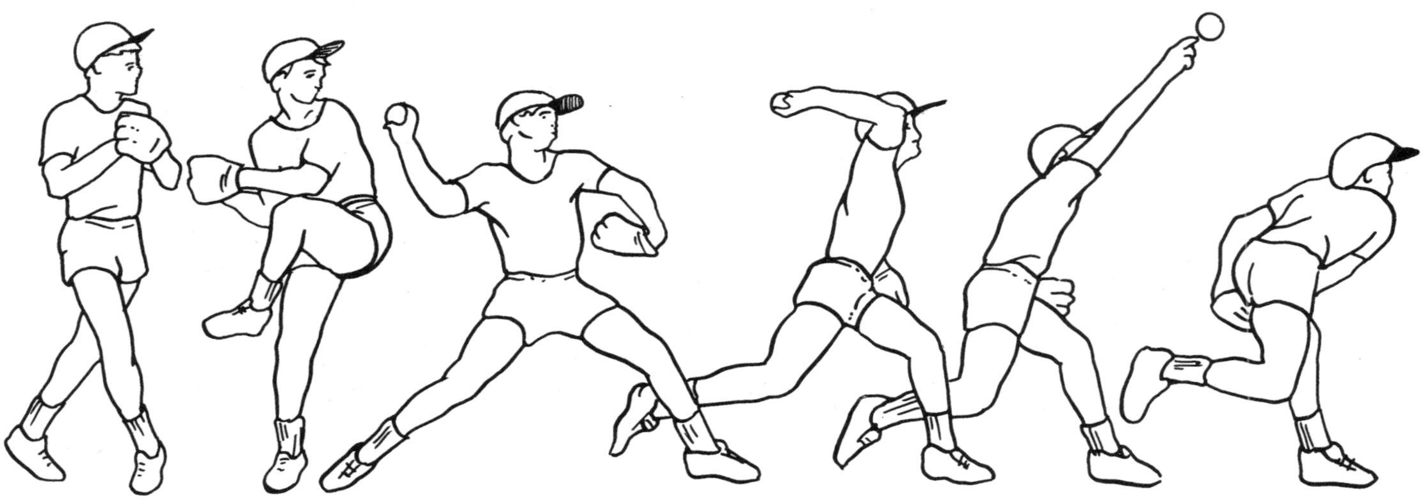

Figure 37.2 The kinetic energy generated during the pitching motion.

ferred downward back to the legs. It has been estimated that over 55% of the kinetic energy and momentum necessary to throw a baseball is generated from the legs and lower trunk (1).

The upper extremity musculature utilized to throw a baseball changes dramatically based on the specific phase of the throw. DiGiovine and coworkers (2) have reported the electromyographic activity of the upper extremity musculature during the pitching motion (see table 37.1). We will briefly summarize the most germane aspects of the EMG activity.

During the windup the EMG activity of the upper extremity is extremely low. During the pitching motion the athlete will pivot on the stance foot to a position parallel with the pitching rubber. The lead leg is then lifted concentrically by the hip flexors while the stance (back) leg is slightly flexed to support the athlete's weight. This position is referred to as the "balanced position" and is a very important position in the synchronicity of body movements during the overhead throw. In this position the body must be vertical; thus, balance, prop-

Table 37.1 EMG of Muscle Groups in the Upper Extremity During Pitching

	No. of pitchers	Windup	Early cocking	Late cocking	Acceleration	Deceleration	Follow-through
Scapular muscles							
Upper trapezius	11	18 ± 16	64 ± 53	37 ± 29	69 ± 31	53 ± 22	14 ± 12
Middle trapezius	11	7 ± 5	43 ± 22	51 ± 24	71 ± 32	35 ± 17	15 ± 14
Lower trapezius	13	13 ± 12	39 ± 30	38 ± 29	76 ± 55	78 ± 33	25 ± 15
Serratus anterior (sixth rib)	11	14 ± 13	44 ± 35	69 ± 32	60 ± 53	51 ± 30	32 ± 18
Serratus anterior (fourth rib)	10	20 ± 20	40 ± 22	106 ± 56	50 ± 46	34 ± 7	41 ± 24
Rhomboids	11	7 ± 8	35 ± 24	41 ± 26	71 ± 35	45 ± 28	14 ± 20
Levator scapula	11	6 ± 5	35 ± 14	72 ± 54	77 ± 28	33 ± 16	14 ± 13
Glenohumeral muscles							
Anterior deltoid	16	15 ± 12	40 ± 20	28 ± 30	27 ± 19	47 ± 34	21 ± 16
Middle deltoid	14	9 ± 8	44 ± 19	12 ± 17	36 ± 22	59 ± 19	16 ± 13
Posterior deltoid	18	6 ± 5	42 ± 26	28 ± 27	68 ± 66	60 ± 28	13 ± 11
Supraspinatus	16	13 ± 12	60 ± 31	49 ± 29	51 ± 46	39 ± 43	10 ± 9
Infraspinatus	16	11 ± 9	30 ± 18	74 ± 34	31 ± 28	37 ± 20	20 ± 16
Teres minor	12	5 ± 6	23 ± 15	71 ± 42	54 ± 50	84 ± 52	25 ± 21
Subscapularis (lower third)	11	7 ± 9	26 ± 22	62 ± 19	56 ± 31	41 ± 23	25 ±18
Subscapularis (upper third)	11	7 ± 8	37 ± 26	99 ± 55	115 ± 82	60 ± 36	16 ± 15
Pectoralis major	14	6 ± 6	11 ± 13	56 ± 27	54 ± 24	29 ± 18	31 ± 21
Latissimus dorsi	13	12 ± 10	33 ± 33	50 ± 37	88 ± 53	59 ± 35	24 ± 18
Elbow and forearm muscles							
Triceps	13	4 ± 6	17 ± 17	37 ± 32	89 ± 40	54 ± 23	22 ± 18
Biceps	18	8 ± 9	22 ± 14	26 ± 20	20 ± 16	44 ± 32	16 ± 14
Brachialis	13	8 ± 5	17 ± 13	18 ± 26	20 ± 22	49 ± 29	13 ± 17
Brachioradialis	13	5 ± 5	35 ± 20	31 ± 24	16 ± 12	46 ± 24	22 ± 29
Pronator teres	14	14 ± 16	18 ± 15	39 ± 28	85 ± 39	51 ± 21	21 ± 21
Supinator	13	9 ± 7	38 ± 20	54 ± 38	55 ± 31	59 ± 31	22 ± 19
Wrist and finger muscles							
Extensor carpi radialis longus	13	11 ± 8	53 ± 24	72 ± 37	30 ± 20	43 ± 24	22 ± 14
Extensor carpi radialis brevis	15	17 ± 17	47 ± 26	75 ± 41	55 ± 35	43 ± 28	24 ± 19
Extensor digitorum communis	14	21 ± 17	37 ± 25	59 ± 27	35 ± 35	47 ± 25	24 ± 18
Flexor carpi radialis	12	13 ± 9	24 ± 35	47 ± 33	120 ± 66	79 ± 36	35 ± 16
Flexor digitorum superficialis	11	16 ± 6	20 ± 23	47 ± 52	80 ± 66	71 ± 32	21 ±11
Flexor carpi ulnaris	10	8 ± 5	27 ± 18	41 ± 25	112 ± 60	77 ± 42	24 ± 18

*Means and standard deviations, expressed as a percentage of the maximal manual muscle test.
Reprinted with permission of DiGiovine NM, Jobe, FW, Pink M, et al. An electromyographic analysis of upper extremity in pitching *J Shoulder Elbow Surg*, 1:15-24, 1992.

rioception, and muscular stability are important attributes in maintaining this posture. The shoulder joint complex musculature becomes active during the early cocking phase. During early cocking the upper trapezius, supraspinatus, deltoid, and serratus anterior muscles exhibit moderately high to moderate levels of EMG activity, respectively (2). Late cocking is characterized by the internal rotators acting eccentrically to control shoulder external rotation. In addition, these muscles are elastically stretched to provide a stretch stimulus to the muscle spindle, provoking a powerful concentric contraction during the next phase of the throw, the acceleration phase. During late cocking the serratus anterior, subscapularis, infraspinatus, teres minor, and pectoralis major muscles exhibit significant EMG activity (2). During arm cocking shoulder joint angular velocity is approximately 1,100°/s (3); maximum anterior shear force is approximately 380 ±90 N and compressive forces 660 ±110 N (4). Thus, approximately 85 lbs of force is acting on the glenohumeral joint in an attempt to sublux the humeral head anteriorly, while approximately 147 lbs of force is compressing the glenohumeral joint during the arm cocking phase. The arm-cocking phase of the pitch takes approximately 0.11 s to complete (4). It has been reported that the shoulder joint may externally rotate in excess of 175° during the late cocking phase/acceleration phase of the throw (5). One must recognize that this is due to the combined motions of the glenohumeral, scapulothoracic, thoracic, and lumbar spine.

Once the arm reaches maximal external rotation, the elbow joint begins to extend and the shoulder joint internally rotates and adducts, initiating the acceleration phase of throwing. This sequence of joint motions (elbow, then shoulder) appears to play a significant role in proper throwing mechanics (5). During the acceleration phase the maximum internal rotation velocity exceeds 7,000°/s (5). This is the fastest human movement. Regardless of what type of pitch is thrown or the style of the thrower (sidearm, overhead, etc) at ball release, the shoulder joint is abducted between 90° to 100° (6). The difference between the "overhead" and "sidearm" thrower is not the amount of shoulder abduction, but rather the degree of lateral tilt of the trunk. During the acceleration phase the subscapularis, latissimus dorsi, and trapezius exhibit high muscular activity. The acceleration phase takes approximately 0.03–0.04 s to complete (4) (see figure 37.3).

After ball release the arm continues to horizontally adduct and extend as the kinetic energy is gradually dissipated through the lower extremity. During arm deceleration the forces at the glenohumeral joint reach high levels. Maximum posterior shear force is 400 ±90 N, while the compressive force is 1090 ±110 N (5). During deceleration the teres minor, lower trapezius, and posterior deltoid musculature act eccentrically to decelerate the arm, resist glenohumeral joint distraction, and dissipate the tremendous forces generated during the throwing motion (2). It takes approximately 0.04 s to complete the deceleration phase(4). The follow-through phase of the pitch is the continuation of the deceleration phase, where joint forces and muscular activity are gradually diminished.

The energy generated during the acceleration phase of throwing must be gradually dissipated after ball release during the deceleration and follow through phases. This usually occurs by the action of the larger body segments and muscles. To reduce the distraction forces that were generated during the deceleration phase, the thrower should exhibit a complete follow-through path that allows the energy and momentum to be dissipated over a longer period of time. Decelerating too quickly or abruptly will result in tremendous forces that may lead to injury.

Consequently, the throwing shoulder complex is subjected to tremendous unnatural stresses. The

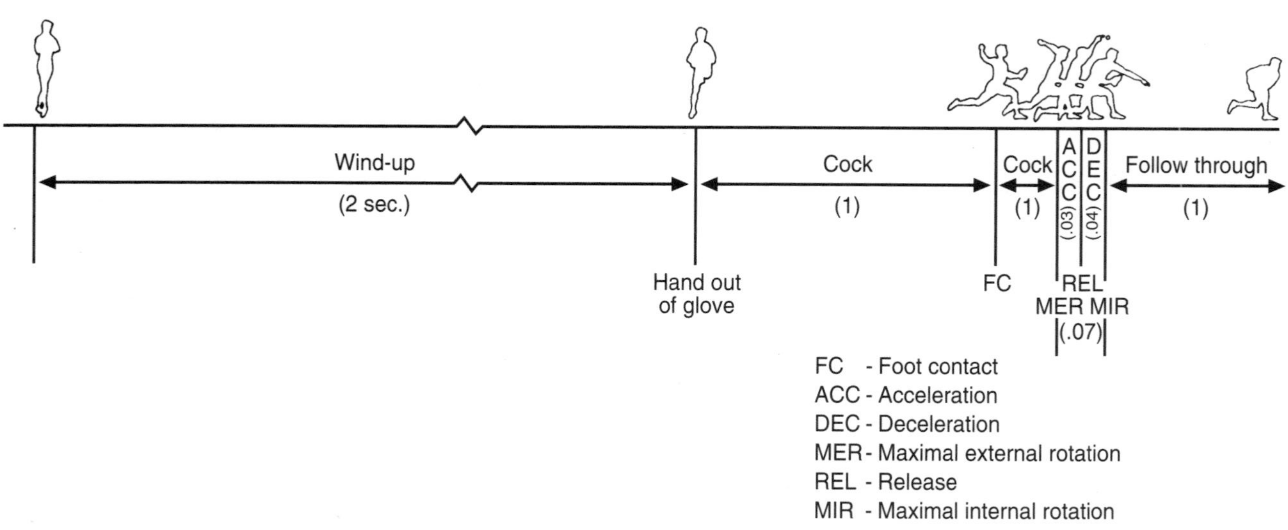

Figure 37.3 Approximate time lengths for the phases of pitching.

thrower's shoulder must be flexible enough to allow the excessive external rotation required to throw a baseball. However, the thrower's shoulder must also be stable enough to prevent subluxation of the shoulder joint. Therefore, there appears to exist a paradox when describing the thrower's shoulder: "the thrower's shoulder must be loose enough to throw but stable enough to prevent subluxation." Functional stability is provided by the joint capsule and the musculature about the shoulder joint complex. The shoulder musculature must act to accelerate the arm and also decelerate or dissipate the forces generated, all while providing dynamic joint stability. Dynamic joint stability is accomplished by coactivation of the stabilizing muscles. Due to the tremendous forces occurring at extremely high angular velocities and the repetitive nature of throwing, the thrower becomes susceptible to a variety of shoulder joint injuries. The most common injuries include overuse tendonitis, capsular hyperlaxity (subluxation), posterior cuff impingement, glenoid labral lesions, and tensile rotator cuff tissue failure.

The Thrower's Shoulder Joint

Upon physical examination of the thrower's shoulder joint, a characteristic pattern becomes obvious. The pitcher usually exhibits excessive external rotation (125–145°) and a significant reduction in internal rotation (45–55°). Brown and coworkers (7) reported that professional pitchers exhibited 132° ±1° of external rotation at 90° of abduction. This was approximately 10° more than the nonthrowing shoulder, and approximately 9° greater than the position players' throwing shoulders. Johnson (8) reported that collegiate pitchers exhibited greater external rotation (128–136°) compared to infielders (109–115°) and outfielders (114–120°). Recently, Bigliani and associates (9) examined the range of motion of 148 professional players, 72 pitchers and 76 position players. The investigators reported that the pitcher's external rotation with the arm abducted to 90° averaged 118° (range 95–145°) on the dominant shoulder. Conversely, the position player's dominant shoulder averaged 109° (range 80–105°). Additionally, the authors noted significantly less internal rotation in the dominant shoulder than in the nondominant shoulder.

Thus, the thrower's shoulder exhibits significant hypermobility of the anterior structures to permit excessive external rotation, whereas the posterior structures appear hypermobile, and often internal rotation is diminished. These changes appear more prominently in the pitcher than in the position player. Additionally, this asymmetrical imbalance in motion may contribute to anterior humeral head migration.

Several investigators have examined the muscular strength in the overhead throwing athlete (10–15), with varying results and conclusions. Wilk and associates (14) have demonstrated that external rotation strength of the pitcher's throwing shoulder is significantly weaker than the nonthrowing shoulder. Conversely, the throwing shoulder's internal rotation strength is significantly stronger than the nonthrowing shoulder. In addition, the throwing shoulder's adduction strength is also significantly stronger than the nonthrowing shoulder (15). Table 37.2 illustrates the muscular strength values in professional baseball pitchers. Magnusson and coworkers (16) studied muscular strength in professional pitchers and compared them to a control group of nonthrowing, nonathletic individuals. In pitchers, the supraspinatus muscle was significantly weaker on the throwing side compared to the nonthrowing side. Pitchers were weaker than the control group for shoulder abduction, external rotation, internal rotation, and the supraspinatus muscle (16).

Due to the excessive glenohumeral joint motion exhibited by the overhead thrower, most frequently the anterior and inferior shoulder joint capsule is lax. This capsular laxity permits excessive range of motion. The hypermobility of the shoulder joint capsule can be appreciated during the stability assessment of the glenohumeral joint, most commonly during the fulcrum test or sulcus test (17). The hypermobility and hyperlaxity in the thrower's shoulder has been referred to as thrower's laxity (18) or acquired laxity (19). Bigliani and coworkers (9) examined the shoulder laxity in 72 professional baseball pitchers and 76 professional position players. The investigators noted a high degree of inferior glenohumeral joint laxity, with 61% of pitchers and 47% of position players exhibiting a positive sulcus sign on the dominant (throwing) shoulder. Additionally, in the players who exhibited a positive sulcus sign on the dominant side, 54% of the

Table 37.2 Unilateral Muscle Ratios in the Throwing Athlete

	Reported Ratio	Goal
ER/IR	62 – 66%	66 – 75%
ABD/ADD	78 – 84%	66 – 72%
ABD/ER	62 – 66%	64 – 69%

pitchers exhibited a positive sulcus sign on the nondominant side; only 45% of position players exhibited a nondominant sulcus sign. Thus, it would appear that baseball players, especially pitchers, exhibit inherent laxity and, with throwing, the laxity generally increases (adaptive response or acquired). Due to thrower's laxity, numerous injuries may develop in the pitcher's shoulder joint complex.

Common Injuries to the Thrower's Shoulder

Injuries to the throwing shoulder can usually be divided into two broad categories: macrotraumatic and microtraumatic injuries. Macrotraumatic injuries are usually acute significant failures in which the athlete remembers injuring the shoulder. In baseball, this injury usually occurs while diving to catch a ball or sliding into a base and may result in a shoulder subluxation or dislocation, fracture, or rotator cuff tear. Conversely, microtraumatic injuries are more common injuries and are usually associated with overuse syndromes, muscular imbalances, and laxity; they have a gradual onset.

The most common overuse injuries are shoulder subluxation and shoulder impingement. Anterior shoulder subluxation is common in pitchers and is caused by the repetitive microtraumatic forces applied to the anterior glenohumeral joint capsule during throwing. Due to the repetitive microtraumatic forces the anterior capsule gradually stretches out and increases susceptibility to various injuries. These injuries include glenoid labrum fraying and tearing (20, 21), undersurface rotator cuff fraying (22, 23), and posterior impingement (24, 25).

The Thrower's Shoulder Paradox

The thrower's shoulder must be lax enough to be able to fully cock the arm. Usually at least 135–140° of external rotation is required. But the shoulder capsule cannot be too loose; otherwise, the static/dynamic restraint is lost and the humeral head would be predisposed to sublux anteriorly during extreme external rotation in late arm cocking. Furthermore, the surrounding musculature of the glenohumeral joint must act to co-contract to produce glenohumeral joint compression, thus creating dynamic joint stability. In addition, specific muscles must work in a synchronized fashion to accelerate the arm while also dynamically stabilizing the glenohumeral joint. This coordinated and synchronized muscle firing, which both creates arm movement and stabilizes the shoulder joint, must occur at extremely fast angular velocities. As previously mentioned, the acceleration phase takes approximately 0.03 s and the deceleration phase approximately 0.04 s. Thus, the paradox: the thrower's shoulder must exhibit significant mobility enabling the throwing motion to occur, but the shoulder must also exhibit dynamic stability, all of which occur at tremendously rapid angular velocities. Additionally, microtraumatic forces applied to shoulder joint may lead to microtraumatic tissue failure and pain, which often cause a loss of muscular strength and dynamic stability.

Gloussman and coworkers (26) examined the EMG activity of the shoulder musculature in individuals with glenohumeral instability during throwing. The investigators noted a marked decrease in EMG activity of the pectoralis major, latissimus dorsi, subscapularis, and serratus anterior muscles during the late cocking phase. Increased activity was noted for the biceps brachii and the supraspinatus muscle. This may suggest a conscious or subconscious compensatory mechanism for the instability.

Gowan (27) compared the EMG activity of the shoulder musculature of amateur pitchers with professional pitchers. Overall, the amateur pitchers exhibited significantly greater EMG activity of specific muscles, particularly the rotator cuff muscles, during the acceleration phase. These findings suggest that the professional pitcher (highly skilled) requires less muscular activity of the stabilizing muscles because of improved throwing efficiency. Several investigators have reported that the unskilled tennis player produces significantly greater EMG activity than the highly skilled player when performing the tennis service motion (29, 38).

Upon physical examination of the healthy thrower's shoulder (during spring training physicals, etc.) we have noticed some other interesting characteristic features. First, pitchers frequently exhibit hypermobility of the scapula of the thoracic wall on the throwing shoulder. The medial border of the scapula lifts or wings off the thoracic wall (medial tilt) during specific motions such as internal rotation and horizontal adduction.

Also, we have noted in some throwers that the glenohumeral joint appeared extremely lax when examined for range of motion and static stability compared to other throwers. Yet some of the excessively lax individuals are asymptomatic and are unaware of the significant laxity or significant "play" in the shoulder joint capsule. This observation is reinforced annually and is seen clinically when treating throwers for injuries to other body parts. Hence, it has led us to believe that other factors contribute to shoulder joint functional stability than merely ligamentous static stability and muscular strength. We believe that some of the other factors are proprioception, kinesthesia, and neuromuscular control. Because of the importance of neuromuscular control in the overhead thrower, we have developed specific exercises and drills that are designed to enhance neuromuscular abilities.

Philosophical Approach to Treatment

Frequently, the terms proprioception and kinesthesia are used interchangeably. Proprioception refers to the conscious and unconscious appreciation of joint position (30). Kinesthesia is the sensation of joint motion or acceleration. The efferent (motor) response to sensory information is termed neuromuscular control (31). There appear to be two motor control mechanisms that interpret efferent information and coordinate efferent responses. Feedforward neuromuscular control involves planning movements based on sensory information from past experiences (32, 33). The feedback process continuously regulates motor control through reflex pathways. Thus, through these mechanisms the subject can adjust the level of muscle activation and muscular stiffness. Furthermore, stiff muscles resist stretching episodes more effectively, have greater muscular tone, and thus provide more effective dynamic stabilization (34). Through proper neuromuscular training in rehabilitation, we believe we can train the subject to preactivate muscles in anticipation of movements and joint loads and also to react to movements or loads that may be potentially harmful. We have referred to this reaction ability as reactive neuromuscular control (35).

The Rehabilitation Program for Throwers

The rehabilitation and training program we use for the overhead thrower utilizes the four elements for neuromuscular control and functional stability, which have been modified from the work of Swanik, Lephart, and associates (36). The four elements include (1) proprioception and kinesthesia, (2) dynamic stabilization, (3) reactive neuromuscular control, and (4) functional activities. We will briefly discuss specific rehabilitation techniques to enhance these four elements in the overhead throwing athlete (see table 37.3).

The nonoperative rehabilitation program utilized for the overhead thrower involves a multiphased approach that is progressive and sequential. The specific goals of each of the four phases of the program are outlined in table 37.4. For the purposes of this paper we will discuss the specific rehabilitation exercises and drills that we utilize to restore functional movement patterns in the overhead thrower.

During the initial phase, one of the primary goals of the rehabilitation program is to normalize shoulder motion, particularly shoulder internal rotation and horizontal adduction. Thus, specific stretches to address posterior rotator cuff and capsular tightness should be performed, to prevent the consequential anterior displacement of the humeral head due to posterior tightness. Another primary goal of this phase is to reestablish baseline dynamic stability as well as restore proprioception and kinesthesia. Lephart and associates (37) have demonstrated significant proprioceptive deficits in patients who have had chronic traumatic anterior shoulder instability. Furthermore, the examiners reported that surgical stabilization of the involved shoulder improved shoulder joint proprioception (37). Voight and coworkers (38) examined the effects of muscle fatigue on shoulder joint proprioception. The investigators reported that shoulder proprioception was diminished in the presence of shoulder muscular fatigue, suggesting that various muscular receptors contribute to proprioception (38). Thus, during this first phase the rehabilitation drills are designed to restore the neurosensory properties of the microtraumatically injured shoulder ligaments in the thrower and enhance the sensitivity of the afferent mechanoreceptors (39).

Specific drills that address the neuromuscular goals during the initial phase are rhythmic stabilization (RS) and reciprocal isometric (RI) contractions for the internal/external rotators of the shoulder. These drills are performed at various degrees of shoulder elevation (see figure 37.4, *a-c*). Additionally, proprioceptive neuromuscular facilitation (PNF) drills are performed in mid range progressing to end range of motion. The PNF pattern we most commonly utilize is the D_2 flex/ext pattern with manual resistance utilizing rhythmic stabilization, slow reversal holds, and reciprocal isometrics (40, 41). The PNF techniques utilize specific skilled sensory input from the clinician to bring about or facilitate a specific movement pattern. The manual techniques allow the clinician the opportunity to increase the patient's awareness of specific movement patterns and reinforce or facilitate weak

Table 37.3 Restoring Proprioception/Kinesthesia/Neuromuscular Control in the Thrower

Elements	Rehabilitation techniques
Baseline dynamic stability and proprioception/kinesthesia	– Static rhythmic stabilization drills – PNF (short arc) (supine) – PNF (full ROM) – PNF, RS, RI, SRH – Joint repositioning – Axial loading or CKE exercise – PNF, RS, RI, SRH (sidelying) – PNF (seated or standing)
Dynamic stability and neuromuscular control	– Dynamic stabilization drills end range – PNF D_2, IR/ER, 90/90 – Selective muscle activation – Biofeedback – Scapula neuromuscular control drills – Plyometrics
Reactive neuromuscular control	– PNF (end range) – Reaction to joint perturbances • PNF (tubing/manual) • 90/90 ER/IR (tubing/manual) • eyes open, closed, single-limb stance – Plyometrics – Endurance muscle training – Throwing drills underweight or overweight ball
Functional motor patterns	– Gradual return to throwing (interval throwing) – Functional drills – Plyometrics

Table 37.4 Rehabilitation Phases and Goals for the Overhead Thrower

Phase one
- Goals: Diminish pain and inflammation
  - Normalize motion
  - Retard muscular atrophy
  - Reestablish dynamic stability
  - Control functional stress/strain

Phase two
- Goals: Progress strengthening program
  - Promote/restore muscular balance
  - Enhance dynamic stability, neuromuscular control
  - Continue flexibility drills

Phase three
- Goals: Aggressive strengthening
  - Enhance reactive neuromuscular control
  - Improve strength, power, endurance
  - Gradual return to throwing

Phase four
- Goals: Return to competitive throwing
  - Continuation of the strength, power, endurance, and neuromuscular program

patterns. The purpose of the RS, SRH, and RI is to facilitate an agonist/antagonist muscular coactivation. Efficient coactivation assists in restoring the balance in the force couples of the shoulder joint, thus enhancing joint congruency and reducing the loads on the static structures. The anticipation of joint loads and stress applied is also beneficial in the restoration of proprioception and kinesthesia. The RS technique applied during D_2 flex/ext exercises are generally employed at 45°, 90°, and 125° of arm elevation.

Other drills include early joint repositioning tasks that enhance conscious proprioceptive and kinesthetic awareness, which will eventually lead to unconscious appreciation of joint position and motion (36). Axial loading exercises or closed kinetic chain (CKS) exercises may also be beneficial. It has been suggested that joint compression maximally stimulates the articular receptors (42). Thus, axial loading drills such as weights shifts, weight bearing on limb, and alternating isometrics (AI) techniques performed in the quadruped, triped, or biped position may be beneficial in restoring proprioception and kinesthesia (43, 44). As the patient improves, the PNF

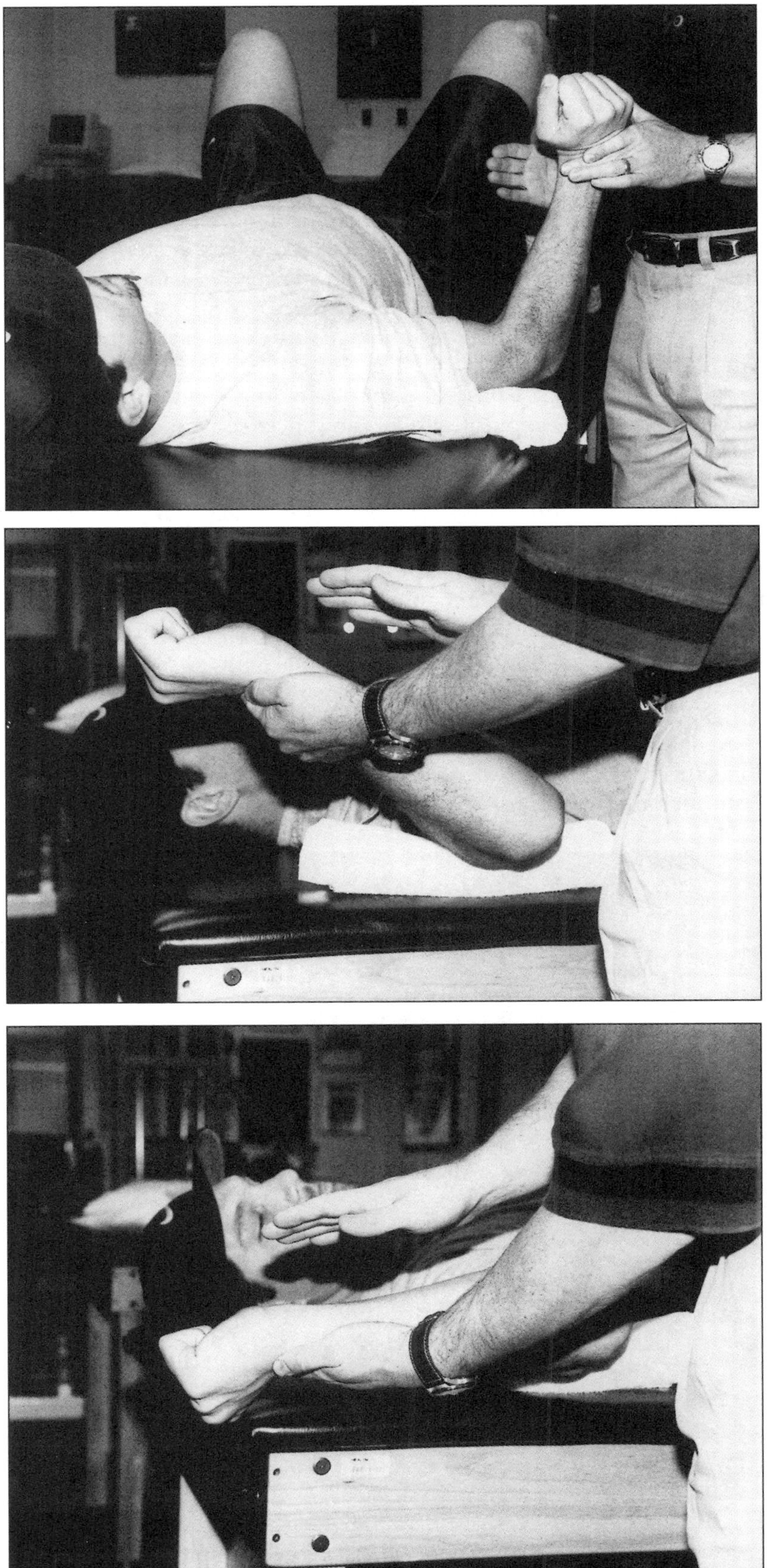

a b c

Figure 37.4 Rhythmic stabilization drills performed at (*a*) 30° of external rotation in the scapula plane (*b*) 45° of external rotation at 90° of abduction, and (*c*) 90° of external rotation at 90° of abduction.

D_2 patterns may be performed in the sidelying position and also in sitting or standing position. By altering position the effects of gravity are changed as well as the tactile stimulus and stability to the scapulae. The primary goal during this initial phase is to reestablish a baseline level of dynamic joint stability and to restore proprioception and kinesthesia awareness.

In phase two of the rehabilitation program, the primary goals are to enhance dynamic stability and to facilitate neuromuscular control. Additionally, the rehabilitation program should attempt to restore muscular balance at the glenohumeral and scapulothoracic joints. During this phase, the extremity is placed in positions of vulnerability (i.e., at end range), and the patient is instructed to dynamically stabilize the joint while manual resistance techniques such as RS and RI are applied. In the overhead thrower, the PNF D_2 pattern and ER/IR at 90° of abduction are frequently utilized positions. Figure 37.5 illustrates end range dynamic stabilization techniques for the shoulder rotators.

Additionally, reeducation of selective muscle activation is necessary for dynamic stabilization and neuromuscular control. Selective muscular activation is also utilized to restore muscular balance and symmetry. In the overhead thrower, the shoulder external rotators, scapular retractors, protractors, and depressors are frequently isolated due to weakness. Biofeedback may assist the athlete in developing muscular coactivation during specific drills. We have established a core exercise program for the overhead throwing athlete that specifically addresses the vital muscles involved in the throwing motion. This program was developed based on the collective EMG research of numerous investigators (45–49). We have referred to the exercise regimen as the "throwers ten program" (see table 37.5) (50).

The scapula provides proximal stability to the shoulder, enabling quality distal segment mobility; it is vital for normal arm function. The scapula acts as a base of support for the glenohumeral joint. Scapulothoracic motion is controlled by several force couples. Traditionally, isotonic exercise techniques were utilized to strengthen the scapular muscles and potentially enhance dynamic stability. Several authors have emphasized the importance of scapular muscular strength and neuromuscular control (51, 52). We have developed specific exercise drills to enhance neuromuscular control of the scapulothoracic joint. These drills are referred to as scapulothoracic neuromuscular control drills and exercises (44). These drills are designed to maximally challenge the scapulothoracic muscular force couples and to stimulate the proprioceptive and kinesthetic awareness at the scapulae.

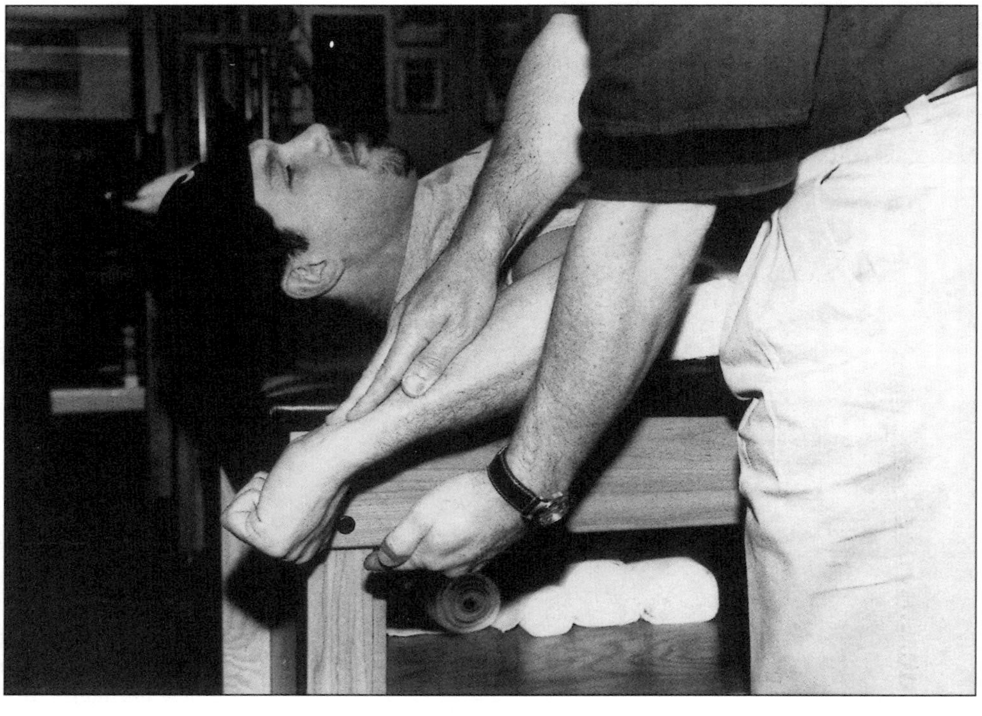

Figure 37.5 Rhythmic stabilization drills performed at end range with the arm in 90° of abduction. The arm is positioned at the end range for shoulder external rotation.

Table 37.5 Throwers Ten Exercise Program

The Throwers Ten Program is designed to exercise the major muscles necessary for throwing. The program's goal is to be an organized and concise exercise program. In addition, all exercises included are specific to the thrower and are designed to improve strength, power and endurance of the shoulder complex musculature.

1. **A: Diagonal Pattern D2 Extension:**
   Involved hand will grip tubing handle overhead and out to the side. Pull tubing down and across your body to the opposite side of leg. During the motion lead with your thumb Perform ____ sets of ____ repetitions ____ times daily.

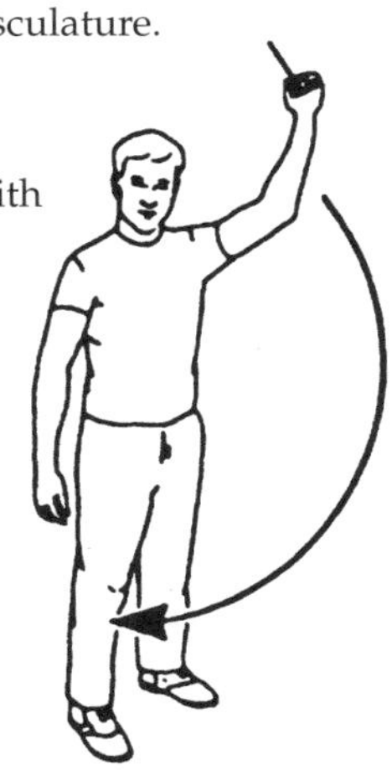

   B: Diagonal Pattern D2 Flexion:
   Gripping tubing handle in hand of involved arm, begin with arm out from side 45° and palm facing backward. After turning palm forward, proceed to flex elbow and bring arm up and over uninvolved shoulder. Turn palm down and reverse to take arm to starting position. Exercise should be performed in controlled manner. Perform ____ sets of ____ repetitions ____ times daily.

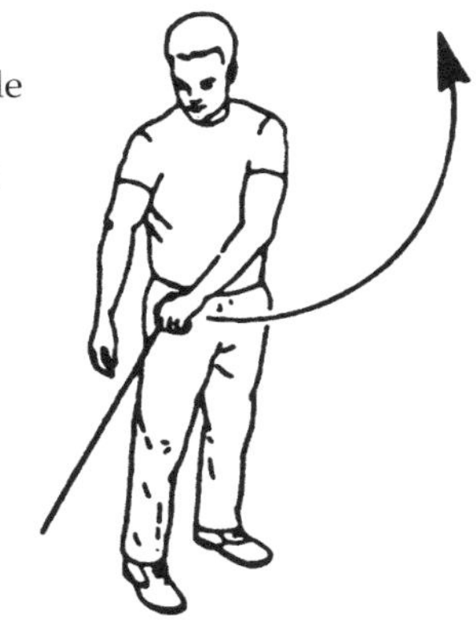

2. **A: External Rotation at 0° Abduction**
   Standing with involved elbow fixed at side, elbow at 90° and involved arm across front of body. Grip tubing handle while the other end of tubing is fixed. Pull out with arm, keeping elbow at side. Return tubing slowly and controlled. Performed ____ sets of ____ repetitions ____ times daily.

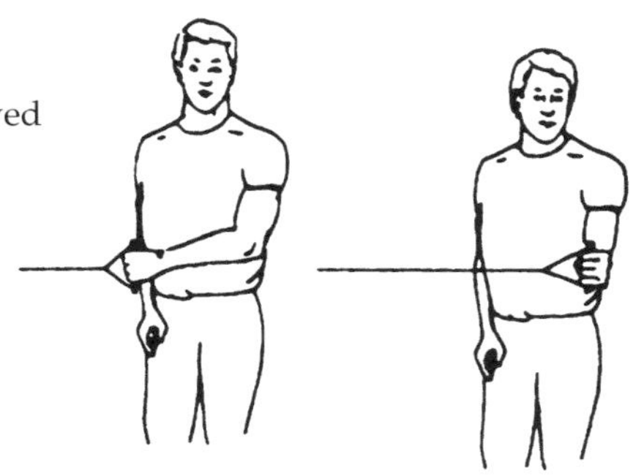

   B: Internal Rotation at 0° Abduction:
   Standing with elbow at side fixed at 90° and shoulder rotated out. Grip tubing handle while other end of tubing is fixed. Pull arm across body keeping elbow at side. Return tubing slowly and controlled. Perform ____ sets of ____ repetitions ____ times daily.

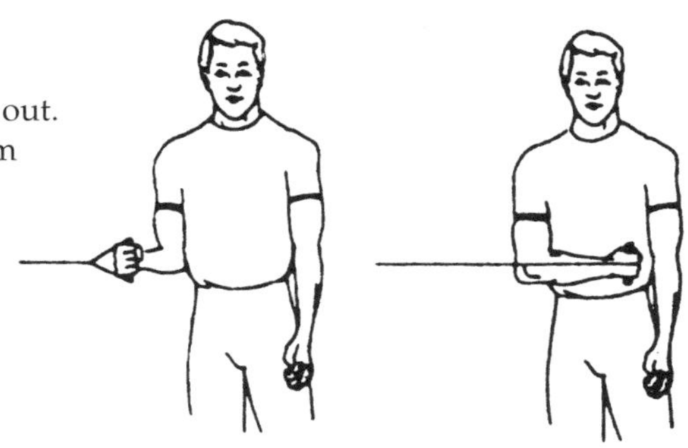

(*cont.*)

C: External Rotation at 90° Abduction:
Stand with shoulder abducted 90° and elbow flexed 90°. Grip tubing handle while the other end is fixed straight ahead, slightly lower than the shoulder. Keeping shoulder abducted, rotate shoulder back keeping elbow at 90°. Return tubing and hand to start postion.

I. ***Slow Speed Sets*** (Slow and Controlled):
Perform ____ sets of ____ repetitions ____ times daily.

II. ***Fast Speed Sets:*** Perform ____ sets of ____ repetitions/ seconds ____ times daily.

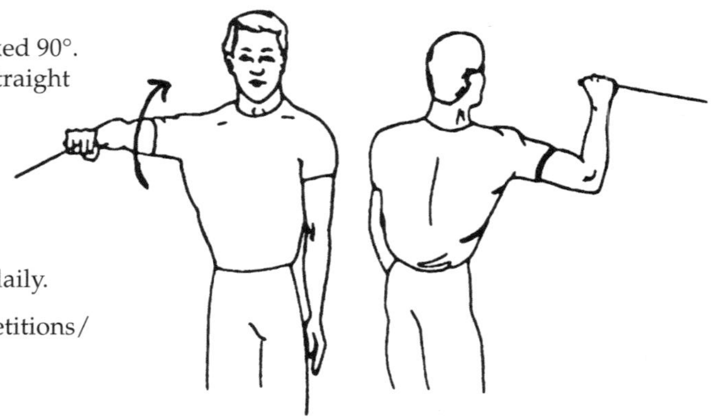

D: Internal Rotation at 90° Abduction:
Stand with shoulder abducted to 90°, externally rotated 90° and elbow bent to 90°. Keeping shoulder abducted, rotate shoulder forward, keeping elbow bent at 90°. Return tubing and hand to start position.

I. ***Slow Speed Sets*** (Slow and Controlled):
Perform ____ sets of ____ repetitions ____ times daily.

II. ***Fast Speed Sets:*** Perform ____ sets of ____ repetitions/ seconds ____ times daily.

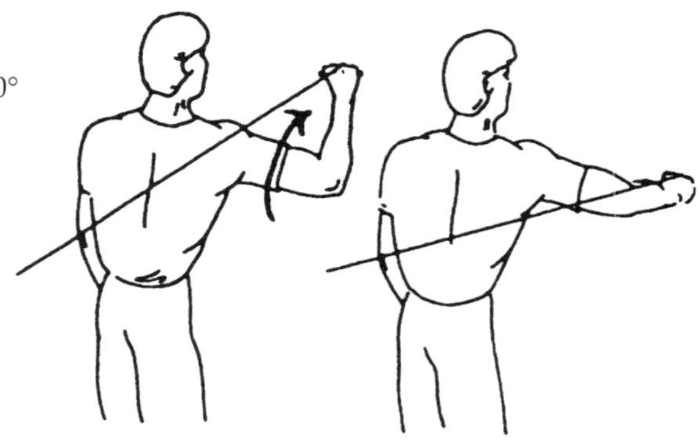

3. **Shoulder Abduction to 90°:**
Stand with arm at side, elbow straight, and palm against side. Raise arm to the side, palm down, until arm reaches 90° (shoulder level). Hold 2 seconds and lower slowly. Perform ____ sets of ____ repetitions ____ times daily.

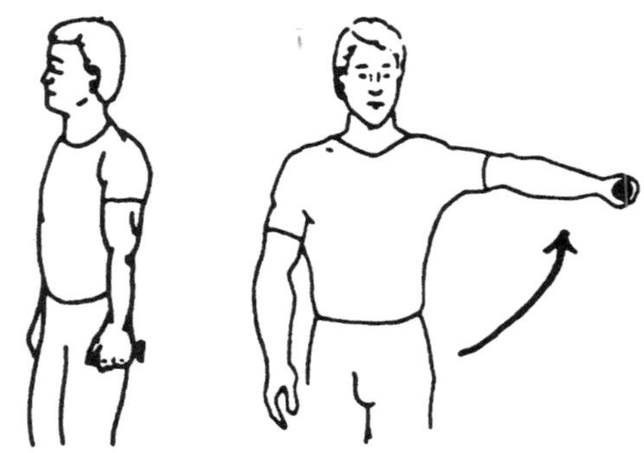

4. **Scaption, Internal Rotation:**
Stand with elbow straight and thumb down. Raise arm to shoulder level at 30° angle in front of body. Do not go above shoulder height. Hold 2 seconds and lower slowly. Perform ____ sets of ____ repetitions ____ times daily.

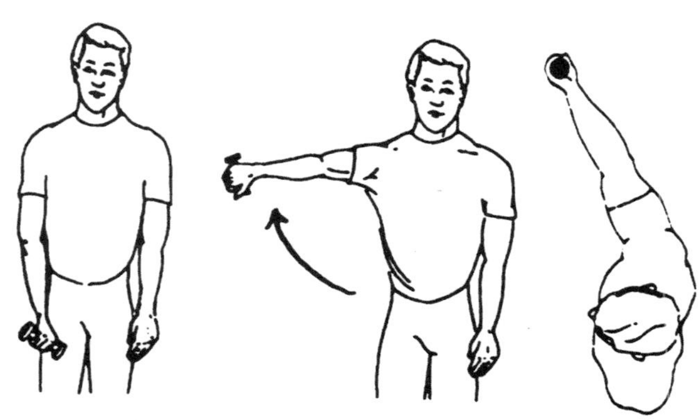

Table 37.5 *(continued)*

5. **A: Prone Horizontal Abduction (Neutral):** Lie on table, face down, with involved arm hanging straight to the floor, and palm facing down. Raise arm out to the side, parallel to the floor. Hold 2 seconds and lower slowly. Perform ____ sets of ____ repetitions ____ times daily.

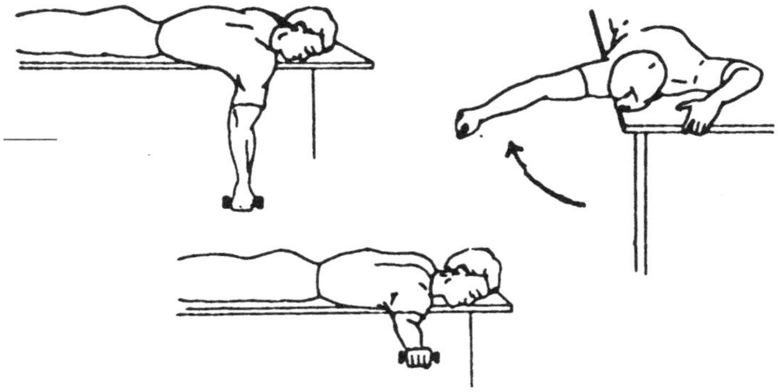

B: Prone Horizontal Abduction (Full ER, 100° ABD): Lie on table, face down, with involved arm hanging straight to the floor, and thumb rotated up (hitchhiker). Raise arm out to the side with arm slightly in front of shoulder, parallel to the floor. Hold 2 seconds and lower slowly. Perform ____ sets of ____ repetitions _____ times daily.

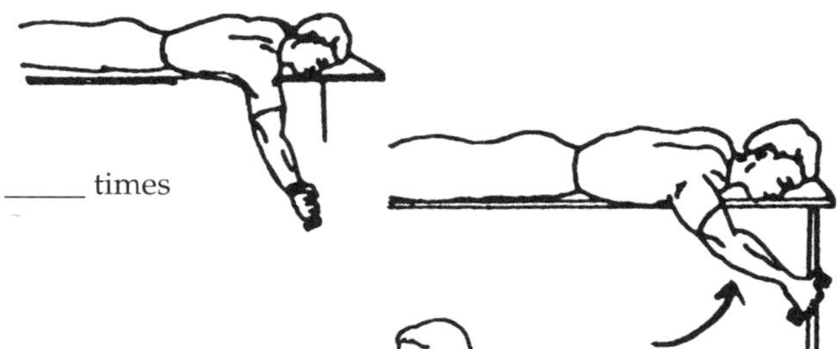

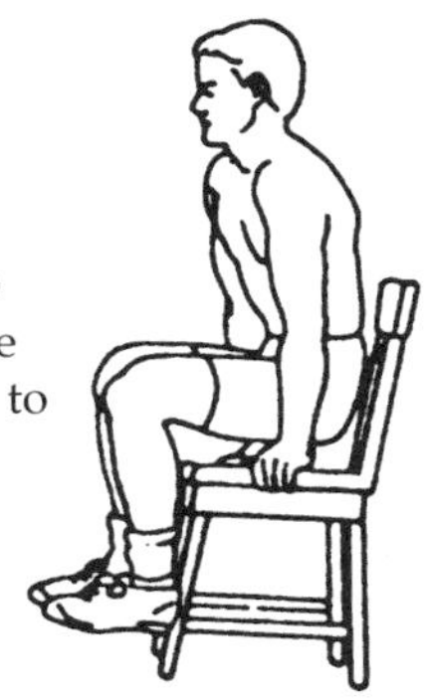

6. **Press-Ups:** Seated on a chair or on a table, place both hands firmly on the sides of the chair or table, palms down and fingers pointed outward. Hands should be placed in line with shoulders. Slowly push downward through the hands to elevate your body.

7. **Prone Rowing:** Lying on your stomach with your involved arm hanging over the side of the table, dumbbell in hand and elbow straight. Slowly raise arm, bending elbow, and bring dumbbell as high as possible. Hold at the top for 2 seconds, then slowly lower. Perform ____ sets of ____ repetitions ____times daily.

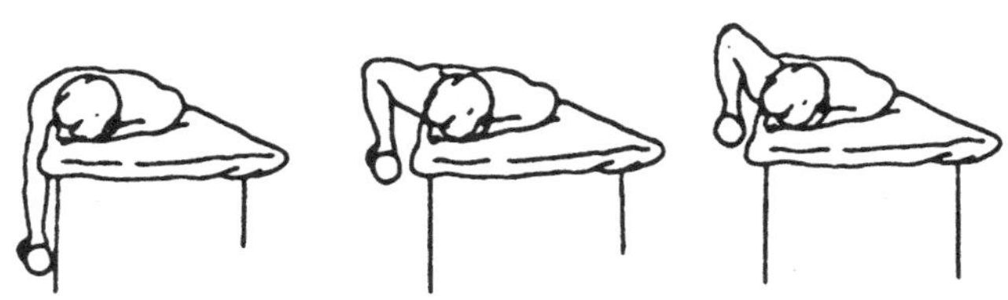

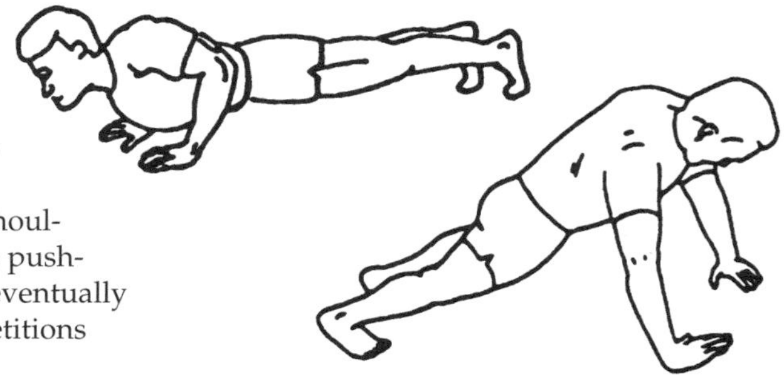

8. **Push-Ups:** Start in the down position with arms in a comfortable position. Place hands no more than shoulder width apart. Push up as high as possible, rolling shoulders forward after elbows are straight. Start with a push-up into wall. Gradually progress to table top and eventually to floor as tolerable. Perform ____ sets of ____ repetitions ____ times daily.

Table 37.5 (*continued*)

9. A: Elbow Flexion:
Standing with arm against side and palm facing inward, bend elbow upward turning palm up as you progress. Hold 2 seconds and lower slowly. Perform ____ sets of ____ repetitions ____ times daily.

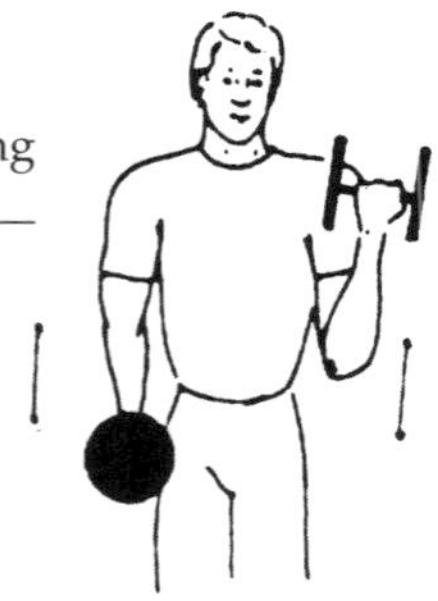

B: Elbow Extension:
Raise involved arm overhead. Provide support at elbow from uninvolved hand. Straighten arm overhead. Hold 2 seconds and lower slowly. Perform ____ sets of ____ repetitions ____ times daily.

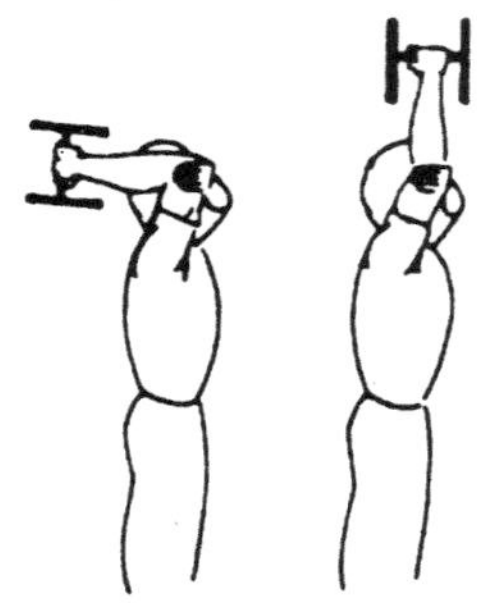

10. A: Wrist Extension:
Supporting the forearm and with the palm facing downward, raise weight in hand as far as possible. Hold 2 seconds and lower slowly. Perform ____ sets of ____ repetitions ____ times daily.

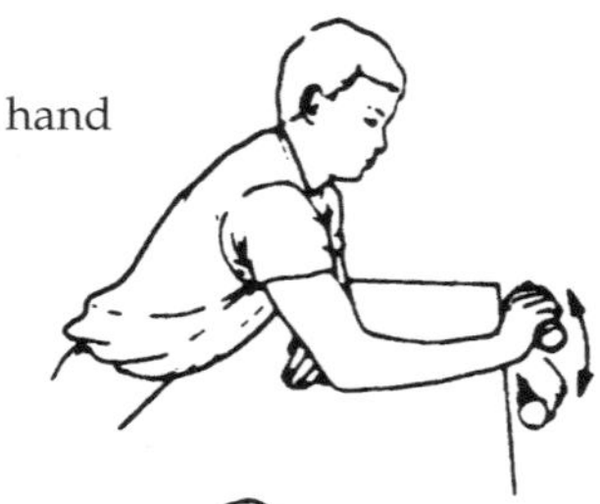

B: Wrist Flexion:
Supporting the forearm and with palm facing upward, lower a weight in hand as far as possible and then curl it up as high as possible. Hold for 2 seconds and lower slowly. Perform ____ sets of ____ repetitions ____ times daily.

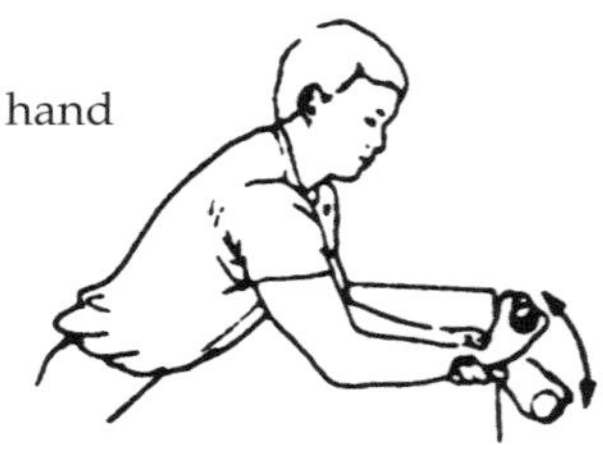

C: Supination:
Forearm supported on table with wrist in neutral position. Using a weight or hammer, roll wrist taking palm up. Hold for a 2 count and return to starting position. Perform ____ sets of ____ repetitions ____ times daily.

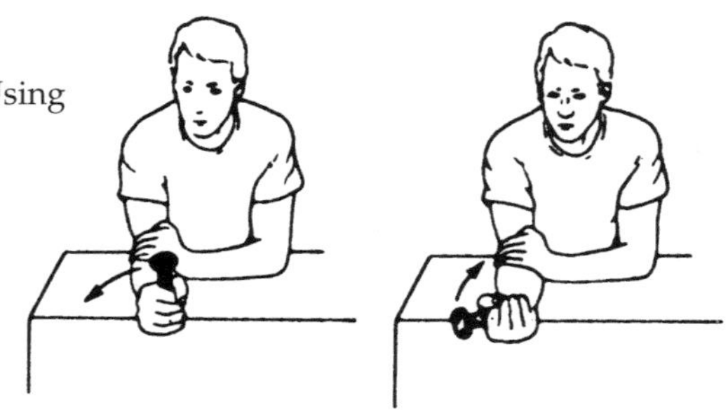

D: Pronation:
Forearm should be supported on a table with wrist in neutral position. Using a weight or hammer, roll wrist taking palm down. Hold for a 2 count and return to starting position. Perform ____ sets of ____ repetitions ____ times daily.

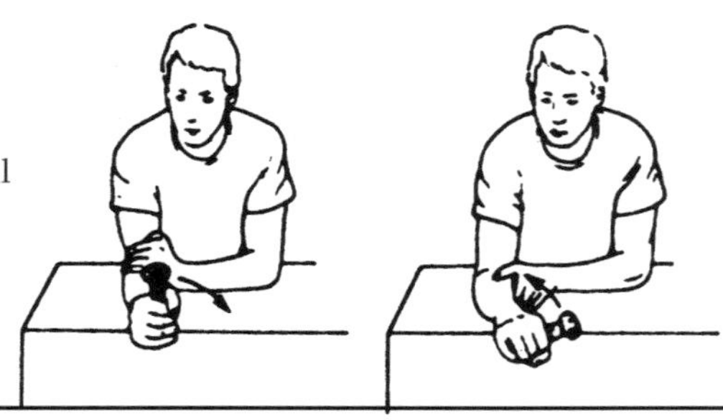

With this technique, the patient is sidelying on the uninvolved arm, as the affected arm is abducted to 90° and internally rotated. The patient's hand is placed on the table to fixate the distal segment and assist in isolating the proximal musculature of the scapula. The patient is instructed to slowly elevate and then depress the scapula against the clinician's manual resistance (see figure 37.6, *a* and *b*). Scapular protraction and retraction are also performed in the same manner. The clinician can utilize a variety of manual techniques such as slow reversal holds, rhythmic stabilization, and timing for emphasis to intensify the dynamic control and kinesthesia of the scapulothoracic joint. The movement progresses from straight planes, to circular movements, to diagonal patterns. The emphasis is on quality not quantity of movement. The author believes this type of neuromuscular training enhances the dynamic joint stability and proprioceptive awareness. A functional stable scapulothoracic articulation is critical for the overhead athlete.

Additionally, plyometrics or stretch-shortening exercises may be utilized to enhance dynamic stability. Plyometric exercise employs three phases, all intended to utilize the elastic and reactive properties of the muscle to generate maximal force production. The first phase is the eccentric phase, where a rapid prestretch is applied to the musculotendinous unit, stimulating the muscle spindle. The second phase is the amortization phase, representing the time between the eccentric and concentric phases. This time should be as short as possible so that the beneficial neurological effects of the prestretch are not lost. The final phase is the resultant concentric contraction. Wilk and associates (53) have established a plyometric exercise program for the overhead thrower. The plyometric program is designed to enhance dynamic stability, improve neuromuscular control, and enhance performance. During the second phase of the rehabilitation program, the suggested plyometric drills are two-handed drills such as the two-handed side-to-side throw, two-handed chest press and two-handed overhead soccer throw. These drills are selected because they are less demanding on the shoulder joint. It is important that a satisfactory level of dynamic stability has been established prior to initiating plyometrics.

In phase three the primary goals are to enhance dynamic stabilization, improve reactive neuromuscular control, and improve power and endurance. Also during this phase we usually initiate a gradu-

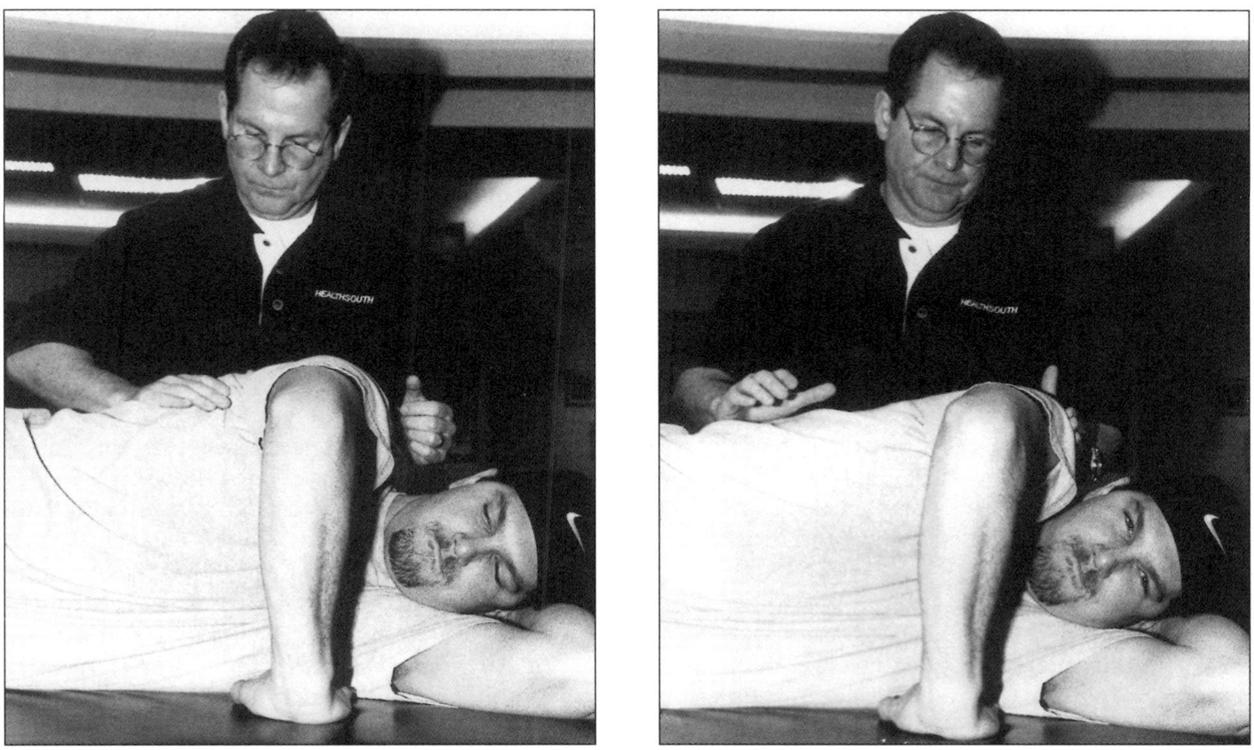

Figure 37.6 Scapular neuromuscular control drills. (*a*) The patient slowly depresses the scapular, (*b*) manual resistance is applied to resist scapular elevation.

ated throwing program. Reactive neuromuscular training focuses on stimulating the reflex pathways from the articular and tenomuscular receptors to skeletal muscle. During these drills, unanticipated joint perturbations are introduced with the goal of enhancing reactive neuromuscular control. Numerous exercise drills can be utilized to create a joint perturbation, and we will briefly discuss a couple of techniques that we prefer.

The first perturbation technique is a PNF technique. The patient is standing with resistance exercise tubing in one hand. The patient will perform a D_2 flexion pattern against the resistance of the tubing and the manual resistance provided by the clinician (see figure 37.7*a*). Once the patient reaches end range, the clinician quickly reverses the manual contact and now attempts to push the patient's arm into further flexion; the patient must react to this overpressure. This quick reversal is followed with reciprocal isometrics performed at end range (see figure 37.7*b*). A similar technique can be performed with the arm abducted to 90°. The patient externally rotates against the resistance of the exercise tubing and the manual resistance of the clinician (see figure 37.7*c*). At end range, the clinician attempts to push the patient's arm into further external rotation, thus creating a joint perturbation to which the patient must react. The patient should perform this reactive neuromuscular control drill first with eyes open, then progress to eyes closed, and finally to standing on a single lower extremity, to enhance core stability.

In addition, weighted plyoballs (Functionally Integrated Technology, California) can be used to create a joint perturbation. In the case of the overhead thrower, the patient is supine with the arm abducted to 90° and the elbow flexed to 90°. The starting position is with the arm externally rotated approximately 60°. The clinician lightly tosses a lightweight (2 lb) plyoball to the patient, and the weight of the ball causes the arm to externally rotate. The patient must react, stabilize, and throw the ball back (see figure 37.8). An exercise progression for this reactive neuromuscular control drill can be found in table 37.6.

As previously mentioned, the author believes that plyometric exercises are excellent to enhance reactive neuromuscular control. In this third phase more aggressive plyometrics are initiated. Plyometric drills we utilize include the one-handed baseball throw, two-handed side throws, two-handed underhand side throws, two-handed setup and soccer throws, plyometric push-ups, and the like (53). The plyometric throwing drills have been proven to be an excellent transitional exercise and training activity prior to initiating an interval throwing program.

Additionally, muscular endurance exercise should be performed in the case of the overhand thrower with shoulder dysfunction. As previously mentioned, Voight and coworkers (38) have documented a relationship between muscular fatigue and diminished proprioception. In addition, Wickiewicz and associates (54) have demonstrated that once the rotator cuff muscles are fatigued the humeral head migrates superiorly when arm elevation is initiated. Thus, these studies illustrate that fatigue of the rotator cuff muscles can lead to a loss of dynamics stability, which allows the humeral head to migrate superiorly. Recently at our institution, Gladstone and coworkers (55) documented in professional baseball pitchers during a game situation that once the shoulder muscles fatigue, the humeral head relocates superiorly. Thus, endurance drills are critical for the overhead thrower. Specific endurance drills we utilize are wall dribbling with a plyoball (figure 37.9), wall arm circles (figure 37.10), wall arm horizontal abduction/adduction movements (figure 37.11), and the versaclimber (56). Other techniques that may be beneficial include throwing an underweight or overweight ball (57–62). These techniques are designed to enhance timing, coordination, and the transfer of kinetic energy.

During phase four the primary goals are a gradual return to throwing, while maintaining the muscular strength and neuromuscular system gains that have been established in the previous three phases. During this phase we utilize a combination of PNF rhythmic stabilization drills, selective muscle activation exercises (throwers ten program), reactive neuromuscular control drills (perturbations), and plyometrics. In addition, an interval throwing program is initiated. The interval throwing program is designed to gradually increase the number of throws and the distance, intensity, and types of throws to facilitate a restoration of normal biomechanics. The interval throwing program is organized into two phases: phase I—a long toss program (from 45 to 180 ft) and phase II—an off-the-mound program for pitchers (50). The goal of this last phase is to enhance sport-specific techniques that reestablish proper biomechanics, thus reducing the chance of re-injury. It may be necessary for a skilled individual to assess the player's throwing mechanics to ensure that proper biomechanics are utilized. This is to prevent further injury.

a

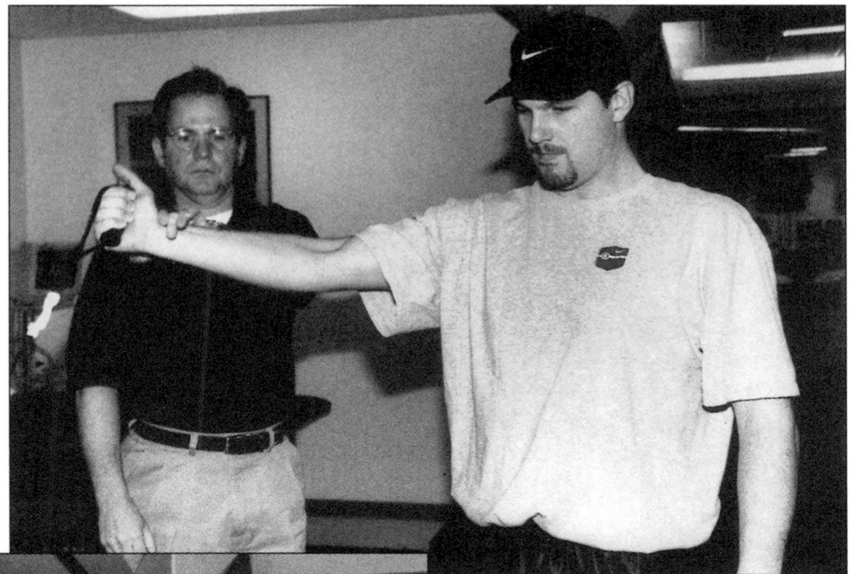

b

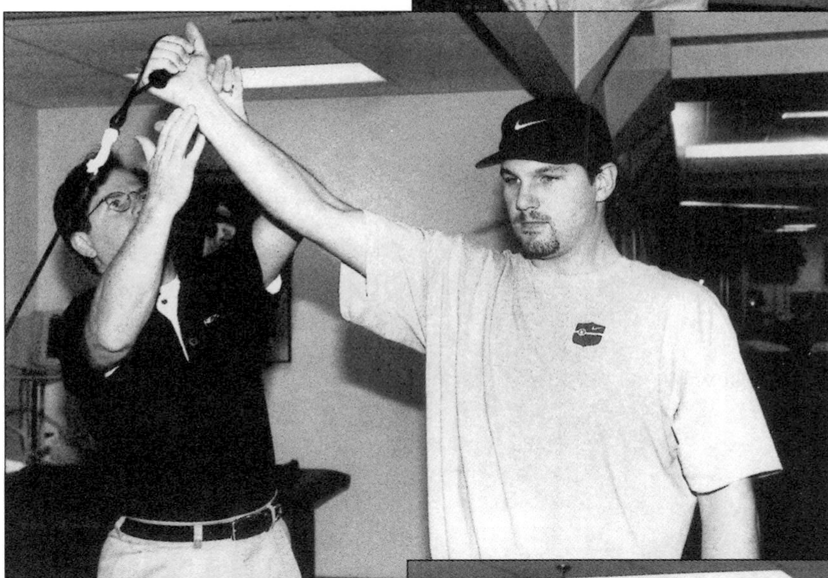

c

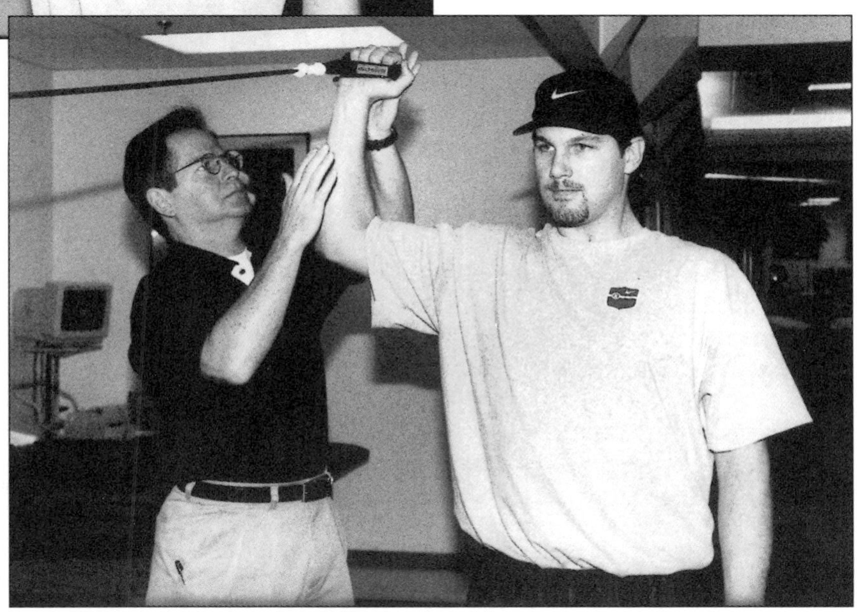

Figure 37.7 Reactive neuromuscular control drills. (*a*) Manual resistance is applied as the patient performs PNF D_2 flexion against the resistance of exercise tubing, (*b*) end range rhythmic stabilization is utilized, (*c*) end range RS applied during ER at 90° abduction.

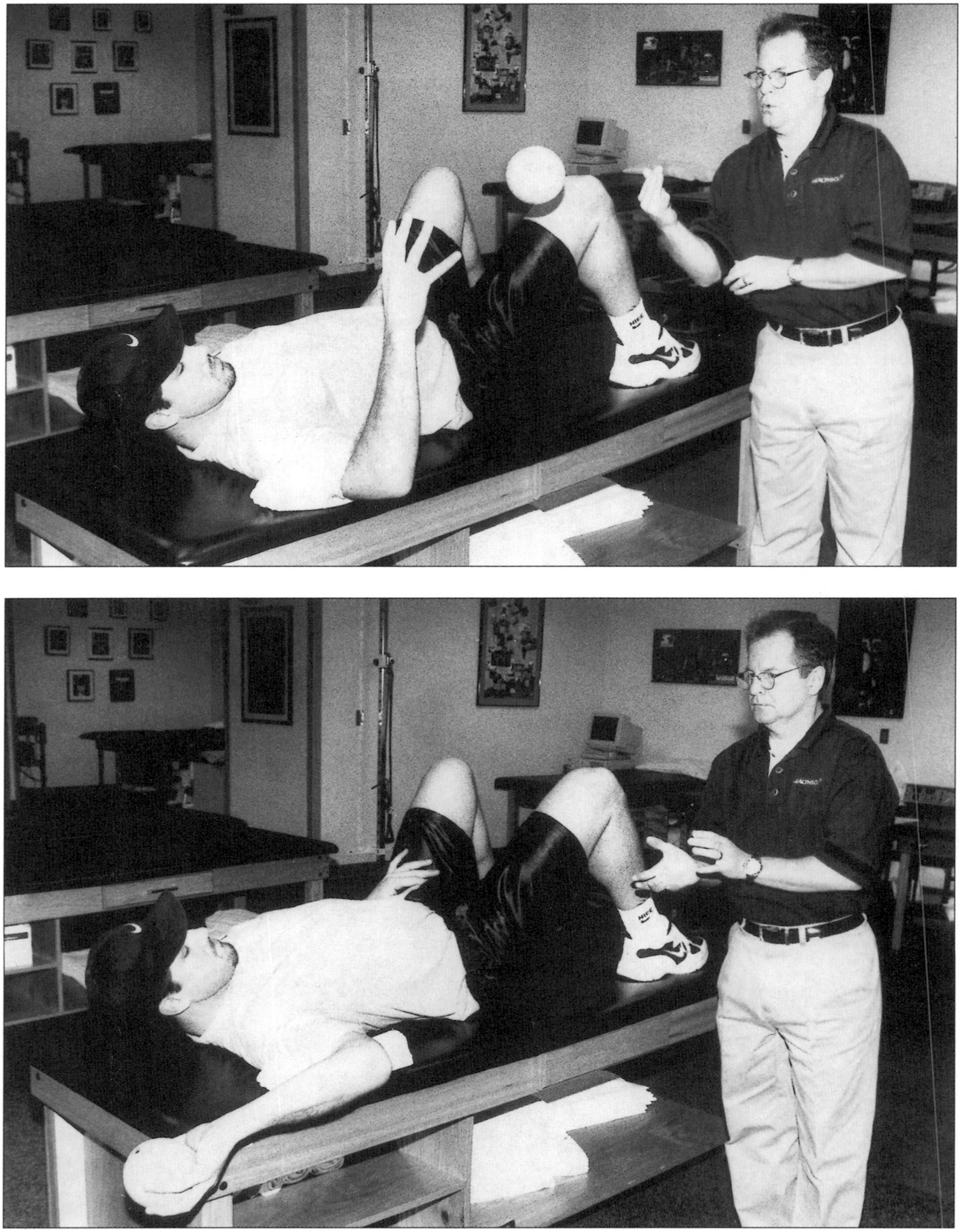

a

b

Figure 37.8 Reactive neuromuscular drill. A plyoball is tossed to create joint perturbation at end range. The patient must react to the perturbation and dynamically stabilize the joint.

Table 37.6 Movement Awareness Drill

Abduction	Movement Awareness Drills
0° abduction	Supine table (arm support)
45° abduction	Standing wall (arm support)
90° abduction	Slightly away from wall (minimal support)
>90° abduction	Standing without support

Functional Testing for the Throwing Athlete

There has been very little research published regarding functional testing for the overhead throwing athlete. Davies (51, 63) has established a functional test that is performed in a clinical setting to determine throwing ability. The test is performed using a 2 lb plyoball and a plyoback or rebounder. The athlete stands 15´ from the plyoback or target (see figure 37.12). The target is 4´ from the floor and the target zone is a 1´ by 1´ square marked on the plyoback. The testing protocol is 3 submaximal warm-ups, followed by 10 maximal warm-ups and 3–30 s throwing tests. To determine results, the number of throws within the target is divided by the total number of throws. Davies also has established some normative data for this functional testing procedure (63). Another test published to evaluate the overhead throw is the Underkofler softball skills test (65). In this test the subject, using a one-step delivery, throws a softball as far as possible. Distance is determined to the nearest inch. The author is unaware of any other functional tests that have been published at this time.

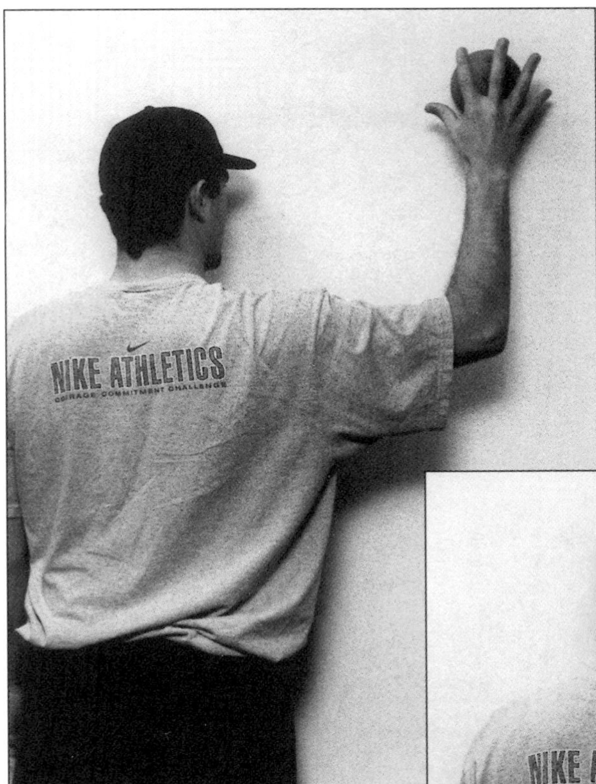

a

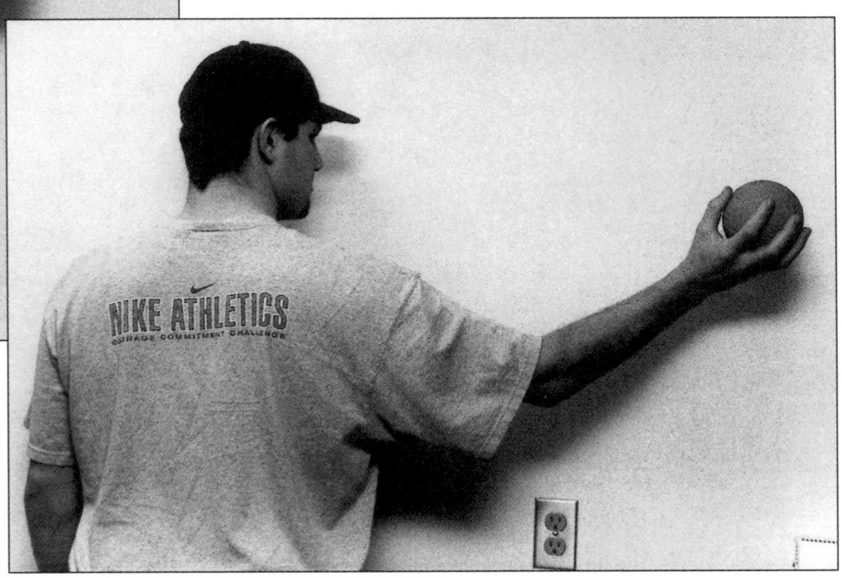

b

Figure 37.9 Endurance drill: plyoball wall dribbling.

Summary

The treatment of shoulder injuries in the throwing athlete has dramatically changed in the past several years. Presently, rehabilitation plays a vital role in the successful outcome after shoulder injuries or surgeries. Due to the excessive forces generated, significantly high muscular activity, and tremendously high angular velocities, the shoulder joint is susceptible to injury. Additionally, the hypermobility of the anterior glenohumeral joint

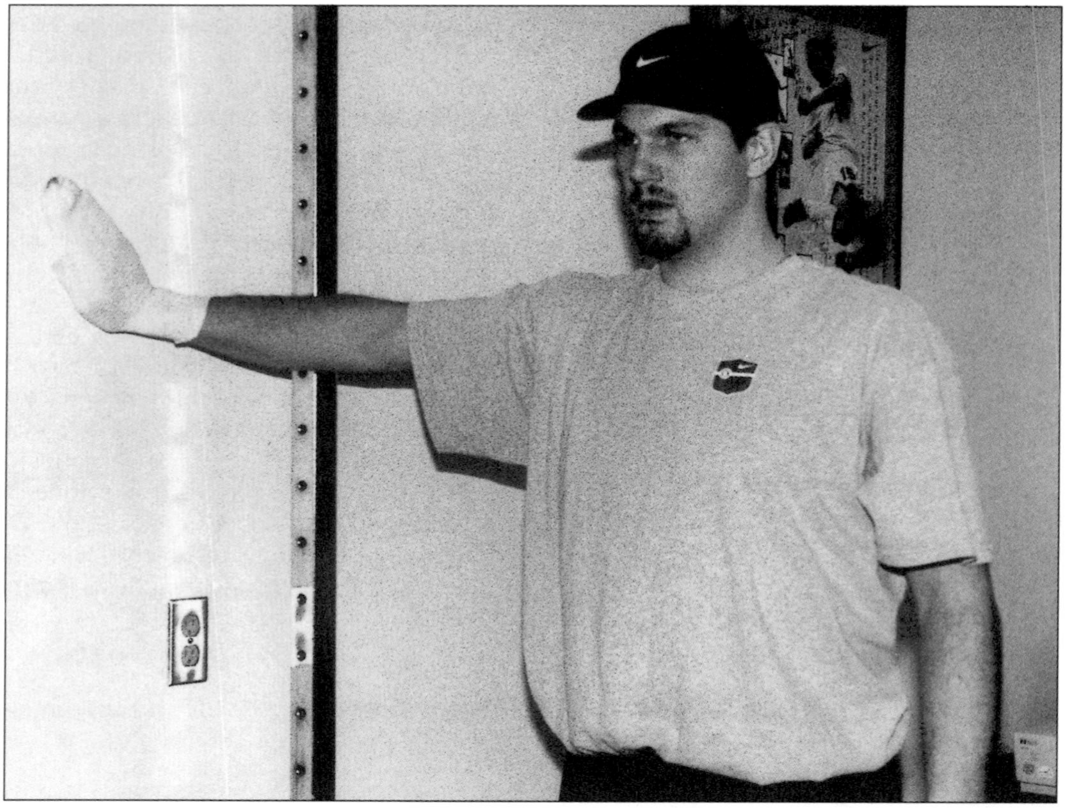

Figure 37.10 Endurance drill: wall air circles.

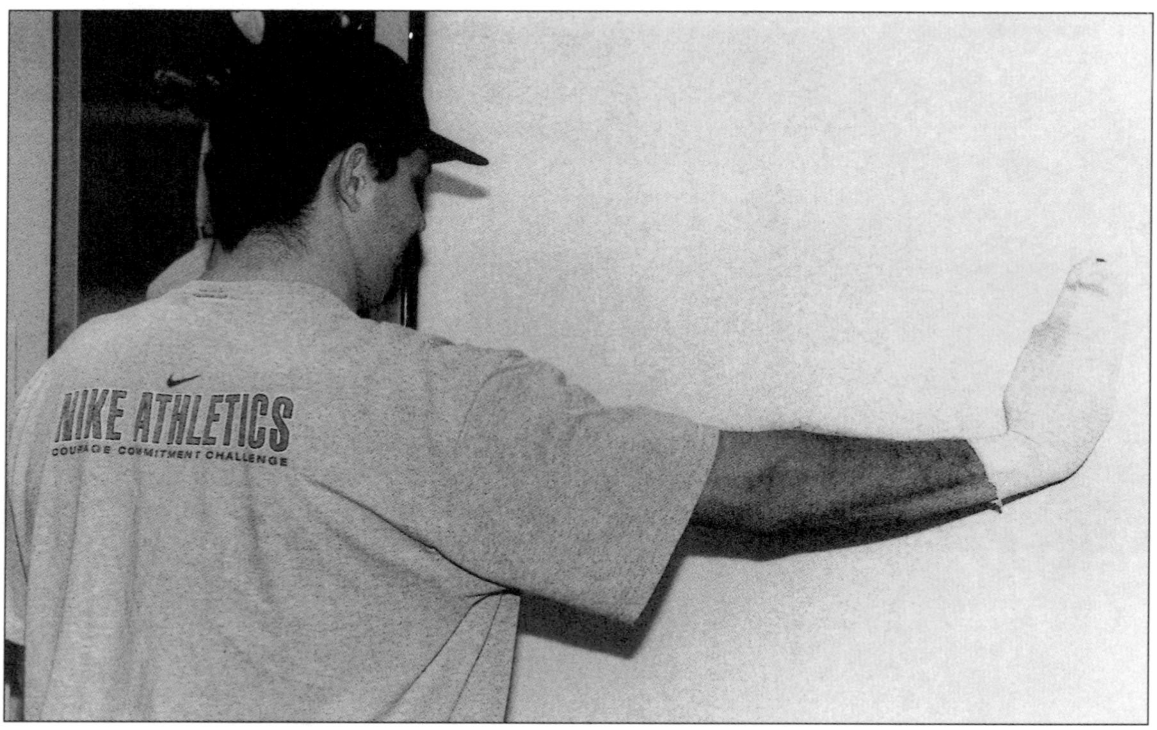

Figure 37.11 Endurance drill: wall arm horizontal abd/add.

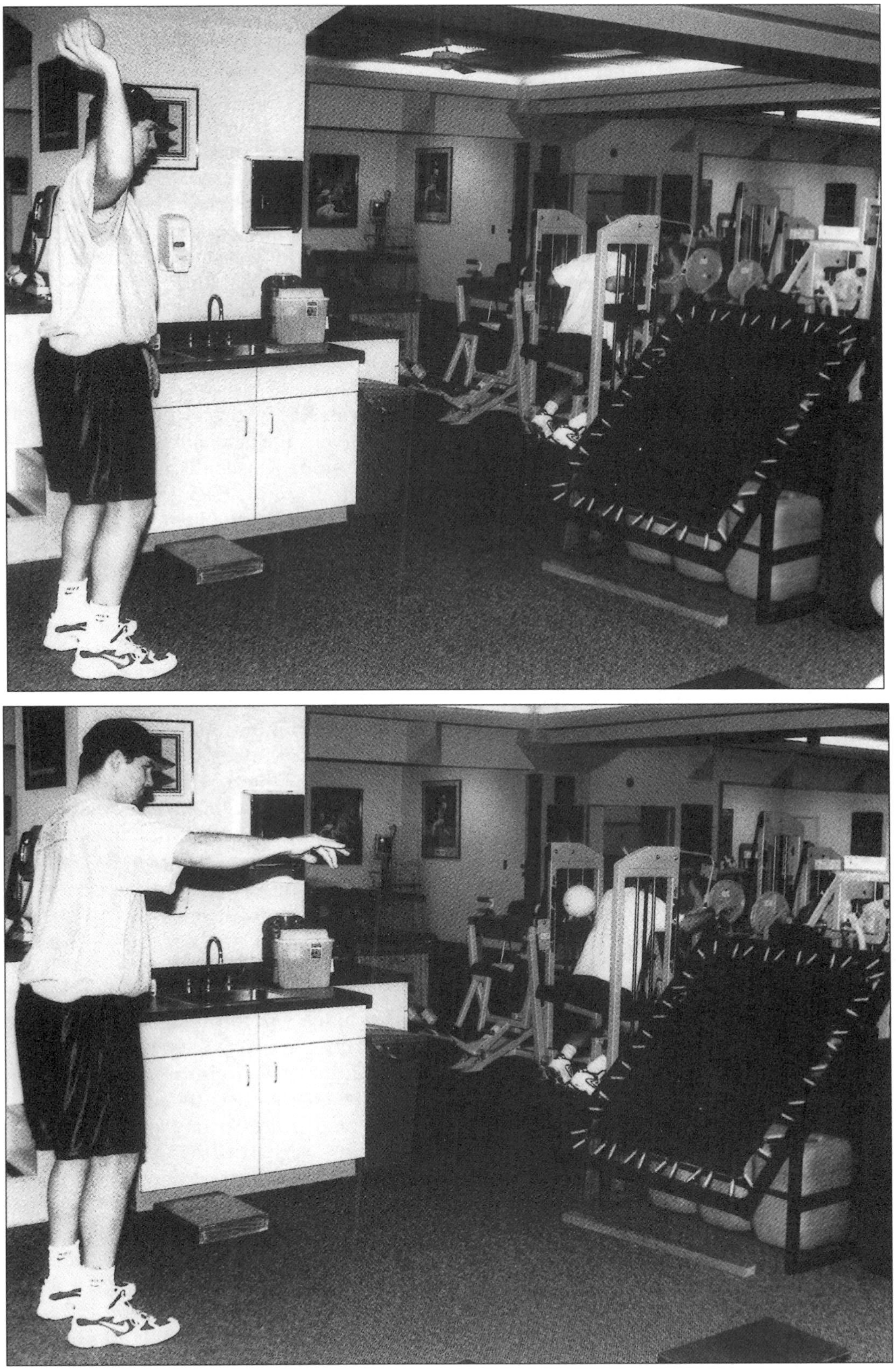

a

b

Figure 37.12 Polysomatic throwing drill. The thrower is performing a baseball throw into a Plyoback using a Plyoball (Functional Integrated Technologies, Watsonville, CA).

capsule contributes significantly to many of the more common shoulder injuries seen in the overhead thrower. In the past the rehabilitation program involved only an isotonic strengthening program; presently, the program incorporates principles of proprioception, kinesthesia, neuromuscular control, plyometrics, and reactive neuromuscular drills. One of the primary goals of the rehabilitation program in the overhead thrower is enhancing dynamic joint stability. The author believes that utilizing a program with the previously mentioned elements will enhance the functional outcome in the overhead throwing athlete.

References

1. Toyoshima S, Hoshikawa T, Miyashita M, et al: Contribution of the body parts to throwing performance. In *Biomechanics IV,* Nelson RC, Morehouse CA (eds). Baltimore: University Park Press, 1974, 169–74.
2. DiGiovine NM, Jobe FW, Pink M, et al: An electromyographic analysis of the upper extremity in pitching. *J Shoulder Elbow Surg* 1: 15–24, 1992.
3. Fleisig GS, Dillman CJ, Andrews JR: Biomechanics of the shoulder during throwing. In *The Athlete's Shoulder,* Andrews JR, Wilk KE (eds). New York: Churchill Livingstone, 1994.
4. Fleisig GS, Escamilla RF, Andrews JR: Biomechanics of throwing. In *Athletic Injuries and Rehabilitation,* Zachazewski JE, Magee DJ, Quillen WS (eds). Philadelphia: Saunders,
5. Fleisig GS, Andrews JR, Dillman CJ, et al: Kinetics of baseball pitching with implications about injury mechanisms. *Am J Sports Med* 23: 233–39, 1995.
6. Dillman CJ: Proper Mechanics of pitching. *Sports Med Update* 5: 15–21, 1990.
7. Brown LP, Niehues SL, Harrah A, et al: Upper extremity range of motion and isokinetic strength of the internal and external shoulder rotators in major league baseball players. *Am J Sports Med* 16: 577–85, 1988.
8. Johnson L: Patterns of shoulder flexibility among college baseball players. *J Ath Trn* 27: 44–49, 1992.
9. Bigliani LU, Codd TP, Connor PM, et al: Shoulder motion and laxity in the professional baseball player. *Am J Sports Med* 25: 609–13, 1997.
10. Alderink GJ, Kuck DJ: Isokinetic shoulder strength of high school and college aged pitchers. *J Orthop Sports Phys Ther* 7: 163–72, 1986.
11. Cook EE, Gray UL, Savinar-Nogue E, et al: Shoulder antagonistic strength ratios: A comparison between college level baseball pitchers and nonpitchers. *J Orthop Sports Phys Ther* 8: 451–61, 1987.
12. Hinton RY: Isokinetic evaluation of shoulder rotational strength in high school baseball pitchers. *Am J Sports Med* 16: 274–79, 1988.
13. Bartlett LR, Storey MD, Simons DB: Measurement of upper extremity torque production and its relationship to throwing speed in the competitive athlete. *Am J Sports Med* 17: 89–91, 1989.
14. Wilk KE, Andrews JR, Arrigo CA, et al: The strength characteristics of internal and external rotator muscles in professional baseball pitchers. *Am J Sports Med* 21: 61–69, 1993.
15. Wilk KE, Andrews JR, Arrigo CA: The abductor and adductor strength characteristics of professional baseball pitchers. *Am J Sports Med* 23(3): 307–11, 1995.
16. Magnusson SP, Gleim GW, Nicholas JA: Shoulder weakness in professional baseball pitchers. *Med Sci Sports Exerc* 26: 5–9, 1994.
17. Wilk KE, Andrews JR, Arrigo CA: The physical examination of the glenohumeral joint: Emphasis on the stabilizing structures. *J Orthop Sports Phys Ther* 25: 380–89, 1997.
18. Wilk KE: The thrower's shoulder: Evaluation and common injuries. Paper presented at the 1997 Advances on the Knee and Shoulder Course. Hilton Head, SC. May 24, 1997.
19. Andrews JR: Clinical examination of the shoulder in the throwing athlete. Paper presented at the 8th annual Injuries in Baseball Course. Birmingham, AL. January 26, 1990.
20. Andrews JR, Carson WG: The arthroscopic treatment of glenoid labrum tears in the throwing athlete. *Orthop Trans* 8: 44–48, 1984.
21. Andrews JR, Kupferman SP, Dillman CJ: Lateral tears in throwing and racquet sports. *Clin Sports Med* 10: 901–909, 1991.
22. Andrews JR, Meister K: Classification and treatment of rotator cuff injuries in the overhead athlete. *J Orthop Sports Phys Ther* 18: 413–19, 1993.
23. Jobe FW, Bradley JP: The diagnosis and nonoperative treatment of shoulder injuries in athletes. *Clin Sports Med* 8: 419–38, 1989.
24. Walch G, Boileau P, Noel E, Donele T: Impingement of the deep surface of the supraspinatus tendon on the glenoid rim: An arthroscopic study. *J Shoulder Elbow Surg* 1: 239–45, 1992.
25. Jobe CM: Evidence linking posterior superior labral impingement and shoulder instability. Paper presented at the American Shoulder and Elbow Surgeons Meeting. Seattle. 1991.

26. Gloussman R, Jobe FW, Tibone JE, et al: Dynamic electromyographic analysis of the throwing shoulder with glenohumeral instability. *J Bone Joint Surg* 70A: 220–26, 1988.
27. Gowan ID: Comparative electromyographic analysis of the shoulder during pitching. *J Sports Med* 15: 586–90, 1987.
28. Van Ghelvwe B, Hebbelinck M: Muscle actions and ground reaction forces in tennis. *Int J Sport Biomech* 2: 88–93, 1986.
29. Miyashita M, Tsunoda T, Sakurai S, et al: Muscular activities in the tennis serve and overhead throw. *Scand J Sports Sci* 2: 52–59, 1980.
30. Mooncastle VS: *Medical physiology* 14th ed. St. Louis: Mosby, 1980.
31. Jonsson HJ, Karrholm J, Elmqvist LG: Kinematics of active knee extensions after tear of the anterior cruciate ligament. *Am J Sports Med* 17: 796–802, 1989.
32. Dunn TG, Gillig SE, Ponser SE, Weil N: The learning process in biofeedback: Is it feedforward or feedback? *Biofeedback Self Reg* 11(2): 143–55, 1986.
33. LaCroix JM: The acquisition of autonomic control through biofeedback: The case against an afferent process and a two process alternative. *Psychophysiol* 18: 573–87, 1981.
34. McNair PJ, Wood GA, Marshall RN: Stiffness of the hamstring muscles and its relationship to function in anterior cruciate deficient individuals. *Clin Biomech* 7: 131–73, 1992.
35. Wilk KE, Arrigo CA: Current concepts in the rehabilitation of the athletic shoulder. *J Orthop Sports Phys Ther* 18: 365–78, 1993.
36. Swanik CB, Lephart SM, Giannantonio FP, Fu FH: Reestablishing proprioception and neuromuscular control in the ACL-injured athlete. *J Sport Rehabil* 6: 182–206, 1997.
37. Lephart SM, Warner JJP, Bursa PA, Fu FH: Proprioception in the shoulder of healthy, unstable, and surgically repaired shoulders. *J Shoulder Elbow Surg* 3: 371–81, 1996.
38. Voight ML, Hardin JA, Blackburn TA, Tippett S, Canner GC: The effects of muscle fatigue on and the relationship of arm dominance to shoulder proprioception. *J Orthop Sports Phys Ther* 23: 348–52, 1996.
39. Lephart SM, Pincivero DM, Giraldo JL, Fu FH: The role of proprioception in the management and rehabilitation of athletic injuries. *Am J Sports Med* 25: 130–37, 1997.
40. Knott M, Voss D: *Proprioceptive neuromuscular facilitation*. New York: Hoeber Medical Division of Harper & Row, 1968, 84–85.
41. Sullivan PE, Markos PA, Minor MD: *An integrated approach to therapeutic exercise: Theory and clinical application*. Reston, VA: Reston. 1982.
42. Clark FJ, Burgess PR: Slowly adapting receptors in cat knee joint: Can they signal joint angle? *J Neurophysiol* 38: 1448–463, 1975.
43. Wilk KE, Arrigo CA, Andrews JR: Closed and open kinetic chain exercises for the upper extremity. *J Sport Rehabil* 5: 88–102, 1996.
44. Wilk KE, Arrigo CA: An integrated approach to upper extremity exercises. *Orthop Phys Ther Clin North Am* 9: 337–60, 1992.
45. Townsend H, Jobe FW, Pink M, Perry J: Electromyographic analysis of the glenohumeral muscles during a baseball rehabilitation program. *Am J Sports Med* 19: 264–69, 1991.
46. Moseley JB, Jobe FW, Pink M, et al: EMG analysis of the scapular muscles during a shoulder rehabilitation program. *Am J Sports Med* 20: 182–134, 1992.
47. Blackburn TA, McLeod WB, White B: EMG analysis of posterior rotator cuff exercises. *J Ath Trn* 25: 40–45, 1990.
48. Jobe FW, Moynes DR: Delineation of diagnostic criteria and rehabilitation program for rotator cuff injuries. *Am J Sports Med* 10: 336–42, 1982.
49. Pappas AM, Zawacki RM: Rehabilitation of the pitching shoulder. *Am J Sports Med* 13: 223–31, 1985.
50. Wilk KE, Andrews JR, Arrigo CA, et al: *Preventive and rehabilitative exercises for the shoulder and elbow* 5th ed. Birmingham, AL: American Sports Medicine Institute, 1997.
51. Davies GJ, Dickoff-Hoffman SD: Neuromuscular testing and rehabilitation of the shoulder complex. *J Orthop Sports Phys Ther* 18: 449–56, 1993.
52. Paine RM: *The role of the scapula in the shoulder.* New York: Churchill Livingstone, 1994, 495–512.
53. Wilk KE, Voight ML, Kerris MA, Gambetta V, Andrews JR: Stretch-shortening drills for the upper extremity: Theory and clinical application. *J Orthop Sports Phys Ther* 17: 225–39, 1993.
54. Wickiewicz TH, Chen SK, Otis JC, Warren RF: Glenohumeral kinematics in a muscle fatigue model: A radiographic study. Paper presented at the 1994 Specialty Day meeting, American Orthopaedic Society for Sports Medicine. New Orleans. February 1994.
55. Gladstone J, Andrews JR, Wilk KE, Chiemlewski T: The effects of muscular fatigue on glenohumeral kinematics in the overhead professional baseball pitcher: A radiographic study. Paper presented at the American Sports Medicine Institute Fellows Research Day. July 12, 1996.

56. Wilk KE, Arrigo CA, Andrews JR: *Functional training for the overhead athlete.* Sports Physical Therapy Home Study Course. LaCrosse, WI. 1995.
57. DeRenne C, Ho K, Blitzblau A: Effects of weighted implement training on throwing. *J Appl Sport Sci Res* 4: 16–19, 1990.
58. Toyoshima S, Miyashita M: Force-velocity relation in throwing. *Res Q* 44: 86–95, 1973.
59. Vasiliev LA: Use of different weights to develop specialized speed-strength. *Soviet Sports Rev* 18: 49–52, 1983.
60. Brose DE, Hanson DL: Effect of overload training on velocity and accuracy of throwing. *Res Q* 38: 528–33, 1967.
61. Egstrom GH, Logan GA, Wallis EL: Acquisition of throwing skill involving projectiles of varying weights. *Res Q* 31: 420–25, 1960.
62. Litwhiler D, Hamm L: Overload: Effect on throwing velocity and accuracy. *Ath J* 53: 64–65, 1973.
63. Davies GJ: *Compendium of isokinetics in clinical usage* 4th ed. Onalaska, WI: S & S, 1992, 445.
64. Collins DR, Hodges PB: *A comprehensive guide to sport skills tests and measurements.* Springfield, IL: Charles C Thomas, 1978, 330–33.
65. Wilk KE, Arrigo CA, Andrews JR: Current concepts: The stabilizing structures of the glenohumeral joint. *J Ortho Sports Phys Ther* 25: 364–79, 1997.

About the Editors

Scott M. Lephart, PhD, ATC, associate professor at the University of Pittsburgh, is director of the internationally recognized Neuromuscular Research Laboratory, one of the first clinical research laboratories dedicated to sports medicine.

Dr. Lephart received the Inaugural New Investigator Award from the National Athletic Trainers' Association Research (NATA) and Education Foundation in 1998. In 1994, he received the Charles Neer Award for Outstanding Basic Science Research from the American Shoulder and Elbow Surgeons Society, the first nonorthopaedic surgeon to receive the honor. In 1999, he received the Distinguished Educator Award from the NATA.

Dr. Lephart is a Fellow with the American College of Sports Medicine and a member of the NATA. He has served as editor of the *Journal of Sport Rehabilitation* since 1996.

He received his PhD in Sports Medicine from the University of Virginia in 1989.

Freddie H. Fu, MD, ScD (Hon.), is the David Silver Professor and Chairman of the Department of Orthopaedic Surgery in the School of Medicine at the University of Pittsburgh. He holds secondary appointments as Professor of Physical Therapy and Health Physical and Recreation Education and serves as the Head Team Physician for the University of Pittsburgh's Athletic Department.

Dr. Fu graduated summa cum laude from Dartmouth College in 1974 and attained his medical degree from the University of Pittsburgh in 1977. He completed his general surgery internship at Brown University before returning to Pittsburgh to complete his residency and an orthopaedic research fellowship. He also completed an A.O. International Fellowship at the Hannover Trauma Center in Germany and an arthroscopic surgery fellowship in East Lansing, Michigan.

Dr. Fu's major research interests are clinical outcomes and biology and biomechanics of the knee and shoulder in sport-related injuries. He has presented at numerous international and national conferences and has written textbooks, book chapters, and research publications. He is a member of and has held offices in several academic organizations, including the prestigious Herodicus Society, the American Shoulder and Elbow Surgeons Society, and the American Orthopaedic Association.

Dr. Fu's efforts in clinical and basic science research have led to more than 70 professional awards, 200 international and 400 national presentations, and editorship of 12 major orthopaedic textbooks. He is the co-author of 60 book chapters on the management of sports injuries and has contributed to more than 150 international research publications.